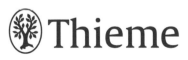

Top 3 Differentials in Radiology

A Case Review

Second Edition

William T. O'Brien, Sr., DO, FAOCR
Director, Pediatric Neuroradiology Fellowship
Cincinnati Children's Hospital Medical Center
Associate Professor of Radiology
University of Cincinnati College of Medicine
Cincinnati, Ohio

Thieme
New York • Stuttgart • Delhi • Rio de Janeiro

Thieme Medical Publishers, Inc.
333 Seventh Avenue
New York, New York 10001

Executive Editor: William Lamsback
Managing Editor: J. Owen Zurhellen IV
Associate Managing Editor: Kenneth Schubach
Developmental Editor: Judith Tomat
Director, Editorial Services: Mary Jo Casey
Editorial Director: Sue Hodgson
Production Editor: Sean Woznicki
International Production Director: Andreas Schabert
International Marketing Director: Fiona Henderson
International Sales Director: Louisa Turrell
Director, Institutional Sales: Adam Bernacki
Senior Vice President and Chief Operating Officer: Sarah Vanderbilt
President: Brian D. Scanlan
Printer: Beltz Grafische Betriebe

Library of Congress Cataloging-in-Publication Data

Names: O'Brien, William T., Sr., editor.
Title: Top 3 differentials in radiology : a case review / [edited by]
    William T. O'Brien, Sr.
Other titles: Top three differentials in radiology
Description: Second edition. | New York : Thieme, [2018] | Includes
    bibliographical references and indexes.
Identifiers: LCCN 2017044158 (print) | LCCN 2017044654 (ebook)
    | ISBN 9781626232792 (E-book) | ISBN 9781626232785
    (paperback : alk. paper)
Subjects: | MESH: Radiography | Diagnosis, Differential |
    Case Reports
Classification: LCC RC78.2 (ebook) | LCC RC78.2 (print) |
    NLM WN 200 | DDC 616.07/572—dc23
LC record available at https://lccn.loc.gov/2017044158

The views expressed in this book are those of the author and contributors, and do not reflect the official policy or position of the United States Government, the Department of Defense, Department of the Army or the Department of the Air Force.

Copyright © 2018 by Thieme Medical Publishers, Inc.

Thieme Publishers New York
333 Seventh Avenue, New York, NY 10001 USA
+1 800 782 3488, customerservice@thieme.com

Thieme Publishers Stuttgart
Rüdigerstrasse 14, 70469 Stuttgart, Germany
+49 [0]711 8931 421, customerservice@thieme.de

Thieme Publishers Delhi
A-12, Second Floor, Sector-2, Noida-201301
Uttar Pradesh, India
+91 120 45 566 00, customerservice@thieme.in

Thieme Publishers Rio de Janeiro, Thieme Publicações Ltda.
Edifício Rodolpho de Paoli, 25º andar
Av. Nilo Peçanha, 50 – Sala 2508,
Rio de Janeiro 20020-906 Brasil
+55 21 3172-2297 / +55 21 3172-1896

ISBN 978-1-62623-278-5

Also available as an e-book:
eISBN 978-1-62623-279-2

Important note: Medicine is an ever-changing science undergoing continual development. Research and clinical experience are continually expanding our knowledge, in particular our knowledge of proper treatment and drug therapy. Insofar as this book mentions any dosage or application, readers may rest assured that the authors, editors, and publishers have made every effort to ensure that such references are in accordance with **the state of knowledge at the time of production of the book.**

Nevertheless, this does not involve, imply, or express any guarantee or responsibility on the part of the publishers in respect to any dosage instructions and forms of applications stated in the book. **Every user is requested to examine carefully** the manufacturers' leaflets accompanying each drug and to check, if necessary in consultation with a physician or specialist, whether the dosage schedules mentioned therein or the contraindications stated by the manufacturers differ from the statements made in the present book. Such examination is particularly important with drugs that are either rarely used or have been newly released on the market. Every dosage schedule or every form of application used is entirely at the user's own risk and responsibility. The authors and publishers request every user to report to the publishers any discrepancies or inaccuracies noticed. If errors in this work are found after publication, errata will be posted at www.thieme.com on the product description page.

Some of the product names, patents, and registered designs referred to in this book are in fact registered trademarks or proprietary names even though specific reference to this fact is not always made in the text. Therefore, the appearance of a name without designation as proprietary is not to be construed as a representation by the publisher that it is in the public domain.

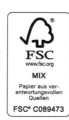

Dedicated in memory of

William E. Shiels II, DO, FAOCR

1954–2015

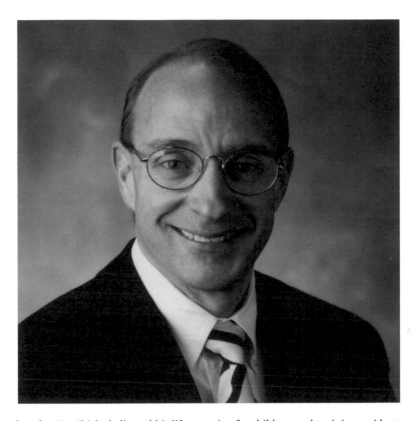

For decades, Dr. Shiels dedicated his life to caring for children and training residents and fellows in the art of pediatric imaging. His pioneering and innovative contributions will certainly outlive his tenure, which was cut far too short. He will be sorely missed but will never be forgotten.

Contents

Preface

It is a distinct pleasure to present the second edition of *Top 3 Differentials in Radiology: A Case Review*. This book is primarily intended for radiology residents and staff physicians who are preparing for board examinations or looking for a refresher in differentials for common and important imaging gamuts. This second edition has new illustrative cases and updated content throughout, while retaining its high-yield format.

The book is organized into 12 core sections based on specific radiology subspecialties. Each section contains a series of common and important imaging gamuts. On the first page of each case, readers are presented with images from a patient whose diagnosis is as yet unknown, along with a clinical history and detailed image legend. The illustrative cases are meant to highlight a key finding or gamut, which is the basis for the case discussion. The second page identifies the key finding, from which a list of differentials is broken down into the "Top 3" and additional differential diagnoses. The discussion section of each case provides a brief review of important imaging and clinical manifestations for all entities on the list of differentials, and imaging pearls are provided at the end of each case to allow for a quick review of key points. The final diagnosis is provided for each case; however, it is by no means the focus of this review book. In fact, many illustrative cases have a final diagnosis which would not be considered in the "Top 3" for the particular gamut.

Instead, the primary aim of the book is to generate and have an understanding of a reasonable list of gamut-based differentials, rather than obtaining the "correct" answer. The final section, titled "Roentgen Classics," contains cases from each of the previous core subspecialty sections that have imaging findings characteristic of a single diagnosis; thus, no differential is presented. A detailed discussion of the final diagnosis follows.

As with the first edition and subspecialty "Top 3" books, it is important to realize that the differentials and discussions are based on the key finding or gamut and not necessarily the illustrative cases that are shown. This is by design, since I felt it would be more high-yield to base the differentials and discussions on the overall gamut/key finding rather than the illustrative case presented. Having an understanding of gamut-based differentials will allow one to subsequently tailor the list of differentials for any case that is shown within the gamut, whereas basing the differentials on the selected images would be limited in terms of future utility.

I sincerely hope that you find the "Top 3" case-based approach enjoyable and useful, and I wish you all the best in your future endeavors.

William T. O'Brien Sr.

Acknowledgments

This book would not have been possible without the contributions of numerous colleagues. First and foremost, I am indebted to the faculty of David Grant USAF Medical Center, the University of California at Davis, Oakland Children's Hospital (where I completed my radiology residency training), and the University of Cincinnati and Cincinnati Children's Hospital Medical Center (where I completed my neuroradiology fellowships). The dedicated staff at these institutions have had a profound impact on my career. Their influence is what inspires me to remain in academics in the hopes of having a similar impact on the next generation of radiologists.

Each of the section editors for this second edition devoted many hours to ensure high quality content in the form of new illustrative cases and updated content throughout, while maintaining the central "Top 3" theme. In many instances, they utilized their own teaching file cases to enhance the contributions of case contributors within their chapter. I am grateful to the chapter editors and contributors for the time and expertise they offered to this project.

Lastly, I would like to thank my family for their continuous love and support, as well as the sacrifices they made during completion of this project. I have been blessed with a wonderful wife, Annie; two sons, Patrick and Liam; and a daughter, Shannon. Annie and I have been together for over two decades, and we could not be more proud of our three incredible children. I am grateful beyond words for the joy that they bring into my life each and every day.

Contributors

M. Jason Akers, MD
Radiology Inc.
Huntington, West Virginia

Karen M. Ayotte, MD
Chief, Pediatric Imaging
David Grant USAF Medical Center
Travis AFB, California

Jasjeet Bindra, MBBS
Associate Professor
Division of Musculoskeletal Imaging
Associate Chair of Education
Associate Program Director, Radiology Residency
Program Director, NMDR Residency
Department of Radiology
University of California Davis
Sacramento, California

Natasha Brasic, MD
Department of Radiology and Biomedical Imaging
University of California, San Francisco
San Francisco, California

Cam Chau, MD
Department of Diagnostic Imaging
UC Davis Medical Center
Sacramento, California

Chloe M. Chhor, MD
Department of Radiology
University of California, San Francisco
San Francisco, California

Boon Chye Ching, MBBS, FRCR (UK), MMED
Diagnostic Imaging
National Cancer Centre
Singapore

Daniel G. Church, MD
Clinical Fellow in Radiology
Lucile Packard Children's Hospital
Stanford, California

Brady S. Davis, DO
Captain, United States Air Force
Department of Diagnostic Imaging
David Grant USAF Medical Center
Travis Air Force Base, California

Matthew R. Denny, MD
San Jose, California

Paul B. DiDomenico, MD
Clinical Instructor of Radiology
Department of Radiology & Biomedical Imaging
Yale University School of Medicine
Staff Radiologist
VA Connecticut Health Care System
New Haven, Connecticut

Adam R. Dulberger, BS
Medical Student
Uniformed Services University
Bethesda, Maryland

Eva Escobedo, MD
Professor of Radiology
University of California Davis Medical Center
Sacramento, California

Hedieh K. Eslamy, MD
Clinical Fellow in Radiology
Lucile Packard Children's Hospital
Stanford, California

Cameron C. Foster, MD
Associate Professor of Nuclear Medicine
Nuclear Medicine Residency Program Director
Director of Clinical Nuclear Medicine and PET
University of California Davis Health
Sacramento, California

Sonia Kaur Ghei, MD
Department of Diagnostic Imaging
University of California Davis Medical Center
Sacramento, California

David D. Gover, MD
Lt. Colonel, United States Air Force
Chief, Vascular and Interventional Radiology
David Grant USAF Medical Center
Travis Air Force Base, California

Philip Granchi, MD
Department of Diagnostic Imaging
University of California Davis Medical Center
Sacramento, California

Bo Yoon Ha, MD
Clinical Fellow in Radiology
Lucile Packard Children's Hospital
Stanford, California

Bang Huynh, MD
Chief, Thoracic Imaging
David Grant USAF Medical Center
Travis Air Force Base, California

Robert A. Jesinger, MD, MSE
Colonel, United States Air Force
Academic Chair, Diagnostic Radiology Residency at David Grant
  USAF Medical Center
Assistant Professor of Radiology, Uniformed Services University
  of the Health Sciences
Travis Air Force Base, California
Associate Clinical Radiology Faculty
University of California Davis
Sacramento, California

Todd M. Johnson, MD
Chief, Abdominal Imaging
David Grant USAF Medical Center
Travis Air Force Base, California

Brian S. Johnston, MD
Breast Imaging and Intervention
Division of Diagnostic Imaging
Banner M.D. Anderson Cancer Center
Gilbert, Arizona

David A. Kephart Jr.
PGY-2, Diagnostic Radiology Christiana Care Health System
Newark, Delaware

Jason S. Kim, BS
Medical Student (MS4)
Uniformed Services University
Bethesda, Maryland

Michael C. Kuo, MD
Clinical Fellow, Abdominal Imaging
University of California Davis Medical Center
Sacramento, California

Grant E. Lattin Jr., MD
Lt. Colonel, United States Air Force
Program Director, Diagnostic Radiology Residency & Body
  Imaging Fellowship
National Capital Consortium, Walter Reed National Military
  Medical Center
Associate Professor, Uniformed Services University of the He-
  alth Sciences
F. Edward Hébert School of Medicine
Bethesda, Maryland

Jessica W.T. Leung, MD, FACR, FSBI
Professor of Diagnostic Radiology
Section Chief of Breast Imaging
MD Anderson Cancer Center
The University of Texas
Houston, Texas

Brian J. Lewis, DO
Major, United States Air Force
Department of Radiology
10th Medical Group
United States Air Force Academy
Colorado Springs, Colorado

John P. Lichtenberger III, MD
Lt. Colonel, United States Air Force
Associate Professor
Department of Radiology
Uniformed Services University of the Health Sciences
Bethesda, Maryland

Shaun Loh, MD, MBA
Department of Diagnostic Imaging
University of California Davis Medical Center
Sacramento, California

Matthew L. Lutynski, DO
Associate Program Director, Transitional Year Internship
Associate Program Director, Radiology Residency
National Capital Consortium
Assistant Professor, Department of Radiology and Radiological
  Sciences
Uniformed Services University of the Health Sciences
Bethesda, Maryland

Michael Mahlon, DO
Chief
Musculoskeletal Imaging and Diagnostic Services
Madigan Army Medical Center
Joint Base Lewis-McChord, Washington
Assistant Professor
The Uniformed Services University of the Health Sciences
Bethesda, Maryland
Consultant Radiologist, ARIS Radiology
Hudson, Ohio

Brent D. McCarragher, MD
Radiology Resident
Walter Reed National Military Medical Center
Bethesda, Maryland

Arash J. Momeni, MD
Department of Diagnostic Imaging
David Grant USAF Medical Center
Travis Air Force Base, California

Mischa Monroe
Medical Student
Uniformed Services University
Bethesda, Maryland

Wayne L. Monsky, MD, PhD
Assistant Professor of Radiology
University of Dalifornia Davis Medical Center
Sacramento, California

Matthew J. Moore, MD
Clinical Instructor in Neuroradiology
University of Cincinnati
Cincinnati, Ohio

Sima Naderi, MD
Assistant Professor of Radiology
University of California Davis Medical Center
Sacramento, California

Contributors

Vicki E. Nagano, MD
Department of Nuclear Medicine
Kaiser Sacramento
Sacramento, California

William T. O'Brien, Sr., DO, FAOCR
Fellowship Program Director, Pediatric Neuroradiology
Cincinnati Children's Hospital Medical Center
Associate Professor of Radiology
University of Cincinnati College of Medicine
Cincinnati, Ohio

James B. Odone, MD
Lt. Colonel, United States Air Force
Staff Radiologist
Diagnostic Imaging Department
Landstuhl Regional Medical Center
Landstuhl, Germany

Eleanor L. Ormsby, MD, MPH
Chief Resident, Diagnostic Imaging
University of California Davis Medical Center
Sacramento, California

Anokh Pahwa, MD
Department of Diagnostic Imaging
University of California Davis Medical Center
Sacramento, California

Chirag V. Patel, MD
Assistant Professor of Radiology
University of California Davis Medical Center and Children's
    Hospital
Sacramento, California

Glade E. Roper, MD
Mineral King Radiology
Visalia, California

Erika Rubesova, MD
Clinical Associate Professor
Lucile Packard Children's Hospital
Stanford University
Stanford, California

Rocky C. Saenz, DO, FAOCR
Vice-Chairman, Department of Radiology
Program Director of Diagnostic Radiology Residency
Clinical Assistant Professor
Michigan State University
Director of MRI & Musculoskeletal Imaging
Beaumont Hospital System, Botsford Campus
Farmington Hills, Michigan

Thomas Ray Sanchez, MD
Chief of Pediatric Radiology
University of California Davis Children's Hospital
Associate Professor
University of California Davis School of Medicine
Sacramento, California

Paul M. Sherman, MD, FACR
Director of Neuroimaging Research
USAF School of Aerospace Medicine
Wright Patterson Air Force Base, Ohio
Associate Professor of Radiology
Uniformed Services University
Bethesda, Maryland

Kamal D. Singh, MD
Chief, Nuclear Medicine
Kaiser West Los Angeles
Los Angeles, California

Arvind Sonik, MD
Department of Diagnostic Imaging
University of California Davis Medical Center
Sacramento, California

Rebecca Stein-Wexler, MD
Professor of Pediatric Radiology
Director, Radiology Residency Program
University of California Davis Medical Center and Children's
    Hospital
Sacramento, California

Corinne D. Strickland, MD
Department of Diagnostic Imaging
University of Arizona College of Medicine
Tucson, Arizona

Joyce F. Sung, MD
Maternal Fetal Medicine Fellow
Lucile Packard Children's Hospital
Stanford, California

Michael A. Tall, MD
Colonel, United States Air Force
Fellowship Program Director, Musculoskeletal Radiology
San Antonio Uniformed Health Education Consortium
San Antonio, Texas

Jeffrey P. Tan, MD
Department of Diagnostic Imaging
48th Medical Group
RAF Lakenheath, United Kingdom

Adrianne K. Thompson, MD
Chief, Body Imaging
Wilford Hall Medical Center
Lackland Air Force Base, Texas

Charles A. Tujo, MD
Diagnostic Radiologist
David Grant Medical Center
Travis Air Force Base, California
Assistant Professor of Radiology
Uniformed Services University
Bethesda, Maryland

Laura J. Varich, MD
Clinical Associate Professor of Radiology
Lucille Packard Children's Hospital
Stanford, California

David J. Weitz, MD
Chief, Ultrasound Imaging
David Grant USAF Medical Center
Travis Air Force Base, California

Ely A. Wolin
Lieutenant Colonel, United States Air Force
Program Director, Diagnostic Radiology Residency
David Grant USAF Medical Center
Travis AFB, California

Charlyne Wu, MD
Department of Diagnostic Imaging
University of California Davis Medical Center
Sacramento, California

Philip Yen, MD
Department of Diagnostic Imaging
University of California Davis Medical Center
Sacramento, California

Adam J. Zuckerman, DO
Clinical Instructor in Neuroradiology
University of Cincinnati
Cincinnati, Ohio

Part 1

Chest and Cardiac Imaging

1

Case 1

Arash J. Momeni

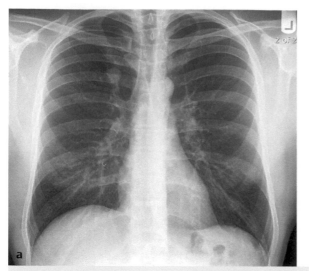 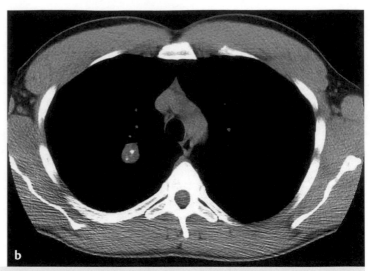

Fig. 1.1 **(a)** Posteroanterior radiograph of the chest demonstrates a solitary pulmonary nodule within the right upper lobe. **(b)** Unenhanced computed tomography (CT) image through the upper chest shows a circumscribed right upper lobe pulmonary nodule with regions of coarse central calcification and small subtle foci of macroscopic fat.

■ Clinical Presentation

Preoperative evaluation, asymptomatic (►Fig. 1.1).

■ Key Imaging Finding

Solitary pulmonary nodule

■ Top 3 Differential Diagnoses:

- **Granuloma**. Granulomas are produced secondary to an infectious or inflammatory process, such as tuberculosis, fungal disease, and vasculitides. They present radiographically as solitary or multiple pulmonary nodules. If benign patterns of calcification are identified (central, diffuse, popcorn, or laminated), no further work-up is necessary. Eccentric, speckled, or amorphous calcifications, however, are suspicious for a neoplastic process until proven otherwise. Calcified hilar and mediastinal lymph nodes are commonly seen with granulomatous disease.
- **Neoplasm**. Both primary lung cancer and metastatic disease may present as a solitary pulmonary nodule or mass (>3 cm). Irregular borders or suspicious calcifications (speckled, eccentric) suggest neoplasm over granulomatous disease. Adenocarcinoma characteristically presents as a solid, part-solid, or ground-glass nodule in a peripheral location and is considered the most common primary malignant lung neoplasm. Squamous cell and small cell carcinomas are associated with smoking and tend to occur centrally. Squamous cell carcinoma has a proclivity to cavitate. Small cell carcinoma typically presents as a perihilar mass with associated lymphadenopathy.
- **Hamartoma**. Hamartomas are composed of normal tissue assembled in a disorganized fashion. They are the most common benign tumor of the lung, accounting for 5 to 10% of solitary pulmonary nodules. Classically, they are well-defined, solitary masses less than 4 cm in diameter. Focal macroscopic fat, in addition to a benign pattern of calcification (such as popcorn calcification), is most helpful in making the diagnosis. Evaluation for fat should rely on visible fat, and not on Hounsfield unit (HU), which may falsely be low from averaging with air.

■ Additional Differential Diagnoses:

- **Round pneumonia**. Typically seen in pediatric patients younger than 8 years, pneumonia may have a rounded mass-like appearance. It is due to centrifugal spread of the rapidly replicating bacteria through the pores of Kohn and canals of Lambert from a single primary focus in the lung.
- **Arteriovenous malformation (AVM)**. AVMs are abnormal communications between a pulmonary or systemic artery and a pulmonary vein. When multiple, nearly 90% are associated with Osler–Weber–Rendu syndrome (hereditary hemorrhagic telangiectasia), characterized by epistaxis, telangiectasia of skin and mucous membranes, and gastrointestinal bleeding. Although usually congenital, AVMs may be acquired in the setting of cirrhosis, trauma, or certain infections. Radiographically, they are well defined. Contrast-enhanced imaging reveals avidly enhancing nodules or masses with an enlarged feeding artery and draining vein. It is critical to prospectively identify AVMs, since inadvertent biopsy can have catastrophic consequences. AVMs are typically treated with embolization (coils or detachable balloons).

■ Diagnosis

Hamartoma

✓ Pearls

- Benign calcification patterns for a pulmonary nodule include central, diffuse, popcorn, or laminated.
- Malignant features include irregular borders, suspicious calcifications, or eccentric soft-tissue mass.
- Evaluation for fat should rely on visible fat, and not on HU, which may falsely be low from averaging with air.

Suggested Readings

Suut S, Al-Ani Z, Allen C, et al. Pictorial essay of radiological features of benign intrathoracic masses. Ann Thorac Med. 2015; 10(4):231–242

Truong MT, Ko JP, Rossi SE, et al. Update in the evaluation of the solitary pulmonary nodule. Radiographics. 2014; 34(6):1658–1679

Case 2

Philip Yen

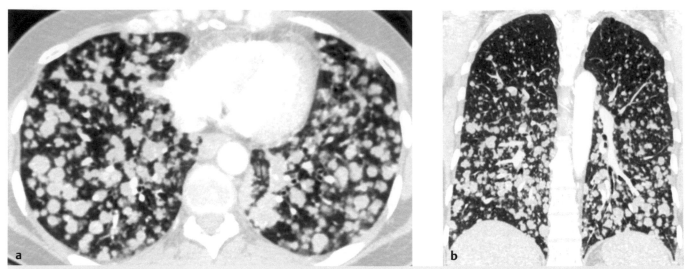

Fig. 2.1 (a) Axial contrast-enhanced computed tomography (CT) shows randomly distributed, well-defined pulmonary nodules. **(b)** Coronal CT shows lower lobe predominance.

■ Clinical Presentation

A 39-year-old woman undergoing treatment for breast cancer (▶Fig. 2.1).

■ Key Imaging Finding

Multiple pulmonary nodules

■ Top 3 Differential Diagnoses

- **Metastatic disease**. The majority of patients with multiple metastatic pulmonary nodules have a known primary malignancy. Although nodules can be found anywhere in the lung as they are primarily spread hematogenously, they tend to be randomly distributed with a lower lobe predominance because of the increased blood flow as compared to the upper lobes. Nodules may vary in size, reflecting separate episodes of metastases or varying growth rates. Nodules can be small and numerous or large "cannon-ball" lesions, which are generally seen with sarcomas and gastrointestinal primary malignancies.
- **Tuberculosis or fungal granulomatous disease**. *Mycobacterium tuberculosis* is an aerobic bacterium that disseminates by inhalation of airborne respiratory droplets. Primary and secondary (reactivation) patterns of pulmonary involvement may be seen. Hematogenous spread of the disease results in multiple 1- to 2-mm nodules dispersed in a random distribution. Common fungal causes of multiple granulomatous nodules include histoplasmosis and coccidioidomycosis, both of which may manifest with a miliary pattern accompanied by hilar and/or mediastinal adenopathy.
- **Septic emboli**. Patients with septic emboli usually have a concomitant history of intravenous (IV) drug abuse, bacterial endocarditis, or other source of systemic infection. Patients present with multiple bilateral nodules that tend to be peripheral in location and well defined. A vessel may be identified coursing directly into the center of a nodule, termed the "feeding vessel sign," thought to represent the hematogenous source of the nodule. However, this sign is not specific for septic emboli, as it may also be seen in metastatic disease.

■ Additional Differential Diagnoses

- **Granulomatosis with polyangiitis (GPA)**. GPA (formerly Wegener granulomatosis) is a vasculitis that affects multiple organs, including the kidneys, upper and lower airways, and lungs. Detection of serological markers such as antineutrophil cytoplasmic antibodies (c-ANCA) frequently aids in diagnosis. Pulmonary manifestations include multiple lung nodules that may range from 2 to 10 cm. These nodules may cavitate and appear thick-walled with air–fluid levels. A history of multiple sinus infections is common.
- **Rheumatoid arthritis (RA)**. Pulmonary involvement of RA occurs after musculoskeletal manifestations. The most common pulmonary manifestation is a pleural effusion. Rheumatoid nodules are not a common presentation of RA, but when they do occur, they can be as small as 2 mm or as large as 5 cm. Nodules may be solitary or multiple and usually are peripheral and well defined. Of particular note is the tendency to disappear with successful therapy as subcutaneous rheumatoid nodules heal.

■ Diagnosis

Metastatic disease

✓ Pearls

- Because of blood flow, hematogenous spread (whether of infection or neoplasm) tends to favor the lower lobes.
- Tuberculosis and fungal infections can have similar imaging features; TB may be primary or secondary.
- Septic emboli occur in patients with IV drug abuse, endocarditis, or systemic infections and may cavitate.
- The majority of RA patients have musculoskeletal manifestations prior to pulmonary involvement.

Suggested Readings

Collins J, Stern EJ. Chest Radiology: The Essentials. Philadelphia, PA: Lippincott Williams & Wilkins; 2008

Walker CM, Abbott GF, Greene RE, Shepard JA, Vummidi D, Digumarthy SR. Imaging pulmonary infection: classic signs and patterns. AJR Am J Roentgenol. 2014; 202(3):479–492

Webb R, Higgins C. Thoracic Imaging: Pulmonary and Cardiovascular Radiology. Philadelphia, PA: Lippincott Williams & Wilkins; 2010

Case 3

Philip Yen and Matthew L. Lutynski

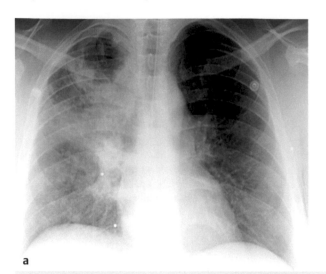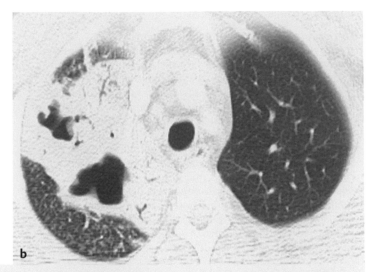

Fig. 3.1 (a) Posteroanterior chest radiograph shows a right upper lobe consolidation with a large right apical cavitation. (b) Contrast-enhanced axial computed tomography (CT) image shows a thick-walled right upper lobe consolidation with two cavitations.

■ Clinical Presentation

A 40-year-old man with fevers, night sweats, hemoptysis, and weight loss (▶Fig. 3.1).

■ Key Imaging Finding

Cavitary pulmonary nodule/mass

■ Top 3 Differential Diagnoses

- **Tuberculosis.** Primary tuberculosis (TB) may be asymptomatic or present with lobar air-space consolidations. Cavitations are unusual in this phase but can occasionally be found. Reactivation disease presents clinically with night sweats, fever, and weight loss. Radiographically, this phase manifests as multiple cavitations reflecting the increased inflammation and necrosis. These are predominantly in the upper lobes where the higher oxygen tension enables the aerobic bacterium to thrive and where lymphatic clearance is less than that of the lower lobes.
- **Fungal disease.** The most common fungal causes of cavitary lesions are the endemic fungi. Histoplasmosis is endemic to the Ohio and Mississippi River valleys. It particularly favors the nitrogen-rich soil found in bat- or avian guano–laden areas such as caves and chicken houses. Coccidioidomycosis is a soil-borne fungus that is endemic to the Southwestern United States and is spread by inhalation. As with reactivation TB, chronic cavitary fungal colonization preferentially involves the upper lobes.
- **Squamous cell carcinoma (primary or metastatic).** Approximately 30% of all primary lung cancers arise from primary squamous cell carcinoma (SCC). It is typically located centrally with involvement of hilar or mediastinal lymph nodes. Patients frequently have a history of smoking. Metastatic SCC originates from either a head and neck primary or cervical cancer in females. SCC commonly cavitates.

■ Additional Differential Diagnoses

- **Pyogenic infection (pulmonary abscess, septic emboli).** *Staphylococcus aureus* is the most common bacterial infection to result in cavitation. It typically causes a widespread consolidation and may lead to cavitation and abscess formation. In the setting of multiple widespread cavities, a source of showering septic emboli should be considered.
- **Granulomatosis with polyangiitis (GPA).** GPA (formerly Wegener granulomatosis) is a multiorgan vasculitis that affects the airways, lungs, and kidneys. Patients present with sinus disease, along with cough and hemoptysis. Serum antineutro-phil cytoplasmic antibodies (c-ANCA) are frequently detected. The most common pulmonary manifestations are multiple lung nodules, followed by air-space consolidations, ground-glass opacities, and thick-walled cavitations.
- **Rheumatoid arthritis (RA).** Although not a common manifestation, RA occasionally can present with well-defined pulmonary nodules, which tend to cavitate. The lesions commonly regress with treatment of the underlying disease process. More frequently, thoracic involvement of RA consists of a pleural effusion.

■ Diagnosis

Reactivation tuberculosis

✓ Pearls

- Cavitation within the upper lobes and superior segment involvement are associated with postprimary TB.
- Histoplasmosis and coccidioidomycosis are the most common fungal pulmonary infections in the United States.
- SCC (primary or secondary) commonly cavitates; primary SCC is associated with smoking.
- GPA is a vasculitis that affects the airways, lungs, and kidneys; pulmonary nodules cavitate.

Suggested Readings

Collins J, Stern EJ. Chest Radiology: The Essentials. Philadelphia, PA: Lippincott Williams & Wilkins; 2008

Walker CM, Abbott GF, Greene RE, Shepard JA, Vummidi D, Digumarthy SR. Imaging pulmonary infection: classic signs and patterns. AJR Am J Roentgenol. 2014; 202(3):479–492

Webb R, Higgins C. Thoracic Imaging: Pulmonary and Cardiovascular Radiology. Philadelphia, PA: Lippincott Williams & Wilkins; 2010

Case 4

John P. Lichtenberger III

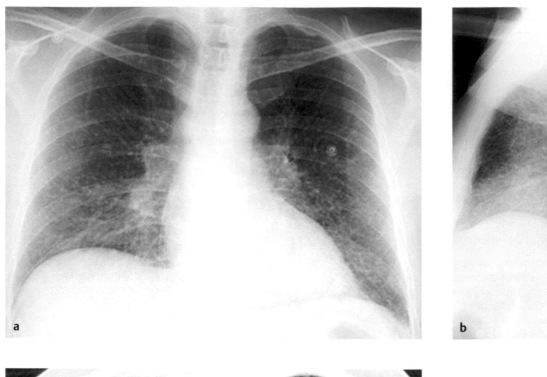

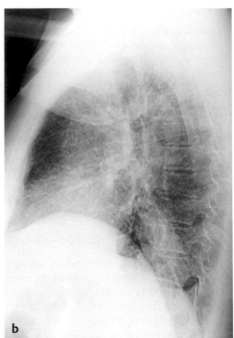

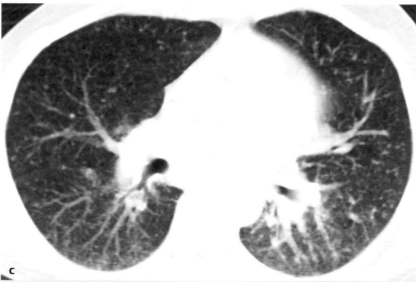

Fig. 4.1 **(a)** Frontal and **(b)** lateral chest radiographs reveal diffuse bilateral tiny nodular densities, along with bilateral hilar fullness. **(c)** Axial computed tomography (CT) image in lung window demonstrates diffuse bilateral 1- to 3-mm miliary nodules in a random distribution.

■ Clinical Presentation

A 28-year-old immunocompromised patient with chronic cough (▶Fig. 4.1).

■ Key Imaging Finding

Miliary pulmonary nodules

■ Top 3 Differential Diagnoses

- **Tuberculosis (TB)**. Pulmonary infection with *Mycobacterium tuberculosis* is classified as primary or reactivation based on clinical and radiographic features. Predominantly, a lower lobe air-space disease, mediastinal lymphadenopathy, and pleural effusions are typical radiographic manifestations of primary infection. Reactivation TB, however, characteristically presents as upper lobe consolidation with regions of cavitation and fibrosis, endobronchial spread with ill-defined centrilobular opacities in a "tree-in-bud" configuration, or hematogenous spread with randomly distributed 1- to 3-mm nodules, referred to as a miliary pattern. The miliary pattern is more common in children, elderly, and immunocompromised patients (HIV, transplant, etc.).

- **Fungal disease**. Fungal infection in the lung encompasses both primary infection in immunocompetent patients (e.g. *Histoplasma, Coccidioides,*blastomycosis) and opportunistic infection in immunosuppressed patients (e.g., *Aspergillus, Candida, Cryptococcus*). Although radiographic features are somewhat organism dependent, disseminated fungal infection can result in a miliary pattern identical to miliary TB. Chronic fungal infections may cavitate.
- **Metastases**. Although hematogenous metastases to the lung may occur with numerous primary malignancies, thyroid carcinoma, renal cell carcinoma (RCC), and melanoma are the most common primary malignancies to produce a miliary pattern of dissemination in the chest.

■ Additional Differential Diagnoses

- **Pneumoconioses**. The pneumoconioses result from inhalation of particulate matter as a result of occupational exposure. Silicosis and coal worker's pneumoconiosis are among the most common entities. Radiographic findings consist of multiple upper lobe fibrotic nodules ranging from 1 to 10 mm in size. When small, the appearance mimics that of miliary disease processes. As the disease progresses, fibrosis ensues and the nodular densities coalesce. Eggshell calcifications may be seen within hilar and mediastinal lymph nodes. A late complication referred to as progressive massive fibrosis presents

radiographically as upper lobe masslike opacities in the setting of underlying fibrosis. Patients are at an increased risk of superinfection, especially TB.
- **Healed varicella**. Acute varicella pneumonia is a severe form of primary infection which occurs primarily in children and pregnant patients. The infection presents as multifocal regions of patchy air-space disease, and affected patients are very ill. Healed varicella presents radiographically as calcified miliary pulmonary nodules in a random distribution.

■ Diagnosis

Fungal disease (coccidioidomycosis)

✓ Pearls

- Miliary spread of TB is most common in children, elderly, and immunocompromised patients.
- Disseminated fungal disease may present with a miliary pattern; chronic fungal disease can cavitate.

- Thyroid carcinoma, RCC, and melanoma are the most common primary neoplasms with a miliary pattern.
- Pneumoconioses result from occupational exposure; eggshell lymph node calcifications may be seen.

Suggested Readings

Collins J, Stern EJ. Chest Radiology: The Essentials. Philadelphia, PA: Lippincott Williams & Wilkins; 2008

Mcloud TC, Boiselle PM. Thoracic Radiology: The Requisites. Philadelphia, PA: Mosby; 2010

Walker CM, Abbott GF, Greene RE, Shepard JA, Vummidi D, Digumarthy SR. Imaging pulmonary infection: classic signs and patterns. AJR Am J Roentgenol. 2014; 202(3):479–492

Case 5

Paul B. DiDomenico

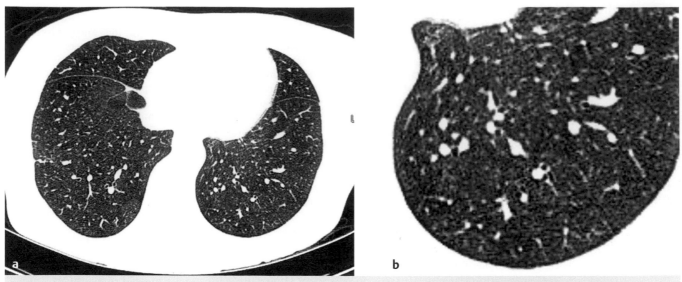

Fig. 5.1 (a) Axial CT image through the chest and (b) coned-down view of the left lower lobe in lung window reveals diffuse bilateral ill-defined centrilobular ground-glass nodules.

■ Clinical Presentation

A 50-year-old woman with cough and shortness of breath (▶ Fig. 5.1).

■ Key Imaging Finding

Centrilobular pulmonary nodules

■ Top 3 Differential Diagnoses

- **Infectious bronchiolitis** (*Mycobacterium avium-intracellulare* **infection [MAI], tuberculosis [TB]**). Infection from both tuberculous and nontuberculous mycobacterial (NTMB) organisms may manifest as numerous small nodular opacities centered on the bronchiole of the secondary pulmonary lobule with sparing of the subpleural space (centrilobular nodules). Numerous species of mycobacteria are ubiquitous in the environment, but *M. avium intracellulare* and *Mycobacterium Kansasii* account for most nontuberculous infections. A pattern of clustered nodules with branching opacities (so-called tree-in-bud pattern) in the lingula and right middle lobe is typical of MAI and is often seen in elderly women; this pattern is termed "Lady Windermere" syndrome. NTMB infections may be indistinguishable from postprimary (reactivation) TB.
- **Hypersensitivity pneumonitis (HP).** Also known as extrinsic allergic alveolitis, HP results from exposure to environmental antigens inhaled as dust particles. Varying sources of organic dusts may result in farmer's lung (moldy hay), bird fancier's lung (avian proteins), or humidifier lung (thermophilic bacteria), which are indistinguishable radiographically. Following exposure, the acute phase may exhibit fine nodular or ground-glass opacities. Centrilobular nodules with ground-glass opacities are typical of the subacute phase of the disease, most often in the mid- to lower lung zones. If exposure continues, there may be progression to end-stage lung disease with fibrosis.
- **Endobronchial spread of tumor.** Metastatic spread of tumors within the chest may take a variety of routes including direct, hematogenous, lymphatic, and endobronchial spread. While hematogenous spread is the most common form of widespread dissemination, endobronchial spread is also possible in late stages of disease and may manifest as centrilobular nodules in any part of the lung.

■ Additional Differential Diagnoses

- **Respiratory bronchiolitis-associated interstitial lung disease (RB-ILD).** RB-ILD is usually seen in smokers 30 to 50 years of age. Findings at computed tomography (CT) include either upper lobe predominance or diffuse centrilobular nodules, representing accumulated pigmented macrophages, with patchy ground-glass opacities.
- **Pneumoconioses.** Silicosis and coal worker's pneumoconiosis result from occupational exposure and present as upper lobe– predominant interstitial lung diseases. Either perilymphatic or centrilobular nodules may be present, which may eventually coalesce to form masslike opacities and potentially calcify. Involved lymph nodes may also calcify peripherally, resulting in a characteristic "eggshell" appearance. Late findings may include masslike fibrosis with peripheral emphysema (progressive massive fibrosis).

■ Diagnosis

Hypersensitivity pneumonitis

✓ Pearls

- Mycobacteria are common causes of infectious bronchiolitis; a "tree-in-bud" appearance is characteristic.
- HP results from exposure to inhaled antigens; centrilobular nodules and ground-glass opacities are typical.
- Endobronchial spread of tumor occurs in late stages of malignancy and may involve any part of the lung.
- RB-ILD is a smoking-related process with diffuse or upper lobe–predominant centrilobular nodules.

Suggested Readings

Collins J. CT signs and patterns of lung disease. Radiol Clin North Am. 2001; 39(6):1115–1135

Walker CM, Abbott GF, Greene RE, Shepard JA, Vummidi D, Digumarthy SR. Imaging pulmonary infection: classic signs and patterns. AJR Am J Roentgenol. 2014; 202(3):479–492

Webb WR, Müller NL, Naidich DP. High-Resolution CT of the Lung. Philadelphia, PA: Lippincott Williams & Wilkins; 2009

Case 6

John P. Lichtenberger III

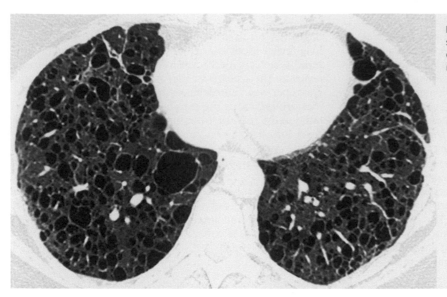

Fig. 6.1 Unenhanced axial CT image of the chest shows numerous bilateral thin-walled cysts, most of which are similar in size. The intervening lung is normal.

■ Clinical Presentation

A 31-year-old woman with a smoking history, chronic cough, and shortness of breath (▶Fig. 6.1).

■ Key Imaging Finding

Cystic lung disease

■ Top 3 Differential Diagnoses

- **Emphysema.** Emphysema is characterized by nonfibrotic enlargement of the airways distal to the terminal bronchioles with destruction of alveolar walls. Computed tomography (CT) further characterizes this process based on the location of these cystic spaces at the lobular level. Centrilobular emphysema involves the central portion of the secondary pulmonary lobule with upper lobe predominance and is highly associated with cigarette smoking. Panlobular emphysema involves the entire lobule and is classically associated with alpha-1 antitrypsin deficiency. Paraseptal emphysema is predominantly subpleural, involving the alveolar ducts and sacs. Bronchiectasis refers to enlargement and thickening of portions of the airways.
- **Lymphangioleiomyomatosis (LAM).** A relatively rare disease affecting women of reproductive age, LAM is characterized by proliferation of smooth muscle cells around bronchioles.

This results in air trapping and characteristic thin-walled lung cysts. The cysts are typically uniform in size. Air trapping predisposes patients to pneumothoraces. A similar process involving the lymphatics results in chylous pleural effusions. LAM may occur as an isolated abnormality or in association with tuberous sclerosis.

- **Pulmonary Langerhans cell histiocytosis (LCH).** Seen predominantly in young and middle-aged adults and almost exclusively in smokers, pulmonary LCH is an idiopathic disease of mature histiocyte proliferation. On imaging, numerous small (<1.0 cm) upper lobe predominant nodules, many of which demonstrate cavitation, are eventually replaced by irregular thin walled cysts of varying sizes. Costophrenic sulci are typically spared. Associated pneumothoraces are common. Occasionally, LCH may progress to interstitial fibrosis and honeycombing.

■ Additional Differential Diagnoses

- **Pneumocystis pneumonia.** The most common cause of diffuse pneumonia in immunocompromised patients, *Pneumocystis* pneumonia classically results in central ground glass opacities with or without reticulonodular interstitial thickening on plain radiographs. CT most commonly demonstrates ground glass opacification with abnormal air spaces, to include thin walled cysts, pneumatoceles, and pneumothoraces, as well as interlobular septal thickening.

- **Lymphocytic interstitial pneumonitis (LIP).** Lymphocytic infiltration of the alveolar septa characterizes lymphocytic interstitial pneumonitis, a lower lobe–predominant hyperplasia of bronchus-associated lymphoid tissue. A reticulonodular interstitial pattern on plain radiographs is better characterized on CT as centrilobular nodules with thin-walled cystic air spaces and regions of ground-glass opacification. LIP is commonly seen in the setting of Sjögren's syndrome and AIDS, particularly in children.

■ Diagnosis

Lymphangioleiomyomatosis

✓ Pearls

- Cysts and emphysema can coexist but are distinct processes; centrilobular emphysema is most common.
- Cysts must be distinguished from bronchiectasis by establishing lack of continuity with the airways.

- LAM occurs almost exclusively in women of child-bearing age; chylous pleural effusions may be seen.
- LCH is seen almost exclusively in smokers and tends to spare the costophrenic sulci.

Suggested Readings

Collins J, Stern EJ. Chest Radiology: The Essentials. Philadelphia, PA: Lippincott Williams & Wilkins; 2008

Koyama M, Johkoh T, Honda O, et al. Chronic cystic lung disease: diagnostic accuracy of high-resolution CT in 92 patients. AJR Am J Roentgenol. 2003; 180(3):827–835

Case 7

William T. O'Brien, Sr.

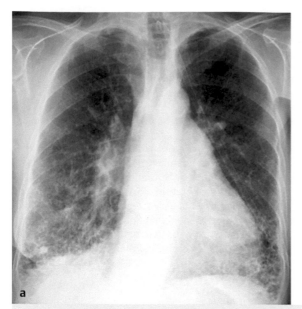 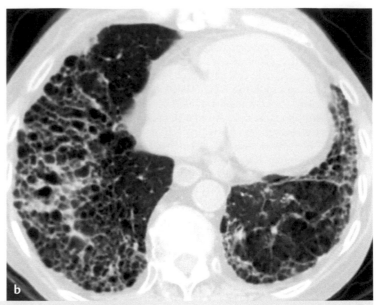

Fig. 7.1 **(a)** Frontal chest radiograph demonstrates coarsened interstitial lung markings predominantly at the lung bases. **(b)** Axial CT image shows traction bronchiectasis and fibrotic changes predominantly in the lower lobes and a dilated, patulous, fluid-filled esophagus.

■ Clinical Presentation

A 50-year-old woman with chronic shortness of breath and difficulty swallowing (►Fig. 7.1).

■ Key Imaging Finding

Lower lobe interstitial lung disease (ILD)

■ Top 3 Differential Diagnoses

- **Usual interstitial pneumonia (UIP)**. UIP is a relatively common cause of chronic fibrosing lung disease. Patients often present with worsening progressive cough and shortness of breath. Plain radiographs reveal increased interstitial markings at the lung bases with normal-to-low lung volumes. On high-resolution computed tomography (HRCT), UIP presents as irregular septal thickening along the peripheral aspect of the lower lobes with subpleural honeycombing and traction bronchiectasis in advanced cases. Occasionally, ground-glass opacities may been seen, which correlate with regions of active alveolitis. Once diagnosed, median survival is approximately 3 years. About 70% of UIP have no identifiable cause are termed idiopathic pulmonary fibrosis (IPF).
- **Collagen vascular diseases**. Collagen vascular diseases include **scleroderma**, **rheumatoid arthritis** (RA), and **systemic lupus erythematosus** (SLE) and involve the lungs to varying degrees. Scleroderma is a systemic process that affects young females and involves many organ systems—the lungs, esophagus, and musculoskeletal system. Pulmonary findings include pneumonitis and ILD with striking lower lobe predominance. HRCT reveals irregular septal thickening and subpleural honeycombing. Secondary findings include a dilated, patulous esophagus. RA is a systemic disease that most severely affects articular surfaces. Pulmonary involvement may be seen in up to 50% of cases. Unilateral pleural effusion is the most common presentation of RA within the chest. Additional manifestations include lower lobe ILD, necrobiotic pulmonary nodules, and pericarditis. Caplan syndrome refers to coal worker's pneumoconiosis superimposed upon RA. SLE is a systemic process that occurs in young females. Pleural and pericardial effusions are the most common manifestation of SLE in the chest.
- **Asbestos-related disease**. Asbestos-related lung disease results from occupational exposure, as can be seen in former shipyard workers and mechanics. The clinical and radiographic manifestations usually present 20 years after the initial exposure. Pleural thickening and pleural plaques are the most common radiographic manifestation and are typically bilateral, involving predominantly the lower thorax. The plaques often calcify. A benign exudative pleural effusion may also occur. Rounded atelectasis is a common finding and presents as a rounded mass, which abuts the pleura in a region of underlying pleural thickening. Vessels can be seen "swirling" into the lesion. HRCT findings include subpleural lines and parenchymal bands extending to the pleura. Lung involvement can include lower lobe septal thickening and subpleural honeycombing. When there is pulmonary fibrosis, it is called asbestosis.

■ Additional Differential Diagnoses

- **Drug toxicity**. Drug toxicity from chemotherapeutic agents or illicit drug abuse may rarely result in predominantly lower lobe ILD characterized by irregular septal thickening and subpleural honeycombing. Other patterns of injury include pulmonary edema, pulmonary hemorrhage, and hypersensitivity pneumonitis. Bleomycin and busulfan are the most common chemotherapeutic agents that cause lower lobe ILD. Amiodarone may also result in lower lobe ILD, along with characteristic dense opacities.

■ Diagnosis

Connective tissue disorder (scleroderma)

✓ Pearls

- UIP is the histologic and imaging descriptor of many diseases; when the cause is unknown, it is called IPF.
- Scleroderma is the most common collagen vascular disease that produces lower lobe fibrosis.
- Asbestos exposure and asbestosis are related but different; asbestosis is defined by interstitial fibrosis.
- Chemotherapeutic agents may predominantly cause lower lobe ILD; amiodarone produces dense opacities.

Suggested Readings

Mueller-Mang C, Grosse C, Schmid K, Stiebellehner L, Bankier AA. What every radiologist should know about idiopathic interstitial pneumonias. Radiographics. 2007; 27(3):595–615

Case 8

Bang Huynh

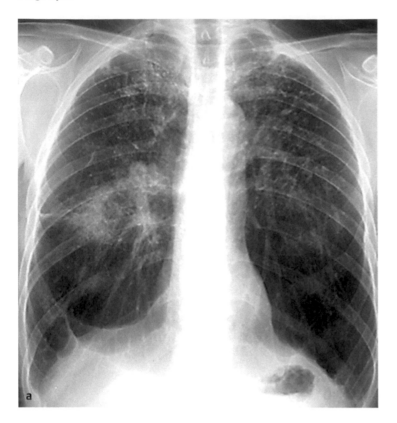
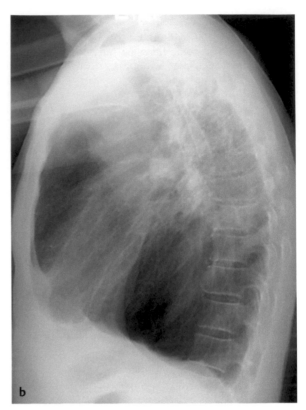

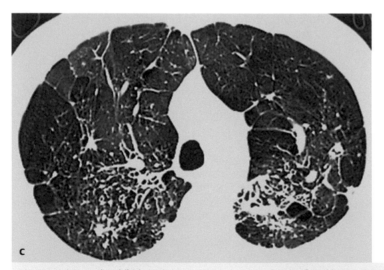

Fig. 8.1 **(a)** Frontal and **(b)** lateral chest radiographs show hyperinflated lungs with narrowing of the mediastinum and flattening of the diaphragm, better seen on the lateral view, as well as superior retraction of the hila. There are coarsened, irregular interstitial markings and countless small nodules predominantly within the upper lobes. A masslike opacity is seen in the right upper lobe extending from the hilum. **(c)** Axial CT image in lung window reveals multiple 2- to 3-mm nodules, interlobular septal thickening with traction bronchiectasis, and scarring with distortion of the normal architecture within the upper lobes.

■ **Clinical Presentation**

Chronic progressive shortness of breath (▶ Fig. 8.1).

■ Key Imaging Finding

Upper lobe interstitial lung disease

■ Top 3 Differential Diagnoses

- **Postprimary tuberculosis (TB)**. Primary TB can have a broad range of presentations but is typically characterized by mediastinal and unilateral hilar lymphadenopathy (sometimes of low attenuation). Parenchymal involvement can range from poorly defined opacities to lobar consolidations. Pleural effusions are not uncommon. Nodal calcification is present in about a third of cases. There is no distribution preference, and cavitation, though possible, is not common. In contrast, postprimary TB favors the posterior segments of the upper lobes or superior segments of the lower lobes primarily because of higher oxygen tension and less efficient lymphatic clearance. Cavitation and fibrosis are distinct features of postprimary TB. Other manifestations of TB include miliary and endobronchial patterns.
- **Sarcoidosis**. Sarcoidosis is a systemic disease of unknown etiology characterized by noncaseating granulomas. Thoracic disease may include mediastinal/hilar and parenchymal involvement. Hilar adenopathy is often bilateral and symmetric. Parenchymal involvement usually consists of countless 2- to 4-mm centrilobular and subpleural (perilymphatic) nodules. There is an upper lobe and peribronchovascular distribution. Sarcoid granulomas can resolve completely; however, they occasionally cause severe and extensive fibrosis that resembles progressive massive fibrosis that is seen in complicated silicosis.
- **Cystic fibrosis (CF)**. CF is a genetic disorder affecting Caucasian children and young adults. The lungs and gastrointestinal tract are most affected with thick secretions from exocrine glands. Pulmonary involvement occurs in more than 90% of patients. Viscous secretions result in upper lobe–predominant mucus plugging, air trapping, bronchial wall thickening, and bronchiectasis.

■ Additional Differential Diagnoses

- **Silicosis/coal worker's (CW) pneumoconiosis**. Pneumoconiosis is a broad term that describes reactions of the lungs to inhaled dust particles. CW pneumoconiosis and silicosis are pathologically different but have very similar radiographic appearances. Silicosis is caused by the inhalation of free silica, a compound associated with mining of heavy metal, sandblasting, and stonework. Patients may present acutely following heavy exposure whereby silicoproteinosis develops or, more commonly, with chronic silicosis from decades of exposure. The chronic form results from cyclic inflammation, resulting in fibrosis with upper lobe predominance. Complicated silicosis is an extreme progression where the fibrosis coalesces into masslike opacities, a process called progressive massive fibrosis.
- **Langerhans' cell histiocytosis (LCH)**. Pulmonary LCH is characterized by abnormal histiocyte proliferation and is seen predominantly in young and middle-aged smokers. Imaging findings include numerous small upper lobe–predominant nodules, many of which cavitate, and irregular cysts of varying sizes. Costophrenic sulci are typically spared. Associated pneumothoraces are common.

■ Diagnosis

Complicated silicosis

✓ Pearls

- Postprimary TB may result in upper lobe cavitary pulmonary nodules and fibrosis.
- Sarcoidosis presents with symmetric hilar adenopathy; perilymphatic pulmonary nodules may also be seen.
- Pulmonary manifestations of CF include upper lobe mucous plugging, air trapping, and bronchiectasis.
- Silicoproteinosis is a unique form of silicosis that is acute and indistinguishable from alveolar proteinosis.

Suggested Readings

Mueller-Mang C, Grosse C, Schmid K, Stiebellehner L, Bankier AA. What every radiologist should know about idiopathic interstitial pneumonias. Radiographics. 2007; 27(3):595–615

Pipavath S, Godwin JD. Imaging of interstitial lung disease. Clin Chest Med. 2004; 25(3):455–465

Pipavath S, Godwin JD. Imaging of interstitial lung disease. Radiol Clin North Am. 2005; 43:589–599

Case 9

Arash J. Momeni

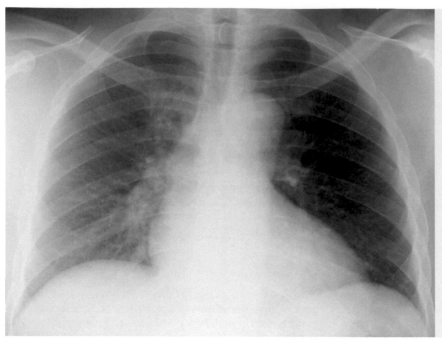

Fig. 9.1 Frontal chest radiograph demonstrates hyperlucency of the left hemithorax. Lung volumes are normal and symmetric.

■ Clinical Presentation

A 40-year-old man with occasional dyspnea on exertion (▶ Fig. 9.1).

■ Key Imaging Finding

Unilateral hyperlucent lung

■ Top 3 Differential Diagnoses That You Cannot Afford to Miss

- **Airway obstruction**. The hallmark of airway obstruction in children is air trapping, which is manifested as failure of the lung to decrease in volume, and subsequently increase in opacification, on expiratory chest radiographs. The mediastinum may shift to the contralateral side. Air trapping occurs when an endobronchial lesion causes a check-valve type of obstruction. In children, this is usually secondary to foreign body aspiration (which may be radiolucent). Expiratory views, decubitus views, and fluoroscopy may be helpful.
- **Pulmonary embolism**. Oligemia of the lung beyond the occluded pulmonary vessel, or the Westermark sign, is a helpful but not commonly encountered sign of pulmonary embolism.

A large unilateral thrombus, whether bland, septic, or neoplastic, can result in a unilateral hyperlucent lung.
- **Pneumothorax**. A pneumothorax results in hyperlucency of the ipsilateral hemithorax and typically presents with central displacement of the visceral pleural line, absence of lung markings distal to the displaced pleural line, and possible contralateral shift of the mediastinum (tension pneumothorax). In a supine patient, a pneumothorax may collect anteromedially, in the nondependent portion of the thorax. This will result in the pneumothorax presenting as lucency in the anteromedial chest rather than as a pleural line. A deep hyperlucent sulcus may also be seen. A tension pneumothorax is a true emergency.

■ Additional Differential Diagnoses

- **Chest wall abnormality**. Several chest wall abnormalities may result in a hyperlucent lung. For example, mastectomy results in relative radiolucency on the side of breast tissue removal. Poland syndrome is characterized by a spectrum of abnormalities ranging from isolated absence of the pectoralis major muscle to additional abnormalities of the ipsilateral extremity, such as syndactyly, brachydactyly, and rib anomalies.
- **Swyer–James syndrome**. Swyer–James syndrome, or MacLeod syndrome, is a form of obliterative bronchiolitis that occurs following an insult, classically viral, to the developing lung. This process affects small bronchi and bronchioles. The portions of the lung ventilated by abnormal airways remain

inflated by collateral air drift. Chest radiographs demonstrate unilateral hyperlucency because of reduced lung perfusion. Air trapping may be seen on expiratory radiographs or high-resolution computed tomography (HRCT). Lung volumes on the affected side may be normal or decreased. On CT, additional findings may include bronchiectasis and attenuated vessels in areas of decreased lung attenuation.
- **Acute asthmatic attack**. Hyperlucency in asthma is secondary to bronchoconstriction and compensatory vasoconstriction of hypoventilated portions of the lung. As this is usually a more central process, findings are commonly bilateral but may be asymmetric.

■ Diagnosis

Chest wall abnormality (Poland syndrome)

✓ Pearls

- Expiratory views, decubitus views, and fluoroscopy may be helpful in evaluating for foreign bodies.
- Always consider pulmonary embolism and pneumothorax (in a supine patient) with a hyperlucent lung.

- Swyer–James syndrome is usually a unilateral process where the affected lung is reduced in size.

Suggested Readings

Collins J, Stern EJ. Chest Radiology: The Essentials. Philadelphia, PA: Lippincott Williams & Wilkins; 2008

Reid L, Simon G. Unilateral lung transradiancy. Thorax. 1962; 17:230–239

Case 10

Bang Huynh

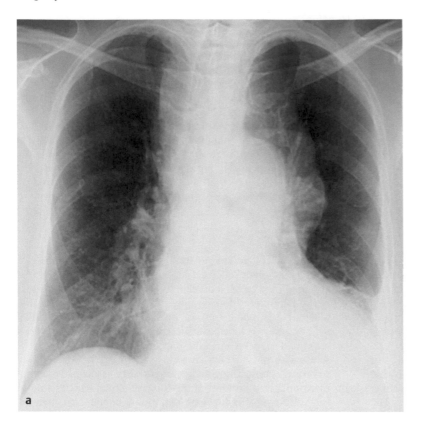
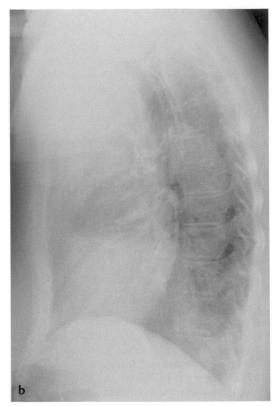
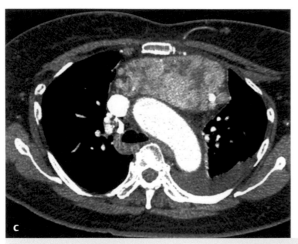
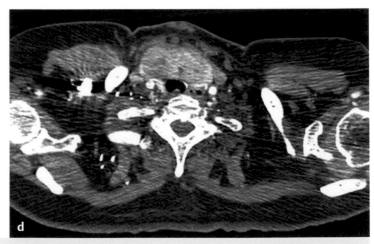

Fig. 10.1 **(a)** Posteroanterior radiograph shows a lobulated mediastinal mass that does not silhouette the aortic arch. **(b)** Lateral radiograph shows that the retrosternal clear space is obscured. **(c,d)** Enhanced axial CT images reveal a heterogeneously enhancing anterior mediastinal mass with coarse foci of calcification **(c)**, which is contiguous with the thyroid gland **(d)**.

■ Clinical Presentation

Employment physical (▶ Fig. 10.1).

■ Key Imaging Finding

Anterior mediastinal mass

■ Top 3 Differential Diagnoses

- **Lymphoma**. Lymphoma is a primary neoplasm of the lympho-reticular system that is divided into two main types: Hodgkin disease (HD) and non-Hodgkin lymphoma (NHL). While HD is the less common of the two types, it is more likely to involve the thorax (up to 85% of HD cases as compared to 40–50% of NHL cases). Of the HD cases with thoracic involvement, nearly all (98%) involve superior mediastinal nodes (i.e., aorticopul-monary window, prevascular, paratracheal). The percentage of superior mediastinal node involvement in HD is so high that normal superior mediastinal nodes in the setting of thoracic involvement make HD unlikely. Calcification does not occur prior to treatment. In HD, the anatomic extent of disease correlates well with prognosis. In contrast, prognosis of NHL is better predicted by histopathologic classification.
- **Thymic lesion**. The normal thymus increases from birth to puberty, after which it begins to involute over a 5- to 15-year period. Thymic tissue is progressively replaced by fat. By the age of 60 years, little thymic tissue remains. Abnormalities of thymic origin can be due to a number of processes. The thymus itself may be abnormally enlarged, as in thymic hyperplasia or thymic rebound, or abnormally infiltrated, as in lymphoid follicular hyperplasia. A number of masses and tumors can arise from the thymus, including thymoma, thymic carcinoma, thymic carcinoid, cysts, lipomas, and lymphoma. Thymomas (most common) most often occur in the third and fourth decades of life and may be associated with myasthenia gravis.
- **Thyroid lesion**. Thyroid masses account for approximately 10% of mediastinal masses. The majority (80%) are in the anterior mediastinum. Mediastinal masses of thyroid origin are almost always contiguous with the thyroid gland. A truly ectopic mediastinal mass without a connection to the thyroid is possible but uncommon. Radiographically, mediastinal thyroid masses often cause tracheal deviation. On computed tomography (CT), normal thyroid tissue has a characteristic appearance, being high attenuation relative to adjacent soft tissue on noncontrast studies and enhancing avidly postcontrast. Calcifications may be present, but in the end, differentiation between goiter and thyroid carcinoma is difficult unless lymphadenopathy, destruction of adjacent structures (e.g., tracheal invasion), or metastases are present.

■ Additional Differential Diagnoses

- **Germ cell neoplasm (GCN)**: GCNs, which account for about 10% of primary mediastinal masses, arise from primitive germ cells that have arrested in the mediastinum during embryologic migration. The majority are located in the anterior mediastinum and present during the second through fourth decades of life. GCNs can be benign or malignant, but the majority (80%) are benign. GCNs include teratomas, seminomas, embryonal carcinoma, yolk sac tumors, choriocarcinoma, and mixed cell types. Imaging findings are broad. Solid and cystic components may be present. Teratomas, which contain elements of all germinal layers, can include skin, hair, fat, and bones if well differentiated.

■ Diagnosis

Thyroid lesion (goiter)

✓ Pearls

- HD presents as noncalcified mediastinal adenopathy involving the anterior and superior mediastinum.
- Thymic lesions include thymomas (most common), invasive thymomas, carcinomas, lipomas, and cysts.
- Thyroid lesions are contiguous with the thyroid gland, result in tracheal deviation, and avidly enhance.
- GCN most commonly presents in the second through fourth decades of life; the majority are benign.

Suggested Readings

Carter BW, Okumura M, Detterbeck FC, Marom EM. Approaching the patient with an anterior mediastinal mass: a guide for radiologists. J Thorac Oncol. 2014; 9(9, Suppl 2):S110–S118

Reed JC. Chest Radiology: Plain Film Patterns and Differential Diagnoses. Philadelphia, PA: Mosby Inc; 2010

Case 11

Bang Huynh

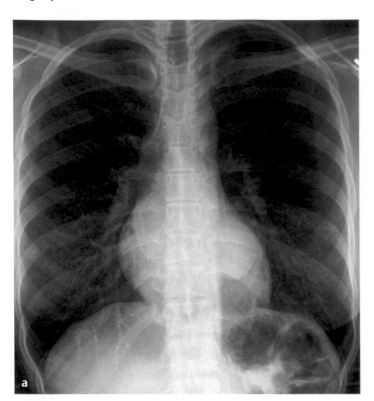
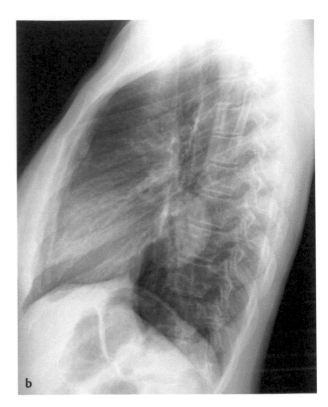
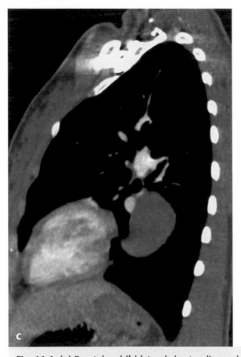
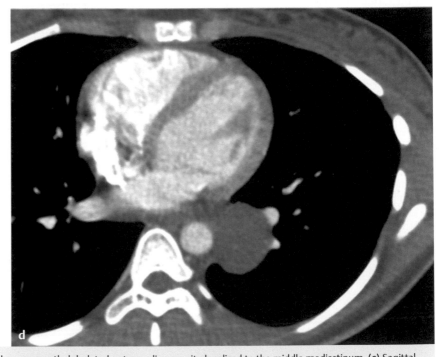

Fig. 11.1 **(a)** Frontal and **(b)** lateral chest radiographs show a smooth, lobulated, retrocardiac opacity localized to the middle mediastinum. **(c)** Sagittal and **(d)** axial CT images in soft-tissue window confirm a well-circumscribed lobulated soft-tissue mass in the middle (visceral) mediastinum.

■ Clinical Presentation

Preemployment physical chest X-ray, asymptomatic (▶Fig. 11.1).

■ Key Imaging Finding

Middle mediastinal mass

■ Top 3 Differential Diagnoses

- **Lymphadenopathy**. Lymphadenopathy is a nonspecific finding that may be reactive or neoplastic in etiology. Lymphoma is high on the differential diagnostic list, and metastasis, particularly if patient has a known primary, must be considered. The pattern and appearance of lymphatic spread in the thorax may vary depending on the causative etiology. There are some secondary features, best evaluated by computed tomography (CT), which may help narrow the differential diagnosis. Low-attenuation nodes may reflect necrosis in the setting of tuberculosis, fungal infection, metastasis, and lymphoma. Enhancing nodes may be seen in the setting of Castleman disease, hypervascular metastases, tuberculosis, and rarely sarcoidosis.
- **Vascular abnormality**. Vascular abnormalities must always be considered initially in the differential of a middle mediastinal mass, particularly if in proximity to the aorta. Possible causes of abnormal aortic and middle mediastinal contours include thoracic aortic aneurysm, penetrating aortic ulcers, and pseudoaneurysms. CT and magnetic resonance imaging (MRI) are helpful in the evaluation of aortic pathology. Aortic aneurysms (diameter > 4 cm) can be described by their shape (fusiform or saccular) and by the extent of wall involvement (true or false aneurysm). Saccular aneurysms are associated with infections and are at high risk for rupture, while fusiform aneurysms are more often associated with atherosclerosis and vasculitis. Pulmonary artery aneurysms are less common causes of middle mediastinal masses. Etiologies include primary and secondary pulmonary artery hypertension, as well as trauma, neoplasm, or infection.
- **Congenital cyst**. Foregut duplication cysts are the most common congenital cysts in the middle mediastinum and result from abnormalities in foregut development. Among the various types, mediastinal bronchogenic cysts are the most common. While they may present in any part of the mediastinum, most are in contact with the tracheobronchial tree and within 5 cm of the carina; thus, most are in the middle mediastinum. On radiographs, they often appear as smooth, sharply circumscribed lobular or round densities. On CT, about half have simple fluid attenuation, while the remainder have varying attenuation, depending on proteinaceous or blood content. When of higher attenuation, they can appear solid, but will not enhance. The wall, if perceptible, is thin unless the cyst is complicated by infection. Rarely, the wall will calcify. Most mediastinal bronchogenic cysts are asymptomatic but can increase in size over time to become symptomatic by compression of adjacent structures. Pericardial cysts are less common and result from failure of fusion of a portion of the pericardium. Most are located at the cardiophrenic angle, right greater than left. Management of congenital cysts tends to be surgical, although more recent options include percutaneous or transbronchial aspiration.

■ Additional Differential Diagnoses

- **Hiatal hernia**. A hiatal hernia is a protrusion of the part of the stomach through the diaphragmatic hiatus. A gas or gas–fluid level may be seen within a hiatal hernia. Radiographically, esophageal carcinoma can mimic a hernia, as both can present with subtle abnormal bowing of the azygoesophageal recess.

■ Diagnosis

Congenital cyst (bronchogenic)

✓ Pearls

- Mediastinal lymphadenopathy is most often due to lymphoma, metastases, infectious process, or sarcoid.
- Vascular enlargement of the thoracic aorta or pulmonary arteries may result in a middle mediastinal mass.
- Bronchogenic duplication cysts are the most common congenital cysts in the middle mediastinum.

Suggested Readings

Carter BW, Tomiyama N, Bhora FY, et al. A modern definition of mediastinal compartments. J Thorac Oncol. 2014; 9(9, Suppl 2):S97–S101

Webb WR, Higgins CB. Thoracic Imaging. Philadelphia, PA: Lippincott Williams & Wilkins; 2010

Case 12

Brent McCarragher and Thomas Ray S. Sanchez

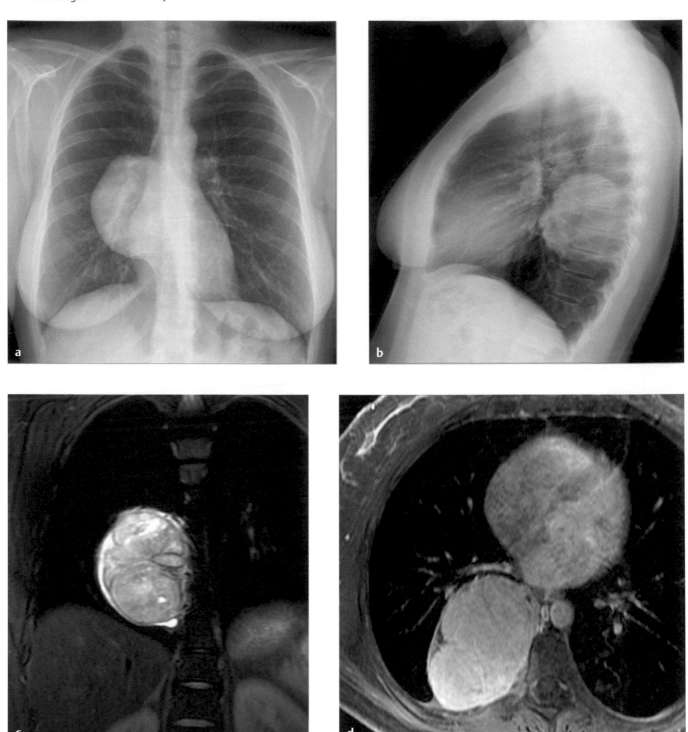

Fig. 12.1 **(a)** Posteroanterior and **(b)** lateral chest radiographs show a well-defined right paraspinal mass, which arises from the posterior mediastinum. **(c)** Coronal T2-weighted image shows a heterogeneous hyperintense right paraspinal solid mass. **(d)** The axial T1 postcontrast image with fat suppression demonstrates a homogenously enhancing right paraspinal mass. There is no evidence of intraspinal extension or bony involvement.

◼ Clinical Presentation

A 34-year-old asymptomatic woman with incidental finding (▶Fig. 12.1).

■ Key Imaging Finding

Posterior mediastinal mass

■ Top 3 Differential Diagnoses

- **Neurogenic tumor**. Neurogenic tumors are the most common posterior (paravertebral) mediastinal masses and are grouped into nerve sheath tumors, sympathetic ganglion cell tumors, and preganglionic tumors. Nerve sheath tumors are the most common and include schwannoma, neurofibroma, and malignant peripheral nerve sheath tumor. Sympathetic ganglion cell tumors include neuroblastoma and ganglioneuroblastomas, often occur in the pediatric population, and are typically aggressive primitive neoplasms of neuroectodermal origin. Concerning imaging characteristics include necrosis, hemorrhage, and the lack of a capsule. Paraganglioma is a rare neuroendocrine tumor which is hypervascular with characteristic flow voids on magnetic resonance imaging (MRI) and a classic salt-and-pepper appearance; however, this not a specific finding. Important imaging findings to consider for all posterior mediastinal masses include vascular encasement, intraspinal extension, rib splaying, and bony erosion.

- **Developmental cyst**. Neurenteric, enteric duplication, and bronchogenic cysts can be grouped together under the heading of bronchopulmonary foregut cysts/malformations. They are difficult to differentiate from one another on imaging and essentially look the same on most imaging studies. They are well-marginated round/oval masses that are cystic in nature (low density on computed tomography [CT] and high intensity on T2-weighted MRI images) and have thin walls. The presence of infection or hemorrhage can result in less characteristic imaging findings that may mimic a solid lesion or abscess. Neurenteric cysts have associated spinal malformations, which, when present, suggest the diagnosis.
- **Lymphoma**. Although the anterior mediastinum is the classic location infiltrated by lymphoma, posterior mediastinal lymph nodes can occasionally be involved as well. Homogenous masses with lobulations and the absence of necrosis or calcification in untreated cases will help differentiate lymphoma from other posterior mediastinal masses.

■ Additional Differential Diagnoses

- **Extramedullary hematopoiesis**. In patients with severe and chronic anemia (often associated with sickle cell disease, thalassemia, or hypersplenism), extramedullary hematopoiesis may occur as a result of the body's attempt to produce more red blood cells. Extramedullary hematopoiesis presents as bilateral but often asymmetric paraspinal masses. Associated findings include trabecular coarsening of the adjacent verte-

brae. Tissue correlation will sometimes be needed to rule out malignancy.
- **Mediastinal hematoma**. Mediastinal widening with associated pleural effusion (more commonly on the left) is the most common sign of mediastinal/vascular injury. Cross-sectional imaging is helpful in identifying the underlying vascular injury.

■ Diagnosis

Schwannoma

✓ Pearls

- Neurogenic tumors represent the most common posterior mediastinal masses.
- Sympathetic ganglion cell tumors occur more commonly in pediatric patients.

- Neuroenteric cysts commonly have associated spinal malformations.
- Extramedullary hematopoiesis often presents as bilateral but asymmetric posterior mediastinal masses.

Suggested Readings

Nakazono T, White CS, Yamasaki F, et al. MRI findings of mediastinal neurogenic tumors. AJR Am J Roentgenol. 2011; 197(4):W643–52

Occhipinti M, Heidinger BH, Franquet E, Eisenberg RL, Bankier AA. Imaging the posterior mediastinum: a multimodality approach. Diagn Interv Radiol. 2015; 21(4):293–306

Case 13

Bang Huynh

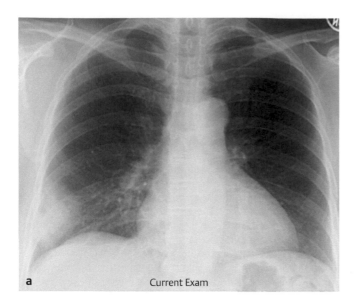

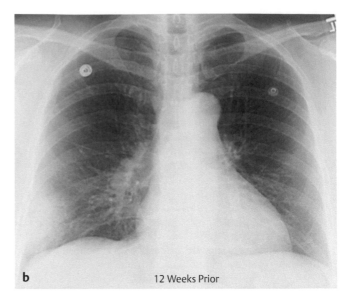

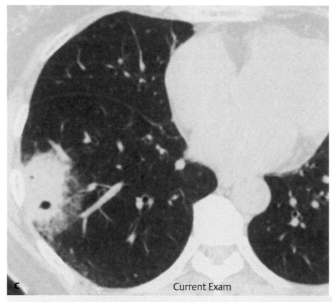

Fig. 13.1 (a) Current posteroanterior (PA) chest radiograph shows a peripheral consolidation within the right lower lobe. (b) PA chest radiograph obtained 12 weeks prior shows a similar finding. (c) Current axial CT image of the chest in lung window confirms a peripheral consolidation in the right lower lobe with a rim of ground-glass opacity and subcentimeter cyst.

■ Clinical Presentation

Follow-up of a suspected pneumonia treated 12 weeks ago (▶ Fig. 13.1).

■ Key Imaging Finding

Chronic air-space disease

■ Top 3 Differential Diagnoses

- **Organizing pneumonia (OP)**. Organization is a histologic process of fibroblast proliferation in the lung and can be thought of as a lung response to injury, most commonly infection. Patients typically present with cough and dyspnea. They are often treated for infectious pneumonia at initial presentation but fail to improve with treatment. When OP is later considered and the patient is treated with steroids, findings may improve. OP is primarily an intra-alveolar process, manifesting with patchy and peribronchial consolidations. There is often a lower lobe predominance with sparing of the subpleural space. In some patients, the distribution can be peripheral, a pattern similar to that seen in chronic eosinophilic pneumonia. Ground-glass opacities are also commonly seen on computed tomography (CT).
- **Lung cancer**. Air-space opacities that persist despite clinical treatment should raise the suspicion of a neoplastic cause. Lung cancer, particularly adenocarcinoma in this case given the associated ground-glass opacity and central pseudocavitation, can cause a chronic air-space opacity and resemble consolidation. Lymphoma may also cause a chronic consolidation, although the more typical presentation in the lung is bilateral nodules and masses.
- **Pulmonary alveolar proteinosis (PAP)**. PAP is a disease characterized by the filling of the alveolar air spaces with protein. In most cases, there is no known etiology, but some cases are thought to be due to exposure to dust (particularly silica). Symptoms are often mild for the degree of radiographic change. On radiographs, PAP manifests as bilateral, diffuse or patchy hazy opacities. On CT, the classic pattern is smooth interlobular septal thickening on a background of ground-glass opacities ("crazy paving"); however, "crazy paving" is not specific to PAP and includes a differential. PAP can also present as patchy ground-glass opacities or consolidations with an abrupt margin separating normal from involved lung.

■ Additional Differential Diagnoses

- **Chronic eosinophilic pneumonia**. Chronic eosinophilic pneumonia is an idiopathic process characterized by alveolar and interstitial infiltration of inflammatory cells. Patients also usually have increased eosinophils in the peripheral blood. Radiographically, homogeneous peripheral consolidations are present, in a pattern reminiscent of "the photographic negative of pulmonary edema." Consolidation may also be patchy, sometimes with an upper lobe predominance. Patients respond rapidly to the administration of steroids.
- **Lipoid pneumonia**. Lipoid pneumonia is the result of chronic aspiration of products that contain oil or fat. On radiographs, there are consolidations with a lower lobe distribution. The classic CT finding is consolidations with low attenuation HU -40 to -100. As this is usually a longstanding process, fibrosis, necrosis, and even cavitations may be present.

■ Diagnosis

Lung cancer (adenocarcinoma)

✓ Pearls

- OP is a common cause of chronic air-space disease; symptoms improve with steroids.
- CT findings associated with PAP are classically described as "crazy paving"; however, this is nonspecific.
- Bronchioloalveolar carcinoma may present as a ground-glass nodule (most common) or chronic air-space disease.
- Chronic eosinophilic pneumonia presents with homogeneous peripheral consolidations.

Suggested Readings

Kligerman SJ, Franks TJ, Galvin JR. From the radiologic pathology archives: organization and fibrosis as a response to lung injury in diffuse alveolar damage, organizing pneumonia, and acute fibrinous and organizing pneumonia. Radiographics. 2013; 33(7):1951–1975

Case 14

John P. Lichtenberger III

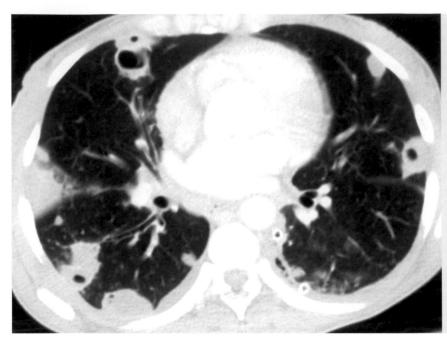

Fig. 14.1 Axial CT of the chest in lung window shows multiple bilateral peripheral consolidations, some of which are cavitary and wedge-shaped.

■ Clinical Presentation

Young adult with cough and shortness of breath (▶Fig. 14.1).

■ Key Imaging Finding

Peripheral air-space disease

■ Top 3 Differential Diagnoses

- **Embolic disease (pulmonary or septic emboli).** While the bronchial circulation may be protective in the more proximal airways, occlusion of distal pulmonary arteries from embolic sources, malignancy, or interstitial edema may lead to focal peripheral pulmonary hemorrhage and infarction. Radiographically, this produces wedge-shaped, peripheral regions of consolidation. Most pulmonary emboli are multiple with a lower lobe predominance and result from deep venous thrombosis. Causes of venous thrombosis are extensive but include trauma, malignancy, hypercoagulable states, and central venous line placement. When infected material is embolized, often a complication of intravenous drug use or endocarditis, septic emboli may cause peripheral consolidations with central cavitation. On computed tomography (CT), septic emboli commonly demonstrate a feeding vessel extending into the peripheral region of consolidation. Hampton's hump refers to a peripheral wedge-shaped opacity along the diaphragm and is highly suggestive of pulmonary embolism. Heart failure is an important predisposing factor for pulmonary infarction in general.

- **Organizing pneumonia (OP).** A nonspecific inflammatory response resulting in alveolar space fibrosis, OP is characterized by focal areas of chronic lower lobe–predominant peripheral consolidation, which often spares the subpleural space. Diffuse and bronchovascular nodules may also be seen. Lung volumes are often normal radiographically.
- **Eosinophilic pneumonia.** Eosinophilic lung disease encompasses a wide range of disorders characterized by tissue or blood eosinophilia and pulmonary involvement, typically differentiated by integrating clinical presentation with imaging findings. While acute eosinophilic pneumonia typically demonstrates a pattern similar to pulmonary edema, chronic eosinophilic pneumonia is suggested by homogeneous peripheral consolidations, which radiographically may be seen as a photographic negative of pulmonary edema. Upper lobe predominance and a protracted course may distinguish chronic eosinophilic pneumonia from other entities, such as Churg–Strauss (granulomatous vasculitis associated with asthma) and Loeffler (eosinophilia and transient and migratory consolidations) syndromes.

■ Additional Differential Diagnoses

- **Pulmonary contusion.** In the setting of trauma, hemorrhage into the alveolar space can result in peripheral nonsegmental consolidations, typically adjacent to sites of thoracic injury along the rib cage. These pulmonary contusions usually resolve rapidly if parenchymal injury is not complicated by pneumatocele, laceration, hematoma, or infection.
- **Alveolar sarcoidosis.** Sarcoidosis most commonly presents as bilateral symmetric hilar and mediastinal lymphadenopathy

with or without parenchymal involvement. The most common parenchymal manifestations include perilymphatic nodules and architectural distortion with an upper lobe predominance. Peripheral consolidations associated with mediastinal and bilateral hilar adenopathy in an asymptomatic patient may be a rare presentation of alveolar sarcoidosis.

■ Diagnosis

Septic emboli

✓ Pearls

- Pulmonary infarcts from emboli may present with peripheral wedge-shaped lower lobe consolidations.
- Eosinophilic pneumonia can present as a photographic negative of pulmonary edema with eosinophilia.

- Pulmonary contusions present as nonsegmental consolidations along the chest wall at sites of injury.

Suggested Readings

Bray TJ, Mortensen KH, Gopalan D. Multimodality imaging of pulmonary infarction. Eur J Radiol. 2014; 83(12):2240–2254

Case 15

John P. Lichtenberger III

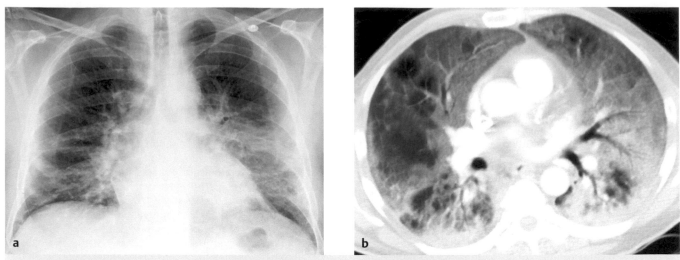

Fig. 15.1 **(a)** Posteroanterior chest radiograph shows lower lung–predominant bilateral patchy air-space opacities. **(b)** Contrast-enhanced axial CT of the chest in lung window shows diffuse ground-glass opacity in a geographic distribution with lobular sparing.

■ Clinical Presentation

Adult man with shortness of breath (►Fig. 15.1).

■ Key Imaging Finding

Ground-glass opacification

■ Top 3 Differential Diagnoses

- **Pulmonary edema**. Pulmonary edema follows a natural progression which involves interstitial edema with Kerley B lines, cephalization of flow, and resultant air-space disease (ground-glass opacities with regions of consolidation). The central and perihilar lungs are involved early with patchy opacities in a batwing configuration. Cardiomegaly and pleural effusions are seen in the setting of cardiogenic pulmonary edema.
- **Infection**. Pneumocystis, cytomegalovirus, and respiratory syncytial virus pneumonias may account for ground-glass opacities, particularly in an immunocompromised patient. Invasive aspergillosis may elicit a ground-glass halo around a focal region of consolidation which represents pulmonary hemorrhage. A panlobular distribution is more typical of *Pneumocystis* pneumonia.
- **Acute respiratory distress syndrome (ARDS)**. Diffuse lung parenchymal injury resulting in pulmonary opacification and hypoxia characterizes ARDS. Common causes of ARDS include trauma, sepsis, toxic inhalation, and near-drowning. Although ARDS remains a clinical diagnosis, the underlying pathology leads to ground-glass opacities with regions of consolidation. The lack of cardiomegaly and pleural effusions helps distinguish this entity from cardiogenic pulmonary edema. Pneumothorax is a frequent complication.

■ Additional Differential Diagnoses

- **Pulmonary hemorrhage**. Air-space disease secondary to pulmonary hemorrhage may manifest as ground-glass opacities, as well as ground-glass nodules. Common etiologies include trauma and vasculitis.
- **Alveolar proteinosis**. An idiopathic disease predominantly affecting middle-aged men, alveolar proteinosis results from chronic accumulation of excessive proteinaceous material in the alveoli. Radiographic features may mimic pulmonary edema, although cardiomegaly and pleural effusions are not characteristic. On computed tomography (CT), ground-glass opacities are distributed geographically with sharp margination and associated smooth septal thickening. Juxtaposition of normal and involved lung parenchyma has been termed "crazy paving," which in and of itself is a nonspecific finding. Treatment consists of bronchoalveolar lavage.
- **Vasculitis**. Perivascular inflammation within the lung secondary to a vasculitic process may appear as ground-glass opacities. Common causes include Wegener granulomatosis and systemic lupus erythematosus. Symptomatic patients are treated with steroids during acute flares.

■ Diagnosis

Infection (*Pneumocystis* pneumonia)

✓ Pearls

- Pulmonary edema progresses from interstitial to air-space disease; cardiomegaly and effusions are typical.
- Atypical infections may present with ground-glass opacities, especially in immunocompromised patients.
- ARDS results from diffuse lung injury; it mimics pulmonary edema but lacks cardiomegaly or effusions.
- Alveolar proteinosis presents with ground-glass opacities and septal thickening; it is treated with lavage.

Suggested Readings

Lichtenberger JP, III, Sharma A, Zachary KC, et al. What a differential a virus makes: a practical approach to thoracic imaging findings in the context of HIV infection--part 1, pulmonary findings. AJR Am J Roentgenol. 2012; 198(6):1295–1304

Park CM, Goo JM, Lee HJ, Lee CH, Chun EJ, Im JG. Nodular ground-glass opacity at thin-section CT: histologic correlation and evaluation of change at follow-up. Radiographics. 2007; 27(2):391–408

Case 16

Arash J. Momeni

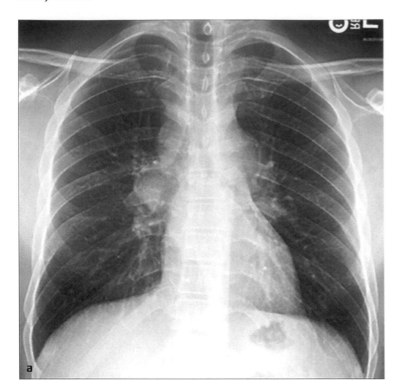
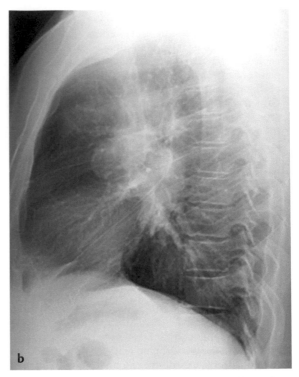

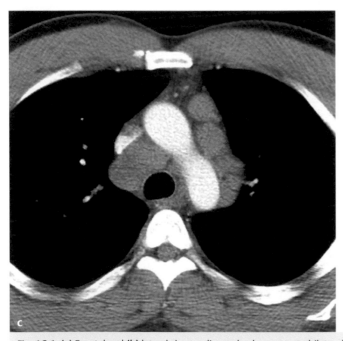
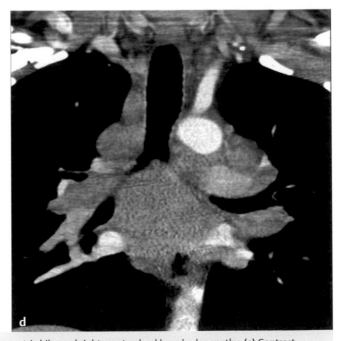

Fig. 16.1 (a) Frontal and (b) lateral chest radiographs demonstrate bilateral symmetric hilar and right paratracheal lymphadenopathy. (c) Contrast-enhanced axial and (d) coronal CT images in soft tissue window confirm bulky bilateral, symmetric hilar and mediastinal adenopathy.

■ Clinical Presentation

A 45-year-old African American man with cough and chronic shortness of breath (▶Fig. 16.1).

■ Key Imaging Finding

Mediastinal/hilar lymphadenopathy

■ Top 3 Differential Diagnoses

- **Infection**. Reactive lymphadenopathy from an infectious etiology, such as bacterial pneumonia, tuberculosis (TB), and fungal disease, is the most common cause of mediastinal lymph node enlargement. Coexistent pulmonary disease, including granuloma formation or air-space disease, is commonly seen. Calcified lymph nodes may be seen in the setting of TB and fungal disease, to include histoplasmosis and coccidioidomycosis. Mycobacterial infection may present with low-attenuation lymph nodes.
- **Lymphoma**. Thoracic involvement of lymphoma is usually associated with Hodgkin disease. It typically presents as superior mediastinal lymphadenopathy, resulting in mediastinal widening on chest radiographs. On computed tomography (CT), lymphoma may present as multiple discrete masses located in known lymph node sites, conglomerate lymphadenopathy, or as an anterior mediastinal mass. Calcification in the absence of treatment is exceedingly rare. Lymphoma is the second most common intrathoracic malignancy associated with HIV infection, in which it is usually aggressive, widely disseminated, and associated with extranodal disease.
- **Sarcoidosis**. Sarcoidosis is a systemic disease of unknown etiology characterized by noncaseating granulomas. It characteristically affects African American patients between 20 and 40 years of age, with women affected more often than men. Lymphadenopathy is the most common intrathoracic manifestation and occurs in 75 to 80% of patients at some point in their illness. The classic pattern is bilateral hilar and right paratracheal nodal enlargement, the so-called 1–2–3 sign. Sarcoidosis may be classified according to its appearance on the chest radiograph as normal (stage 0), lymphadenopathy only (stage I), nodal enlargement and parenchymal disease (stage II), parenchymal disease only (stage III), and end-stage pulmonary fibrosis (stage IV).

■ Additional Differential Diagnoses

- **Metastatic disease**. Primary neoplasms may present with mediastinal or hilar lymph node enlargement. Neoplasms prone to mediastinal or hilar metastases include lung, breast, and head and neck carcinomas; genitourinary tract neoplasms; and melanoma.
- **Pneumoconioses**. Pneumoconioses are a set of occupational diseases caused by inhalation of dust particles, including coal and silica. In addition to upper lobar parenchymal disease, scarring, and subpleural micronodules, silicosis and coal worker's pneumoconiosis characteristically present with calcified hilar and mediastinal lymph nodes in a characteristic "eggshell" configuration. These patients are prone to superimposed infection, especially TB, as well as an increased risk of developing lung cancer.

■ Diagnosis

Sarcoidosis

✓ Pearls

- Reactive lymphadenopathy is common with infection; nodes may calcify with TB and fungal disease.
- Absence of superior mediastinal lymphadenopathy makes Hodgkin disease an unlikely consideration.
- Sarcoidosis classically presents with right paratracheal and bilateral hilar lymphadenopathy ("1–2–3" sign).
- Pneumoconioses are occupational diseases that present with calcified nodes in an "eggshell" pattern.

Suggested Readings

Criado E, Sánchez M, Ramírez J, et al. Pulmonary sarcoidosis: typical and atypical manifestations at high-resolution CT with pathologic correlation. Radiographics. 2010; 30(6):1567–1586

Whitten CR, Khan S, Munneke GJ, Grubnic S. A diagnostic approach to mediastinal abnormalities. Radiographics. 2007; 27(3):657–671

Case 17

Bang Huynh

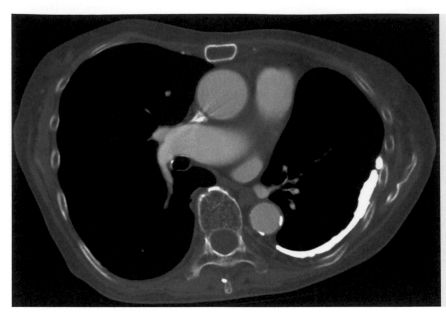

Fig. 17.1 Axial CT image through the chest in bone window shows unilateral thick uniform pleural calcification along the posterior pleural surface of the left hemithorax. The ipsilateral hemithorax is small compared to the right.

■ Clinical Presentation

Withheld (▶Fig. 17.1).

■ Key Imaging Finding

Calcified pleural disease

■ Top 3 Differential Diagnoses

- **Asbestos-related pleural disease**. Manifestations of asbestos exposure include pleural plaques, pleural thickening, and pleural effusions. Of these, pleural plaques are the most common. Plaques develop 10 to 20 years after exposure. On computed tomography (CT), plaques have a "squared" profile. Calcifications are seen in about 20% of cases, typically of the parietal surface. Most cases tend to be bilateral, but are not necessarily symmetric. The apices and costophrenic sulci are often spared. As a side note, asbestos exposure, asbestosis, and mesothelioma may be related, but are distinct entities. Asbestosis is the interstitial pulmonary fibrosis that occurs as a result of asbestos exposure, and mesothelioma is a pleural-based malignancy.
- **Fibrothorax**. Fibrothorax is the result of an organizing pyothorax, hemothorax, or effusion. If extensive enough, it can cause lung restriction. Pleural calcifications can develop in the setting of fibrosis, regardless of the cause. Calcifications are often seen in patients with healed tuberculosis, prior bacterial empyema, or prior hemothorax. Unlike plaques related to asbestos exposure, fibrothorax tends to be unilateral.
- **Iatrogenic (pleurodesis)**. Talc pleurodesis is the intentional creation of fibrosis for symptomatic malignant pleural effusions, chylous effusions, or recurrent spontaneous pneumothoraces. As with other causes of pleural fibrosis, calcification can occur. Talc pleurodesis can mimic true pleural calcification by the accumulation of talc in the pleural space. In such instances, deposits of high-density talc can coat the visceral and parietal surface. If an effusion is present, a variant of the "split pleura" sign may be present.

■ Diagnosis

Fibrothorax (secondary to prior tuberculous pleuritis)

✓ Pearls

- Asbestos-related pleural disease usually develops 10 to 20 years after onset of exposure.
- Asbestos-related pleural plaques tend to be bilateral but are usually asymmetric.
- Fibrothorax presents as pleural calcifications and restriction in a patient with prior infection or hemorrhage.
- Talc pleurodesis is utilized to treat recurrent pleural effusions or pneumothoraces.

Suggested Readings

Choi J-A, Hong KT, Oh Y-W, Chung MH, Seol HY, Kang E-Y. CT manifestations of late sequelae in patients with tuberculous pleuritis. AJR Am J Roentgenol. 2001; 176(1):441–445

Murray JG, Patz EF, Jr, Erasmus JJ, Gilkeson RC. CT appearance of the pleural space after talc pleurodesis. AJR Am J Roentgenol. 1997; 169(1):89–91

Case 18

Brent McCarragher and Thomas Ray S. Sanchez

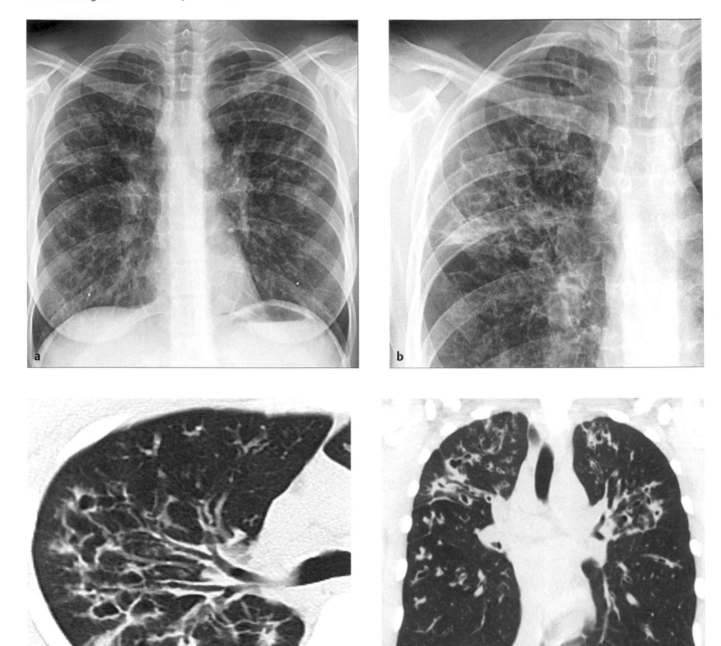

Fig. 18.1 **(a)** Posteroanterior radiograph of the chest shows diffuse peribronchial thickening in an upper lobe distribution. **(b)** Coned-down view of the RUL demonstrates thickened and dilated bronchi as well as foci of parenchymal cysts. **(c)** Coned-down axial CT image through the right upper lobe (RUL) in lung window shows diffuse bronchiectasis with dilated and thickened airways and mucus plugging of the distal airways giving rise to the "signet ring sign" with the dilated bronchial diameter greater than the accompanying blood vessel. **(d)** Coronal CT image in lung window reveals dilated and thickened bronchioles with a lack of distal tapering, the "tram-track" sign, in an upper lobe distribution.

■ Clinical Presentation

A 22-year-old woman with history of chronic cough, asthmalike symptoms, and severe sinusitis (▶Fig. 18.1).

■ Key Imaging Finding

Bronchiectasis

■ Top 3 Differential Diagnoses

- **Postinfectious.** The most common cause of bronchiectasis is postinfectious, resulting from poorly treated or necrotizing infections, including bacterial, viral, and mycobacterial etiologies. The end result is peribronchial injury, impaired clearance of secretions, and further colonization by pathogenic agents. Tuberculosis typically involves the upper lobes; *Mycobacterium avium* complex characteristically affects the lingula and right middle lobe (RML) in older women (Lady Windermere syndrome). Recurrent aspiration often affects the lower lobes, while Swyer–James syndrome presents with focal increased lucency because of air trapping.
- **Cystic fibrosis.** Cystic fibrosis is an autosomal recessive disorder of abnormal chloride transport affecting the lungs, reproductive tract, and pancreas. It primarily affects Caucasian children and results in decreased life expectancy. Abnormal inflammatory mediators cause large amounts of proteases to be released, which result in tissue destruction and bronchiectasis. Additionally, viscous secretions cause mucus plugging, leading to bacterial infections, chronic inflammation, and peribronchial injury reminiscent of postinfectious bronchi-

ectasis. The upper lobes are asymmetrically affected likely secondary to increased intrinsic clearance of the lower lobes. Computed tomography (CT) reveals cystic and cylindrical bronchiectasis with bronchial wall and interstitial thickening, nodular mucoid impaction, dilated bronchioles compared to the adjacent pulmonary artery ("signet ring sign"), and diffuse bronchiolitis ("tree-in-bud" nodularity).
- **Allergic bronchopulmonary aspergillosis (ABPA).** ABPA is a type of hypersensitivity reaction to *Aspergillus fumigatus*. Individuals with ABPA have recurrent asthma exacerbations, elevated immunoglobulin E (IgE) levels, eosinophilia, and skin reactivity to *A. fumigatus*. Imaging reveals recurrent alveolar infiltrates with diffuse bronchiectasis. CT findings include tree-in-bud nodularity and diffuse bronchial wall thickening with a central and upper lobe predominance. Mucous bronchial impaction of the central dilated bronchi results in the characteristic "finger-in-glove" opacities, which are typically of increased attenuation secondary to iron and manganese fungal debris (>70 HU).

■ Additional Differential Diagnoses

- **Obstructive lesion.** Focal bronchiectasis may represent a postobstructive process that is most often due to an underlying endobronchial mass, foreign body, or stricture. Retained secretions and decreased clearance result in an environment prone to infectious colonization and airway injury with bronchiectasis.

- **Primary ciliary dyskinesia.** Primary ciliary dyskinesia is autosomal recessive disorder of cilia motility, resulting in poor mucociliary clearance, chronic infections, and bronchiectasis. Kartagener syndrome is a variant of this disease characterized by sinusitis, bronchiectasis, infertility, and situs inversus.

■ Diagnosis

Cystic fibrosis

✓ Pearls

- Lady Windermere syndrome occurs in older women with chronic RML/lingula infection and bronchiectasis.
- Cystic fibrosis is primarily a disease of Caucasians with upper lobe–predominant bronchiectasis.

- Central bronchiectasis with mucous plugging ("finger-in-glove") is characteristic of ABPA.
- Focal bronchiectasis may be postobstructive because of an endobronchial mass, foreign body, or stricture.

Suggested Readings

Cantin L, Bankier AA, Eisenberg RL. Bronchiectasis. AJR Am J Roentgenol. 2009; 193(3):W158–71

Milliron B, Henry TS, Veeraraghavan S, Little BP. Bronchiectasis: mechanisms and imaging clues of associated common and uncommon diseases. Radiographics. 2015; 35(4):1011–1030

Case 19

Paul B. DiDomenico and Brent McCarragher

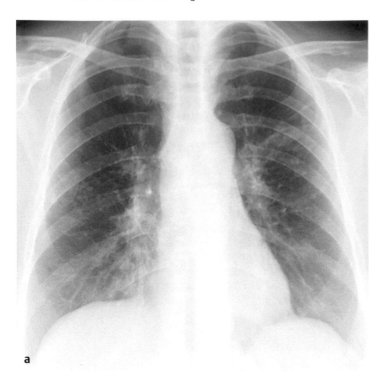
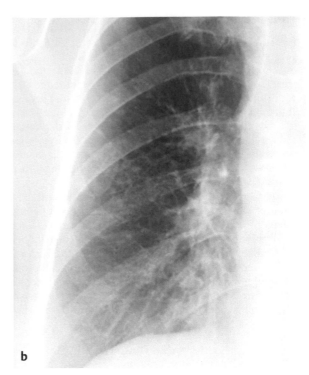
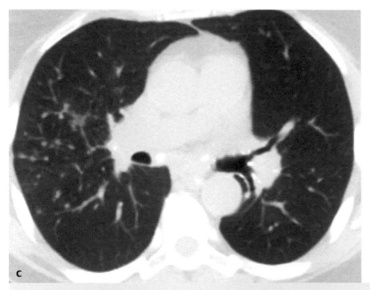

Fig. 19.1 (a) Frontal and (b) coned-down chest radiographs demonstrate reticular and nodular densities in the right midlung. (c) Axial CT image in lung window reveals multiple peribronchovascular and subpleural nodules in a perilymphatic distribution.

■ Clinical Presentation

Young adult man with fatigue (▶Fig. 19.1).

■ Key Imaging Finding

Perilymphatic pulmonary nodules

■ Top 3 Differential Diagnoses

- **Sarcoidosis**. Sarcoidosis is a systemic disease characterized by noncaseating granulomas. The lungs are the most commonly involved organ system. Chest radiographs may demonstrate upper lobe–predominant interstitial disease that most often has a reticulonodular pattern. On high-resolution computed tomography (CT), the interstitial appearance is that of multiple 1- to 5-mm nodules in a peribronchovascular and subpleural (perilymphatic) distribution with irregular interlobular septal thickening and regions of architectural distortion. Additional imaging findings may include enlarged hilar and mediastinal lymph nodes (common), alveolar opacities, and fibrotic changes with peripheral honeycombing in late-stage disease.
- **Lymphangitic spread of tumor**. Lymphangitic carcinomatosis refers to neoplastic infiltration of the pulmonary lymphatics. Pulmonary lymphatic involvement may result from direct spread of an adjacent primary tumor, retrograde extension of nodal disease, or lymphatic extension of hematogenous metastases. A perilymphatic nodular pattern is characteristic and is most often unilateral or bilateral but asymmetric. Pleural effusions may also be seen. Common tumors prone to lymphangitic spread include bronchogenic, breast, renal, gastrointestinal, and thyroid carcinomas, as well as melanoma.
- **Pneumoconioses**. Silicosis and coal worker's pneumoconiosis result from occupational exposure and present as upper lobe–predominant interstitial lung diseases, owing to decreased lymphatic clearance of the upper lobes. Either perilymphatic or centrilobular nodules may be present, which may eventually coalesce to form masslike opacities that may calcify. Involved lymph nodes may also calcify peripherally, resulting in a characteristic "eggshell" appearance. Late findings may include masslike fibrosis with peripheral emphysema (progressive massive fibrosis).

■ Additional Differential Diagnoses

- **Lymphoproliferative disorder**. Lymphoproliferative disorders, including lymphoma, posttransplant lymphoproliferative disorder (PTLD), and lymphoid interstitial pneumonitis (LIP), may manifest as a perilymphatic pulmonary nodular pattern. Correlation with clinical history is helpful as PTLD occurs in up to 8% of lung transplant patients, and LIP is associated with HIV/AIDS in children and with Sjögren's syndrome in adults.

■ Diagnosis

Sarcoidosis

✓ Pearls

- Parenchymal involvement of sarcoidosis can manifest as multiple bilateral perilymphatic nodules.
- Lymphangitic carcinomatosis presents most commonly as a unilateral perilymphatic nodular pattern.
- Pneumoconioses are inhalational diseases which may reveal perilymphatic or centrilobular nodules.
- Lymphoproliferative disorders (lymphoma, PTLD, and LIP) most often occur in predisposed patients.

Suggested Readings

Shroff G, Konopka K, Chiles C. Perilymphatic pulmonary nodules: definition, differential diagnosis, and demonstration of the "pipe-cleaner" sign. Contemp Diagn Radiol. 2013; 36(6):1–5

Case 20

John P. Lichtenberger, III

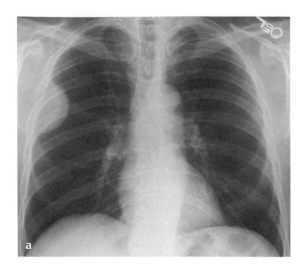

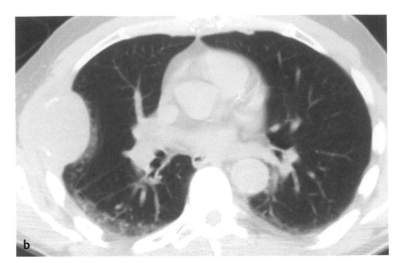

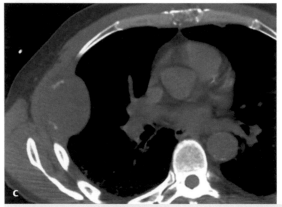

Fig. 20.1 **(a)** Posteroanterior radiograph of the chest shows a smooth, peripheral, well-demarcated mass with a broad base and obtuse angles with respect to the chest wall indicating an extrapulmonary origin. Subtle rib erosive changes are present. **(b,c)** Axial unenhanced CT images of the chest in lung and bone window confirm the extrapulmonary location of the mass with a smooth interface with lung parenchyma. Rib erosive changes are better seen on CT.

■ Clinical Presentation

Dyspnea and chest pain (▶Fig. 20.1).

■ Key Imaging Finding

Pleural-based mass

■ Top 3 Differential Diagnoses

- **Pleural metastases.** The most common neoplasm of the pleura is metastatic disease, usually from adenocarcinoma of the lung and breast, lymphoma, or invasive thymoma. While effusion is the most common presentation of metastatic pleural disease, metastases can also cause both diffuse pleural thickening and pleural seeding with nodular thickening and plaques. The metastatic foci may involve the pleura directly or extend into the pleura from chest wall involvement, to include the ribs. Irregular pleural thickening and chest wall invasion/erosive changes are suggestive of an aggressive process.
- **Empyema.** Defined as pulmonary parenchymal infection extending to the pleural surface, empyema is most frequently the result of bacterial pneumonia, recent surgery, or trauma. Important complications include bronchopleural fistulae and fibrous loculation. Drainage into the chest wall, termed empyema necessitatis, is most often seen in tuberculosis, although other considerations include fungal infection in immunocom-

promised patients, as well as malignancy. Radiographically, loculated collections with obtuse margins may be lenticular and compress the adjacent lung. Air–fluid levels may be seen in both empyema and lung abscess. However, pleural collections tend to have different sizes and configurations on frontal and lateral projections, while parenchymal abscesses typically have a similar appearance on frontal and lateral views.
- **Mesothelioma.** Although rare, mesothelioma is the most common primary pleural neoplasm and is associated with prior asbestos exposure. Radiologic features suggesting mesothelioma include irregular, nodular pleural thickening (>1 cm), involvement of the mediastinal pleura, volume loss of the involved hemithorax, and calcification. Pleural effusions are also relatively common. Mesothelioma and pleural metastases, however, are not reliably differentiated based solely on imaging findings.

■ Additional Differential Diagnoses

- **Fibrous tumor of the pleura.** Localized fibrous tumor of the pleura is a solitary, lobular, encapsulated tumor arising from either the visceral (80%) or parietal pleural. These tumors may be quite large at presentation and, when pedunculated, may demonstrate pathognomonic positional mobility. Important associated clinical features include hypertrophic osteoarthropathy (HOA) and episodic hypoglycemia. Characteristics findings on computed tomography (CT) include contrast enhancement, heterogeneity related to central necrosis, and/or

hemorrhage. Fibrous content may result in low signal intensity on T1 and T2 magnetic resonance imaging (MRI) sequences.
- **Fibrothorax.** Etiologies of focal or diffuse fibrosis of the pleura include hemothorax, tuberculous or pyogenic empyema, asbestos-related pleural disease, and inflammatory conditions such as rheumatoid effusions. Pleural thickening in fibrothorax is usually less than 1 cm and may calcify; the mediastinal pleural is usually spared.

■ Diagnosis

Pleural metastases

✓ Pearls

- Metastases are the most common pleural neoplasm; look for chest wall involvement/erosive changes.
- Empyemas often result from bacterial infection; bronchopleural fistulae and loculations are complications.

- Mesothelioma is the most common primary pleural malignancy and is associated with asbestos exposure.
- Fibrous tumors of the pleura may be large and pedunculated; HOA and episodic hypoglycemia may occur.

Suggested Readings

Nickell LT, Jr, Lichtenberger JP, III, Khorashadi L, Abbott GF, Carter BW. Multimodality imaging for characterization, classification, and staging of malignant pleural mesothelioma. Radiographics. 2014; 34(6):1692–1706

Case 21

John P. Lichtenberger III

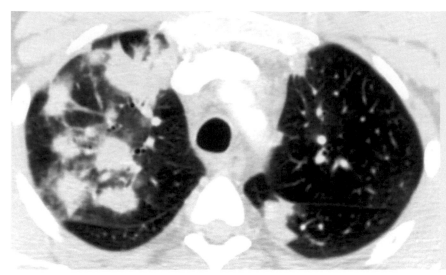

Fig. 21.1 Axial computed tomography (CT) of the chest in lung window shows asymmetric bilateral confluent opacities in a peribronchovascular distribution.

■ Clinical Presentation

A 40-year-old HIV-positive patient with shortness of breath, fever, and nonproductive cough (▶Fig. 21.1).

■ Key Imaging Finding

Parenchymal disease in an HIV patient

■ Top 3 Differential Diagnoses

- *Pneumocystis* **pneumonia (PCP)**. HIV patients with CD4 counts below 200 are at increased risk of acquiring PCP; it is the most common opportunistic infection in this population. The disease course is indolent with patients presenting with several weeks of dyspnea, fever, and cough. The most common imaging findings are confluent regions of ground-glass opacities with or without reticulonodular septal thickening. Cysts may be present in up to one-third of cases.
- **Tuberculosis (TB)**. The clinical and radiographic findings of TB in the HIV population depend largely on the CD4 count. In patients with a CD4 count above 200, the findings are similar to reactivation TB in immunocompetent hosts, to include upper lobe consolidations with cavitation and centrilobular pulmonary nodules in a "tree-in-bud" configuration. In patients with CD4 counts below 200, the findings are more reflective of primary TB, to include lower lobe consolidations, lymphadenopathy, and pleural effusion.
- **Fungal infection**. Histoplasmosis and coccidioidomycosis infection in the HIV population consists predominantly of a miliary pattern because of hematogenous dissemination of disease. With severe infection, pulmonary consolidations may occur.

■ Additional Differential Diagnoses

- **Invasive aspergillosis**. Invasive aspergillosis is an aggressive infection (mortality rate, 70–90%) that presents with multiple pulmonary nodules and surrounding ground-glass halo secondary to hemorrhage. Cavitation is common. An "air crescent" sign is seen in the recovery or healing phase.
- **Kaposi sarcoma**. Kaposi sarcoma is the most common AIDS-related malignancy in the United States. Nearly all patients with Kaposi sarcoma have skin involvement. Pulmonary involvement consists of nodular peribronchovascular septal thickening, as well as lymphadenopathy and pleural effusions.
- **Pulmonary lymphoma**. AIDS-related lymphoma is of the non-Hodgkin variant and typically presents as multiple nodules or masses (up to 5 cm). Less common radiographic manifestations include air-space consolidation or reticulonodular septal thickening. Lymphocytic interstitial pneumonia (LIP) is a lymphoproliferative disorder that may rarely evolve into lymphoma. LIP presents in immunocompromised patients as centrilobular pulmonary nodules, smooth or nodular septal thickening, and ground-glass opacities.

■ Diagnosis

Kaposi sarcoma

✓ Pearls

- PCP is the most common opportunistic infection in HIV; ground-glass opacities are most often seen.
- In immunocompromised patients, TB most often presents with air-space disease, miliary nodules, and lymphadenopathy.
- Invasive aspergillosis presents as nodules with a ground-glass halo; "air crescent" sign occurs with healing.
- Pulmonary involvement of Kaposi sarcoma is usually preceded by cutaneous or visceral involvement.

Suggested Readings

Lichtenberger JP, III, Sharma A, Zachary KC, et al. What a differential a virus makes: a practical approach to thoracic imaging findings in the context of HIV infection--part 1, pulmonary findings. AJR Am J Roentgenol. 2012; 198(6):1295–1304

Marchiori E, Müller NL, Soares Souza A, Jr, Escuissato DL, Gasparetto EL, Franquet T. Pulmonary disease in patients with AIDS: high-resolution CT and pathologic findings. AJR Am J Roentgenol. 2005; 184(3):757–764

Case 22

Bang Huynh

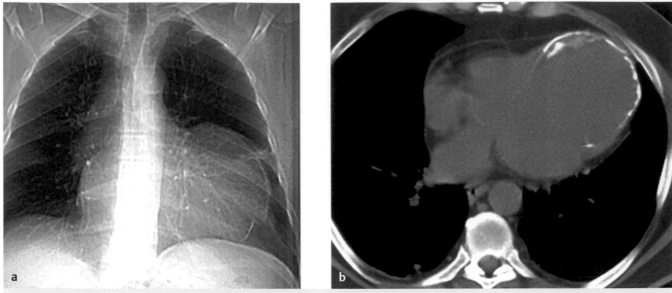

Fig. 22.1 **(a)** Scout CT image shows an abnormally enlarged left ventricular contour with a rim of peripheral calcification. **(b)** Unenhanced CT image of the chest in soft-tissue window reveals a wide-neck left ventricular outpouching with myocardial calcifications.

■ Clinical Presentation

Adult man with chest pain (▶Fig. 22.1).

■ Key Imaging Finding

Abnormal left ventricular contour

■ Top 3 Differential Diagnoses

- **True left ventricular aneurysm**. A true ventricular aneurysm is the result of a myocardial infarction. Unlike false aneurysms (which are contained ruptures), true aneurysms have a true myocardial wall. The wall can be thinned and akinetic or dyskinetic with paradoxical bulging during systole. As is the case with scarring of any cause, it can partially calcify. Most true aneurysms involve the anterolateral wall or apex of the left ventricle. A more reliable distinguishing feature from false aneurysms, however, is the presence of a wide neck (>50% of the aneurysm diameter) that is typically seen with true aneurysms. Most true aneurysms are treated medically unless they are felt to cause arrhythmias or exacerbate heart failure. Thrombus may form in the aneurysm, requiring more aggressive management, as left-sided emboli may result in systemic end-arterial occlusions.

- **False left ventricular aneurysm**. A false ventricular aneurysm is a pseudoaneurysm that maintains communication with the ventricular cavity. It represents a rupture of the myocardium that is contained by pericardial adhesions and hematoma and is a rare complication of myocardial infarction. Differentiation between a true and false aneurysm is important, because false aneurysms have a propensity to rupture. For that reason, false aneurysms are usually resected. A progressively enlarging abnormal ventricular contour should alert to the possibility of an expanding false aneurysm. False aneurysms tend to occur on the posterior or diaphragmatic surface of the heart, but the location alone is not a reliable discriminator. On computed tomography (CT) or magnetic resonance imaging (MRI), the more reliable finding is a narrow neck (<50% of the aneurysm diameter).

- **Pericardial cyst/mass**. Pericardial cysts or masses should be included in the differential diagnosis of an abnormal cardiac contour on radiographs. On CT or MRI, a pericardial mass or cyst should be readily distinguishable from a ventricular aneurysm. Pericardial cysts are usually fluid attenuation on CT. Occasionally, proteinaceous fluid can cause it to be of higher attenuation. On MRI, pericardial cysts follow fluid signal characteristics. When proteinaceous, the fluid can be high signal on T1-weighted sequences. A pericardial mass will be morphologically different from an aneurysm. Gradient echo and postcontrast imaging are helpful in distinguishing thrombus from tumor.

■ Additional Differential Diagnoses

- **Calcific pericarditis**. Calcific pericarditis is mentioned not because it results in a ventricular contour abnormality but because the associated pericardial calcifications can mimic calcifications in infarcted or aneurysmal myocardium on radiographs. Tuberculosis is a relatively common cause of pericardial calcifications. Other causes include viral and uremic pericarditis.

■ Diagnosis

True ventricular aneurysm

✓ Pearls

- True aneurysms involve all myocardial layers, have a wide neck, and commonly involve the cardiac apex.
- False aneurysms are contained ruptures which commonly occur along the diaphragmatic cardiac surface.
- Pericardial cysts and masses may produce an abnormal cardiac contour on radiographs.
- Calcific pericarditis results from TB, viral, or uremic pericarditis and may mimic ventricular calcifications.

Suggested Readings

Konen E, Merchant N, Gutierrez C, et al. True versus false left ventricular aneurysm: differentiation with MR imaging--initial experience. Radiology. 2005; 236(1):65–70

Webb WR, Higgins CB. Thoracic Imaging. Philadelphia, PA: Lippincott Williams & Wilkins; 2005

Case 23

Bang Huynh

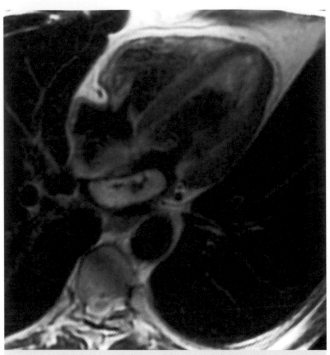

Fig. 23.1 Four-chamber double inversion recovery T2-weighted MR image shows a T2-hyperintense left atrial mass with an apparent stalklike attachment to the interatrial septum.

■ Clinical Presentation

Mass discovered on echocardiography performed for palpitations (▶Fig. 23.1).

■ Key Imaging Finding

Cardiac mass

■ Top 3 Differential Diagnoses

• **Thrombus**. Thrombus represents the most common cardiac mass and should be the leading differential of a nonenhancing cardiac filling defect. Left ventricular thrombi are usually associated with ventricular aneurysms; left atrial thrombi are often associated with atrial fibrillation. While often seen on computed tomography (CT), magnetic resonance imaging (MRI) is the modality of choice for distinction between a thrombus and tumor. Tumors enhance, while thrombi do not. MRI signal characteristics can be helpful, particularly on gradient echo (GRE), where thrombi tend to be low in signal. That said, myxomas can also be dark on GRE, and fresh thrombi may not yet be low signal on GRE. Thrombi in the left chambers can embolize to cause stroke or end-organ ischemia/infarct.

• **Metastases**. Cardiac metastases are far more common than primary cardiac neoplasms. Melanoma, leukemia, and lymphoma are frequent culprits, but any malignancy can find its way to the heart, for example, breast and lung carcinoma. Routes to the heart include hematogenous seeding, lymphatic spread, or direct extension. MRI is helpful in revealing extent and location and thus helps in assessing resectability.

• **Benign primary cardiac neoplasm**. While far less common than metastases, benign primary cardiac tumors are more common than malignant primary cardiac tumors by a ratio of 4:1. Although benign in the sense that they do not metastasize or locally invade, they can still cause significant morbidity and mortality by interfering with normal cardiac function. Such masses can cause arrhythmias, abnormal myocardial contraction/relaxation, and obstruction of normal coronary flow. Among the benign cardiac primaries, myxomas are the most common and typically occur in young to middle-aged adults (more common in women). Myxomas are usually in the left atrium (70%), pedunculated, and attached to the interatrial septum. They can be large and cause symptoms secondary to outflow obstruction or systemic emboli. On gradient cine MR images, myxomas are hypointense; they are isointense to cardiac muscle on T1 sequences and heterogeneously enhance. Calcifications may be seen. Rhabdomyomas are the most common primary benign cardiac neoplasm in children and are associated with tuberous sclerosis. Rhabdomyomas more commonly originate along the interventricular septum and may be multiple.

■ Additional Differential Diagnoses

• **Malignant primary cardiac neoplasm**. About 20% of primary cardiac tumors are malignant. Of those, sarcomas are the most common, followed by primary cardiac lymphomas. While the absence of aggressive features does not exclude malignancy, the presence of the following features makes malignancy likely: irregular margins, disruption of normal boundaries (extension into vessels and/or outside of heart into mediastinum), central necrosis, multichamber involvement, pericardial effusion, or metastases.

■ Diagnosis

Cardiac thrombus

✓ Pearls

• Thrombus is the most common cardiac mass; left-sided thrombi can embolize, causing end-organ ischemia.
• Metastases are by far the most common cardiac neoplasms; MRI helps determine the extent of disease.

• Myxomas are the most common benign primary cardiac neoplasms in adults (rhabdomyomas in children).
• Malignant primary cardiac tumors are the least common neoplasms; sarcomas are the most common type.

Suggested Readings

Lichtenberger JP, III, Reynolds DA, Keung J, Keung E, Carter BW. Metastasis to the heart: a radiologic approach to diagnosis with pathologic correlation. AJR Am J Roentgenol. 2016; 4:1–9

Case 24

Bang Huynh

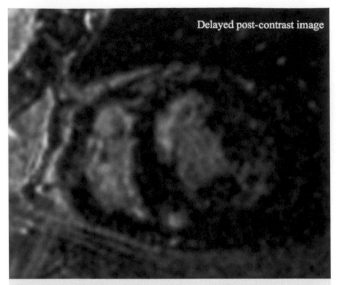

Fig. 24.1 Short-axis myocardial delayed enhancement MR image shows subendocardial enhancement in the left anterior descending coronary artery distribution.

■ Clinical Presentation

Adult man with chest pain (▶ Fig. 24.1).

■ Key Imaging Finding

Delayed myocardial enhancement

■ Top 3 Differential Diagnoses

- **Infarction/Scar**. Use of gadolinium chelates in cardiac magnetic resonance imaging (MRI) includes assessment of early perfusion (first pass) and delayed enhancement pattern. Delayed images are typically acquired 8 to 10 minutes postinjection. Normal myocardium enhances early, while infracted myocardium or scar tissue demonstrates delayed enhancement. The distinction between viable and nonviable myocardium is important for clinical decisions. Viable tissue, such as hibernating or stunned myocardium, does not have delayed enhancement. In contrast, infarcted tissue enhances in a delayed fashion. The delayed enhancement is typically subendocardial or transmural in a coronary artery vascular distribution. The extent of mural scarring is important as well; in general, myocardial scarring or fibrosis involving more than 50% of the wall thickness is unlikely to recover contractile function following revascularization.
- **Myocarditis**. Myocarditis refers to inflammation of the myocardium resulting from a large variety of causes, ranging from infections, drugs, and toxins to systemic diseases. The specific cause often remains unknown. Like infarctions, myocarditis can result in delayed myocardial enhancement. Unlike infarcts, however, the enhancement tends to involve the midportion of the myocardium, rather than subendocardial or transmural involvement. Additionally, myocarditis often does not correspond to a coronary artery vascular distribution. The enhancement pattern of myocarditis has been described as becoming less intense and more diffuse over a period of weeks to months. That said, the distinction between myocarditis and infarction often cannot be made by imaging alone.
- **Cardiac neoplasm**. Metastases to the heart are far more common than primary cardiac tumors. Cardiac neoplasms (metastatic or primary) usually enhance and sometimes have delayed enhancement. The presence and pattern of delayed enhancement are usually not helpful in characterizing the histology of the mass. Morphologic features of the mass and clinical history help distinguish cardiac neoplasms from other etiologies of delayed myocardial enhancement.

■ Additional Differential Diagnoses

- **Infiltrative disease**. Amyloidosis is perhaps the most common infiltrative disease process involving the myocardium. It is caused by deposition of fibril proteins and can result in a restrictive cardiomyopathy. In addition to causing cardiac dysfunction, MRI in setting of amyloidosis can reveal areas of delayed enhancement. The delayed enhancement is often diffuse and heterogeneous and does not correspond to a vascular distribution. Glycogen storage diseases may have similar findings. Abnormal enhancement can also be seen with other infiltrative processes, such as sarcoidosis and lymphoma, which typically reveal more focal regions of heterogeneous delayed myocardial enhancement.

■ Diagnosis

Infarction/scar

✓ Pearls

- Infarction presents as subendocardial or transmural delayed enhancement in a vascular distribution.
- Myocarditis typically involves the midportion of the myocardium and does not follow a vascular territory.
- Cardiac masses may demonstrate delayed enhancement but will be masslike in a nonvascular distribution.
- Infiltrative diseases cause restrictive physiology and diffuse or focal delayed heterogeneous enhancement.

Suggested Readings

Araoz PA, Eklund HE, Welch TJ, Breen JF. CT and MR imaging of primary cardiac malignancies. Radiographics. 1999; 19(6):1421–1434

Vogel-Claussen J, Rochitte CE, Wu KC, et al. Delayed enhancement MR imaging: utility in myocardial assessment. Radiographics. 2006; 26(3):795–810

Case 25

Bang Huynh

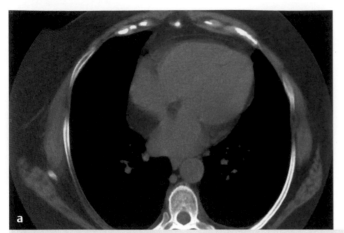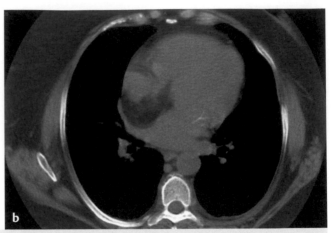

Fig. 25.1 (a, b) Unenhanced axial CT images in soft-tissue window demonstrate fat attenuation within the interatrial septum with sparing of the fossa ovalis.

■ Clinical Presentation

History withheld (▶ Fig. 25.1).

■ Key Imaging Finding

Cardiac wall fat

■ Top 3 Differential Diagnoses

- **Lipoma**. Lipomas are soft masses composed of encapsulated mature adipose cells. As such, they have attenuation on computed tomography (CT) and signal characteristic on magnetic resonance imaging (MRI) identical to subcutaneous fat. On MRI, lipomas will have high signal on T1 sequences; the signal will suppress with fat saturation. Most are homogenous and occasionally contain thin septations. Lipomas do not enhance following the administration of intravenous contrast. Common locations are the right atrium and atrial septum.
- **Lipomatous hypertrophy of the interatrial septum (LHIS)**. Despite having a fat composition similar to lipomas, this is a distinct entity. Unlike lipomas, lipomatous hypertrophy is not encapsulated. Instead, the fat insinuates the interatrial septum around the fossa ovalis. It is not a true neoplasm. Associated symptoms include supraventricular arrhythmias.
- **Arrhythmogenic right ventricular dysplasia (ARVD)**. ARVD is a cardiomyopathy of unknown etiology characterized by fibrofatty infiltration of the right ventricular myocardium. Important MRI findings include right ventricular wall motion abnormalities (either focal or global), myocardial delayed enhancement, wall thinning, and focal aneurysm. Clinically, ARVD is associated with arrhythmias and sudden death in otherwise healthy patients. Diagnosis of ARVD is based on a combination of major and minor criteria. MRI alone is not sufficient for making the diagnosis but provides important information regarding the right ventricular wall motion, myocardial thinning, dilatation, and fibrofatty replacement.

■ Diagnosis

Lipomatous hypertrophy of the interatrial septum

✓ Pearls

- Lipomas are well-encapsulated lesions that most commonly occur in the right atrium and atrial septum.
- LHIS may present with supraventricular arrhythmias.
- ARVD results in right ventricular wall abnormalities, including fibrofatty replacement.
- ARVD is associated with arrhythmias and sudden cardiac death in otherwise healthy patients.

Suggested Readings

Attili AK, Chew FS. Imaging of cardiac masses and myocardial disease: self-assessment module. AJR Am J Roentgenol. 2007; 188(6, Suppl):S21–S25

Gaerte SC, Meyer CA, Winer-Muram HT, Tarver RD, Conces DJ, Jr. Fat-containing lesions of the chest. Radiographics. 2002; 22(Spec No):S61–S78

Case 26

Jason Kim

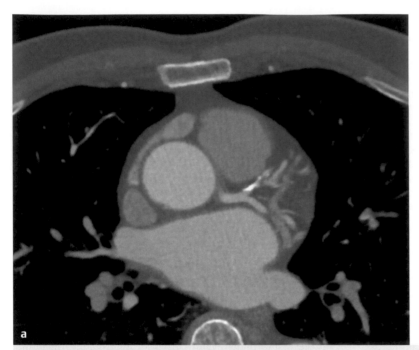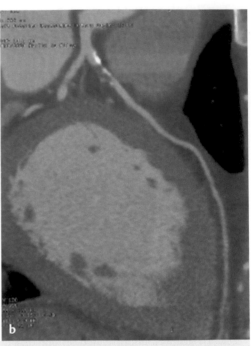

Fig. 26.1 **(a)** Axial image from cardiac-gated coronary CT angiography demonstrates calcified and noncalcified atherosclerotic plaque in the proximal left anterior descending artery (LAD) resulting in severe stenosis. **(b)** Curved planar reformatted image of the LAD shows the severe proximal LAD stenosis relative to the left main coronary artery and the distal LAD.

■ Clinical Presentation

A 72-year-old man with chest pain (▶Fig. 26.1).

■ Key Imaging Finding

Coronary artery disease

■ Top 3 Differential Diagnoses

- **Atherosclerosis**. Atherosclerosis is the pathologic process of obstructive plaque formation in vascular lumens. It is associated with risk factors, including middle or advanced age, hyperlipidemia, hypertension, and cigarette smoking. Contrast luminography via invasive angiography is the historical gold standard imaging technique for diagnosing stenosis, with the added benefit of pressure measurements across stenotic regions and the possibility of immediate intervention. Computed tomography (CT) coronary angiography and magnetic resonance (MR) angiography are useful tests for patients with low to intermediate pretest probability of coronary artery disease. Cross-sectional imaging has the added benefit of noninvasively detecting small regions of noncalcified plaque and positive remodeling. "Significant stenosis" is defined as >50% stenosis of the vessel diameter.
- **Coronary artery aneurysm**. Coronary artery aneurysm is an abnormal focal dilatation in a coronary artery. Etiologies include poststenotic dilatation secondary to atherosclerosis, bacterial inoculation of vessel wall, vasculitis such as Kawasaki disease, and trauma/iatrogenic aneurysms from catheter-based interventions. Most patients are asymptomatic, and clinical manifestations are generally due to the underlying cause of the aneurysm and the development of ischemia or cardiac dissection. An aneurysm is typically characterized as having a diameter that exceeds normal adjacent coronary segments and involves less than 50% of the length of the vessel.
- **Anomalous coronary arteries**. Approximately 1 to 2% of the general population has anomalous coronary artery anatomy, which ranges from benign to life-threatening variants. Clinically significant anomalies include atresia, origin from the pulmonary artery, fistulas, and interarterial course. Interarterial course refers to traversal between the pulmonary artery and aorta with or without a slitlike orifice and is associated with sudden cardiac death. Surgical repair remains controversial but may be justified in patients with symptoms of ischemia irrespective of other causes.

■ Additional Differential Diagnoses

- **Coronary artery dissection**. Coronary artery dissection can occur spontaneously or may be iatrogenic, and can precipitate acute myocardial infarction, causing 0.1 to 0.4% of acute coronary syndromes. Spontaneous coronary artery dissection is associated with fibromuscular dysplasia, postpartum state, and connective tissue disorders. Coronary angiography may show an intimal flap with contrast dissecting along the vessel wall. Associated stenosis or occlusion may mimic atherosclerosis. Long and diffuse narrowing on angiography can also indicate intramural hematoma.

■ Diagnosis

Atherosclerosis

✓ Pearls

- Significant coronary artery stenosis is defined as >50% stenosis of vessel diameter.
- Coronary artery aneurysms involve short segments with a diameter that exceeds normal artery segments.
- An interarterial coronary artery travels between the pulmonary artery and aorta and may be life-threatening.
- Coronary artery dissection may be detected by an intimal flap and stenosis on coronary angiography.

Suggested Readings

Bastarrika G, Lee YS, Huda W, Ruzsics B, Costello P, Schoepf UJ. CT of coronary artery disease. Radiology. 2009; 253(2):317–338

Tarkin JM, Dweck MR, Evans NR, et al. Imaging atherosclerosis. Circ Res. 2016; 118(4):750–769

Case 27

Adam Dulberger

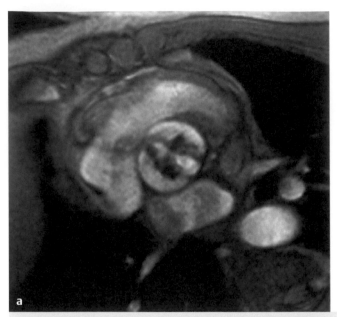
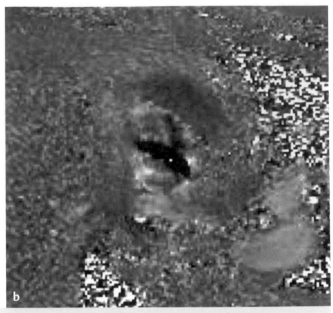

Fig. 27.1 **(a)** Steady-state free precession MRI short axis at the aortic valve shows thickened, irregular aortic valve leaflets with slitlike opening of the valve orifice. **(b)** Phase-contrast image of the aortic valve with velocity encoding (VENC) of 350 cm/s shows fish-mouth morphology of flow through the aortic valve. Tiny focus of white in the otherwise black flow indicates aliasing with a peak velocity greater than 350 cm/s.

■ Clinical Presentation

An 18-year-old man with heart murmur (▶Fig. 27.1).

■ Key Imaging Finding

Aortic valve disease

■ Top 3 Differential Diagnoses

- **Aortic stenosis**. Aortic stenosis (AS) refers to partial obstruction of blood flow across the aortic valve and is most commonly caused by congenital disease (i.e., bicuspid aortic valve), acquired causes (i.e., degenerative calcifications), or both. Symptoms of AS usually develop gradually after a 10- to 20-year asymptomatic latent period. The classic triad of AS symptoms includes angina, dyspnea, and syncope. Although echocardiography is the preferred imaging modality for initial assessment and longitudinal evaluation of patients with valvular disease, magnetic resonance imaging (MRI) provides more thorough anatomic and quantitative evaluation. While spin-echo MRI is more useful for visualizing detailed anatomic changes, cine gradient echo (GRE) MRI may be used to measure the size and extent of the stenotic jet into the ascending aorta, in order to determine the severity of AS.
- **Aortic regurgitation (AR)**. AR refers to diastolic flow of blood from the aorta across the aortic valve and into the left ventricle, and is caused by incompetent closure of the aortic valve. Rheumatic heart disease is the most common cause of AR in the developing world, while aortic root dilation is most commonly responsible in developed nations. Severe AR may lead to palpitations, angina, and symptoms of heart failure (i.e., dyspnea on exertion and orthopnea). Infective endocarditis may cause acute valve destruction and lead to rapid development of insufficiency symptoms. As with AS, MRI may also be used to provide a more detailed quantification of the severity of AR compared to echocardiography by assessing the dephasing jets across the aortic valve.
- **Aortic valve replacement**. Symptomatic patients with severe AS or AR often undergo valve replacement, for which several techniques exist. Classically, the valve is replaced through an open surgical technique (median sternotomy) and the patient is placed on a cardiopulmonary bypass machine during the surgery. Alternatively, transarterial aortic valve replacement (TAVR) is a less invasive technique in which a mechanical valve is placed at the site of the diseased valve through a catheter. Currently, in the United States, TAVR is reserved for patients at high risk for open-heart surgery. MRI is useful in evaluating for complications after aortic valve replacement.

■ Additional Differential Diagnoses

- **Bicuspid aortic valve**. Bicuspid aortic valve (as opposed to the normal three-valve leaflets) is the most common congenital heart disease, caused by abnormal fusion of two of the aortic valve leaflets. The estimated incidence of a bicuspid valve in the general population is thought to be roughly 2% and is twice as common in males as in females. A bicuspid aortic valve may lead to the development of AS and/or AR. MRI is especially useful in assessment of the dynamic motion of heavily diseased bicuspid valves, for which echocardiography may provide limited utility. On cross-sectional imaging, the bicuspid valve demonstrates a characteristic "fish-mouth" appearance.

■ Diagnosis

Bicuspid aortic valve with AS

✓ Pearls

- MRI provides more thorough evaluation of aortic disease (AS or AR) compared to echocardiography.
- Aortic valve replacement may be performed through an open or minimally invasive (TAVR) technique.
- Bicuspid aortic valve demonstrates a characteristic "fish-mouth" appearance.

Suggested Readings

Bennett CJ, Maleszewski JJ, Araoz PACT. CT and MR imaging of the aortic valve: radiologic-pathologic correlation. Radiographics. 2012; 32(5):1399–1420

Cawley PJ, Maki JH, Otto CM. Cardiovascular magnetic resonance imaging for valvular heart disease: technique and validation. Circulation. 2009; 119(3):468–478

Case 28

Mischa Monroe

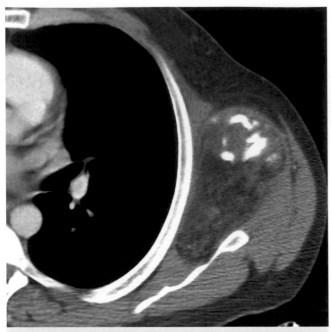

Fig. 28.1 Axial contrast-enhanced CT image shows a large, oblong left chest wall mass with fat attenuation, soft-tissue components, and calcification.

■ Clinical Presentation

A 35-year-old man with painful chest wall mass (▶Fig. 28.1).

■ Key Imaging Finding

Chest wall mass

■ Top 3 Differential Diagnoses

- **Metastatic disease**. Metastatic disease is the most common cause of chest wall malignancy. The most common primary tumors leading to metastasis include breast, lung, prostate, and melanoma. Metastases can arise through three pathways: hematogenous, lymphatic, or direct invasion. Computed tomography (CT) is the modality of choice for imaging chest wall lesions because of its optimal spatial resolution and differentiation of osseous and soft-tissue masses. Multiple chest wall masses in the presence of known or suspected malignancy are highly suspicious for metastatic disease.
- **Fatty tumor**. Lipomas, composed almost entirely of mature fat cells within a fibrous capsule, are the most common benign tumors of soft tissue, occurring in 1% of the population. They are most frequently observed on the trunk and arms. Lipomas present as soft, painless subcutaneous nodules. Liposarcoma is a malignancy of fat cells with soft-tissue components and often presents as a painful enlarging mass. Findings that are atypical for lipoma include greater than 60 years of age

at presentation and soft-tissue septa that are greater than 2 mm in thickness. Findings suspicious for liposarcoma include soft-tissue components greater than 2 cm and an overall mass size greater than 10 cm. Oftentimes, the distinction between an atypical lipoma and liposarcoma may need to be made via image-guided biopsy or excision.
- **Rib tumor**. The most common benign chest wall tumor is osteochondroma, which accounts for one-third to one-half of all benign bony lesions. The most common malignant chest wall tumor is chondrosarcoma, which accounts for one-third of malignant bone tumors. On imaging, osteochondromas present as pedunculated masses on the rib surface with a medullary cavity that is contiguous with the lesion. While radiography is often the initial imaging study for a painful bone lesion followed by CT, magnetic resonance imaging (MRI) is best to evaluate for soft-tissue invasion and bone marrow edema. Clinically, a symptomatic growing mass would favor chondrosarcoma over osteochondroma.

■ Additional Differential Diagnoses

- **Chest wall Infection**. Infection of the chest wall often results from extension of an existing intrathoracic or spine infection. Other less common routes of chest wall infection include trauma, surgery, and hematogenous spread. Empyema may decompress into the chest wall, termed empyema necessitans. On imaging, fluid and phlegmon from within the intrathoracic infection may be seen passing the rib wall and extending into the subcutaneous soft tissues.
- **Elastofibroma dorsi**. Elastofibroma dorsi is an infrascapular fibrous tissue mass with fatty streaks found deep to latissi-

mus dorsi and serratus anterior muscles. It presents with a 5:1 female-to-male ratio and an average age at diagnosis of 65 to 70 years. In autopsy series, most of these tumors are bilateral; however, in unilateral cases, it is more common on the right. The sensation of scapular clicking is a common symptom. On T1 and T2 MRI sequences, the fibrous component will appear isointense to muscle and internal streaks of fat will be hyperintense.

■ Diagnosis

Metastatic disease

✓ Pearls

- Differentiating lipoma from liposarcoma may require image-guided biopsy or excision.
- Metastases are the most common chest wall tumor; chondrosarcoma is the most common primary malignancy.

- Elastofibroma dorsi often presents with scapular clicking, and is more common in elderly women.

Suggested Readings

Lichtenberger JP, III, Carter BW, Abbott GF. Pitfalls in imaging of the chest wall. Semin Roentgenol. 2015; 50(3):251–257

Case 29

Matthew L. Lutynski

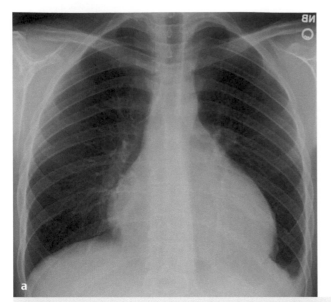
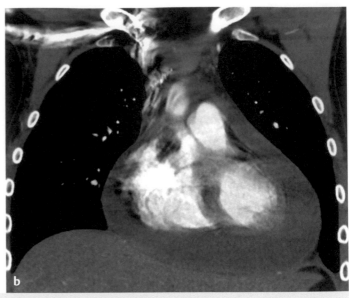

Fig. 29.1 **(a)** Frontal chest radiograph shows an enlarged cardiac silhouette and trace left pleural effusion. The cardiac silhouette has a "water bottle" configuration. **(b)** Contrast-enhanced coronal CT image reveals a large pericardial effusion.

■ Clinical Presentation

A 21-year-old man presenting to the emergency room after 3 weeks of chest pain (►Fig. 29.1).

■ Key Imaging Finding

Enlarged cardiac silhouette

■ Top 3 Differential Diagnoses

- **Cardiomyopathy**. Cardiomegaly is the general imaging feature observed in cardiomyopathy. The specific chamber involvement and degree of dysfunction (typically quantified by left ventricular ejection fraction) are key data points a radiologist can provide to the clinician evaluating for multiple possible etiologies. Subtypes include dilated cardiomyopathy (ischemic or nonischemic), hypertrophic cardiomyopathy, restrictive cardiomyopathy, arrhythmogenic right ventricular cardiomyopathy/dysplasia, and unclassified. Contrast-enhanced cardiac magnetic resonance imaging (MRI) can play a key role in diagnosis and surveillance of disease. Heart failure with pulmonary edema often presents with cardiomegaly, cephalization of flow, Kerley B lines, and pleural effusions.

- **Pericardial effusion**. When the pericardial space distends with fluid, it can make the cardiac silhouette appear enlarged in a "water bottle" configuration. The lateral radiograph may also demonstrate an "Oreo cookie" or fat pad sign, created by the radiopaque effusion separating the radiolucent pericardial and epicardial fat. While multiple etiologies exist, some of the more common causes of pericardial effusion include myocardial infarction (Dressler's syndrome), left ventricular heart failure, renal failure, infection (such as viral and tuberculosis), and autoimmune disease (such as rheumatoid arthritis and systemic lupus erythematosus). When rapidly occurring or if the volume is significant, the effusion can impair cardiac output and produce cardiac tamponade. Imaging findings suggestive of cardiac tamponade include collapse of the right atrium, straightening of the interventricular septum, and dilated vena cava.

- **Mediastinal mass**. Uncommonly, the appearance of an enlarged cardiac silhouette can result from an underlying mediastinal mass (e.g., Hodgkin lymphoma, thymic lesion, thyroid lesion, germ cell neoplasm, pericardial cyst, cardiac mass). Cross-sectional imaging readily identifies the mass as the cause of the underlying cardiac silhouette enlargement on radiographs.

■ Additional Differential Diagnoses

- **Valvular heart disease**. Chronic aortic and mitral valve regurgitation or severe aortic stenosis can produce left ventricular dilation, which can lead to the enlarged cardiac silhouette. MRI provides a thorough evaluation of valvular heart disease.

■ Diagnosis

Pericardial effusion with cardiac tamponade (Coxsackie B virus)

✓ Pearls

- Congestive heart failure presents with cardiomegaly and pulmonary edema with pleural effusions.

- Pericardial effusion may produce a "water bottle" appearance; looks for signs of cardiac tamponade.
- MRI provides a thorough evaluation of valvular heart disease.

Suggested Readings

Boxt LM, Abbara S. Cardiac Imaging: The Requisites. Philadelphia, PA: Elsevier, Inc.; 2016

Wang ZJ, Reddy GP, Gotway MB, Yeh BM, Hetts SW, Higgins CB. CT and MR imaging of pericardial disease. Radiographics. 2003; 23(Spec No):S167–S180

Case 30

David A. Kephart Jr.

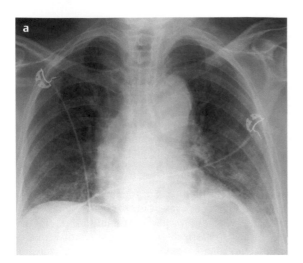
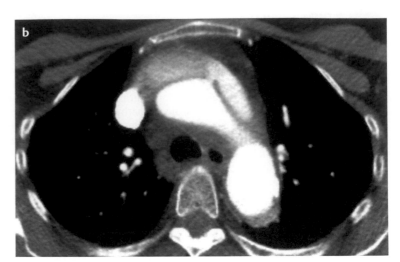
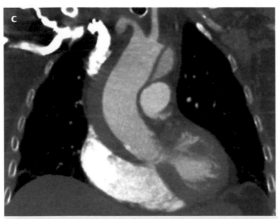

Fig. 30.1 (a) Anteroposterior chest radiograph shows widening of the upper mediastinum and abnormal contour of the aortic arch with displacement of atherosclerotic calcifications. **(b)** Axial contrast-enhanced CT image shows focal intimal defect in the anterolateral ascending aorta with active hemorrhage. **(c)** Coronal reformatted contrast-enhanced CT image reveals the extent of abnormality, extending to the level of the aortic valve annulus.

■ Clinical Presentation

An 84-year-old woman with chest pain, diaphoresis, and near-syncope (▶Fig. 30.1).

■ Key Imaging Finding

Acute aortic syndrome (AAS)

■ Top 3 Differential Diagnoses

- **Aortic dissection (AD)**. AD is the most common acute aortic disorder. Associated risk factors include hypertension, advanced age, atherosclerosis, previous cardiac surgery, and connective tissue diseases. Classically, patients present with acute tearing chest pain, although sharp chest pain is the most common presenting complaint. Computed tomography (CT) is the most commonly used imaging modality owing to its wide availability, speed, and high sensitivity. AD is characterized by a tear of the intimal layer of the aorta causing an inflow of blood into the media, forming a true and a false lumen separated by an intimomedial flap. The classic intimomedial flap is seen in two-thirds of cases on contrast-enhanced images. The false lumen is usually larger in diameter and may contain thrombus. AD is classified as Type A with involvement of the ascending aorta and Type B in which only the descending aorta is involved. Untreated Type A dissection has a mortality rate of 20% at 24 hours and 50% within 1 month. Surgical repair of the ascending aorta is currently the treatment of choice. Type B dissection is generally managed conservatively with antihypertensive medication.
- **Intramural hematoma (IMH)**. IMHs account for fewer than 6% of cases of AAS. IMH is defined as bleeding of the vasa va-sorum in the medial layer of the aorta without an intimal tear. A hyperattenuating crescent region within the aortic wall on unenhanced CT images with no subsequent contrast enhancement is the hallmark of IMH (crescent sign). IMH can be due to either spontaneous rupture of the vasa vasorum of the aortic wall or a penetrating atherosclerotic ulcer. IMH can extend, progress, regress, or reabsorb. Up to half of patients progress to classic AD; regression is seen in up to one-third of cases. Management of IMH is similar to AD.
- **Penetrating atherosclerotic ulcer**. Penetrating atherosclerotic ulcer is an atheromatous plaque that disrupts the intimal layer of the aortic wall with subsequent extension into the media. The mid-descending thoracic aorta is most commonly involved. Patients who become hemodynamically symptomatic are treated either surgically by grafting of the affected area or with endovascular therapy (descending aorta involvement). Conservative management, often in asymptomatic patients, involves antihypertensive therapy with close imaging follow-up, especially within the first 30 days of presentation, because of its relatively poor prognosis.

■ Additional Differential Diagnoses

- **Intra-aortic blood pool**. Intramural blood pool (IBP) is described as localized contrast medium–filled pool inside an IMH. Communication between the contrast medium–filled pool and the true lumen is absent or has an orifice less than 2 mm in diameter. In addition, distal connection with the intercostal artery or lumbar artery can be observed. IBPs should be differentiated from ulcerlike projection because IBPs are associated with a more favorable outcome and most IBPs show complete resorption over time.

■ Diagnosis

Type A aortic dissection

✓ Pearls

- Type A AD involves the ascending aorta; Type B dissections only involve the descending aorta.
- IMH presents as a crescent-shaped region of increased aortic wall attenuation on CT with no enhancement.
- Penetrating ulcers result from disruption of the intimal layer because of an atheromatous plaque.

Suggested Readings

Chiu KW, Lakshminarayan R, Ettles DF. Acute aortic syndrome: CT findings. Clin Radiol. 2013; 68(7):741–748

Ridge CA, Litmanovich DE. Acute aortic syndromes: current status. J Thorac Imaging. 2015; 30(3):193–201

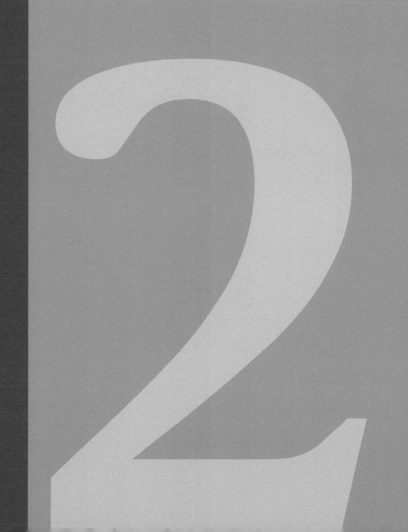

Part 2

Gastrointestinal Imaging

Case 31

Robert A. Jesinger

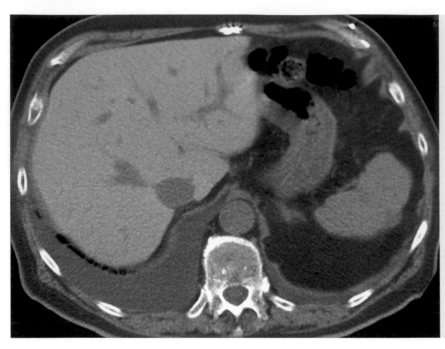

Fig. 31.1 Unenhanced computed tomography (CT) image of the liver demonstrates diffuse increased attenuation (>80 HU). Small layering bilateral pleural effusions are noted, as is metallic artifact along the anterior chest wall.

■ Clinical Presentation

A 65-year-old man with recurrent congestive heart failure (CHF) (▶Fig. 31.1).

■ Key Imaging Finding

Hyperdense liver

■ Top 3 Differential Diagnoses

- **Iron deposition**. Iron deposition in the liver, commonly in the reticuloendothelial system, can be seen as a consequence of increased oral intake, multiple blood transfusions (usually in the setting of dialysis or chronic anemia), ineffective erythropoiesis (thalassemia, sideroblastic anemia), or from the more rare disorder of primary hemochromatosis. Hepatic enlargement, increased parenchymal attenuation (HU > 80), and cirrhotic liver morphology can be key visual markers, as can laboratory markers of impaired hepatic function. Careful detection of liver masses is important because of increased risk of hepatocellular carcinoma. Classic magnetic resonance imaging (MRI) features of iron deposition include decreased hepatic parenchymal signal intensity on T2-weighted imaging sequences because of the superparamagnetic effect of iron. Decreased myocardial and pancreatic parenchymal T2 signal intensity is a classic MRI feature in primary hemochromatosis, while decreased T2 signal intensity in the spleen is characteristic of secondary hemochromatosis.

- **Amiodarone therapy**. Amiodarone is an antiarrhythmic medication that is 40% iodine by weight. It has primary hepatic and biliary metabolism and is slowly excreted into bile by the liver. Hence, chronic amiodarone therapy increases hepatic parenchymal attenuation; normalization occurs over weeks to months after the medication is discontinued. In addition to a hyperdense liver, amiodarone therapy is associated with lower lobe pulmonary interstitial lung disease (ILD), as well as focal pulmonary infiltrates with characteristic increased attenuation.

- **Glycogen storage disease**. There are multiple subtypes of glycogen storage disease, many of which can result in decreased liver density similar to hepatic steatosis. Types I (von Gierke) and IV, however, are subtypes that are associated with increased hepatic attenuation. Type IV in particular may result in cirrhosis with an increased incidence of hepatocellular carcinoma. Unlike hemochromatosis, the classic MRI feature is increased hepatic parenchymal signal on T1-weighted imaging sequences.

■ Additional Differential Diagnoses

- **Gold therapy**. Intramuscular gold therapy was commonly used to treat patients with rheumatoid arthritis until approximately the 1990s. Agents with less toxicity are now routinely used as disease-modifying agents for rheumatoid arthritis in place of gold therapy. Chronic accumulation of gold salts results in a hyperdense liver.

- **Thorotrast**. Thorotrast is a radioactive material (alpha emitter) that was used as a contrast agent for several decades (1920–1950s). The agent is taken up by the reticuloendothelial system, resulting in dense opacities within the liver, spleen, and lymph nodes. There is an increased risk of malignancy, especially angiosarcoma.

■ Diagnosis

Amiodarone therapy

✓ Pearls

- Primary hemochromatosis affects **p**ancreas, while **s**econdary hemochromatosis affects **s**pleen.
- Amiodarone may cause a hyperdense liver, high attenuation pulmonary infiltrates, and ILD.

- Hepatoma and angiosarcoma may arise in the setting of a hyperdense liver.

Suggested Readings

Lim RP, Tuvia K, Hajdu CH, et al. Quantification of hepatic iron deposition in patients with liver disease: comparison of chemical shift imaging with single-echo T2*-weighted imaging. AJR Am J Roentgenol. 2010; 194(5):1288–1295

Federle MP, Jeffrey RB, Woodward PJ, Borhani A. Diagnostic Imaging: Abdomen. 2nd ed. Philadelphia, PA: Lippincott Williams & Wilkins; 2009

Guyader D, Gandon Y, Deugnier Y, et al. Evaluation of computed tomography in the assessment of liver iron overload. A study of 46 cases of idiopathic hemochromatosis. Gastroenterology. 1989; 97(3):737–743

Tani I, Kurihara Y, Kawaguchi A, et al. MR imaging of diffuse liver disease. AJR Am J Roentgenol. 2000; 174(4):965–971

Case 32

Robert A. Jesinger

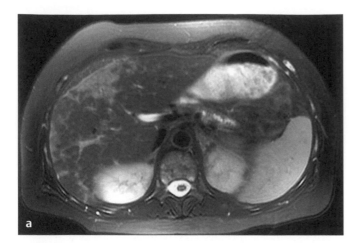 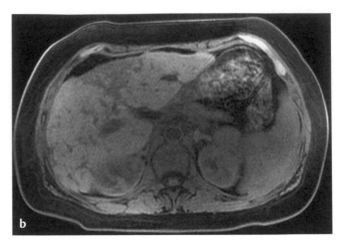

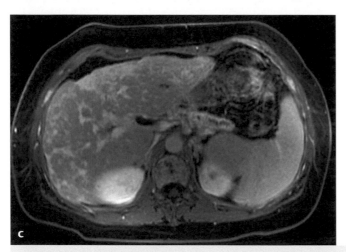

Fig. 32.1 (a) Axial T2-weighted MR image with fat suppression demonstrates a nodular liver contour with capsular retraction and numerous confluent wedge-shaped foci of increased signal intensity peripherally. These regions are low in signal intensity on **(b)** T1-weighted fat suppressed image and **(c)** demonstrate heterogeneous enhancement post gadolinium.

■ Clinical Presentation

A 67-year-old woman with chronic liver enzyme elevation and a history of breast cancer (▶ Fig. 32.1).

■ Key Imaging Finding

Nodular liver contour

■ Top 3 Differential Diagnoses

- **Cirrhosis**. Cirrhosis is a chronic liver disease characterized by hepatic fibrosis and regenerative hepatic nodules. Common causes include alcohol (micronodular cirrhosis), chronic viral hepatitis (macronodular cirrhosis), autoimmune hepatitis, and chronic metabolic conditions (primary biliary cirrhosis, primary hemochromatosis, Wilson disease, alpha-1 AT deficiency). Imaging findings include nodular liver surface contour, distorted hepatic architecture with atrophy, and stigmata of portal hypertension (enlarged main portal vein with slow flow, flow reversal or occlusion; varices, splenomegaly, gallbladder/bowel wall thickening, and ascites). Magnetic resonance imaging (MRI) of liver nodules helps distinguish regenerative nodules (low T2 signal) from neoplastic nodules (high T2 signal). The use of gadoxetate disodium can help in distinguishing or characterizing hepatic lesions because of hepatocyte phase of imaging.
- **Treated metastases**. Chemotherapy treatment of liver metastases (commonly from breast, lung, and colorectal cancer) can result in scarring of hepatic tumor implants. Liver parenchyma, between these areas of scarring, can be normal or regenerative. The overall imaging appearance simulates macronodular cirrhosis, and hence is referred to as "pseudocirrhosis." Correlation with appropriate history is helpful.
- **Budd–Chiari syndrome**. Chronic hepatic venous occlusive disease can result in a nodular liver contour, usually as a consequence of regenerative nodules. In chronic Budd–Chiari syndrome, these nodules are usually small, multiple, and hypervascular, and the number of nodules is often underestimated on computed tomography (CT). Large regenerative hypervascular nodules may be seen and are usually hyperintense on T1 MRI sequences. There is no evidence that large regenerative nodules degenerate into malignancy. A central scar in nodules greater than 1 cm can be seen. Caudate hypertrophy occurs as a result of its separate venous drainage into the inferior vena cava, which may simulate a dominant nodule.

■ Additional Differential Diagnoses

- ***Schistosoma japonicum***. *S. japonicum*, a major cause of hepatic schistosomiasis, is highly associated with hepatic fibrosis. Calcified eggs along the portal tracts produce the pathognomonic "turtleback" calcification. The size and shape of the liver can be preserved, but fibrosis and portal tract calcification often result in a nodular liver contour.
- **Confluent hepatic fibrosis**. Confluent hepatic fibrosis may occur in the setting of chronic liver disease. The most common appearance is a wedge-shaped hypodense region on CT which extends from the hilum. The anterior segment of the right hepatic lobe and medial segment of the left hepatic lobe are the most common sites of involvement. There is overlying capsular retraction and little or no enhancement.

■ Diagnosis

Treated breast metastases (pseudocirrhosis)

✓ Pearls

- MRI helps distinguish regenerative (low T2 signal) from neoplastic (high T2 signal) liver nodules.
- Pseudocirrhosis is most commonly seen with treated breast, lung, and colorectal metastases.

- The "turtleback" appearance of the liver is most commonly associated with schistosomiasis.

Suggested Readings

Brancatelli G, Federle MP, Grazioli L, Golfieri R, Lencioni R. Benign regenerative nodules in Budd-Chiari syndrome and other vascular disorders of the liver: radiologic-pathologic and clinical correlation. Radiographics. 2002; 22(4):847–862

Dodd GD, III, Baron RL, Oliver JH, III, Federle MP. Spectrum of imaging findings of the liver in end-stage cirrhosis: part I, gross morphology and diffuse abnormalities. AJR Am J Roentgenol. 1999; 173(4):1031–1036
Saenz RC. MRI of benign liver lesions and metastatic disease characterization with gadoxetate disodium. J Am Osteopath Coll Radiol. 2012; 1(4):2–9

Case 33

Robert A. Jesinger

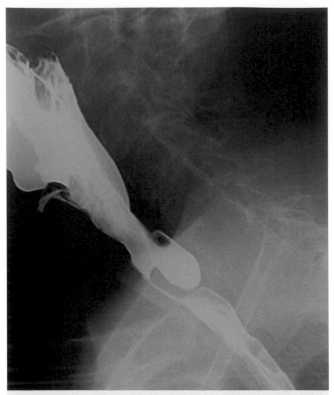

Fig. 33.1 Lateral view from an upper gastrointestinal examination demonstrates a large contrast-filled outpouching along the posterior aspect of the cervical esophagus.

■ **Clinical Presentation**

A 75-year-old woman with difficulty swallowing (▶Fig. 33.1).

■ Key Imaging Finding

Esophageal diverticulum

■ Top 3 Differential Diagnoses

- **Proximal esophageal pulsion diverticulum**. Pulsion diverticula of the esophagus are thought to develop because of increased intraluminal pressure combined with focal areas of weakness in the esophageal wall. The more common **Zenker diverticulum** is a midline defect that occurs in the posterior cervical esophagus *above the level* of the cricopharyngeal muscle (upper esophageal sphincter). Zenker diverticulum occurs through Killian's dehiscence, which is at the junction of the cricopharyngeal and inferior pharyngeal constrictor muscles. A **Killian–Jamison diverticulum** is a lateral defect that occurs in the cervical esophagus *at the level* of the cricopharyngeal muscle. Both typically occur in older patients, and presenting complaints include dysphagia, halitosis, and intermittent coughing from aspiration. An additional proximal pulsion diverticulum is the **lateral hypopharyngeal diverticulum**, which occurs more cephalad within the hypopharynx. These are commonly seen in older patients with chronic obstructive pulmonary disease, as well as at a younger age in occupations such as glassblowers and wind instrument musicians. They are associated with laryngoceles.

- **Distal esophageal pulsion diverticulum**. Diverticula in the distal esophagus (lower 6–10 cm), termed epiphrenic diverticula, usually occur in the setting of an underlying esophageal motility disorder (e.g., achalasia, diffuse esophageal spasm). Most patients have minimal symptoms, but surgical diverticulectomy is indicated in severely symptomatic patients.

- **Midesophageal traction diverticulum**. Diverticula of the midesophagus commonly develop by "traction" effects from an inflammatory process within the adjacent mediastinum (e.g., tuberculosis, histoplasmosis). Midesophageal diverticula can also be seen in the spectrum of foregut duplications/malformations or in the postsurgical setting after tracheoesophageal fistula repair.

■ Additional Differential Diagnoses

- **Intramural pseudodiverticulosis**. Intramural pseudodiverticulosis is a rare condition in which numerous 1- to 4-mm saccular outpouchings form within the esophageal wall secondary to inflammatory dilatation of esophageal submucosal glands. Most patients have an associated motility disorder or underlying esophageal strictures.

■ Diagnosis

Proximal esophageal pulsion diverticulum (Zenker diverticulum)

✓ Pearls

- Zenker diverticulum is a posterior midline defect that occurs above the level of the cricopharyngeal muscle.
- Killian–Jameson is a lateral defect that occurs at the level of the cricopharyngeal muscle.

- Mediastinal inflammatory processes that cause scarring can create an esophageal traction diverticulum.

Suggested Readings

Duda M, Serý Z, Vojácek K, Rocek V, Rehulka M. Etiopathogenesis and classification of esophageal diverticula. Int Surg. 1985; 70(4):291–295

Federle MP, Jeffrey RB, Woodward PJ, Borhani A. Diagnostic Imaging: Abdomen. 2nd ed. Philadelphia, PA: Lippincott Williams & Wilkins; 2009

Sydow BD, Levine MS, Rubesin SE, Laufer I. Radiographic findings and complications after surgical or endoscopic repair of Zenker diverticulum in 16 patients. AJR Am J Roentgenol. 2001; 177(5):1067–1071

Case 34

Eleanor L. Ormsby

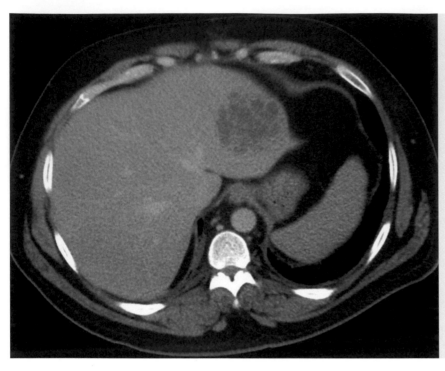

Fig. 34.1 Axial contrast enhanced computed tomography (CT) image demonstrates a relatively ill-defined, 5 cm, hypodense, multilocular mass in the left lobe of the liver. The rim and septations within the lesion have similar density to surrounding hepatic parenchyma.

■ Clinical Presentation

A 43-year-old man with history of epigastric pain (▶Fig. 34.1).

■ Key Imaging Finding

Solitary hypodense, hypovascular liver mass

■ Top 3 Differential Diagnoses

- **Hepatic cyst**. Hepatic cysts are thought to be congenital lesions arising from developmental defects of the biliary ducts. They are well circumscribed with very thin or imperceptible walls. They rarely cause symptoms and typically do not result in abnormal liver function tests. Simple cysts do not enhance.
- **Solitary metastasis**. The most common appearance of hepatic metastases on computed tomography (CT) is a low-density lesion with respect to the liver parenchyma. There may be a degree of peripheral rim enhancement. Calcifications may be seen in mucinous adenocarcinomas of the colon, stomach, or ovary. Hypovascular metastatic masses are best seen on portal venous phase images. Smaller lesions may fill in on delayed images.

- **Hepatic abscess**. Hepatic abscesses are most commonly pyogenic usually from ascending cholangitis, hematogenous spread, or direct extension from adjacent sites of infection. They may also occur as a complication after surgery or traumatic events involving the liver. Hepatic abscesses are hypodense with peripheral enhancement. Pyogenic abscesses are commonly multilocular. Amebic abscesses appear similar to pyogenic abscesses but tend to be unilocular. They are common worldwide and have a tendency to rupture. Echinococcal infection (hydatid cyst) can be very large with rimlike calcification. Daughter cysts within the larger cyst are pathognomonic. Mycotic abscesses are typically multiple and small.

■ Additional Differential Diagnoses

- **Peripheral cholangiocarcinoma**. Intrahepatic cholangiocarcinomas are hypodense on arterial and portal venous phase imaging and characteristically demonstrate delayed (>10 minutes) peripheral to central enhancement. Overlying capsular retraction is due to fibrosis. The masses tend to be infiltrative with irregular borders. Biliary ductal dilatation is common peripheral to the tumor.

- **Biliary cystadenoma**. Biliary cystadenomas are uncommon, multilocular, well-defined cystic masses arising from the bile ducts. They typically occur in middle-aged women who complain of chronic abdominal pain. The cyst wall may enhance. Malignant transformation to cystadenocarcinoma can occur.

■ Diagnosis

Hepatic abscess (pyogenic)

✓ Pearls

- Delayed imaging with intravenous contrast is helpful in differentiating hepatic cysts from hypodense metastases.
- Amebic abscesses in the liver are fairly common worldwide and have a tendency to rupture.

- Delayed imaging (>10 minutes) is helpful in the diagnosis of cholangiocarcinoma.

Suggested Readings

Engelbrecht MR, Katz SS, van Gulik TM, Laméris JS, van Delden OM. Imaging of perihilar cholangiocarcinoma. AJR Am J Roentgenol. 2015; 204(4):782–791

Qian LJ, Zhu J, Zhuang ZG, Xia Q, Liu Q, Xu JR. Spectrum of multilocular cystic hepatic lesions: CT and MR imaging findings with pathologic correlation. Radiographics. 2013; 33(5):1419–1433

Case 35

Robert A. Jesinger

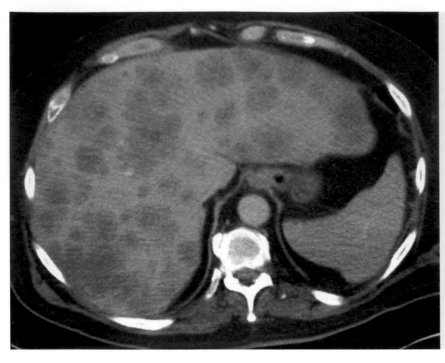

Fig. 35.1 Contrast-enhanced axial computed tomography (CT) image of the liver demonstrates multiple hypoattenuating hepatic lesions with a few regions of internal and peripheral enhancement.

■ Clinical Presentation

A 58-year-old man with weakness and weight loss (▶Fig. 35.1).

■ Key Imaging Finding

Multiple hypoattenuating hepatic lesions

■ Top 3 Differential Diagnoses

- **Hepatic cysts**. Small isolated hepatic cysts are commonly seen on routine abdominal computed tomography (CT) and ultrasound. Hepatic cysts are well-circumscribed, homogeneous masses of near-water attenuation value (-20 to +20 HU) that show no enhancement after intravenous (IV) contrast administration. When multiple hepatic cysts are seen, polycystic kidney and/or liver disease, biliary hamartomas, and Caroli disease should be considered. Caroli disease is characterized by dilated biliary ducts surrounding an enhancing portal vein and hepatic artery, which is referred to as the central dot sign. When a large solitary liver cyst is noted, hepatic cystadenoma, biloma, and/or hydatid cyst should be considered. Usually, hepatic cysts are not associated with biliary obstruction, nor is spontaneous cyst rupture common.
- **Metastatic disease**. Liver metastases rank second to lymph node metastases in cancer patients. Virtually any primary malignant neoplasm can produce liver metastases, but the most common primary tumor sites include the colon, lung, breast, stomach, and pancreas. In children, the most common primary tumors producing hypoattenuating liver metastases include neuroblastoma, Wilms tumor, and leukemia. Most metastatic lesions enhance after IV contrast administration, but their visual conspicuity usually results from normally enhancing adjacent liver parenchyma. Surgical resection of isolated metastatic liver lesions has been found to increase survival time in certain cancers (e.g., colon cancer).
- **Multiple hepatic abscesses**. Hepatic abscesses are relatively rare, but when encountered, they typically fall into three categories: pyogenic (80%), amebic (10%), and fungal (10%). Historically, pyogenic hepatic abscesses were found in the setting of appendicitis, but currently, diverticulitis and sepsis are more common causes. Amebic abscesses are prone to rupture. Imaging findings include thick-walled, hypoattenuating liver masses with internal septations, peripheral lesion enhancement, and gas in up to 20% of cases. Untreated liver abscesses have a high mortality rate. However, image-guided catheter drainage has improved mortality rates significantly.

■ Additional Differential Diagnoses

- **Cholangiocarcinoma**. A rare cancer of the bile ducts, cholangiocarcinomas typically present as multiple hypoattenuating infiltrative lesions, paralleling the bile ducts and causing biliary obstruction. Risk factors include primary sclerosing cholangitis, parasitic liver flukes (e.g., *Clonorchis sinensis*), choledochal anomalies, and prior thorotrast exposure. Delayed enhancement (beyond 10 minutes) is a key distinguishing feature. Most patients present late, when curative surgical resection is contraindicated.

■ Diagnosis

Metastatic disease (pancreatic adenocarcinoma)

✓ Pearls

- Hepatic cysts are well-circumscribed, homogeneous masses of near-water attenuation.
- Multiple irregularly shaped hypoattenuating lesions in the liver are concerning for metastases.
- Delayed enhancement (beyond 10 minutes) is important in diagnosing hepatic cholangiocarcinomas.

Suggested Readings

Federle MP, Jeffrey RB, Woodward PJ, Borhani A. Diagnostic Imaging: Abdomen. 2nd ed. Philadelphia, PA: Lippincott Williams & Wilkins; 2009

Mortelé KJ, Ros PR. Cystic focal liver lesions in the adult: differential CT and MR imaging features. Radiographics. 2001; 21(4):895–910

Case 36

Chirag V. Patel

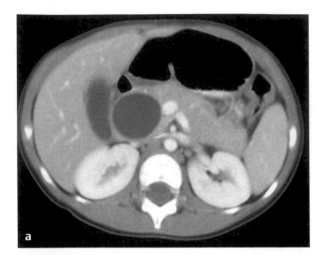 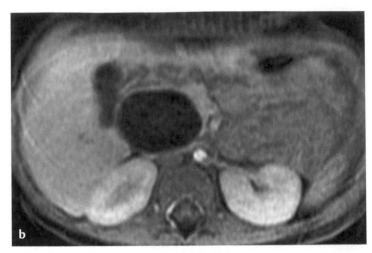

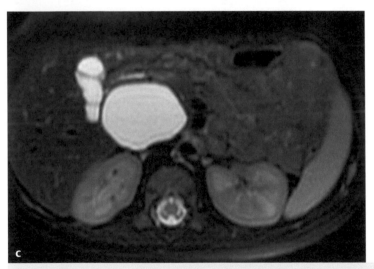 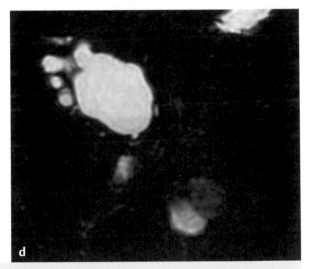

Fig. 36.1 **(a)** Axial contrast-enhanced CT image demonstrates a cystic mass in the right upper quadrant medial to the gallbladder. **(b)** Axial postcontrast T1, **(c)** axial T2, and **(d)** coronal MRCP in a different patient with right upper quadrant abdominal mass, showing cystic dilatation of extrahepatic biliary ducts.

■ Clinical Presentation

A 3-year-old boy with early satiety and intermittent postprandial emesis (►Fig. 36.1).

■ Key Imaging Finding

Right upper quadrant (RUQ) cystic mass in a child

■ Top 3 Differential Diagnoses

- **Choledochal anomaly**. Congenital cystic enlargement of the bile ducts is referred to as a choledochal anomaly. Choledochal cysts are classified into five different types. Type 1 is the most common, accounting for 80 to 90% of cases, and represents cystic or fusiform dilatation of the common bile duct (CBD). Most choledochal cysts become symptomatic in the first decade of life with a palpable RUQ mass, jaundice, and pain being the classic triad of symptoms. Presentation is more insidious in older children and adults. On imaging, demonstration of cystic or fusiform dilatation of the extrahepatic bile duct is enough for diagnosis. However, magnetic resonance cholangiopancreatography (MRCP) or endoscopic retrograde cholangiopancreatography (ERCP) may be of further help in preoperative evaluation. Types 2 through 5 consist of a CBD diverticulum, a choledochocele, intra- and extrahepatic ductal dilatation, and intrahepatic ductal dilatation (Caroli disease), respectively.
- **Pancreatic pseudocyst**. Pseudocyst is the most common cystic lesion of pancreas in children, accounting for 75% of all cystic lesions. Blunt trauma and pancreatitis are the most common etiologies. The diagnosis on imaging is based on the exclusion of communication with the biliary ducts (choledochal cyst) and bowel (enteric duplication cyst or diverticulum) and demonstrating true intrapancreatic location of the cystic lesion. In the absence of a history of acute pancreatitis, careful evaluation for septation or papillary growth should be undertaken to rule out a rare cystic pancreatic malignancy. Correlation for a history of trauma (accidental or nonaccidental) should always be considered.
- **Gastrointestinal (GI) duplication cyst/diverticulum**. GI duplication cysts can occur anywhere in the GI tract; however, the stomach and duodenum are rare locations, while the ileum and esophagus are the most common locations. Diverticula commonly occur within the duodenum. Demonstration of continuity of the cyst with the GI tract and visualization of gut signature on ultrasound (US) aids in diagnosis. There may be fluid-debris levels.

■ Additional Differential Diagnoses

- **Ovarian cystic lesion**. Ovarian cystic lesions can sometimes present as an abdominal mass. When large, demonstrating the ovarian origin may be difficult. In girls younger than 17 years, cystic ovarian teratoma is the most common cystic lesion. Mature cystic teratoma is the most common subtype (90%) and demonstrates fat and/or calcification within a predominantly cystic mass. Simple ovarian cysts also may occur in children, especially in the prenatal and postnatal period while under maternal estrogen stimulation.
- **Mesenteric cyst**. Mesenteric cysts represent lymphangiomas localized to the mesentery. On US, they are seen as single or multiple cysts with thin imperceptible walls and may or may not have septations. On computed tomography (CT), the attenuation coefficients of the cystic content range from water density to fat density, depending on the proportion of chylous component. They are usually homogenous. When complicated by infection or hemorrhage, the cysts can show atypical features, with thick walls and inhomogeneous cystic content.

■ Achalasia

Choledochal anomaly (type 1)

✓ Pearls

- Fusiform dilation of the extrahepatic CBD is the most common choledochal anomaly.
- Diagnosis of pancreatic pseudocyst in a child requires assessment for a history of trauma or pancreatitis.
- Duplication cysts are commonly contiguous with the bowel and have gut signature on US.

Suggested Readings

Chavhan GB, Babyn PS, Manson D, Vidarsson L. Pediatric MR cholangiopancreatography: principles, technique, and clinical applications. Radiographics. 2008; 28(7):1951–1962

Santiago I, Loureiro R, Curvo-Semedo L, et al. Congenital cystic lesions of the biliary tree. AJR Am J Roentgenol. 2012; 198(4):825–835

Case 37

Shaun Loh

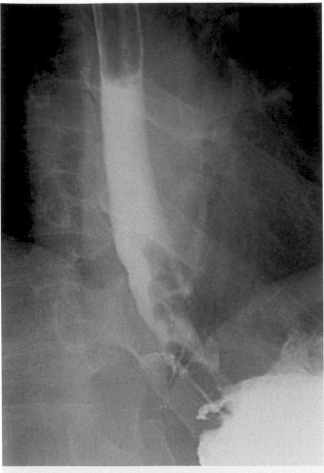

Fig. 37.1 Esophagram demonstrates tortuous longitudinal submucosal filling defects in the distal esophagus.

■ Clinical Presentation

A 40-year-old man with a 2-week history of "food sticking" in his throat (►Fig. 37.1).

■ Key Imaging Finding

Esophageal submucosal masses/thickened folds

■ Top 3 Differential Diagnoses

• **Varices**. Varices are a common sequela of portal hypertension, often secondary to chronic liver disease. They are classified according their pathophysiology as either uphill or downhill varices. Uphill varices are more common and involve the distal portion of the esophagus. They form as a result of portal hypertension, where increased pressures cause upward flow of blood from the portal vein through collateral flow through the azygous vein to the superior vena cava (SVC). Uphill varices commonly cause gastrointestinal bleeding. Downhill varices, on the other hand, are rarer and involve the proximal esophagus. An obstruction of the SVC results in downward flow through the azygous vein to the inferior vena cava and portal vein. Common causes of SVC obstruction include lung cancer, mediastinitis, retrosternal goiters, or thymomas. Downhill varices may present with symptoms of SVC syndrome, including facial, periorbital, or neck swelling. On an esophagram, varices appear as longitudinal, serpentine, radiolucent filling defects, which vary in size with changes in patient positioning and phase of respiration. Cross-sectional imaging reveals avid enhancement of varices.

• **Reflux esophagitis**. The inflammatory changes and submucosal edema in esophagitis may appear as thickened, tortuous folds, much like varices. The thickened folds in the setting of esophagitis, however, will remain fixed in appearance in contradistinction to varices. An adequate clinical history combined with endoscopy will readily differentiate between the two.

• **Varicoid esophageal carcinoma**. Esophageal carcinoma is a common malignancy of the gastrointestinal tract. Advanced esophageal carcinomas may present as infiltrating, polypoid, ulcerative, or varicoid lesions. The varicoid-type lesion is the least common subtype and appears on esophagrams as thickened, rigid, serpentine, longitudinal filling defects because of the submucosal spread of tumor. They are frequently confused for varices but differ in that varicoid tumors have fixed configurations and do not change their appearance in response to esophageal peristalsis, respiratory maneuvers, or repositioning of the patient. Diagnosis is confirmed with endoscopic biopsy.

■ Additional Differential Diagnoses

• **Lymphoma**. Lymphoma rarely involves the esophagus, but when it does, signs of lymphoma are seen in other parts of the body. Most cases of esophageal lymphoma result from contiguous spread along the gastric cardia or fundus. When lymphoma infiltrates in a submucosal fashion, it produces fixed, tortuous, longitudinal folds. Endoscopic biopsy confirms the diagnosis.

■ Diagnosis

Esophageal varices

✓ Pearls

• Portal hypertension causes uphill esophageal varices, while SVC obstruction causes downhill varices.
• Esophageal varices vary in size and appearance with patient positioning; they enhance avidly.

• Reflux esophagitis may present with mucosal abnormalities and thickened folds.
• Varicoid esophageal carcinoma is the least common tumor subtype but may mimic varices.

Suggested Readings

Federle MP, Jeffrey RB, Woodward PJ, Borhani A. Diagnostic Imaging: Abdomen. 2nd ed. Philadelphia, PA: Lippincott Williams & Wilkins; 2009
Kim YJ, Raman SS, Yu NC, To'o KJ, Jutabha R, Lu DS. Esophageal varices in cirrhotic patients: evaluation with liver CT. AJR Am J Roentgenol. 2007; 188(1):139–144

Matsumoto A, Kitamoto M, Imamura M, et al. Three-dimensional portography using multislice helical CT is clinically useful for management of gastric fundic varices. AJR Am J Roentgenol. 2001; 176(4):899–905

Case 38

Paul B. DiDomenico

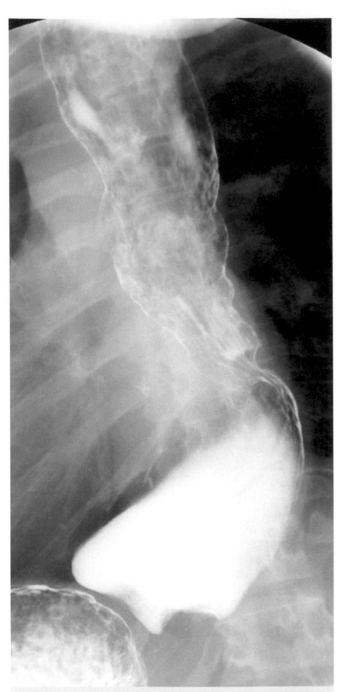

Fig. 38.1 A slightly oblique frontal view from an esophagram reveals a dilated esophagus that tapers to a "bird's beak" appearance distally at the gastroesophageal (GE) junction.

■ Clinical Presentation

Patient with chronic dysphagia (▶Fig. 38.1).

■ Key Imaging Finding

Esophageal dilatation

■ Top 3 Differential Diagnoses

- **Achalasia**. Achalasia is a disease of the myenteric plexus of the esophagus which results in failure of relaxation of the lower esophageal sphincter (LES). Persistent contraction of the LES results in smooth distal tapering with a classic "bird's beak" appearance, proximal dilatation on barium esophagram, and diminished or absent peristalsis. Primary (idiopathic) achalasia is thought to be due to degeneration of the myenteric plexus, while secondary achalasia results from destruction of the plexus by infiltrating tumor or infections such as Chagas' disease or fungal infection. Treatment options include calcium channel blockers, pneumatic dilatation, or Heller myotomy.
- **Scleroderma**. Scleroderma is a collagen vascular disease in which smooth muscle becomes fibrotic. This affects the distal two-thirds of the esophagus, which is lined by smooth muscle, resulting in dysmotility and dilatation. The LES becomes incompetent, and there is patulous dilation of the gastroesophageal (GE) junction, which may help distinguish this disorder from achalasia. The resulting chronic reflux, however, may cause a peptic stricture that may mimic achalasia.
- **Esophageal/gastric carcinoma**. Malignancy of either the distal esophagus or gastric cardia may cause mass effect at the GE junction, resulting in a tapered narrowing of the lower esophagus with dysmotility and dilatation. Irregularity of the mucosa, "shouldering" mass effect, and correlation with history may suggest malignancy, although final diagnosis would be made via endoscopy and biopsy.

■ Additional Differential Diagnoses

- **Esophagitis with stricture**. Longstanding reflux, often with a coexisting hiatal hernia, may result in a peptic stricture at the distal esophagus with narrowing of a short distal segment seen on barium esophagram. Esophageal motility is usually normal, and there is minimal dilatation of the esophagus.
- **Postsurgical changes (vagotomy)**. Vagotomy has been reported as a secondary cause of achalasia due to neuronal damage or fibrosis at the GE junction. These changes result in focal narrowing of the distal esophagus with proximal dilatation.

■ Diagnosis

Achalasia

✓ Pearls

- Smooth tapering of the distal esophagus on esophagram ("bird's beak") is a key finding in achalasia.
- Scleroderma often scars the distal esophagus, resulting in a patulous GE junction and chronic reflux.
- Irregular tapering of the distal esophagus on esophagram is a concerning finding for carcinoma.

Suggested Readings

Levine MS, Rubesin SE. Diseases of the esophagus: diagnosis with esophagography. Radiology. 2005; 237(2):414–427

Woodfield CA, Levine MS, Rubesin SE, Langlotz CP, Laufer I. Diagnosis of primary versus secondary achalasia: reassessment of clinical and radiographic criteria. AJR Am J Roentgenol. 2000; 175(3):727–731

Case 39

Eleanor L. Ormsby

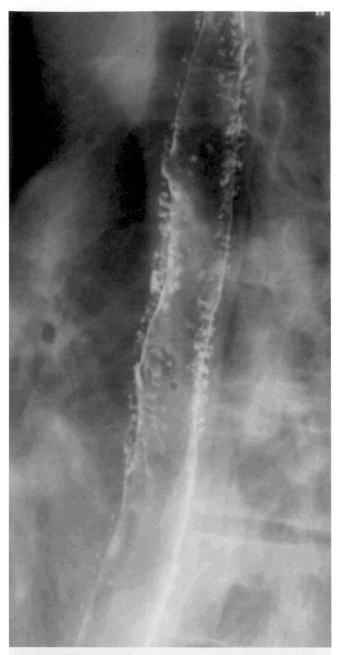

Fig. 39.1 Oblique image from an esophagram demonstrates multiple contrast outpouchings along the midesophageal wall, consistent with intramural pseudodiverticula.

■ Clinical Presentation

A 42-year-old man with odynodysphagia (▶ Fig. 39.1).

■ Key Imaging Finding

Esophageal pseudodiverticula

■ Top 3 Differential Diagnoses

- **Reflux esophagitis**. Pseudodiverticula are flask-shaped outpouchings of contrast filling dilated mucous glands in the esophageal wall. They are the sequela of chronic irritation and esophagitis. Reflux esophagitis usually affects the distal esophagus as a result of irritation of esophageal mucosa by gastric acid. Esophagram demonstrates thickened distal folds, ulcers (which are usually linear), benign strictures (which classically begin immediately above the GE junction), and/or intramural pseudodiverticula. Hiatal hernias are commonly associated with gastroesophageal reflux.
- **Candida esophagitis**. Candida is often cultured in esophageal pseudodiverticulosis, likely due to chronic esophagitis. It is most commonly seen in immunosuppressed patients, especially in the setting of AIDS. Patients with esophageal stasis, such as those with achalasia or scleroderma, are also at risk for developing Candida esophagitis. Esophagram may demonstrate diffuse mucosal nodularity and ulceration, longitudinally oriented plaques, and pseudodiverticula.
- **Superficial spreading carcinoma**. Superficial spreading carcinoma is an unusual form of squamous cell carcinoma, which is characterized by small plaquelike mucosal nodularities on esophagram. Focal necrosis and ulceration can also be seen, as can pseudodiverticula. Endoscopic biopsy confirms the diagnosis.

■ Additional Differential Diagnoses

- **Drug-induced esophagitis**. In most patients with drug-induced esophagitis, there is no underlying esophageal disease. A wide range of drugs can cause esophagitis, including tetracycline, ascorbic acid, and iron sulfate. Esophagram may show single or multiple shallow ulcerations with possible associated fold thickening at the level of the aortic arch or the distal esophagus where a transient delay in the passage of bolus occurs. Occasionally, pseudodiverticula may occur. Repeat esophagrams usually demonstrate complete healing following withdrawal of the medication.

■ Diagnosis

Candida esophagitis

✓ Pearls

- Transmural inflammation in the esophagus may dilate mural glands and result in pseudodiverticula.
- Candidiasis presents in immunosuppressed patients with mucosal plaques and pseudodiverticula.
- Endoscopy is performed to exclude superficial spreading carcinoma in the setting of pseudodiverticula.

Suggested Readings

Lee SS, Ha HK, Byun JH, et al. Superficial esophageal cancer: esophagographic findings correlated with histopathologic findings. Radiology. 2005; 236(2):535–544

Levine MS, Moolten DN, Herlinger H, Laufer I. Esophageal intramural pseudodiverticulosis: a reevaluation. AJR Am J Roentgenol. 1986; 147(6):1165–1170

McGettigan MJ, Menias CO, Gao ZJ, Mellnick VM, Hara AK. Imaging of drug-induced complications in the gastrointestinal system. Radiographics. 2016; 36(1):71–87

Case 40

Robert A. Jesinger

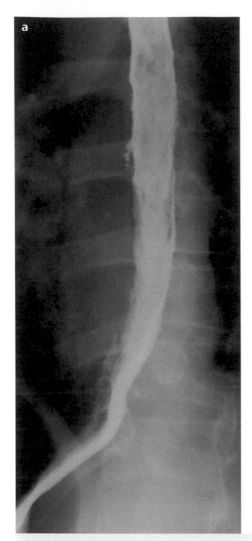
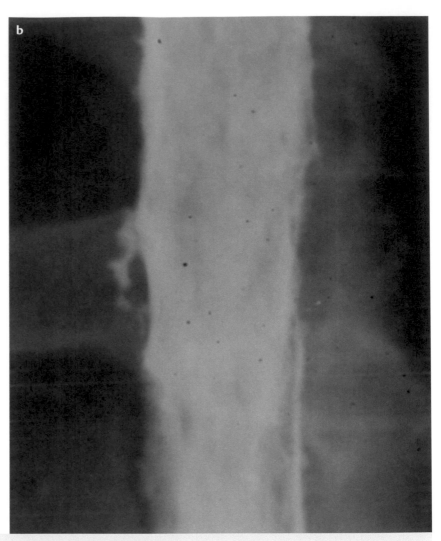

Fig. 40.1 (a) Single-contrast fluoroscopic image and (b) coned-down view of the esophagus from a barium swallow examination demonstrate a large midesophageal ulcer, as well as additional smaller ulcerations and thickening of the longitudinal folds.

■ Clinical Presentation

A 35-year-old man with chest pain and odynodysphagia (▶Fig. 40.1).

■ Key Imaging Finding

Esophageal ulcers

■ Top 3 Differential Diagnoses

- **Reflux esophagitis.** Erosions and ulcerations can form in the distal esophagus as a result of irritation of esophageal mucosa from gastric acid. Key imaging findings of esophageal inflammation include longitudinal fold thickening, pooling of contrast in mucosal erosions or ulcers, poor peristalsis, and poor esophageal distension in the region of inflammation. Midesophageal strictures may be seen in severe chronic reflux. Careful visual assessment for Barrett's metaplasia, hiatal hernia, and reflux on fluoroscopy can aid in assessment.
- **Viral esophagitis (CMV, HIV, HSV).** Discrete ulcers against otherwise normal background mucosa are the hallmark of viral esophagitis. Viral esophagitis typically occurs in immunosuppressed patients, especially in the setting of human immunodeficiency virus (HIV). Herpes simplex virus (HSV)

ulcers tend to be multiple, small, discrete, and focal, while ulcers caused by cytomegalovirus (CMV) and HIV are typically large. Although imaging characteristics may suggest the underlying source of ulceration, serology or biopsy is often used for definitive diagnosis and treatment.
- **Drug-induced esophagitis.** Esophageal injury and ulceration may occur from ingested medications if the tablets become trapped in the esophageal lumen. Typically, esophageal dysmotility or an obstructing lesion is present with subsequent ulcer formation from prolonged direct contact with the esophageal mucosa. Common medications that can cause mucosal injury include antimicrobial medications (doxycycline, tetracycline, clindamycin), anti-inflammatory medications, and supplements (potassium chloride, vitamin C).

■ Additional Differential Diagnoses

- **Caustic esophagitis.** Caustic esophagitis is the consequence of contact injury usually with an alkaline substance. Numerous household and garden chemicals (alkalis), when ingested, can cause both superficial and deep liquefaction necrosis in the esophagus, leading to ulceration and long segment scarring. Acid burns are less frequently encountered and typically lead to less severe superficial mucosal burns.
- **Esophageal carcinoma.** Malignancy should always be considered in the differential diagnosis of mucosal irregularity and ulceration. Both primary squamous cell carcinoma and adenocarcinoma in the setting of Barrett's metaplasia can ulcerate. Aggressive midesophageal malignancies can erode into the tracheobronchial tree, resulting in fistula formation. Metastases and lymphoma may also mimic esophageal carcinoma.

■ Diagnosis

Viral esophagitis (HSV)

✓ Pearls

- Mucosal ulcers, fold thickening, poor peristalsis, and poor distensibility are key findings in esophagitis.
- HSV typically causes multiple small ulcers; CMV and HIV commonly present as large ulcers.

- Contact injury from prolonged retention of certain medications in the esophagus can cause a focal ulcer.
- Esophageal carcinoma and lymphoma should always be considered as a potential cause for an ulcer.

Suggested Readings

Federle MP, Jeffrey RB, Woodward PJ, Borhani A. Diagnostic Imaging: Abdomen. 2nd ed. Philadelphia, PA: Lippincott Williams & Wilkins; 2009

McGettigan MJ, Menias CO, Gao ZJ, Mellnick VM, Hara AK. Imaging of drug-induced complications in the gastrointestinal system. Radiographics. 2016; 36(1):71–87

Young CA, Menias CO, Bhalla S, Prasad SR. CT features of esophageal emergencies. Radiographics. 2008; 28(6):1541–1553

Case 41

Brian S. Johnston

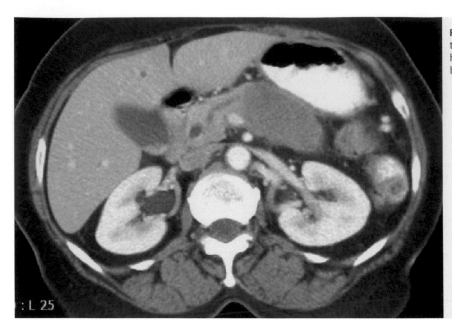

Fig. 41.1 Contrast-enhanced axial computed tomography (CT) image demonstrates a solid, oval, hypodense mass at the junction of the pancreatic body and tail with proximal ductal dilatation.

■ Clinical Presentation

A 51-year-old man with vague abdominal discomfort (▶ Fig. 41.1).

■ Key Imaging Finding

Solid pancreatic mass

■ Top 3 Differential Diagnoses

- **Pancreatic adenocarcinoma**. Ductal epithelial adenocarcinoma is the most common primary tumor of the pancreas and typically occurs in older males. This malignancy grows in an infiltrative manner with poorly defined margins, often mimicking pancreatitis. Vascular encasement of the superior mesenteric vessels essentially makes the disease unresectable. Imaging findings include a hypovascular solid pancreatic mass with distal pancreatic ductal dilatation and parenchymal atrophy. Overall, prognosis is typically poor.
- **Islet cell tumor**. In contrast to pancreatic adenocarcinoma, islet cell tumors (and their metastases) are typically hypervascular, especially when small. Larger lesions often show more heterogeneous attenuation and enhancement because of central cystic degeneration, necrosis, fibrosis, and/or calcification. Peritumoral neovascularity is common, while vascular encasement and narrowing are not typically seen. The tumors are classified by the hormones they produce. Insulinoma is the most common subtype and is most often benign. Gastrinoma, nonfunctioning islet cell tumor, glucagonoma, VIPoma, and somatostatinoma represent less common subtypes of islet cell tumors that tend to have more malignant characteristics. Gastrinoma results in hypersecretion of gastric acid and results in multiple gastric and duodenal (typically postampullary) ulcers. They are commonly associated with Zollinger–Ellison syndrome. Islet cell tumors may be seen as part of multiple endocrine neoplasia syndrome type 1. In general, syndromic islet cell tumors tend to present earlier with homogeneous hypervascularity because of their symptomatology, whereas nonsyndromic or nonsecreting cases tend to present late, often with metastases and a more heterogeneous imaging appearance.
- **Solid and papillary epithelial neoplasm (SPEN)**. SPEN, more recently referred to as solid pseudopapillary tumor (SPT) of the pancreas, is a rare pancreatic tumor that is mostly seen in young women. Imaging findings include a large, well-circumscribed noncalcified mass, usually containing both solid and cystic areas. Necrosis and hemorrhage are common. These neoplasms have a good prognosis after resection. In young children, pancreatoblastoma can have a similar appearance.

■ Additional Differential Diagnoses

- **Lymphoma**. Lymphoma may involve the pancreas, typically from local spread of the non-Hodgkin variant. Associated abdominal or pelvic lymphadenopathy is typically present, which would support the diagnosis. Vascular encasement is less common in contrast to adenocarcinoma.
- **Metastases**. Colorectal and gastric malignancies most commonly involve the pancreas by local invasion. More distant metastases often originate from renal cell carcinoma (~50% of cases), melanoma, lung, and breast cancer. Metastatic disease involving peripancreatic lymph nodes can simulate a primary pancreatic tumor.

■ Diagnosis

Pancreatic adenocarcinoma

✓ Pearls

- A pancreatic mass encasing and narrowing adjacent vessels is pathognomonic of cancer.
- The most common hypervascular islet cell tumor of the pancreas is an insulinoma.
- SPEN is a rare solid and cystic pancreatic tumor that occurs in young women.
- Hypervascular pancreatic metastases include melanoma, breast cancer, and renal cell carcinoma.

Suggested Readings

Lewis RB, Lattin GE, Jr, Paal E. Pancreatic endocrine tumors: radiologic-clinico-pathologic correlation. Radiographics. 2010; 30(6):1445–1464

Saenz R. Pancreatic mass. J Am Osteopath Coll Radiol. 2012; 1(4):38–40

Case 42

Brian S. Johnston

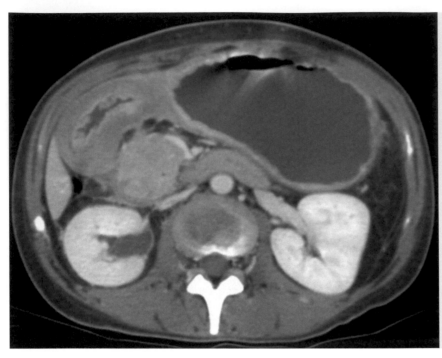

Fig. 42.1 Contrast-enhanced axial computed tomography (CT) image through the upper abdomen demonstrates diffuse circumferential antral wall thickening with narrowing of the gastric lumen. A large nodal mass is seen posterior to the gastric antrum.

■ Clinical Presentation

A 45-year-old woman with weight loss and heartburn (▶ Fig. 42.1).

■ Key Imaging Finding

Linitis plastica

■ Top 3 Differential Diagnoses

- **Gastric carcinoma**. Diffuse infiltrative gastric wall thickening, in association with a rigid, contracted, narrowed stomach ("linitis plastica" appearance), is the second most common appearance for gastric carcinoma after focal irregular wall thickening with ulceration. Poorly differentiated tumor types and poor prognoses are often found in association with the "linitis plastica" type of gastric carcinoma. Key imaging findings include gastric antral wall thickening with possible fundal sparing, absent peristalsis, and loss of normal gastric fold pattern.
- **Metastatic disease**. A common presentation of gastric metastases is diffuse infiltrative wall thickening, with breast and lung cancer representing the most common primary neoplasms. The infiltrative tumor results in a rigid, contracted stomach. Pancreatic adenocarcinoma can invade the distal stomach by contiguous spread, also producing the "linitis plastica" appearance.
- **Lymphoma**. Primary gastric lymphoma accounts for fewer than 15% of gastric malignancies. Secondary gastric involvement, however, is not uncommon in systemic lymphomas, especially the non-Hodgkin variant. Diffuse infiltration of the tumor results in a desmoplastic response and subsequent gastric luminal rigidity and narrowing.

■ Additional Differential Diagnoses

- **Crohn disease**. Severe gastric involvement with Crohn disease can produce a rigid, contracted, narrowed distal stomach, which is referred to as the "ram's horn" appearance. By the time the stomach is involved with Crohn disease, there is typically more pronounced small bowel (usually terminal ileum) and/or colonic involvement as well.

■ Diagnosis

Metastatic disease (breast cancer)

✓ Pearls

- Linitis plastica is the second most common appearance of gastric carcinoma.
- Diffuse infiltrative metastatic breast and lung cancer may produce linitis plastica.
- Lymphoma in the gastric wall is often secondary to diffuse systemic disease involvement.
- Postinflammatory scarring of the distal stomach in Crohn disease is termed the "ram's horn" appearance.

Suggested Readings

Chen CY, Jaw TS, Wu DC, et al. MDCT of giant gastric folds: differential diagnosis. AJR Am J Roentgenol. 2010; 195(5):1124–1130

Federle MP, Jeffrey RB, Woodward PJ, Borhani A. Diagnostic Imaging: Abdomen. 2nd ed. Philadelphia, PA: Lippincott Williams & Wilkins; 2009

Halpert RD. Gastrointestinal Imaging: The Requisites. 3rd ed. Philadelphia, PA: Elsevier; 2006

Case 43

Robert A. Jesinger

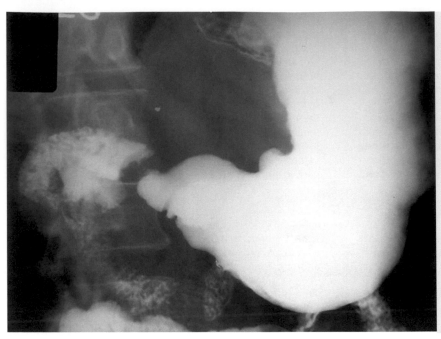

Fig. 43.1 Single-contrast fluoroscopic image from an upper gastrointestinal examination demonstrates a focal smooth outpouching of contrast along the lesser curvature of the stomach. The contrast collection extends beyond the margins of the stomach wall.

■ Clinical Presentation

A 34-year-old man with epigastric pain (▶ Fig. 43.1).

■ Key Imaging Finding

Gastric ulcer

■ Top 3 Differential Diagnoses

- **Peptic ulcer disease**. Benign gastric ulcers typically occur in the gastric antrum and appear as a contrast "outpouching" beyond the margin of the gastric wall. The margins of the ulcer are smooth, and the adjacent fold pattern is typically normal. *Helicobacter pylori* infection has been found to be a major causative factor. Nonsteroidal anti-inflammatory drugs are another but less common cause of benign gastric ulcers.
- **Gastric carcinoma**. Focal gastric wall thickening with ulceration is the most common presentation of gastric carcinoma. Malignant gastric ulcers may occur anywhere within the stomach but most commonly are located in the antrum. In cont-

rast to benign ulcers, malignant ulcers appear as a contrast "inpouching" because of contrast filling an ulcerated gastric mass. The margins of the ulcer are irregular and nodular. Diagnosis is confirmed with endoscopic biopsy.
- **Lymphoma**. Primary gastric lymphoma accounts for fewer than 15% of gastric malignancies. Secondary gastric involvement, however, is not uncommon in systemic disease (e.g., non-Hodgkin lymphoma). Gastric lymphoma may mimic both the diffuse infiltrative type (linitis plastica) and the focal ulcerative variant of gastric adenocarcinoma.

■ Additional Differential Diagnoses

- **Metastatic disease**. A mural gastric mass with central ulceration may be secondary to metastatic disease. The more common primary neoplasms include breast, lung, and malignant melanoma. Pancreatic adenocarcinoma can involve the distal stomach (usually distal greater curvature) by contiguous spread, and central ulceration of the invading mass can occur.
- **Zollinger–Ellison syndrome**. Zollinger–Ellison syndrome consists of multiple gastric and duodenal (classically postbulbar) ulcers secondary to marked gastric hypersecretion cau-

sed by a gastrinoma. The majority of gastrinomas occur within the pancreas (islet cell tumors), but 15% can be found in the duodenum. An association with multiple endocrine neoplasia I occurs in 25% of cases. Clinical features of gastric hypersecretion and diarrhea mimic Ménétrier disease. The majority of gastrinomas (60%) are malignant with a propensity for early liver and lymph node metastases. Hepatic metastases are hypervascular.

■ Diagnosis

Peptic ulcer disease

✓ Pearls

- Contrast "outpouching" suggests a benign gastric ulcer, while "inpouching" suggests a malignant ulcer.
- Ulcer margin and adjacent fold pattern are important in distinguishing benign from malignant ulcers.

- Postbulbar duodenal ulcers are highly suspicious of being caused by Zollinger–Ellison syndrome.

Suggested Readings

Chen CY, Jaw TS, Wu DC, et al. MDCT of giant gastric folds: differential diagnosis. AJR Am J Roentgenol. 2010; 195(5):1124–1130

Federle MP, Jeffrey RB, Woodward PJ, Borhani A. Diagnostic Imaging: Abdomen. 2nd ed. Philadelphia, PA: Lippincott Williams & Wilkins; 2009

Rubesin SE, Levine MS, Laufer I. Double-contrast upper gastrointestinal radiography: a pattern approach for diseases of the stomach. Radiology. 2008; 246(1):33–48

Case 44

Robert A. Jesinger

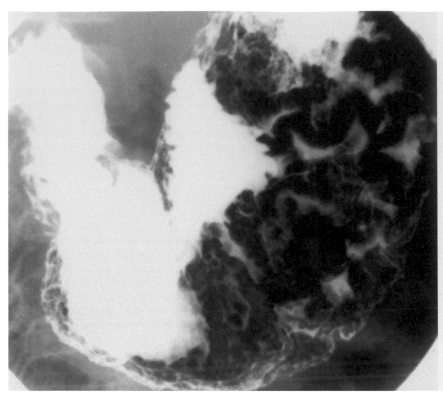

Fig. 44.1 Fluoroscopic image of the stomach from an upper gastrointestinal examination demonstrates marked gastric fold thickening in the regions of the fundus and antrum of the stomach.

■ Clinical Presentation

A 45-year-old man with weight loss, abdominal pain, and diarrhea (►Fig. 44.1).

■ Key Imaging Finding

Gastric fold thickening

■ Top 3 Differential Diagnoses

- **Gastritis**. Chronic inflammation is the most common cause of gastric fold thickening. Common causes include *Helicobacter pylori* infection, nonsteroidal anti-inflammatory drugs, alcohol abuse, and hypersecretion of acid. Secondary imaging findings to suggest gastritis as the cause of gastric fold thickening include small mucosal ulcerations, thickening of the area gastricae in the distal stomach, and decreased gastric peristalsis.
- **Gastric carcinoma**. Focal gastric wall thickening, in association with irregular thickened folds and ulceration, is the most common appearance for gastric carcinoma. There is overlap to the imaging features of gastritis and gastric carcinoma, which may delay diagnosis. Endoscopy with biopsy is often required for definitive diagnosis. Gastric carcinoma may metastasize to the liver (most common). Ovarian metastases (Krukenberg tumors) tend to occurs late and in more advanced cases.
- **Lymphoma**. Primary gastric lymphoma accounts for fewer than 15% of gastric malignancies. Secondary gastric involvement, however, is not uncommon in systemic lymphomas (e.g., non-Hodgkin lymphoma). Focal nodular gastric fold thickening secondary to lymphoma can produce an exaggerated desmoplastic reaction and simulate gastric carcinoma.

■ Additional Differential Diagnoses

- **Metastatic disease**. Focal irregular gastric fold thickening may be secondary to metastatic disease. The more common primary neoplasms include breast and lung cancer. Pancreatic adenocarcinoma can involve the distal stomach (usually distal greater curvature) by contiguous spread.
- **Ménétrier disease**. Hyperplastic hypersecretory gastropathy is a rare condition of uncertain etiology that can affect adults and children. Findings include thickened proximal gastric folds in association with hypersecretion of mucus, protein loss, and low gastric acid output. Enlarged proximal gastric folds and dilution of barium on fluoroscopy secondary to hypersecretion of fluid are key imaging findings. There is an increased risk of gastric cancer which should prompt periodic cancer screening. Severe cases have been treated with partial gastrectomy.

■ Diagnosis

Ménétrier disease

✓ Pearls

- Chronic gastritis is the most common cause for gastric fold thickening (*H. pylori* screening needed).
- Gastric cancer or metastatic breast and lung cancer may present with nodular gastric fold thickening.
- Patients with Ménétrier disease are at increased risk for gastric cancer.

Suggested Readings

Chen CY, Jaw TS, Wu DC, et al. MDCT of giant gastric folds: differential diagnosis. AJR Am J Roentgenol. 2010; 195(5):1124–1130

Friedman J, Platnick J, Farruggia S, Khilko N, Mody K, Tyshkov M. Ménétrier disease. Radiographics. 2009; 29(1):297–301

Rubesin SE, Furth EE, Levine MS. Gastritis from NSAIDS to Helicobacter pylori. Abdom Imaging. 2005; 30(2):142–159

Case 45

Brian S. Johnston

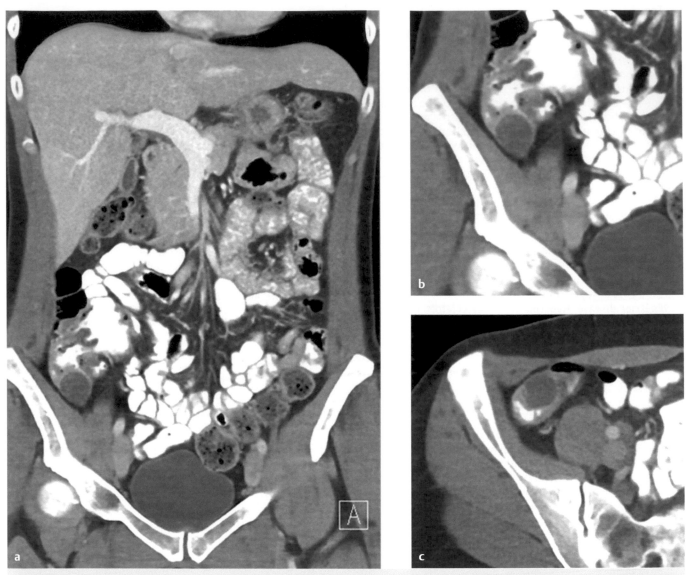

Fig. 45.1 **(a)** Coronal reformatted, **(b)** coronal coned-down, and **(c)** axial coned-down contrast-enhanced (oral and intravenous) axial CT images through the right lower quadrant demonstrate a circumscribed hypodense cecal mass.

■ Clinical Presentation

A 50-year-old man with right lower quadrant (RLQ) abdominal pain (▶Fig. 45.1).

■ **Key Imaging Finding**

Cecal mass

■ **Top 3 Differential Diagnoses**

- **Appendicitis/appendiceal abscess**. An obstructed, dilated appendix or an encapsulated abscess due to perforated appendicitis can present as a focal cecal mass on imaging. Key findings include nonenhancing fluid (pus), fat stranding from inflammation, and an obstructing appendicolith. Careful visual and clinical analysis for rupture is important as emergent surgery is typically avoided after rupture in favor of percutaneous management. Focal calcification usually represents an appendicolith, which can occasionally be seen in the dependent portion of an abscess after perforation.
- **Cecal/appendiceal carcinoma**. Imaging findings in cecal adenocarcinoma depend upon the extent of invasion. As the cecum usually allows for significant tumor growth before development of symptoms (e.g., obstruction), neoplasms in this region are typically large at the time of presentation with transmural invasion, pericolonic adenopathy, and occasionally distant metastases. Pericolonic fat stranding is uncommon, as is desmoplastic reaction, which is a finding that is more commonly seen with carcinoid tumor.
- **Mucocele of the appendix**. Mucocele of the appendix is a descriptive term for an appendix which is distended by mucus. Appendiceal dilatation > 15 mm increases suspicion for a mucocele. Causes include mucinous cystadenoma or cystadenocarcinoma, mucosal hyperplasia, and mucous retention cyst. A mucocele can also occur secondary to occlusion of the appendiceal lumen by an intrinsic or extrinsic benign or malignant mass. Computed tomography (CT) imaging findings include a typically well-encapsulated cystic mass occasionally with mural calcification. Ultrasound shows a simple-to-minimally complex cyst in the region of the appendix. Most appendix mucoceles are asymptomatic, but rupture can lead to pseudomyxoma peritonei.

■ **Additional Differential Diagnoses**

- **Lymphoma**. Although colonic lymphoma is relatively rare, the most common site of involvement is the cecum. The cecum can also be secondarily involved from direct spread of lymphoma from the terminal ileum, which is a common site of lymphomatous involvement. Imaging findings mimic those of cecal adenocarcinoma. Non-Hodgkin lymphoma predominates in adults; Burkitt lymphoma is a subtype more commonly seen in children and young adults.
- **Adnexal mass**. RLQ pain or mass effect in females is commonly due to ovarian or adnexal pathology. These processes may involve or abut the cecum, mimicking a cecal-origin mass. Common etiologies include simple or complex ovarian cysts, endometriosis, tubo-ovarian abscesses, and benign or malignant ovarian neoplasms.

■ **Diagnosis**

Mucocele of the appendix

✓ **Pearls**

- Periappendiceal inflammation or abscess can present as a focal cecal mass.
- Cecal carcinomas are typically large at presentation because of delayed onset of obstructive symptoms.
- Rupture of a mucocele of the appendix leads to pseudomyxoma peritonei.

Suggested Readings

Beydoun T, Kreuer S. Cystic right lower quadrant mass. J Am Osteopath Coll Radiol. 2012; 1(4):32–34

Federle MP, Jeffrey RB, Woodward PJ, Borhani A. Diagnostic Imaging: Abdomen. 2nd ed. Philadelphia, PA: Lippincott Williams & Wilkins; 2009

Kim SH, Lim HK, Lee WJ, Lim JH, Byun JY. Mucocele of the appendix: ultrasonographic and CT findings. Abdom Imaging. 1998; 23(3):292–296

Case 46

Robert A. Jesinger

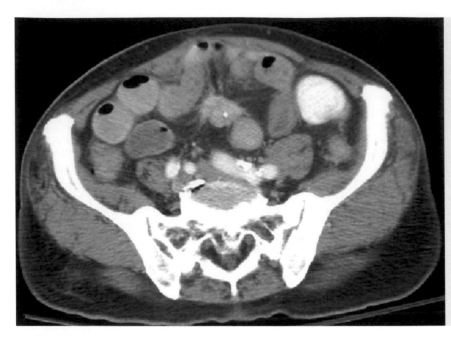

Fig. 46.1 Contrast-enhanced axial computed tomography (CT) image through the lower abdomen demonstrates an ill-defined, solid enhancing mass in the small bowel mesentery with a small calcification. There is retraction of mesenteric vessels toward the mass suggestive of a desmoplastic reaction.

■ Clinical Presentation

A 38-year-old man with chronic abdominal pain (▶Fig. 46.1).

■ Key Imaging Finding

Mesenteric mass

■ Top 3 Differential Diagnoses

- **Metastatic disease**. Metastatic disease to the bowel mesentery can occur via direct spread (pancreatic and colon carcinoma), hematogenous dissemination (breast and lung carcinoma), lymphatic spread (lymphoma), or peritoneal seeding (gastric and ovarian carcinoma). Enhanced computed tomography (CT) is the modality of choice for assessing number of lesions, margins (round vs. irregular), internal components (soft tissue, fluid, calcification, etc.), and enhancement characteristics, as well as identification of the primary source of neoplasm.
- **Carcinoid tumor**. Gastrointestinal carcinoid tumor is a slow-growing hypervascular lesion arising from neuroendocrine cells within the bowel. Mesenteric involvement incites a desmoplastic response, resulting in a spiculated mesenteric mass with intense reactive scarring. Calcifications are visible in up to 70% of cases. Mesenteric involvement is typically secondary with the primary neoplasm most commonly within the appendix or ileum. While the primary lesion is often occult, CT or magnetic resonance (MR) enterography and somatostatin receptor scintigraphy are the best modalities to localize the primary mass.
- **Desmoid tumor/fibrosing mesenteritis**. Mesenteric desmoid tumors consist of focal regions of masslike fibrosis. They are most commonly associated with familial adenomatous polyposis and cranial osteomas (Gardner syndrome). CT reveals a circumscribed or stellate soft-tissue mesenteric mass. Larger lesions may undergo central necrosis, and calcification may be seen posttreatment. A related entity referred to as fibrosing mesenteritis is similar to desmoid tumor both radiographically and pathologically; however, it occurs in the absence of familial adenomatous polyposis and is a diagnosis of exclusion.

■ Additional Differential Diagnoses

- **Reactive lymphadenopathy**. Reactive lymphadenopathy may present as a mesenteric mass and is typically due to an infectious process within the abdomen. Although virtually any abdominal infection may result in conglomerate lymphadenopathy, *Mycobacterium* (tuberculosis [TB] and *Mycobacterium avium-intracellulare* infection [MAI]) and *Tropheryma whipplei* (Whipple disease) are particularly prone to lymph node enlargement. In particular, these infectious agents result in characteristic lymphadenopathy with central low attenuation.
- **Abdominal mesothelioma**. Abdominal mesothelioma arises from the serosal lining of the peritoneal cavity and is associated with a history of asbestos exposure. Classic CT findings include ascites and serosal soft-tissue masses, mimicking peritoneal carcinomatosis. Correlation with chest imaging for pleural thickening and calcification is helpful in establishing the diagnosis, although peritoneal involvement may occur in the absence of pleural disease.

■ Diagnosis

Carcinoid tumor

✓ Pearls

- Masses in the bowel mesentery should prompt a careful search for a primary tumor or polyp syndrome.
- Carcinoid tumor incites a desmoplastic reaction and commonly calcifies.
- Mesenteric adenopathy with central low attenuation is concerning for TB, MAI, and Whipple disease.
- Reactive adenopathy can be related to routine gastroenteritis, but lymphoma should always be considered.

Suggested Readings

Lattin GE, Jr, O'Brien WT, Duncan MD, Peckham S. Sclerosing mesenteritis. Appl Radiol. 2007; 36(5):40–41

Levy AD, Rimola J, Mehrotra AK, Sobin LH. From the archives of the AFIP: benign fibrous tumors and tumorlike lesions of the mesentery: radiologic-pathologic correlation. Radiographics. 2006; 26(1):245–264

Sheth S, Horton KM, Garland MR, Fishman EK. Mesenteric neoplasms: CT appearances of primary and secondary tumors and differential diagnosis. Radiographics. 2003; 23(2):457–473, quiz 535–536

Case 47

Paul B. DiDomenico

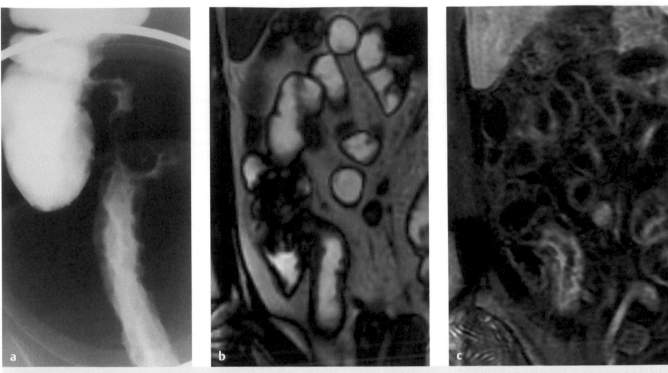

Fig. 47.1 Two patients with the same diagnosis. **(a)** Spot compression view of the right lower quadrant from a small bowel follow-through study in Patient A demonstrates irregularity and thickening of the terminal ileum with stricture formation. **(b)** Coned-down coronal high-resolution T2 MR image (FIESTA) in Patient B shows bowel wall thickening involving the terminal ileum with luminal narrowing. **(c)** Coned-down coronal postcontrast T1 image with fat suppression in Patient B shows abnormal bowel wall thickening and enhancement of the terminal ileum.

■ **Clinical Presentation**

Diarrhea and abdominal pain (▶Fig. 47.1).

■ Key Imaging Finding

Terminal ileal wall thickening

■ Top 3 Differential Diagnoses

• **Inflammatory bowel disease**. Of the two main types of idiopathic inflammatory bowel disease (ulcerative colitis and Crohn disease), Crohn disease characteristically involves the terminal ileum, causing transmural inflammation, thickening, and deep fissuring ulcers. Proliferation of mesenteric fat ("creeping fat") may cause the bowel loops to appear separated on a small bowel follow-through study. Fistulas and sinus tracts are a hallmark of the disease secondary to transmural involvement, and skip (discontinuous) lesions are characteristic. These findings are in contrast to those of ulcerative colitis, which is characterized by continuous involvement of the colon beginning distally and progressing proximally. Ulcerative colitis may cause dilatation of the distal ileum, termed "backwash" ileitis, in approximately 25% of cases.

• **Infection**. Certain infections have a predilection for the terminal ileum, among them *Salmonella*, *Campylobacter*, *Yersinia*, and *Mycobacterium tuberculosis*. Immunosuppressed patients (HIV/AIDS) are also at increased risk for opportunistic infection from *Cryptosporidium* and *Cytomegalovirus* (CMV). Imaging features of these infections are generally nonspecific, and the diagnosis is usually made through stool analysis, mucosal biopsy, and/or response to empiric antimicrobial therapy.

• **Lymphoma**. Non-Hodgkin lymphoma affects the small bowel in approximately one-third of cases, with the ileum being the most common site of involvement. Imaging appearance is variable; however, lymphoma typically manifests as nodular/polypoid or diffuse infiltrative small bowel wall thickening. When the terminal ileum is involved, the bowel wall may be thickened with a narrow lumen, resembling Crohn disease.

■ Additional Differential Diagnoses

• **Ischemia**. Ischemia of the superior mesenteric artery territory can result in bowel wall thickening because of edema and occasionally hemorrhage. There may be gas in the bowel wall (pneumatosis), which may also be seen in the mesenteric and portal venous system on CT imaging. Intravenous contrast material may aid in visualization of the site of occlusion because of clot or atherosclerotic disease.

• **Metastatic disease**. Metastatic spread of carcinoma can involve the terminal ileum through direct spread or peritoneal spread (gastrointestinal or genitourinary primary neoplasms) and hematogenous dissemination (malignant melanoma, lung or breast carcinoma). Metastatic spread to the small bowel is less common than primary small bowel lymphoma.

■ Diagnosis

Crohn disease

✓ Pearls

• Crohn disease classically involves the distal ileum, with chronic inflammation leading to strictures/fistulae.
• CMV or *Cryptosporidium* involvement of the terminal ileum should prompt an evaluation for HIV.

• Nodular ileal wall thickening is concerning for malignancy, including lymphoma and metastatic disease.

Suggested Readings

Furukawa A, Saotome T, Yamasaki M, et al. Cross-sectional imaging in Crohn disease. Radiographics. 2004; 24(3):689–702

Thoeni RF, Cello JP. CT imaging of colitis. Radiology. 2006; 240(3):623–638

Case 48

Robert A. Jesinger

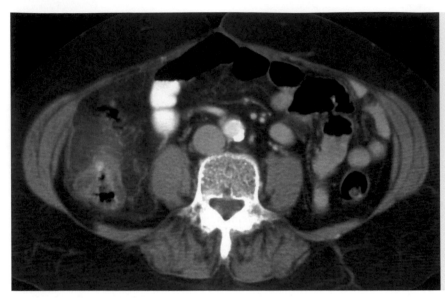

Fig. 48.1 Contrast-enhanced axial computed tomography (CT) image through the abdomen demonstrates eccentric, circumferential wall thickening of the right colon with pericolonic fat stranding.

■ Clinical Presentation

A 52-year-old woman with abdominal pain (▶Fig. 48.1).

■ Key Imaging Finding

Colonic wall thickening

■ Top 3 Differential Diagnoses

• **Infectious colitis**. Infectious colitis is the most common cause of focal bowel wall thickening and is frequently the sequela of diverticulitis. Most cases are caused by gram-negative bacteria. Immunosuppressed patients are not only susceptible to typical infectious causes of colitis, but also prone to severe atypical infections, especially in the setting of neutropenia (neutropenic colitis). Antibiotic therapy may occasionally alter the normal bacterial flora of the colon, allowing for overgrowth of *Clostridium difficile*, which is the causative organism of pseudomembranous colitis. Classic imaging findings of infectious colitis include colonic air–fluid levels, wall thickening, and increased mucosal enhancement.

• **Inflammatory bowel disease**. Crohn disease and ulcerative colitis (UC) are idiopathic conditions leading to transmural (Crohn) or mucosal (UC) bowel wall inflammation. UC begins in the rectum and progresses proximally without skip lesions; Crohn disease, on the other hand, may involve any portion of the gastrointestinal tract from the esophagus to the anus (most commonly the terminal ileum) and routinely demonstrates skip lesions. Early imaging findings reveal mucosal inflammation ("granular" mucosal appearance, edematous haustra). Diffuse bowel wall thickening is typically a later finding. Strictures and fistulas are seen in Crohn disease secondary to transmural involvement, while chronic UC often leads to fixed colonic dilatation ("lead pipe" appearance). Both entities may involve the terminal ileum—Crohn disease results in strictures, while UC results in dilatation because of backwash ileitis. Patients with UC have an increased risk (up to 10%) of colon cancer.

• **Colon carcinoma**. Colon carcinoma may present as focal short segment bowel wall thickening and pericolonic fatty infiltration, mimicking colitis. Secondary findings that suggest underlying malignancy include regional lymphadenopathy and distant metastases, most commonly within the liver. Appropriate cancer screening (e.g., colonoscopy) should be confirmed.

■ Additional Differential Diagnoses

• **Ischemic colitis**. Ischemic bowel disease is commonly the result of atherosclerotic or embolic disease, but may also occur in the setting of hypoperfusion. Watershed areas (splenic flexure) are the most susceptible regions to decreased blood flow. Enhanced computed tomography (CT) is ideal for assessment of bowel wall enhancement and mesenteric artery patency. Complications include bowel necrosis, which may lead to pneumatosis and portal venous gas.

■ Diagnosis

Infectious colitis

✓ Pearls

• Infection, ischemia, and inflammatory conditions are common causes for colonic wall thickening.
• Ischemic bowel necrosis may lead to pneumatosis, portal venous gas, and sepsis.

• Colonoscopy and biopsy is often used to help exclude malignancy in the setting of bowel wall thickening.

Suggested Readings

Boyd SK, Cameron-Morrison JD, Hobson JJ, et al. CT Imaging of large bowel wall thickening. J Am Osteopath Coll Radiol. 2016; 5(2):14–22

Thoeni RF, Cello JP. CT imaging of colitis. Radiology. 2006; 240(3):623–638

Case 49

Eleanor L. Ormsby

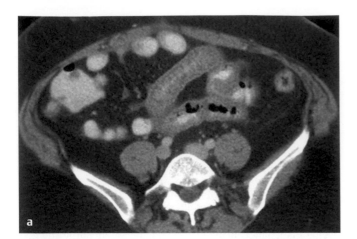
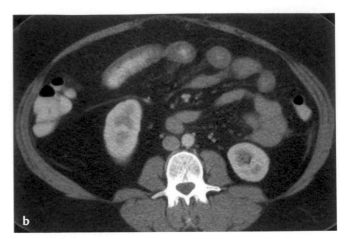
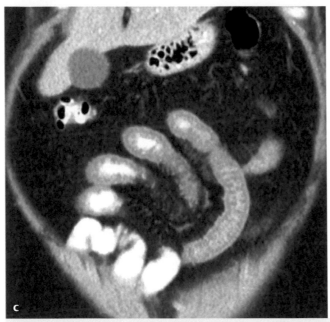

Fig. 49.1 (a, b) Axial and **(c)** coronal reformatted contrast-enhanced (oral and intravenous) CT images show several small bowel loops with marked wall thickening and enhancement along the mucosal and serosal surfaces with relative decreased central bowel wall attenuation.

■ **Clinical Presentation**

Abdominal pain (▶Fig. 49.1).

■ Key Imaging Finding

Small bowel wall thickening

■ Top 3 Differential Diagnoses

- **Crohn disease**. Crohn disease presents with irregularly thickened folds associated with mucosal ulceration (early) and strictures (late). The findings are usually seen in the terminal ileum. The "string sign" has been used to describe marked segmental narrowing of bowel loops. In contrast to ulcerative colitis, lesions in Crohn disease can be scattered in the small bowel ("skip lesions"), with normal bowel interposed between involved segments. On computed tomography (CT), bowel wall thickening and mesenteric stranding are the most common findings. The fibrofatty proliferation seen in the mesentery is referred to as "creeping fat."
- **Lymphoma**. Small bowel lymphoma can occur with or without predisposing factors, such as immunodeficiency syndromes, celiac sprue, or Crohn disease. There are different types of imaging findings, including nodular bowel wall thickening, bowel wall infiltration with loss of bowel markings, and intraluminal polypoid masses. There may be associated luminal narrowing or characteristic aneurysmal dilatation, which is more common with diffuse infiltration.
- **Bowel wall edema**. Bowel wall edema may result from a variety of etiologies, including ischemia, vasculopathy, hypoproteinemia, and angioedema. Ischemia may be due to decreased arterial flow or venous congestion or associated with inflammatory processes as is seen with radiation enteritis. Hypoproteinemia results from liver or kidney disease with hypoalbuminemia. Angioedema may be inherited, acquired, or drug-induced due to angiotensin-converting enzyme inhibitor (ACEI) or nonsteroidal anti-inflammatory drug therapy. Imaging studies demonstrate bowel wall and fold thickening most often involving the small bowel. Mural stratification may be seen with enhancing mucosal and serosal layers with interposed edematous bowel wall.

■ Additional Differential Diagnoses

- **Small bowel hemorrhage**. Small bowel is the most common site of intramural hemorrhage and may be due to trauma, mesenteric ischemia, vasculitis, coagulopathy, anticoagulant medication, or Henoch–Schönlein purpura. Short segment, uniformly thickened small bowel folds with "stack-of-coins" appearance are the typical finding. Appropriate clinical history helps differentiate the underlying cause.
- **Metastases**. Metastases to the small bowel commonly present as multiple masses with nodular bowel wall thickening, which may result in fold tethering or ulceration. Metastases can be from intraperitoneal seeding, hematogenous spread, lymphatic spread, or direct extension from a contiguous neoplasm.
- **Whipple disease**. Whipple disease is a rare, chronic, systemic disease caused by a bacterial infection (gram-positive bacilli with PAS stain). Patients present with chronic diarrhea, arthralgias, and malabsorption. Thickened proximal small bowel folds with micronodularity (1–2 mm) and low-density mesenteric lymphadenopathy are characteristic findings.

■ Diagnosis

Bowel wall edema (angioedema secondary to ACEI)

✓ Pearls

- Mucosal ulceration, mesenteric fibrofatty proliferation, and strictures are key findings in Crohn disease.
- In the setting of trauma, small bowel fold or wall thickening is concerning for hemorrhage.
- Bowel wall edema may be seen with ischemia, vasculopathy, hypoproteinemia, or angioedema.

Suggested Readings

Ishigami K, Averill SL, Pollard JH, McDonald JM, Sato Y. Radiologic manifestations of angioedema. Insights Imaging. 2014; 5(3):365–374

Macari M, Balthazar EJ. CT of bowel wall thickening: significance and pitfalls of interpretation. AJR Am J Roentgenol. 2001; 176(5):1105–1116

Case 50

Shaun Loh

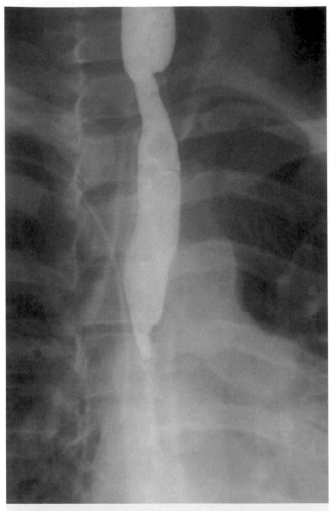

Fig. 50.1 Single contrast frontal esophagram image demonstrates a long segment of abrupt narrowing involving the mid esophagus, which persisted on further imaging.

■ Clinical Presentation

A 40-year-old man with dysphagia (▶ Fig. 50.1).

■ Key Imaging Finding

Esophageal stricture

■ Top 3 Differential Diagnoses for Short-Segment Strictures

- **Reflux esophagitis.** Reflux esophagitis is one of the most common causes of esophageal strictures. The stricture typically appears as an area of smooth, tapered narrowing in the distal esophagus. Asymmetric scarring can occur, resulting in a more eccentric stricture. Sacculations may be present between multiple strictures.
- **Drug-induced stricture.** The two most common agents implicated in drug-induced esophagitis, tetracycline and doxycycline, typically cause superficial ulceration that heals without stricture formation. Other drugs such as quinidine, potassium chloride, alendronate, and nonsteroidal anti-inflammatory drugs (NSAIDs) may cause larger ulcerations and strictures in the proximal to midesophagus. Tablet medications may lodge in the esophagus because of extrinsic compression from

adjacent structures such as the aortic arch or left mainstem bronchus.
- **Esophageal carcinoma.** Squamous cell carcinoma accounts for approximately 80% of all cases of esophageal cancer. Risk factors include smoking, alcohol, caustic ingestions, achalasia, and Plummer–Vinson syndrome. Adenocarcinoma from Barrett's esophagitis comprises the majority of the remaining cases. The most common finding is a fixed narrowing of the esophageal lumen. The tumor may also appear as an annular constricting lesion causing a long-segment stricture with prominent shoulders. Another pattern is that of a polypoid intraluminal filling defect. Prognosis is poor, with a 5-year survival rate of 5%.

■ Top 3 Differential Diagnoses for Long-Segment Strictures

- **Iatrogenic (nasogastric tube [NGT]).** NGTs prevent the lower esophageal sphincter from closing, allowing the acidic gastric contents to bathe the lumen of the distal esophagus. Mucosal injury and stricture formation can ensue. Strictures are most commonly seen with prolonged NGT placement.
- **Caustic ingestion.** Ingestion of strong acids or more commonly bases causes long, symmetric esophageal strictures, usually months to years after the initial injury. The stricture may

appear "threadlike" with a diffuse long segmental narrowing, irregular contours, and ulcerations. Treatment entails either esophageal dilation or esophagectomy. There is an increased risk of malignancy after the initial injury.
- **Radiation changes.** Radiation changes occur within the radiotherapy field during the treatment of thoracic and cervical neoplasms. The strictures are often long, smooth, concentric, and tapered.

■ Diagnosis

Caustic ingestion (lye)

✓ Pearls

- Strictures from reflux esophagitis commonly are seen as smooth areas of narrowing in the esophagus.
- Tablet medications may lodge in the esophagus and incite ulceration and stricture formation.

- Irregular areas of esophageal stricturing are concerning for esophageal carcinoma.
- Prolonged NGT placement can result in mucosal injury to the esophagus and stricture formation.

Suggested Readings

Luedtke P, Levine MS, Rubesin SE, Weinstein DS, Laufer I. Radiologic diagnosis of benign esophageal strictures: a pattern approach. Radiographics. 2003; 23(4):897–909

Case 51

Robert A. Jesinger

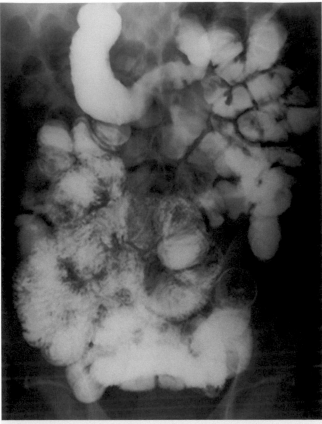

Fig. 51.1 Single-contrast small bowel follow-through image demonstrates dilatation of small bowel loops with reversal of the jejunal and ileal fold pattern.

■ Clinical Presentation

A 29-year-old man with weight loss and chronic abdominal pain (▶Fig. 51.1).

■ Key Imaging Finding

Small bowel dilatation

■ Top 3 Differential Diagnoses

• **Small bowel obstruction**. Small bowel dilatation (>3 cm diameter), air–fluid levels, and prominent thinned folds are key findings in mechanical small bowel obstruction. Common causes include focal adhesions, hernia, intussusception, volvulus, and obstructing mass (lymphoma). Abdominal radiographs and enhanced computed tomography (CT) are standard in the initial evaluation and help guide the need for surgical intervention. Obstruction may be complete or partial. In complete obstruction, a transition point may be found with decompression of bowel loops beyond the level of obstruction. Closed loop obstructions are considered a surgical emergency because of the increased risk of ischemic necrosis and subsequent perforation. Clinically, patients present with nausea and vomiting and demonstrate high-pitched bowel sounds on auscultation.

• **Adynamic ileus**. Adynamic ileus results in bowel dilatation secondary to a lack of peristalsis. In comparison to mechanical obstruction, ileus usually results in fluid-filled loops of small and large bowel without a transition point or decompression of distal bowel loops. Common causes of ileus include medica-

tions (analgesics, anticholinergics, etc.), neurological insult, or inflammatory or infectious processes. Focal ileus may be seen adjacent to sites of inflammation, such as in the setting of pancreatitis or appendicitis. Clinically, bowel sounds are decreased or absent because of lack of peristalsis.

• **Celiac sprue**. Celiac sprue is an autoimmune disorder caused by a hypersensitivity to wheat gluten, resulting in damage to the mucosal lining of the small intestine. Clinical symptoms are related to malabsorption and hypersecretion of fluid. Fluoroscopic findings include small bowel dilatation, reversal of the jejunal and ileal fold patterns ("ilealization of the jejunum" and "jejunization of the ileum"), and dilution of barium due to hypersecretion. Transient intussusceptions are commonly seen, which may further increase small bowel dilatation. Patients with celiac sprue are at increased risk for the development of malignancies, including lymphoma and adenocarcinoma. Diagnosis is confirmed with duodenal biopsy, along with various serological studies. Approximately 70% of patients have symptomatic improvement within 2 weeks of starting a gluten-free diet.

■ Additional Differential Diagnoses

• **Scleroderma**. Scleroderma is a chronic disease thought to represent a type of autoimmune dysfunction which results in excessive deposition of collagen in various organ systems. The deposition of collagen within the small bowel results in diffu-

se scarring. Radiographic manifestations include small bowel dilatation with crowding of folds ("hidebound" bowel), as well as antimesenteric small bowel pseudosacculations.

■ Diagnosis

Celiac sprue

✓ Pearls

• When a transition point is seen, diagnosis is mechanical bowel obstruction.
• Bowel dilation from mural scarring can be seen in scleroderma and celiac sprue.

• Patients with celiac sprue often have reversal of fold patterns and are at increased risk for malignancy.

Suggested Readings

Furukawa A, Yamasaki M, Furuichi K, et al. Helical CT in the diagnosis of small bowel obstruction. Radiographics. 2001; 21(2):341–355

Scholz FJ, Afnan J, Behr SC. CT findings in adult celiac disease. Radiographics. 2011; 31(4):977–992

Case 52

William T. O'Brien, Sr.

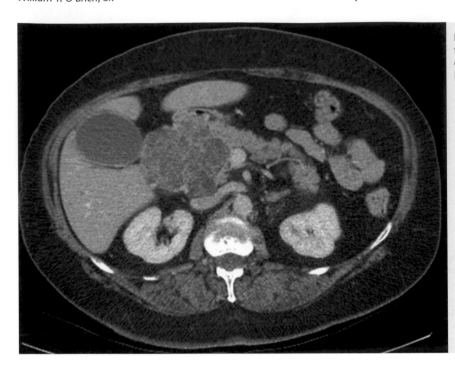

Fig. 52.1 Contrast-enhanced axial computed tomography (CT) image through the upper abdomen demonstrates a multiloculated cystic lesion with thin internal septations within the head of the pancreas.

▪ Clinical Presentation

A 42-year-old woman with early satiety and abdominal discomfort with meals (▶Fig. 52.1).

■ Key Imaging Finding

Cystic pancreatic lesion

■ Top 3 Differential Diagnoses

- **Pancreatic pseudocyst**. Pancreatic pseudocysts are the most common cystic pancreatic lesions, accounting for approximately 90% of all cases, and are a complication of pancreatitis. Although they may be found throughout the abdomen, they occur most frequently within the pancreatic parenchyma. Pseudocysts are contained within a fibrous capsule, and they may be unilocular or multilocular. The cystic components have a high amylase content. Some of these lesions may communicate with the pancreatic duct. Pseudocysts should be suspected in a patient with a history or secondary imaging findings of prior pancreatitis.
- **Mucinous cystadenoma**. Mucinous cystadenomas have malignant potential and are commonly found in middle-aged women. They contain large (>2 cm) mucin-containing cysts and are most commonly seen in the tail of the pancreas. Peripheral calcifications may be seen in approximately 20% of cases. On magnetic resonance imaging (MRI), the lesions are hyperintense on T2-weighted sequences and have a variable appearance on T1 depending on the amount of mucin. The more mucin, the brighter the signal intensity on T1-weighted sequences. These lesions cannot be differentiated from a malignant mucinous cystadenocarcinoma on imaging; therefore, these lesions are usually resected.
- **Serous cystadenoma**. Serous cystadenomas are benign pancreatic neoplasms that usually occur in middle-aged to elderly women. These are most commonly located in the pancreatic head. The lesions consist of numerous small cysts (<2 cm) with thin intervening septations (honeycomb appearance). Central calcifications are seen in up to a half of cases. There is a very small risk of malignancy (<5%); the vast majority of these lesions can be safely followed with imaging. There is an association with von Hippel–Lindau syndrome.

■ Additional Differential Diagnoses

- **Intraductal papillary mucinous neoplasm (IPMN)**. Unlike mucinous and serous cystadenomas, IPMNs communicate with the pancreatic duct. They occur equally in males and females and typically present in the sixth decade. They may affect the main duct with segmental or diffuse ductal dilatation, or they can affect side branches and mimic mucinous or serous cystadenomas. On endoscopy, mucous can be seen emanating from the ampulla. The lesions will fill with contrast on endoscopic retrograde cholangiopancreatography (ERCP).
- **Solid and papillary epithelial neoplasm (SPEN)**. SPEN, more recently referred to as solid pseudopapillary tumor (SPT) of the pancreas, is an uncommon malignant pancreatic neoplasm that characteristically occurs in young women (often in the third decade). They are composed of cystic and solid components and predominantly occur in the pancreatic tail. Cystic components may be complex because of hemorrhage. The malignant nature of these lesions necessitates surgical resection.

■ Diagnosis

Serous cystadenoma

✓ Pearls

- Pancreatic pseudocysts secondary to pancreatitis account for the majority of cystic pancreatic lesions.
- Mucinous cystadenomas have large cysts most commonly in the pancreatic tail.
- Serous cystadenomas have multiple small cysts most commonly in the head of the pancreas.
- IPMNs communicate with the pancreatic duct.

Suggested Readings

Saenz R. Pancreatic mass. J Am Osteopath Coll Radiol. 2012; 1(4):38–40

Theoni R. Pancreatic neoplasms. J Am Osteopath Coll Radiol. 2012; 1(4):10–22

Case 53

Rocky Saenz

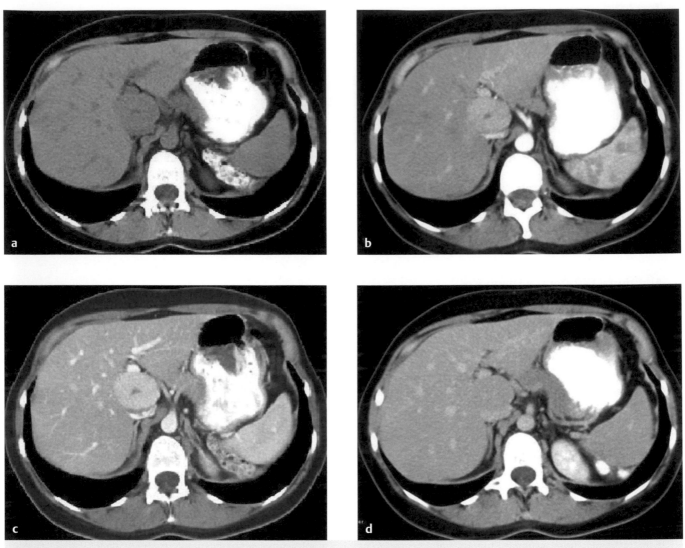

Fig. 53.1 (a) Unenhanced axial CT image demonstrates an isodense mass within the caudate lobe with a central region of low density. (b) The mass demonstrates homogeneous increased enhancement on arterial phase imaging with a central hypodense scar. (c) On venous phase imaging, the mass is isodense to surrounding hepatic parenchyma with maintenance of the central hypodense scar. (d) On delayed imaging, the central scar fills in on with the entire lesion now isodense to surrounding hepatic parenchyma.

■ Clinical Presentation

A 34-year-old woman with vague abdominal discomfort
(►Fig. 53.1).

■ Key Imaging Finding

Liver mass with central scar

■ Top 3 Differential Diagnoses

- **Hemangioma.** Hemangiomas are the most common benign hepatic lesion. The classic imaging findings are initial discontinuous peripheral nodular enhancement in the arterial phase with delayed central filling. Smaller hemangiomas may demonstrate flash-filling during the arterial phase, while larger lesions may have central regions of fibrosis or cystic changes. On magnetic resonance imaging (MRI), hemangiomas are hyperintense on T2-weighted and hypointense on T1-weighted imaging with similar enhancement patterns as seen with computed tomography (CT). On ultrasound, most hemangiomas are well-circumscribed hyperechoic lesions.
- **Focal nodular hyperplasia (FNH).** FNH is an uncommon hepatic lesion that typically presents in young females (75%). The lesion is composed of hepatocytes and classically contains a central low-density scar. On arterial phase imaging, there is homogeneous enhancement of the lesion with a low-density central scar, which fills in on delayed imaging. The central scar is hyperintense on T2-weighted MRI. Since FNH is composed of hepatocytes, it may demonstrate uptake of sulfur colloid (other hepatic lesions demonstrate cold defects) on scintigraphy, although this exam has been somewhat supplanted by MRI. Hepatocyte-specific MR contrast agents with delayed imaging are >95% specific in distinguishing FNH from other hepatic lesions.
- **Hepatocellular carcinoma (HCC).** HCC is the most common primary hepatic malignancy with an increased incidence in patients with chronic liver disease. Patients may present with a single lesion, multiple lesions, or diffuse hepatic involvement. The lesions are typically hypodense and demonstrate increased arterial phase enhancement because of blood supply from the hepatic artery. Portal or hepatic vein invasion is common. Diagnosis can be difficult in cirrhosis with regenerating nodules. MRI can be helpful in these instances since HCC typically displays increased T2 signal intensity. Clinically, HCC is associated with elevated alpha-fetoprotein. **Fibrolamellar HCC** is a rare variant that also occurs in younger patients. The lesion demonstrates peripheral arterial phase enhancement with a central low-density scar that does not fill in on delayed imaging (in contrast to FNH). The central scar in fibrolamellar HCC is hypointense on T2-weighted imaging, while the central scar in FNH is hyperintense on T2-weighted imaging.

■ Additional Differential Diagnoses

- **Hepatic adenoma.** Hepatic adenomas are benign lesions predominantly seen in women (90%). Most often, they are solitary but may occasionally be multiple, especially in patients with glycogen storage disease. Hepatic adenomas have an increased frequency and risk of rupture with the use of oral contraceptives. Adenomas are typically hypervascular; internal hemorrhage can lead to heterogeneity.
- **Hypervascular metastases.** Hypervascular metastases are usually multiple but may occasionally present as a solitary mass. Tumors that classically result in hypervascular metastases include melanoma, renal cell carcinoma, choriocarcinoma, thyroid, carcinoid, pancreatic islet cell tumors, and sarcomas.

■ Diagnosis

Focal nodular hyperplasia

✓ Pearls

- Hemangiomas demonstrate peripheral, nodular, enhancement on arterial phase imaging.
- A hypervascular hepatic lesion within a cirrhotic liver is HCC until proven otherwise.
- Hepatic adenomas are associated with oral contraceptives and are prone to hemorrhage.

Suggested Readings

Kamel IR, Lawler LP, Fishman EK. Comprehensive analysis of hypervascular liver lesions using 16-MDCT and advanced image processing. AJR Am J Roentgenol. 2004; 183(2):443–452

Saenz RC. MRI of benign liver lesions and metastatic disease characterization with gadoxetate disodium. J Am Osteopath Coll Radiol. 2012; 1(4):2–9

Case 54

Brian J. Lewis

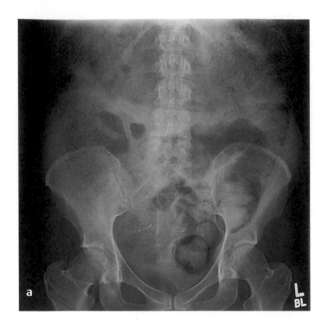

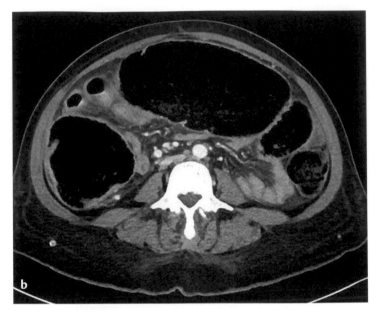

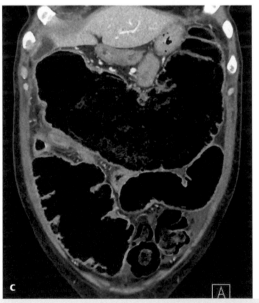

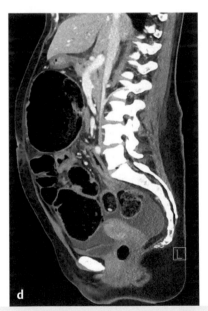

Fig. 54.1 **(a)** Frontal radiograph of the abdomen demonstrates marked colonic distention, most prominent within the transverse colon, with formed stool throughout. **(b)** Axial, **(c)** coronal, and **(d)** sagittal contrast-enhanced CT images of the abdomen and pelvis reveal marked colonic distention with mucosal irregularity and wall thinning, adjacent fat stranding and thickened bowel loops, and free fluid within the pelvis **(d)**. Incidental tubal ligation postprocedural changes are visualized within the pelvis **(a)**.

■ Clinical Presentation

A 50-year-old woman with abdominal pain and distension (►Fig. 54.1).

■ Key Imaging Finding

Large bowel dilatation

■ Top 3 Differential Diagnoses

- **Large bowel obstruction (LBO).** Colon cancer is the most common cause of LBO, accounting for over half of cases. The sigmoid colon and splenic flexure are the most common tumor locations that result in obstruction. Masses large enough to cause luminal obstruction may demonstrate shouldering and central necrosis with infiltration of pericolonic fat, which can mimic diverticulitis with abscess. Pericolonic lymph nodes measuring ≥1 cm in short axis are suspicious for metastases. Recurrent bouts of diverticulitis with stricture formation are less common cause of colonic obstruction. Adhesions, which are a common cause of small bowel obstruction, are an additional infrequent cause of LBO. Regardless of the underlying etiology, perforation is an uncommon but emergent complication, typically occurring in the setting of a severely dilated cecum.
- **Volvulus.** Volvulus refers to the twisting of bowel with resultant obstruction and dilatation of the affected large bowel. Sigmoid volvulus is most common in elderly patients with a redundant and mobile colon, while cecal and transverse colon volvuli are more likely to occur secondary to a congenital defect in the mesentery resulting in increased mobility. The "coffee bean" sign is seen in both cecal and sigmoid volvuli radiographically and refers to an apposed loop of dilated bowel likened to the appearance of a coffee bean. The "bird's beak" sign results from smooth tapering of bowel at the point of obstruction, reminiscent of a bird's beak. Specific to sigmoid volvulus, the "inverted U" sign refers to a dilated loop of sigmoid colon pointing to the right upper quadrant. Computed tomography (CT) often demonstrates the whirl sign with spiraling of collapsed bowel and vessels at the point of obstruction.
- **Colonic pseudo-obstruction (Ogilvie's syndrome).** Colonic pseudo-obstruction refers to large bowel dilatation without a mechanical cause or abrupt transition. It most often affects older patients who are fairly ill with a wide range of underlying medical conditions. While the exact etiology remains uncertain, it is thought to result from decreased parasympathetic activity. Gradual transition near the splenic flexure may be seen. Cecal ischemia and perforation are the most feared complications.

■ Additional Differential Diagnoses

- **Toxic megacolon.** Toxic megacolon refers to severe and potentially life-threatening dilatation of the colon resulting from underlying colitis, most commonly pseudomembranous colitis or inflammatory bowel disease (IBD). CT demonstrates large bowel dilatation (transverse colon > 6 cm), mucosal irregularity, wall thickening with thumb-printing, or thinning with an ahaustral pattern. The risk of perforation increases significantly with greater than 12 cm of cecal dilatation. When suspected, barium enema should be avoided in the setting of toxic megacolon because of increased risk of perforation.

■ Diagnosis

Toxic megacolon (as a complication of IBD)

✓ Pearls

- Colon cancer is the most common cause of LBO.
- The coffee bean (cecal or sigmoid) or inverted U (sigmoid) signs are seen radiographically with volvuli.
- Ogilvie's syndrome affects older patients who are ill; gradual transition at the splenic flexure may be seen.
- Toxic megacolon results from an underlying colitis; when suspected, barium enema should be avoided.

Suggested Readings

Jaffe T, Thompson WM. Large-bowel obstruction in the adult: classic radiographic and CT findings, etiology, and mimics. Radiology. 2015; 275(3):651–663

Thoeni RF, Cello JP. CT imaging of colitis. Radiology. 2006; 240(3):623–638

Case 55

Shaun Loh

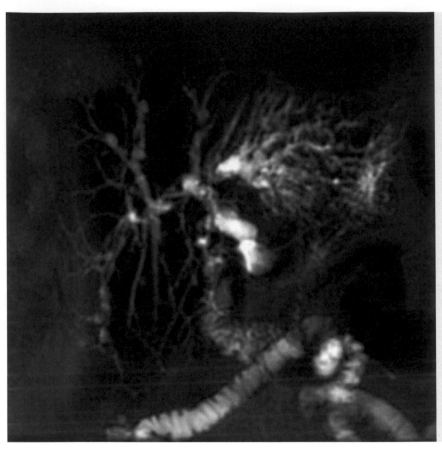

Fig. 55.1 Maximum intensity projection (MIP) image from a magnetic resonance cholangiopancreatography (MRCP) study demonstrates a "string-of-beads" appearance with an alternating pattern of dilated and strictured intrahepatic bile ducts.

■ Clinical Presentation

A 45-year-old woman with jaundice (▶Fig. 55.1).

■ Key Imaging Finding

Intrahepatic biliary ductal strictures

■ Top 3 Differential Diagnoses

- **Primary sclerosing cholangitis (PSC).** PSC is a chronic idiopathic inflammatory disease involving the bile ducts, which may progress to biliary ductal destruction, cholestasis, biliary cirrhosis, and cholangiocarcinoma. It is highly associated with ulcerative colitis. Classic findings include a "string-of-beads" appearance with an alternating pattern of dilation and stenosis of the intrahepatic (IHBD) and extrahepatic bile ducts (EHBD). Diverticular outpouchings of the biliary tree on cholangiography are pathognomonic. Hypertrophy of the caudate lobe occurs in more advanced cases of PSC. Periportal fibrosis may occur and appears on magnetic resonance imaging (MRI) as areas of decreased periportal signal on T1 with increased signal on T2-weighted imaging.
- **Ascending cholangitis.** Ascending cholangitis is a bacterial infection of an obstructed biliary system. Patients may present with Charcot's triad: pain, fever, and jaundice. Choledocholithiasis and strictures from prior surgery may result in biliary obstruction with biliary stasis and infection. The IHBD and EHBD are frequently dilated with high-density purulent bile and thickened walls. Left untreated, complications such as liver abscesses, sepsis, and even death may occur.
- **Acquired immunodeficiency syndrome cholangiopathy.** This cholangiopathy results from strictures caused by AIDS-related opportunistic infections, usually *Cytomegalovirus* (CMV) or *Cryptosporidium*. It is characterized by multiple intrahepatic biliary strictures, distal ampullary stenosis, or cholecystitis. The common bile duct is often involved with irregular areas of thickening and/or ulcerations. MRI reveals asymmetric IHBD and EHBD ductal dilatation with pericholecystic inflammatory changes. On magnetic resonance cholangiopancreatography (MRCP), an alternating pattern of high-signal biliary ductal dilatation and intrahepatic and extrahepatic biliary strictures may be present. Prognosis is poor as the cholangiopathy presents in late-stage AIDS.

■ Additional Differential Diagnoses

- **Neoplasm:** Neoplasms, such as **cholangiocarcinoma** and **metastases**, are another cause of intrahepatic biliary strictures. In cholangiocarcinoma, long strictures and prestenotic ductal dilatation with wall thickening may be the only findings. Malignant strictures may also result from pancreatic or ampullary carcinomas, as well as metastatic disease from colorectal cancer, lung cancer, breast cancer, and lymphoma.
- **Posttransplant arterial ischemia:** Intrahepatic biliary strictures may occur after liver transplantation and are thought to be secondary to hepatic artery occlusion and ischemia. The IHBD are dilated with additional narrowed segments. Doppler ultrasound may show signs of hepatic artery occlusion or stenosis (such as a tardus/parvus waveform).

■ Diagnosis

Primary sclerosing cholangitis

✓ Pearls

- PSC is characterized by a "string-of-beads" appearance of the IHBDs.
- Biliary strictures may be seen as either a cause or complication of ascending cholangitis.

- Care must be taken to assess for cholangiocarcinoma or metastases in the setting of a focal biliary stricture.
- Hepatic artery occlusion complicating liver transplantation leads to biliary necrosis with strictures.

Suggested Readings

Bilgin M, Balci NC, Erdogan A, Momtahen AJ, Alkaade S, Rau WS. Hepatobiliary and pancreatic MRI and MRCP findings in patients with HIV infection. AJR Am J Roentgenol. 2008; 191(1):228–232

Vitellas KM, Keogan MT, Freed KS, et al. Radiologic manifestations of sclerosing cholangitis with emphasis on MR cholangiopancreatography. Radiographics. 2000; 20(4):959–975, quiz 1108–1109, 1112

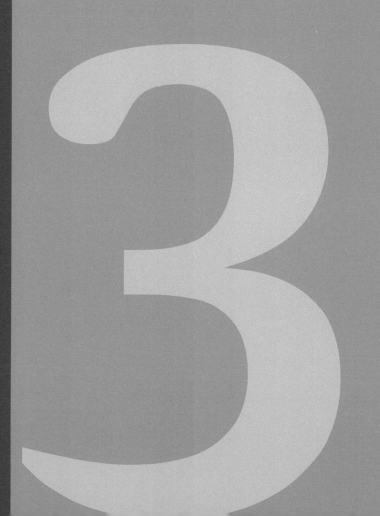

Part 3

Genitourinary Imaging

Case 56

Todd M. Johnson

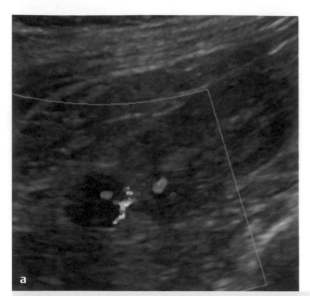 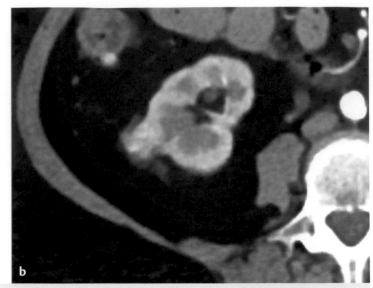

Fig. 56.1 **(a)** Longitudinal color Doppler ultrasound (US) image of the right kidney shows an exophytic hypoechoic upper pole solid mass with internal flow. **(b)** Contrast-enhanced axial computed tomography (CT) image shows a corresponding enhancing exophytic renal mass with surrounding fat stranding. *Images courtesy of Dell Dunn, MD.*

■ Clinical Presentation

A 58-year-old woman with renal insufficiency and hematuria
(▶ Fig. 56.1).

■ Key Imaging Finding

Solid renal mass

■ Top 3 Differential Diagnoses

- **Renal cell carcinoma (RCC)**. RCC is a hypervascular malignant renal neoplasm that arises from tubular epithelium. Although RCC usually presents as a solid, exophytic cortical tumor, it may be cystic. Cystic forms typically have multiple thick septations; enhancing nodules in a cystic lesion are highly suspicious for RCC (Bosniak IV). Smaller lesions are best visualized in the nephrographic phase. Infiltrative RCC can invade the renal pelvis, simulating transitional cell carcinoma (TCC). If complicated by necrosis or hemorrhage, central low density may mimic the central scar of oncocytoma.
- **Oncocytoma**. Oncocytoma is a benign renal tumor that accounts for only about 7% of renal neoplasms. It occurs in older patients (seventh decade) with a male predominance. On contrast-enhanced computed tomography (CT), typically a large (average 7 cm), circumscribed, solid enhancing lesion is present which can have a central scar. This central scar can mimic the central necrosis seen in RCC. On angiography, oncocytomas demonstrate a spoke wheel pattern of enhancement correlating to their arterial supply. Definitive differentiation from RCC can only be made by pathologic diagnosis.
- **Angiomyolipoma (AML)**. AML is a benign tumor of the kidney composed of variable amounts of vascular elements, smooth muscle, and adipose tissue. Gross fat and lack of calcifications in a renal lesion are virtually diagnostic of AML. Although there is no malignant potential, lesions composed predominately of vascular elements and smooth muscle can show enhancement and are indistinguishable from RCC by imaging (because of the nonvisualization of fat). Usually AML is sporadic and solitary; multiple AMLs are associated with tuberous sclerosis.

■ Additional Differential Diagnoses

- **Transitional cell carcinoma**. TCC is a uroepithelial neoplasm that usually arises from the bladder; a smaller portion (<10%) originates from the renal pelvis or calyces. TCC that infiltrates the kidney causes enlargement with preservation of shape. It is relatively hypovascular and ill-defined, demonstrating only mild enhancement.
- **Lymphoma**. Renal lymphoma most often presents as multiple bilateral hypodense renal masses; however, it can also present as a solitary hypodense mass which may simulate a cyst on ultrasound or present as diffuse infiltration of the renal parenchyma. The presence of associated lymphadenopathy is helpful in suggesting the diagnosis.

■ Diagnosis

Renal cell carcinoma

✓ Pearls

- RCCs are hypervascular tumors; smaller lesions are best visualized in the nephrographic phase.
- The central scar of oncocytoma may be indistinguishable from central necrosis in RCC.
- AMLs are benign lesions composed of macroscopic fat, vascular elements, and smooth muscle.
- AMLs with a paucity of fat can mimic RCC.

Suggested Readings

Silverman SG, Mortele KJ, Tuncali K, Jinzaki M, Cibas ES. Hyperattenuating renal masses: etiologies, pathogenesis, and imaging evaluation. Radiographics. 2007; 27(4):1131–1143

Zhang J, Lefkowitz RA, Ishill NM, et al. Solid renal cortical tumors: differentiation with CT. Radiology. 2007; 244(2):494–504

Case 57

James B. Odone

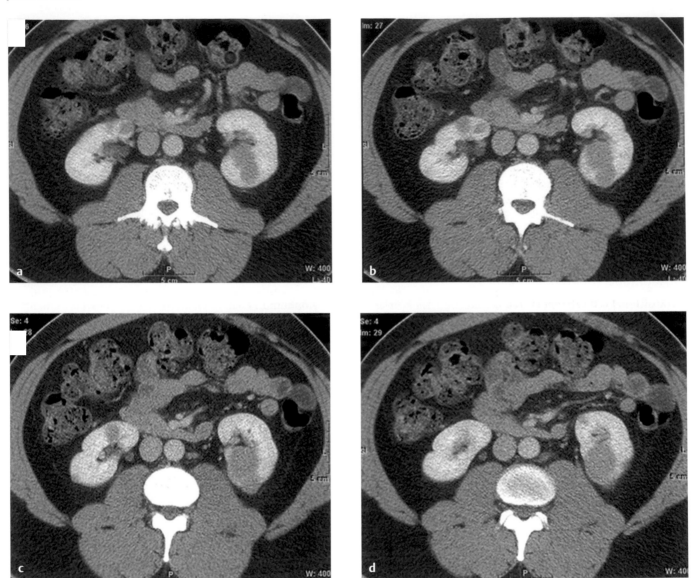

Fig. 57.1 (a-d) Sequential contrast-enhanced axial CT images through the kidneys demonstrate multiple hypodense solid renal masses.

■ **Clinical Presentation**

A 38-year-old man with weight loss and low-grade fever
(►Fig. 57.1).

■ Key Imaging Finding

Multiple bilateral renal lesions/masses

■ Top 3 Differential Diagnoses

- **Lymphoma**. Primary renal lymphoma is rare; however, secondary involvement is common in patients with a known history of lymphoma. The most common pattern of renal involvement is that of multiple bilateral homogeneous hypodense parenchymal masses. Accompanying perirenal lymphadenopathy is relatively common and may provide a diagnostic clue on initial imaging. Less common manifestations of renal lymphoma include a solitary renal mass or diffuse infiltration of the renal parenchyma, which leads to reniform enlargement.
- **Renal infection**. Pyelonephritis is a clinical diagnosis with imaging typically performed to evaluate for complications. Early pyelonephritis may present as a striated nephrogram or focal, triangular area of decreased enhancement. Early abscess formation may mimic solid renal masses. The lesions are typ-

ically hypodense and cortically based. Perinephric stranding is a common secondary finding. Patients are febrile with leukocytosis on urinalysis. Immunosuppressed patients are at increased risk for multifocal renal involvement, especially in the setting of AIDS and IV drug abuse.
- **Renal cell carcinoma (RCC)**. RCC most commonly presents as a solitary hypervascular renal mass; however, multifocal involvement may be seen in a small number of patients, especially those with von Hippel–Lindau (VHL) syndrome. There is an increased incidence of RCC in patients with acquired cystic renal disease of dialysis and those with VHL. The papillary form of RCC may present with hypoenhancing masses. Local spread includes adjacent lymph nodes, as well as direct spread through the ipsilateral renal vein into the inferior vena cava.

■ Additional Differential Diagnoses

- **Angiomyolipomas**. Angiomyolipomas are benign hamartomas composed of vessels, soft tissue, and gross fat. On computed tomography (CT) or magnetic resonance imaging (MRI), visualization of macroscopic fat within a renal lesion is diagnostic of an angiomyolipoma. They are typically solitary and commonly occur in young to middle-aged females; however, multiple lesions may be seen in the setting of tuberous scle-

rosis. Although usually found incidentally, lesions >4 cm are prone to hemorrhage, necessitating intervention.
- **Metastases**. Other than lymphoma, metastatic disease to the kidneys is uncommon. Neoplasms prone to renal metastases include melanoma, lung cancer, and breast cancer, as well as soft-tissue and osseous sarcomas.

■ Diagnosis

Lymphoma

✓ Pearls

- Renal lymphoma may present as bilateral hypodense renal masses; accompanying LAD is a helpful clue.
- Pyelonephritis has a variety of imaging appearances; perinephric stranding is a common associated finding.

- Multifocal RCC typically is seen in association with syndromes, especially VHL.
- Multiple AMLs are seen with tuberous sclerosis; larger lesions are prone to hemorrhage.

Suggested Readings

Dunnick NR. Textbook of Uroradiology. 3rd ed. Philadelphia, PA: Lippincott Williams & Wilkins; 2001

Silverman SG, Mortele KJ, Tuncali K, Jinzaki M, Cibas ES. Hyperattenuating renal masses: etiologies, pathogenesis, and imaging evaluation. Radiographics. 2007; 27(4):1131–1143

Case 58

James B. Odone

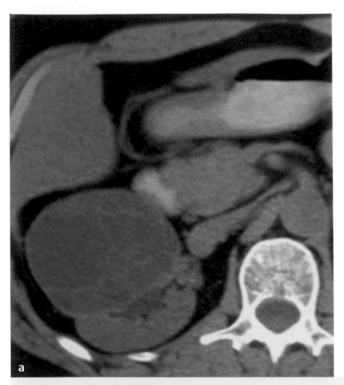 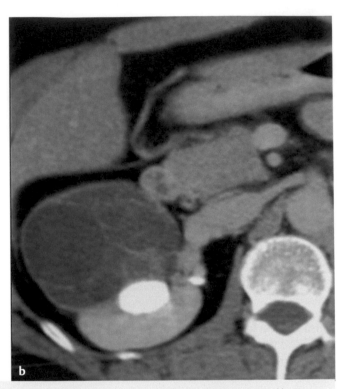

Fig. 58.1 Coned-down axial CT images of the right kidney **(a)** pre- and **(b)** post-IV contrast administration demonstrate a complex cystic renal lesion with multiple thickened enhancing septations.

■ Clinical Presentation

A 49-year-old woman with flank pain (▶Fig. 58.1).

■ Key Imaging Finding

Cystic renal mass

■ Top 3 Differential Diagnoses

- **Complex renal cyst**. Simple renal cysts demonstrate simple fluid attenuation on computed tomography (CT) and do not contain septations, calcifications, or internal debris (Bosniak I). Multiple cysts can be incidental or associated with various syndromes. Complicated or complex cysts are usually the result of hemorrhage or infection, which changes the imaging appearance (Bosniak II). Complex cysts may have internal debris, clot, calcification, or septations. The Bosniak classification is used to determine whether these lesions can be managed medically or surgically (Bosniak III and IV).
- **Cystic neoplasm**. A malignant cystic neoplasm should be considered if a cystic lesion is expansile and/or exhibits suspicious imaging characteristics, such as wall calcification, thickened septations, or enhancement. In an adult, the most frequently encountered cystic malignancy is renal cell carcinoma (RCC; approximately 20% of all RCC), while in a child Wilms tumor

is the most common cystic malignancy. In either case, surgical resection is a necessity. Both RCC and Wilms tumor have a propensity for renal vein invasion and subsequent inferior vena cava propagation, which should be evaluated during presurgical staging.
- **Multilocular cystic nephroma (MLCN)**. MLCN is a rare benign neoplasm that arises from the metanephric blastema. It is often difficult, if not impossible, to distinguish MLCN from malignant processes, such as cystic RCC or cystic Wilms tumors. The age distribution is bimodal with half of the cases seen in young males in the first decade of life and half arising in middle-aged women. The classic description is that of a complex cystic mass with enhancing septations which extends into the renal pelvis. It is typically classified as a Bosniak class III or IV lesion, which necessitates surgical resection. Hemorrhage or calcification is uncommon.

■ Additional Differential Diagnoses

- **Multicystic dysplastic kidney (MCDK) (focal)**. MCDK results from failure of the ureteral bud to induce maturation of the metanephric blastema into nephrons. Most commonly, MCDK affects an entire kidney which is replaced by a nonfunctioning cystic mass. Over time, the mass involutes and may eventually calcify. In the focal form, a portion of the kidney is dysplastic with a cystic mass, while the remainder of the kidney is rela-

tively normal. On CT, there is a nonenhancing cystic mass with multiple septations.
- **Abscess**. Renal abscesses may present as heterogeneously enhancing cystic parenchymal masses. There is usually associated perinephric fat stranding, although this finding is nonspecific. Patients often have a history of fever, pyuria, and flank pain. Follow-up imaging should be performed to exclude an underlying lesion.

■ Diagnosis

Multilocular cystic nephroma

✓ Pearls

- Complex renal cysts are classified and managed with the Bosniak classification.
- Cystic renal tumors are classically RCC in adults and Wilms tumor in children.

- MLCN has a bimodal age distribution and characteristically herniates into the renal pelvis.

Suggested Readings

Hartman DS, Choyke PL, Hartman MS. From the RSNA refresher courses: a practical approach to the cystic renal mass. Radiographics. 2004; 24(Suppl 1):S101–S115

Case 59

William T. O'Brien, Sr.

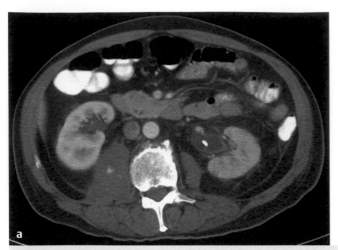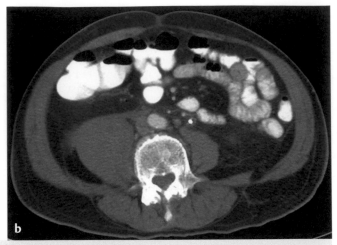

Fig. 59.1 **(a)** Contrast-enhanced axial CT image through the level of the kidneys demonstrates enlargement of the right psoas muscle with a focal region of contrast extravasation, consistent with active hemorrhage. **(b)** An axial image through the lower abdomen reveals inferior extension of the asymmetric right psoas muscle enlargement, as well as surrounding retroperitoneal fat stranding. Incidental note is made of a left ureteral stent on both CT images.

■ Clinical Presentation

A 58-year-old man with prior left ureteral stent and new right-sided flank pain (▶Fig. 59.1).

■ Key Imaging Finding

Retroperitoneal mass

■ Top 3 Differential Diagnoses

- **Retroperitoneal hemorrhage**. Retroperitoneal hemorrhage may result from a variety of causes, including trauma, coagulopathy, aortic aneurysm rupture, or hemorrhage from an underlying mass. Acute hemorrhage will be mildly hyperdense on unenhanced computed tomography (CT). Contrast is routinely given to evaluate for active extravasation. Traumatic hemorrhage usually involves the aorta or renal vessels, while abdominal aortic aneurysms may rupture spontaneously. Hemorrhage from coagulopathy is typically intramuscular with muscle enlargement, heterogeneous density, and fat stranding. Retroperitoneal neoplasms prone to hemorrhage include renal cell carcinoma (most common), angiomyolipoma, and adrenal neoplasms.
- **Lymphadenopathy**. Retroperitoneal lymphadenopathy is usually the result of lymphoma, but may also be due to metastatic disease (pancreatic, renal, or testicular neoplasms) or an infectious process. Non-Hodgkin lymphoma accounts for the vast majority of cases involving the abdomen and retroperitoneum. Lymphoma presents as large soft-tissue masses that displace the aorta anteriorly from the spine, a useful discriminator from other retroperitoneal processes. Posttreatment, lymph nodes may calcify.
- **Retroperitoneal abscess**. Retroperitoneal abscesses result from either hematogenous spread of an occult bacteremia to paraspinal musculature or direct extension from vertebral osteomyelitis. *Staphylococcus aureus* is the most common organism, followed by *Mycobacterium tuberculosis*. Imaging features consist of rim-enhancing fluid collections with surrounding edema. MR is helpful in evaluating for spinal involvement. Treatment includes percutaneous or surgical drainage of fluid collections, as well as intravenous antibiotics.

■ Additional Differential Diagnoses

- **Retroperitoneal fibrosis**. Retroperitoneal fibrosis is a rare disorder that is most commonly idiopathic but may be secondary to drugs or processes that result in a desmoplastic response. On imaging, retroperitoneal fibrosis demonstrates a soft-tissue mass around retroperitoneal structures with medial displacement of the ureters. The process may extend superiorly into the mediastinum. Ureter or vascular compression is common. Associated conditions include primary sclerosing cholangitis, orbital pseudotumor, and thyroiditis.
- **Retroperitoneal sarcoma**. Retroperitoneal sarcomas are classified by tissue type with liposarcoma being the most common. They are malignant neoplasms that are often large (>10 cm) at the time of presentation. On imaging, retroperitoneal liposarcomas are composed of fat, soft tissue, and occasionally calcification. Soft-tissue components demonstrate mild enhancement. When large, retroperitoneal sarcomas displace bowel and the renal collecting system, and they are prone to hemorrhage.

■ Diagnosis

Retroperitoneal hemorrhage (intramuscular hematoma with active extravasation)

✓ Pearls

- Retroperitoneal hemorrhage and abscesses commonly present with paraspinal muscle involvement.
- Non-Hodgkin lymphoma is the most common neoplastic cause of retroperitoneal lymphadenopathy.

- Retroperitoneal fibrosis presents as a soft-tissue mass with medial displacement of the ureters.
- Liposarcoma is the most common retroperitoneal sarcoma; it is prone to hemorrhage.

Suggested Readings

Lenchik L, Dovgan DJ, Kier R. CT of the iliopsoas compartment: value in differentiating tumor, abscess, and hematoma. AJR Am J Roentgenol. 1994; 162(1):83–86

Nishino M, Hayakawa K, Minami M, Yamamoto A, Ueda H, Takasu K. Primary retroperitoneal neoplasms: CT and MR imaging findings with anatomic and pathologic diagnostic clues. Radiographics. 2003; 23(1):45–57

Case 60

Paul B. DiDomenico

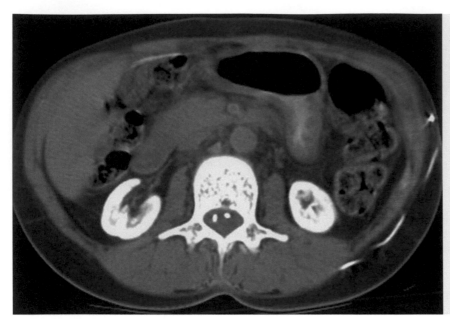

Fig. 60.1 Unenhanced axial computed tomography (CT) image through the kidneys demonstrates dense calcification of the entire renal cortex bilaterally. Regions of calcification are also seen within the spinal canal.

■ Clinical Presentation

Renal insufficiency and history of bowel surgery (▶ Fig. 60.1).

■ Key Imaging Finding

Cortical nephrocalcinosis

■ Top 3 Differential Diagnoses

- **Acute renal cortical necrosis**. Acute cortical necrosis is the most common cause of cortical nephrocalcinosis and may result from severe acute hypotension (due to shock, sepsis, or hemorrhage). Nephrotoxic drugs such as amphotericin B or ingested toxins such as ethylene glycol can also damage the cortex, resulting in cortical nephrocalcinosis.
- **Chronic glomerulonephritis**. Chronic glomerulonephritis is the second most common cause of cortical nephrocalcinosis. The pathophysiology is chronic inflammatory destruction of glomeruli within the renal cortex with resultant dystrophic calcification. There will often be marked renal atrophy with a smooth renal contour. Biopsy is required to determine the un-

derlying cause, such as diabetic nephropathy, lupus nephritis, and membranous glomerulonephritis.
- **Oxalosis**. Hyperoxaluria can occur in both primary and secondary forms. The primary (inherited autosomal recessive) form is rare and usually fatal early in life. The secondary (enteric) form is more common and is related to altered bile acid metabolism from resection or chronic disease of the small bowel, as in Crohn disease. The resulting increased urinary secretion of oxalates may cause calcium oxalate renal stones, medullary nephrocalcinosis or, less commonly, cortical nephrocalcinosis.

■ Additional Differential Diagnoses

- **Chronic transplant rejection**. A patient with a renal transplant may have some degree of chronic rejection, causing cortical necrosis and dystrophic calcification. This diagnosis would be supported by the presence of a kidney in the right lower quadrant (RLQ), the most common location for a transplant.

- **Alport syndrome**. Alport syndrome is a rare syndrome of hereditary nerve deafness and nephritis, and there are case reports of cortical nephrocalcinosis from the associated chronic renal disease.

■ Diagnosis

Oxalosis

✓ Pearls

- Acute cortical necrosis may be caused by severe acute hypotension or drug toxicity.
- Chronic glomerulonephritis may result in smooth renal atrophy and cortical nephrocalcinosis.

- Oxalosis (primary or more commonly secondary) may result in cortical or medullary nephrocalcinosis.
- Chronic transplant rejection may result in cortical nephrocalcinosis; look for a RLQ transplant kidney.

Suggested Readings

Dyer RB, Chen MY, Zagoria RJ. Abnormal calcifications in the urinary tract. Radiographics. 1998; 18(6):1405–1424

Case 61

William T. O'Brien, Sr.

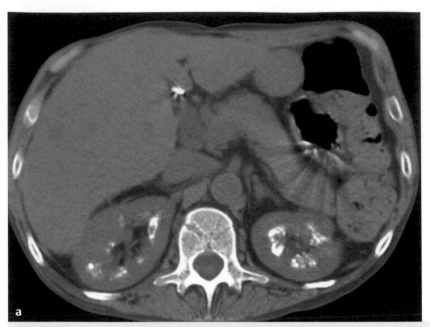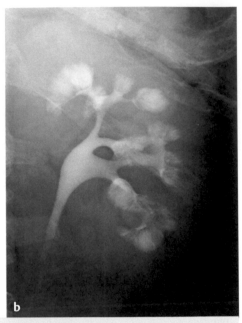

Fig. 61.1 (a) Unenhanced axial CT image through the kidneys demonstrates symmetric bilateral medullary calcifications. (b) Frontal coned-down view of the left kidney from an IVP reveals contrast within the collecting and a striated "paintbrush" appearance of the medullary pyramids.

■ Clinical Presentation

A 38-year-old man with mild renal insufficiency (▶Fig. 61.1).

■ Key Imaging Finding

Medullary nephrocalcinosis

■ Top 3 Differential Diagnoses

- **Hypercalcemia**. Hypercalcemia from a variety of etiologies, including hyperparathyroidism, paraneoplastic syndromes, and sarcoidosis, is a common cause of bilateral symmetric medullary nephrocalcinosis. The abundance of serum calcium that must be filtered by the kidneys results in precipitation of calcium deposits within the renal pyramids. Chronic hypercalcemia results in chronic renal failure, so the kidneys are usually smaller in size. Imaging studies demonstrate bilateral symmetric calcifications within the renal pyramids.
- **Medullary sponge kidney (MSK)**. MSK is a common cause of medullary nephrocalcinosis. The disorder is characterized by idiopathic ectasia of the renal tubules, resulting in urinary stasis and stone formation. Most cases are noted incidentally, but patients may suffer from recurrent urolithiasis or pyelonephritis. MSK is usually bilateral and segmental with sparing of a portion of the renal pyramids. On plain radiographs or computed tomography (CT), macroscopic chunky calcifications will be noted along the renal pyramids. Classic findings on intravenous pyelogram (IVP) include the "growing calculus" sign secondary to contrast filling the dilated tubules around the stones, and the striated, "paintbrush" appearance of the renal pyramids. Although usually an isolated finding, MSK may be associated with hemihypertrophy syndromes.
- **Renal tubular acidosis (RTA)**. Type 1 or distal RTA results in both medullary nephrocalcinosis and urolithiasis secondary to hypercalciuria. In this disorder, there is a citrate deficiency, which results in an inability to adequately acidify the urine at the distal tubule. The body responds by releasing a large amount of calcium into the urine, causing hypercalciuria. Over a period of time, chronic renal insufficiency ensues; therefore, the kidneys may be symmetrically decreased in size.

■ Additional Differential Diagnoses

- **Papillary necrosis**. Papillary necrosis may rarely result in medullary nephrocalcinosis, most commonly when associated with analgesic nephropathy from overuse of nonsteroidal anti-inflammatory medications. Analgesic nephropathy also causes chronic renal insufficiency, so the kidneys are typically small with irregular margins. Radiographic findings include those associated with papillary necrosis, to include ureteral filling defects and the "lobster-claw" and "ball-on-a-tee" configuration of the renal pyramids on IVP, as well as findings associated with MSK (calcifications along the renal pyramids).
- **Lasix**. Chronic use of diuretics, specifically Lasix, in newborns may result in medullary nephrocalcinosis, which appears radiographically as calcifications in the region of the renal pyramids. The radiographic findings often resolve over a period of time once the medication is discontinued.
- **Tuberculosis**. Renal tuberculosis may rarely result in medullary nephrocalcinosis. Unlike other causes of nephrocalcinosis, tuberculosis is usually focal and unilateral at sites of previous pyelonephritis. Inflammation of the urothelium results in infundibular stenosis, urinary stasis, and scarring of the overlying parenchyma. Bilateral involvement is unusual.

■ Diagnosis

Medullary sponge kidney

✓ Pearls

- Adult medullary nephrocalcinosis results from hypercalcemia, MSK, or RTA Type 1.
- MSK classically has a "paintbrush" appearance of the renal pyramids on IVP.
- Chronic Lasix therapy in newborns may result in medullary nephrocalcinosis.

Suggested Readings

Dyer RB, Chen MY, Zagoria RJ. Abnormal calcifications in the urinary tract. Radiographics. 1998; 18(6):1405–1424

Dyer RB, Chen MY, Zagoria RJ. Classic signs in uroradiology. Radiographics. 2004; 24(Suppl 1):S247–S280

Case 62

Chirag V. Patel

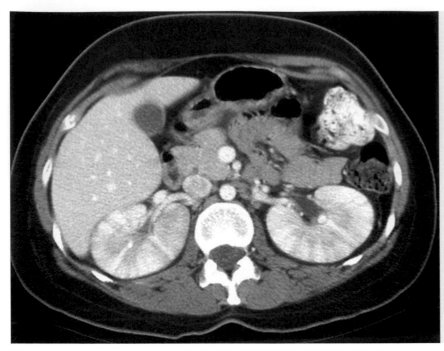

Fig. 62.1 Contrast-enhanced axial CT image demonstrates a bilateral striated nephrogram and mild diffuse renal enlargement.

■ Clinical Presentation

A 41-year-old man with urosepsis (▶Fig. 62.1).

■ Key Imaging Finding

Striated nephrogram

■ Top 3 Differential Diagnoses

- **Pyelonephritis**. Acute pyelonephritis results from bacterial invasion of renal parenchyma. Most cases are diagnosed by typical clinical presentation and laboratory studies. Imaging is warranted in cases of atypical presentations and in the setting of worsening or refractory symptoms despite adequate medical therapy to evaluate for obstruction or abscess formation. Computed tomography (CT) is the imaging modality of choice and may reveal a striated nephrogram, with multiple linear or wedge-shaped regions of hypoperfusion. The focal areas of low attenuation result from edema and microvascular occlusion. Although commonly unilateral, a bilateral striated nephrogram may be seen in the setting of pyelonephritis if both kidneys are involved.
- **Urinary obstruction**. Acute urinary obstruction is most commonly due to ureteral calculi. Patients present with colicky abdominal pain, dysuria, and hematuria. Ultrasound and/or unenhanced CT is the preferred imaging modality. Contrast-enhanced CT (CT urogram) can be used in cases of obstruction demonstrated on noncontrast studies without an identifiable radio-opaque calculus within the ureter, and may be helpful in identifying neoplastic causes of ureteral or renal obstruction. The classic finding in acute urinary obstruction is delayed onset of a progressively dense nephrogram which may be associated with hydronephrosis, hydroureter, and diffuse enlargement of the affected kidney. A striated nephrogram may occasionally be encountered.
- **Renal vein thrombosis (RVT)**. The most common cause of RVT is nephrotic syndrome; in children, dehydration and sepsis are common etiologies. Other less common causes include renal neoplasms, trauma, and other acquired or inheritable hypercoagulable states. Imaging studies will show diffuse enlargement of the affected kidney with thrombus in the renal vein and possibly extension into the inferior vena cava. Common features on CT include prolonged corticomedullary differentiation, delayed or prolonged parenchymal opacification, and delayed or absent pyelocalyceal visualization. Occasionally, a striated nephrogram is encountered.

■ Additional Differential Diagnoses

- **Renal contusion**. Interstitial edema resulting from renal contusion can produce a focal striated appearance in the nephrographic phase. The imaging appearance can mimic other etiologies of a striated nephrogram, especially focal pyelonephritis. A history of trauma or appreciation of injuries to adjacent organs aids in establishing the correct diagnosis.
- **Hypotension**. Hypotension and subsequent hypoperfusion of the kidneys (as well as other organs) can be seen in the setting of trauma, aortic dissection, placental abruption, or other etiologies of shock. The most common imaging finding is bilateral persistent nephrograms. A striated nephrogram is a less frequent manifestation of hypotension.

■ Diagnosis

Bilateral acute pyelonephritis

✓ Pearls

- Pyelonephritis, urinary obstruction, RVT, and contusions usually result in unilateral striated nephrograms.
- Urinary obstruction may present as a persistent nephrogram or a striated nephrogram.
- RVT most often results from nephritic syndrome; trauma and hypercoagulable states are less common.

Suggested Readings

Wolin EA, Hartman DS, Olson JR. Nephrographic and pyelographic analysis of CT urography: differential diagnosis. AJR Am J Roentgenol. 2013; 200(6):1197–1203

Case 63

Charles A. Tujo

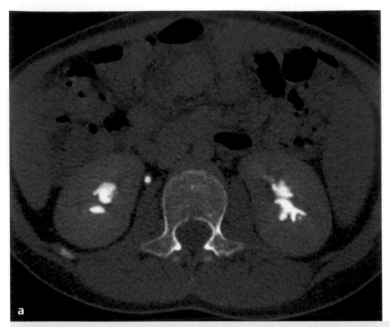 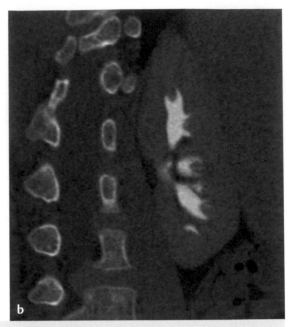

Fig. 63.1 (a) Axial and (b) reformatted coned-down coronal delayed images from a contrast-enhanced computed tomography (CT) of the abdomen demonstrate abnormal collections of contrast within the renal papillae, consistent with papillary necrosis.

■ Clinical Presentation

An 8-year-old boy with chronic renal insufficiency (▶Fig. 63.1).

■ Key Imaging Finding

Papillary necrosis

■ Top 3 Differential Diagnoses

• **Diabetes**. Diabetes is the most common cause of papillary necrosis. It is often associated with urinary tract infection and renal insufficiency or impairment. Diabetes results in small vessel ischemic disease, which affects the renal papillae. Papillary necrosis presents as abnormal contrast patterns involving the renal pyramids, to include the "lobster claw" and "ball-on-tee" appearances. Ureteral filling defects may be seen with sloughed papillae. The findings are usually bilateral, and may be asymmetric.
• **Analgesic nephropathy**. Caused by excessive intake of analgesics, analgesic nephropathy occurs most commonly in middle-aged women. The analgesics reach high concentrations in the renal medulla and lead to necrosis of the renal papillae. Findings are usually bilateral, and may be asymmetric.
• **Pyelonephritis**. Renal infection, especially tuberculosis (TB), can result in papillary necrosis. The exact mechanism is difficult to determine, as associated diabetes and/or obstruction may contribute to the development of pyelonephritis. The most common organism to cause pyelonephritis is *Escherichia coli*; however, *E. coli* infrequently causes papillary necrosis. Infection with TB leads to vasculitis and ultimately vascular insufficiency, which results in papillary necrosis. Findings are typically unilateral.

■ Additional Differential Diagnoses

• **Sickle cell anemia**. The deformation of red blood cells that sludge through small arteries results in medullary ischemia and ultimately papillary necrosis. This process is exacerbated by the hypertonic and hypoxic environment of the renal medulla. Findings are usually bilateral and may be asymmetric.
• **Urinary obstruction**. Obstruction of the urinary tract leads to increased pressure in the renal papilla and decreased perfusion, which ultimately results in papillary necrosis. Depending on the etiology of the obstruction, the process may be unilateral or bilateral. Treatment is focused on relieving the source of obstruction.
• **Renal vein thrombosis**. Renal vein thrombosis is typically the result of a hypercoagulable state, especially in the setting of nephritic syndrome. Venous obstruction leads to renal edema and resultant ischemia. Eventually, papillary necrosis may occur. Treatment is focused on preserving renal perfusion utilizing thrombolysis and treatment of the underlying disorder. Findings are typically unilateral.

■ Diagnosis

Pyelonephritis (TB)

✓ Pearls

• Diabetes is the most common cause of papillary necrosis and is typically bilateral.
• Analgesic nephropathy occurs most often in middle-aged women; findings are usually bilateral.
• Pyelonephritis, especially TB, can result in papillary necrosis; findings are most commonly unilateral.
• Sickle cell anemia results in medullary ischemia with resultant papillary necrosis; it is typically bilateral.

Suggested Readings

Jung DC, Kim SH, Jung SI, Hwang SI, Kim SH. Renal papillary necrosis: review and comparison of findings at multi-detector row CT and intravenous urography. Radiographics. 2006; 26(6):1827–1836

Sheth S, Fishman EK. Multidetector row CT of the kidneys and urinary tract: techniques and applications of the benign diseases. Radiographics. 2004; 24(2):e20

Case 64

Michael Kuo

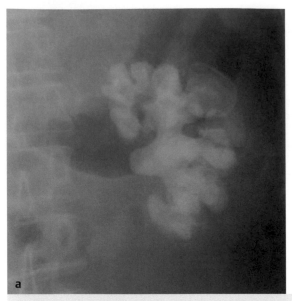 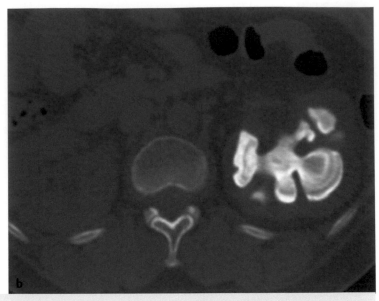

Fig. 64.1 **(a)** Magnified frontal radiographic view of the abdomen demonstrates a large branching calculus throughout the left renal collecting system. **(b)** Axial unenhanced computed tomography (CT) image through the abdomen confirms the large calculus with a "staghorn" branching pattern. *Images courtesy of Todd M. Johnson, MD.*

■ Clinical Presentation

An adult man with history of urolithiasis and renal insufficiency (▶ Fig. 64.1).

■ Key Imaging Finding

Staghorn calculus

■ Top 3 Differential Diagnoses

- **Xanthogranulomatous pyelonephritis (XGP).** XGP is a chronic renal infection characterized by parenchymal destruction and replacement by lipid-laden macrophages. It most commonly occurs in older women. The most common offending organisms include *Escherichia coli* and *Proteus mirabilis*. The entity presents with a centrally obstructing calculus in the majority of patients. The affected kidney is usually nonfunctional. Perirenal fibrofatty proliferation, poor excretion of contrast, and perinephric extension are secondary findings that suggest the diagnosis of XGP, which is best seen on computed tomography (CT). Treatment usually requires nephrectomy.
- **Pyonephrosis with obstructing stone.** Patients with a large obstructing calculus and pyonephrosis are acutely ill with flank pain and fever. The dilated collecting system is filled with purulent material. This is best seen with ultrasound with mobile debris and layering of low-amplitude echoes in a hydronephrotic kidney. The most common organism is *E. coli*. Complications include abscess formation and progression to septic shock. Urgent percutaneous decompression of the infected collecting system is necessary, as this entity has a 25 to 50% mortality rate if untreated.
- **Calcified neoplasm.** Transitional cell carcinoma (TCC) and renal cell carcinoma (RCC) are far less common causes of calcified renal lesions. Only about 2% of TCC calcify, while up to 10% of RCC may contain calcifications. RCC presents as an intraparenchymal mass; TCC presents within the collecting system/renal pelvis. Calcifications are most commonly amorphous but may also appear in a curvilinear, dense, or diffuse pattern. An associated prominent soft tissue or cystic mass is commonly identified on cross-sectional imaging.

■ Diagnosis

Xanthogranulomatous pyelonephritis

✓ Pearls

- XGP presents with a staghorn calculus in most cases (>90%), along with a large nonfunctioning kidney.
- An obstructed urinary collecting system with secondary infection is a urologic emergency.
- TCC and RCC present with amorphous calcifications in the minority of cases.

Suggested Readings

Dyer RB, Chen MY, Zagoria RJ. Classic signs in uroradiology. Radiographics. 2004; 24(Suppl 1):S247–S280

Case 65

Todd M. Johnson

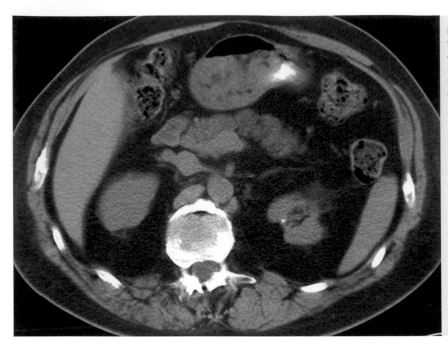

Fig. 65.1 Axial unenhanced computed tomography (CT) image through the abdomen demonstrates focal cortical defects involving the upper pole of the left kidney, one of which along the posteromedial margin has an adjacent small calcification.

■ Clinical Presentation

An elderly man with longstanding renal insufficiency (▶ Fig. 65.1).

■ Key Imaging Finding

Renal cortical defect

■ Top 3 Differential Diagnoses

- **Reflux nephropathy**. Although sterile reflux can result in renal scarring, scarring is usually secondary to underlying infection, with *Escherichia coli* representing the most common organism. Up to half of patients with reflux nephropathy will have evidence of renal scarring; patients with more severe reflux have a higher prevalence of developing renal scarring. Scarring tends to favor the upper and lower renal poles. Calyceal dilatation and distortion can be seen underlying the renal scar.
- **Chronic pyelonephritis**. Pyelonephritis most commonly occurs in adult women. Patients typically present with fever, urinary urgency and frequency, and flank pain. Chronic pyelonephritis occurs more frequently in diabetic patients and results in cortical scarring with underlying dilated calices. *E. coli* is the most common organism. Renal size is decreased, which may mimic chronic global renal infarction. The contralateral kidney may demonstrate compensatory hypertrophy.
- **Renal infarct**. Renal infarction may be global or focal. With global infarction, there is decreased renal size and usually compensatory hypertrophy of the contralateral kidney. Embolic infarction typically results in multiple bilateral defects. Thrombotic or traumatic infarction is usually unilateral with a segmental or subsegmental defect. In the acute setting, a wedge-shaped region of nonenhancing renal parenchyma is seen. The cortical rim sign, in the subacute phase, can be seen in up to 50% of patients because of intact collateral circulation, which results from preserved capsular or subcapsular perfusion.

■ Additional Differential Diagnoses

- **Vasculitis**. Vasculitis results in multiple bilateral wedge-shaped regions of decreased perfusion. Parenchymal scarring with capsular retraction may occur, in addition to microaneurysm formation. Etiologies include polyarteritis nodosa, lupus, and drug abuse.
- **Partial nephrectomy**. Nephron-sparing surgery for renal cell carcinoma (RCC) can be performed to preserve renal function in select patients with limited disease or in those in which complete nephrectomy would be contraindicated. Appropriate clinical history or secondary postoperative findings would be helpful to establish this diagnosis.

■ Diagnosis

Chronic pyelonephritis

✓ Pearls

- Reflux nephropathy scarring favors the upper and lower renal poles.
- Chronic pyelonephritis and renal infarction can both result in decreased renal size.

- Renal infarct may demonstrate the cortical rim sign because of preserved capsular perfusion.

Suggested Readings

Craig WD, Wagner BJ, Travis MD. Pyelonephritis: radiologic-pathologic review. Radiographics. 2008; 28(1):255–277, quiz 327–328

Kawashima A, Sandler CM, Corl FM, et al. Imaging of renal trauma: a comprehensive review. Radiographics. 2001; 21(3):557–574

Case 66

Michael Kuo

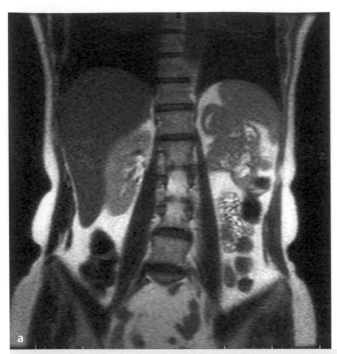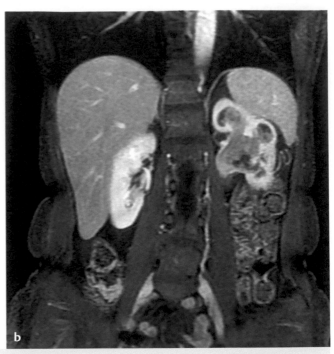

Fig. 66.1 **(a)** T2 coronal MR image shows an iso- to hypointense left renal pelvic mass with associated caliectasis. **(b)** Coronal T1 delayed postcontrast MR image shows a heterogeneously enhancing (precontrast T1 image not shown) soft-tissue mass within the left renal pelvis that extends into the proximal ureter and calices.

■ Clinical Presentation

A 55-year-old woman with hematuria (▶ Fig. 66.1).

■ Key Imaging Finding

Renal pelvic mass

■ Top 3 Differential Diagnoses

- **Transitional cell carcinoma**. Transitional cell carcinoma (TCC) makes up 90% of renal pelvic uroepithelial cancers. It most commonly occurs within the bladder (90%), followed by the renal pelvis and proximal ureter. Single or multiple soft-tissue filling defects can be seen with stippled, serrated, or frondlike surface irregularities. Once a mass is seen within the urinary collecting system, the remainder of the urothelium must be examined to evaluate for synchronous disease. Upper tract TCC has a high association (up to 40%) with development of bladder TCC. When located within the ureter, the classic sign on intravenous pyelogram (IVP) is the "goblet sign"—a cup-shaped contrast collection distal to an intraluminal filling defect of the ureter. TCC within the renal pelvis may obstruct the infundibulum, resulting in the "amputated calyx" sign. Treatment of renal and ureteral TCC includes total nephroureterectomy and bladder cuff excision.
- **Multilocular cystic nephroma (MLCN)**. MLCN is a benign renal neoplasm originating from the metanephric blastema.

MLCN appears as a multilocular cystic mass, which characteristically herniates into the renal pelvis. The cystic mass exhibits a capsule with thin internal septa, both of which may enhance. MLCN occurs most commonly in boys younger than 5 years and in older women in the fifth and sixth decades. Surgical excision is the standard treatment, since MLCN is characterized as a Bosniak class III or IV complex cystic mass and is difficult to distinguish from multilocular cystic renal cell carcinoma (RCC) or Wilms tumor.

- **Medullary carcinoma**. Renal medullary carcinoma is a rare renal tumor arising in calyceal transitional epithelium. This highly aggressive tumor is seen in young African American patients with sickle cell trait. The mass is centrally located and infiltrative, while preserving the renal shape. The prognosis is very poor with mean survival of 15 weeks. If there are no metastases, nephrectomy is the treatment.

■ Additional Differential Diagnoses

- **Renal cell carcinoma**. RCC is a malignant tumor arising from tubular epithelium. RCCs are usually hypervascular solid cortical renal masses; however, they can occasionally be cystic masses that have enhancing septa, calcification of septa, or tumor capsule. Rarely, they may involve the renal pelvis, especially when large. Papillary RCC, which makes up 10 to 15% of RCC, is hypovascular and can easily be mistaken for a cyst on all imaging modalities. Evaluation requires particular attention for renal vein and inferior vena cava tumor extension. Radical nephrectomy is the standard treatment.

■ Diagnosis

Transitional cell carcinoma

✓ Pearls

- Upper tract TCC has a high association (up to 40%) with development of bladder TCC.
- TCC most commonly affects the urinary bladder, followed by the renal pelvis and ureter.

- MLCN has a bimodal age distribution and classically herniates into the renal pelvis.
- Medullary carcinoma arises from the collecting system epithelium in patients with sickle cell trait.

Suggested Readings

Dyer R, DiSantis DJ, McClennan BL. Simplified imaging approach for evaluation of the solid renal mass in adults. Radiology. 2008; 247(2):331–343

Wong-You-Cheong JJ, Wagner BJ, Davis CJ, Jr. Transitional cell carcinoma of the urinary tract: radiologic-pathologic correlation. Radiographics. 1998; 18(1):123–142, quiz 148

Case 67

Todd M. Johnson

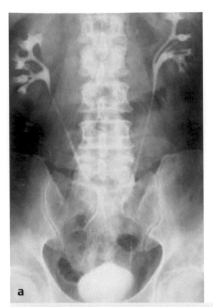 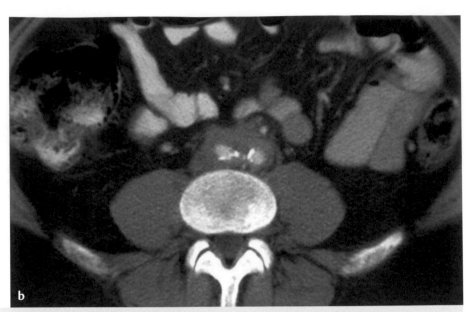

Fig. 67.1 **(a)** Frontal projection from an intravenous pyelogram (IVP) shows medial deviation of the distal ureters. **(b)** Contrast-enhanced computed tomography (CT) image through the lower abdomen demonstrates soft tissue predominantly along the anterior and lateral margins of the common iliac arteries. The opacified and medially deviated ureters are identified with the left ureter approximating the soft tissue density anterolaterally.

■ Clinical Presentation

A 55-year-old man with flank pain (▶Fig. 67.1).

■ Key Imaging Finding

Medial deviation of the ureters

■ Top 3 Differential Diagnoses

• **Retroperitoneal fibrosis**. Retroperitoneal fibrosis is an inflammatory process that typically affects older patients (50–60 years old) with a male predilection. It is most commonly idiopathic (Ormond disease) but may also be secondary to medications (especially migraine therapy), abdominal aortic aneurysms (AAA), neoplasms, and radiation therapy. It has associations with other systemic manifestations, such as mediastinitis, sclerosing cholangitis, and thyroiditis, which has led to a proposed autoimmune basis. Retroperitoneal fibrosis typically presents with an irregular, ill-defined mass centered at the aortic bifurcation. The fibrotic component compresses and medially deviates the ureters. In severe cases, ureteral obstruction may occur. Variable enhancement can be present on computed tomography (CT) depending on the degree of edema and active inflammation. In the chronic setting, fibrosis predominates, which will have low signal intensity on T1 and T2 magnetic resonance imaging (MRI) sequences.

• **Psoas muscle hypertrophy**. In athletic individuals, psoas muscle hypertrophy may result in medial deviation of the ureters because of the normal close anatomic relationship. Cross-sectional imaging can readily differentiate psoas muscle hypertrophy from other causes of medial deviation of the ureters.

• **Pelvic lipomatosis**. Pelvic lipomatosis is an idiopathic condition of increased unencapsulated fat within the pelvis. It occurs more commonly in middle-aged African American males. Compression of the pelvic hollow viscus, including the bladder and rectum, can occur. The distal ureters are medially deviated because of compression of the urinary bladder. In severe cases, ureteral obstruction may occur. Pelvic lipomatosis can be associated with cystitis glandularis.

■ Additional Differential Diagnoses

• **Postoperative**. Several surgical procedures may lead to postoperative medial deviation of the ureters. Common surgical procedures include retroperitoneal lymph node dissection (such as part of the treatment plan for testicular cancer), anterior abdominopelvic resections, and pelvic floor reconstructions. The distal ureters are most often affected.

• **Retrocaval ureter**. A retrocaval ureter occurs secondary to abnormal persistence of the right subcardinal vein. As a result of this anomaly, the right ureter deviates medially and passes posterior to the inferior vena cava (IVC) at approximately the L3/L4 level. Compression may result in proximal ureteral obstruction. Cross-sectional imaging such as CT urography can readily discern the variant location of the right ureter relative to the IVC.

■ Diagnosis

Retroperitoneal fibrosis

✓ Pearls

• Retroperitoneal fibrosis may be idiopathic or secondary to medications, AAA, neoplasms, or radiation.
• Pelvic lipomatosis is most common in African American males and is associated with cystitis glandularis.

• Retrocaval ureter results in medial deviation of the right ureter and may result in proximal obstruction.

Suggested Readings

Craig WD, Fanburg-Smith JC, Henry LR, Guerrero R, Barton JH. Fat-containing lesions of the retroperitoneum: radiologic-pathologic correlation. Radiographics. 2009; 29(1):261–290

Cronin CG, Lohan DG, Blake MA, Roche C, McCarthy P, Murphy JM. Retroperitoneal fibrosis: a review of clinical features and imaging findings. AJR Am J Roentgenol. 2008; 191(2):423–431

Case 68

Todd M. Johnson

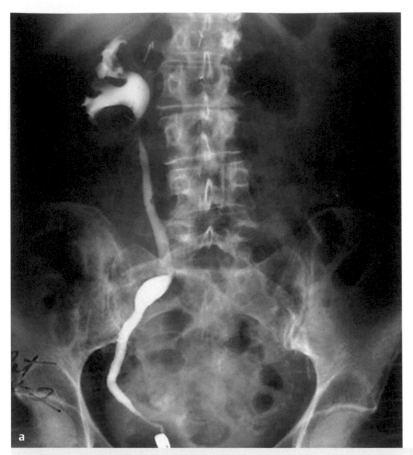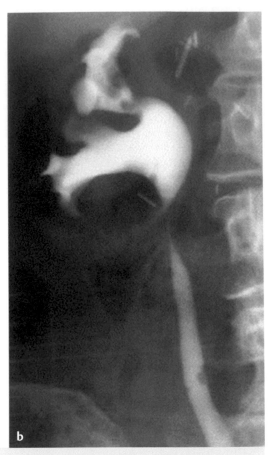

Fig. 68.1 (a) Retrograde pyelogram of the right ureter and **(b)** coned-down view of the right renal pelvis demonstrate multiple subcentimeter circumscribed filling defects.

■ Clinical Presentation

A 53-year-old woman with history of chronic urinary tract infections (▶ Fig. 68.1).

■ **Key Imaging Finding**

Ureteral filling defects

■ **Top 3 Differential Diagnoses**

• **Transitional cell carcinoma (TCC).** TCC is the most common of urothelial tumors (90–95%), and the urinary bladder is most commonly affected. If TCC is discovered in the upper urinary tract, the risk of spread into the urinary bladder is approximately 20 to 40%. Conversely, bladder TCC is associated with upper tract involvement in approximately 2 to 4%. Carcinogen exposures associated with TCC include aromatic amines (smoking and rubber/dye industry) and cyclophosphamide. Multifocal papillary TCC may mimic other disorders including ureteritis cystica and malakoplakia.

• **Radiolucent calculi.** Radiolucent stones can cause filling defects in the collecting system. Uric acid and xanthine stones occur in patients with malignancy on chemotherapy (marked cytolysis) and in gout. Other radiolucent stones include matrix (protein) and indinavir stones. Cystine stones may be faintly radiopaque.

• **Blood clot.** Blood clots may occur within the renal collecting system secondary to trauma, renal calculi, or an underlying mass, such as renal cell or TCC. The blood clots may form round, oval, or irregular mobile filling defects, or they may form a cast of the collecting system/ureter. When large, obstruction may occur.

■ **Additional Diagnostic Considerations**

• **Pyeloureteritis cystica.** Pyeloureteritis cystica is a benign condition associated with chronic urinary tract infection/mucosal irritation, resulting in urothelial metaplasia. It may affect the renal pelvis, ureter, or bladder. Multiple small, round or oval filling defects are seen projecting into the collecting system lumen. The lesions can have a scalloped appearance when viewed in profile. No known malignant potential exists.

• **Fungus ball.** Candida is the most common fungus to involve the urinary tract. Infection typically occurs in immunosuppressed patients (diabetes, transplant, chemotherapy, steroids, etc.) and in patients with indwelling catheters or stents. Radiologic manifestations include multiple mobile radiolucent filling defects.

• **Metastases.** Metastases to the upper tract most commonly arise from a breast carcinoma or melanoma. True metastatic involvement may be intramural or lymphatic (periureteral). Manifestations on pyelography include multiple filling defects and strictures.

■ **Diagnosis**

Pyeloureteritis cystica

✓ **Pearls**

• TCC is the most common urothelial tumor and may be multifocal; it is important to inspect the bladder.
• Radiolucent stones include those composed of uric acid, xanthine, and indinavir.

• Pyeloureteritis cystica is associated with chronic inflammation and has no known malignant potential.
• Fungus balls typically occur in immunocompromised patients; candida is the most common organism.

Suggested Readings

Kawashima A, Vrtiska TJ, LeRoy AJ, Hartman RP, McCollough CH, King BF, Jr. CT urography. Radiographics. 2004; 24(Suppl 1):S35–S54, discussion S55–S58

Case 69

James B. Odone

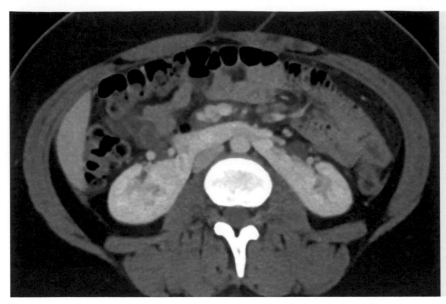

Fig. 69.1 Contrast-enhanced computed tomography (CT) image through the lower abdomen reveals medial deviation of the inferior pole of both kidneys with renal parenchyma extending across midline in continuity with the contralateral kidney. *Image courtesy of Dell Dunn, MD.*

■ Clinical Presentation

A 21-year-old woman with vague abdominal and pelvic pain (▶Fig. 69.1).

■ Key Imaging Finding

Renal migration anomaly

■ Top 3 Differential Diagnoses

- **Horseshoe kidney.** Horseshoe kidney is the most common congenital renal anomaly with an incidence of 1 in every 400 live births. There is increased risk of a horseshoe kidney in Turner and Ellis–van Creveld syndrome. Fusion typically occurs at the lower poles with subsequent arrest of cranial migration, because of restriction at the inferior mesenteric artery. As a result, the kidneys are lower within the abdomen and the inferior renal poles appear more medial than expected on plain film radiography. The interconnecting isthmus may be fibrotic or composed of functioning renal parenchyma. Associated renal anomalies include ureteropelvic junction (UPJ) obstruction and duplication anomalies. Patients are more susceptible to trauma, obstruction, reflux, urinary tract infections, and stone formation. Wilms tumor is two to eight times more common in children with a horseshoe kidney.
- **Crossed fused ectopia**. Crossed fused ectopia is an uncommon congenital anomaly. Usually, the left kidney crosses midline and fuses with the inferior pole of the right kidney. The anomaly is thought to be related to an abnormally situated umbilical artery. Intravenous urography (IVU) will reveal an absent nephrogram in the expected renal fossa and fused renal parenchyma on the contralateral side. The ureters usually insert normally on the bladder; however, vascular supply to the ectopic kidney is typically anomalous. As with horseshoe kidney, patients are more susceptible to trauma, obstruction, reflux, urinary tract infections, and stone formation.
- **Ectopic kidney.** Isolated renal ectopia, typically resulting in a pelvic kidney, has a prevalence of approximately 1 in 1,000 live births. On imaging with IVU, the pelvic kidney may be difficult to identify if it is overlying the sacrum, with the main clue being an empty renal fossa. The ectopic kidney usually has an anomalous blood supply with the renal artery originating from the ipsilateral iliac artery. Complications include UPJ obstruction, vesicoureteral reflux (VUR), and urinary stasis with stone formation. Associated contralateral renal anomalies include agenesis and ectopia.

■ Additional Differential Diagnoses

- **Renal duplication.** Although supernumerary kidneys are extremely rare, a duplex kidney is a common congenital anomaly and occurs along a spectrum from partial to complete duplication. In most cases, the affected kidney will have two ureters—one for the upper pole moiety and one for the lower pole moiety. The lower pole ureter inserts into the bladder normally, while the ectopic upper pole ureter inserts inferomedially (Weigert–Meyer rule). The upper pole moiety is prone to obstruction (commonly due to an ureterocele at the ectopic insertion site) and the lower pole moiety is prone to reflux.

■ Diagnosis

Horseshoe kidney

✓ Pearls

- Horseshoe kidney and renal ectopia are susceptible to injury in blunt abdominal trauma.
- In crossed fused renal ectopia, the ureters insert normally in the bladder.
- Ectopic kidney may be associated with UPJ obstruction, VUR, and urinary stasis with stone formation.
- A duplex kidney is prone to obstruction (upper pole) and reflux (lower pole).

Suggested Readings

Cohen HL, Kravets F, Zucconi W, Ratani R, Shah S, Dougherty D. Congenital abnormalities of the genitourinary system. Semin Roentgenol. 2004; 39(2):282–303

Case 70

Todd M. Johnson

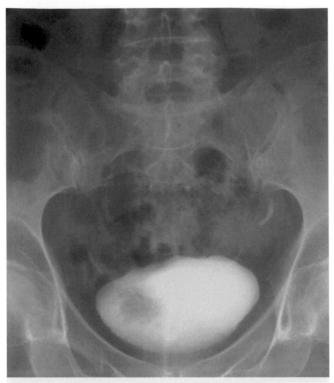

Fig. 70.1 Coned-down view of the pelvis from an IV urogram (IVU) demonstrates an irregular filling defect within the right lateral bladder.

■ Clinical Presentation

A 60-year-old man with gross hematuria (▶ Fig. 70.1).

■ Key Imaging Finding

Bladder filling defect

■ Top 3 Differential Diagnoses

- **Transitional cell carcinoma (TCC).** TCC is the most common of urothelial tumors (90–95%), and the urinary bladder is the most common site of involvement. Carcinogen exposures associated with TCC include aromatic amines (smoking and rubber/dye industry) and cyclophosphamide. Other less common malignant bladder tumors include squamous cell carcinoma (SCC) and adenocarcinoma. SCC is associated with chronic infection or inflammation; adenocarcinoma is the most common malignant tumor in urachal remnants.
- **Fungus ball.** Candida is the most common fungus to involve the urinary tract. Infection typically occurs in immunosup-

pressed patients (diabetes, transplant, chemotherapy, steroids, etc.) and in patients with indwelling catheters or stents. Radiographic manifestations include mobile radiolucent filling defects within the collecting system.
- **Blood clot.** Blood clots may occur within the renal collecting system secondary to trauma, renal calculi, or hemorrhage from an underlying mass, such as renal cell or TCC. Blood clots may form round, irregular, mobile filling defects, or they may form a cast of the collecting system.

■ Additional Differential Diagnoses

- **Radiolucent calculi.** Radiolucent stones can cause filling defects in the collecting system. Uric acid and xanthine stones occur in patients with malignancy on chemotherapy (marked cytolysis) and in gout. Other radiolucent stones include matrix (protein) and indinavir stones. Cystine stones may be faintly radiopaque.
- **Extrinsic compression.** Pelvic masses may cause extrinsic impression on the bladder, which can simulate an intraluminal

filling defect on intravenous urogram (IVU). Common causes include retroperitoneal adenopathy, metastatic disease, or direct extension of a pelvic neoplasm (cervical, prostate, colon, uterine). More benign pelvic masses such as ovarian cysts or abscesses may also produce similar findings. Cross-sectional imaging can usually distinguish a primary bladder mass from extrinsic compression.

■ Diagnosis

Transitional cell carcinoma

✓ Pearls

- TCC is the most common of urothelial tumors; the bladder is the most common site involved.
- Adenocarcinoma occurs within urachal remnants; SCC occurs with chronic inflammation.

- Mobile filling defects within the bladder may be due to fungal infection, blood clot, or stones.
- Candida is the most common fungus to involve the renal collecting system.

Suggested Readings

Raman SP, Fishman EK. Bladder malignancies on CT: the underrated role of CT in diagnosis. AJR Am J Roentgenol. 2014; 203(2):347–354

Wong-You-Cheong JJ, Woodward PJ, Manning MA, Sesterhenn IA. From the Archives of the AFIP: neoplasms of the urinary bladder: radiologic-pathologic correlation. Radiographics. 2006; 26(2):553–580

Case 71

Paul B. DiDomenico

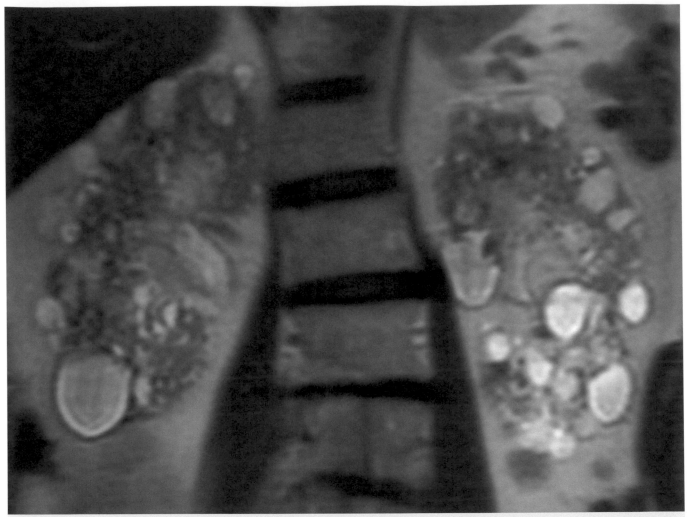

Fig. 71.1 Coronal T2 MR image shows numerous bilateral renal cysts of various sizes and with varying signal intensities, suggesting proteinaceous debris in portions of the cysts. The kidneys are enlarged. *Image courtesy of Dell Dunn, MD.*

■ Clinical Presentation

A 61-year-old man with renal failure (▶Fig. 71.1).

■ Key Imaging Finding

Bilateral renal cysts

■ Top 3 Differential Diagnoses

- **Autosomal dominant polycystic kidney disease (ADPKD).** The presence of multiple bilateral renal cysts of varying size suggests the diagnosis of ADPKD. The kidneys are usually massively enlarged in later stages of the disease, and patients may present with flank pain from mass effect. Cysts of other abdominal organs often coexist, with up to 75% of patients having simple cysts in the liver. Less commonly, there may be cysts in the pancreas, spleen, adnexa, or lungs, and up to 15% of patients will have aneurysms of the cerebral arteries. ADPKD does not confer an increased risk of malignancy (renal cell carcinoma [RCC]) until after initiation of dialysis.
- **End-stage renal disease (hemodialysis).** Patients with chronic renal failure may develop multiple bilateral renal cysts in the setting of hemodialysis. Usually, the kidneys will be relatively atrophic, and extrarenal cysts do not occur as a consequence of this disease, but may be present because of other causes. It is important to be aware that up to 7% of hemodialysis patients will develop RCC, although these cancers have low metastatic potential.
- **von Hippel–Lindau disease (VHL).** VHL disease causes cysts in multiple abdominal organs, including bilateral renal cysts in 75% of cases; however, there is a higher propensity (50%) for coexisting pancreatic cysts as compared to ADPKD. Additionally, up to 40% of patients with VHL develop RCCs and 15% develop pheochromocytomas. Many other neoplasms may be present as well, including cerebellar and spinal hemangioblastomas, retinal angiomas, hepatic adenomas, pancreatic islet cell tumors, and cystadenomas of the epididymis.

■ Additional Differential Diagnoses

- **Tuberous sclerosis.** Renal involvement of tuberous sclerosis is classically described as bilateral angiomyolipomas (AMLs); however, bilateral renal cysts without AMLs have been described in children with this disease. The well-known "clinical triad" presentation includes adenoma sebaceum, seizures, and mental retardation. Imaging findings include subcortical and periventricular calcified hamartomas, subependymal giant cell astrocytomas at the foramen of Monro, pulmonary lymphangiomyomatosis with chylous effusions, cardiac rhabdomyomas, and skeletal osteomas.

■ Diagnosis

Autosomal dominant polycystic kidney disease

✓ Pearls

- ADPCKD patients are at increased risk for RCC after initiation of dialysis.
- Acquired cystic renal disease in chronic renal failure results in small kidneys.
- Renal lesions associated with VHL include renal cysts and RCC.
- Tuberous sclerosis may present with multiple renal cysts or AMLs.

Suggested Readings

Wood CG, III, Stromberg LJ, III, Harmath CB, et al. CT and MR imaging for evaluation of cystic renal lesions and diseases. Radiographics. 2015; 35(1):125–141

Case 72

Todd M. Johnson

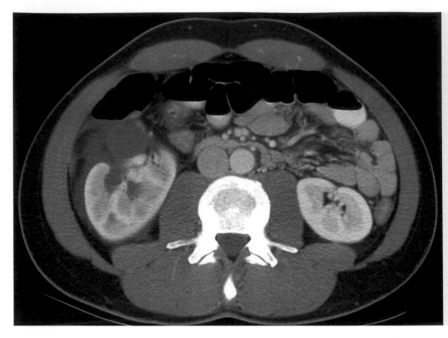

Fig. 72.1 Intravenous and oral contrast-enhanced axial CT image through the level of the kidneys demonstrates fluid and fat stranding within the right perinephric space. There is asymmetric enlargement of the right kidney.

■ Clinical Presentation

A 37-year-old man with right flank pain (▶Fig. 72.1).

■ Key Imaging Finding

Perinephric fluid collection

■ Top 3 Differential Diagnoses

- **Perinephric hemorrhage**. Blunt or penetrating abdominal trauma may result in renal laceration that may be associated with perinephric hemorrhage. Iatrogenic perinephric hemorrhage may occur in the setting of biopsy or following extracorporeal shock wave lithotripsy for nephrolithiasis. Traumatic laceration is graded based on size and severity utilizing the American Association for the Surgery of Trauma (AAST) scale (extension into the renal pelvis and vascular injury upgrade the staging). In the absence of known trauma, follow-up imaging is required to evaluate for underlying malignancy, to exclude renal cell carcinoma (RCC) and angiomyolipoma (AML). RCC is the most common primary renal malignancy, is hypervascular, and is prone to hemorrhage. AMLs have abnormal networks of vasculature and associated aneurysms, which may hemorrhage, especially when large (>4 cm).
- **Urine leak/urinary extravasation**. A urine leak or urinary extravasation may occur in the setting of trauma or obstruction. Trauma can result in lacerations which extend into the renal collecting system or avulsion of the ureteropelvic junction (UPJ). In either case, urine will collect in the perinephric space and other retroperitoneal compartments. To differentiate from hemorrhage, delayed imaging should be performed in the excretory phase (5-minute delay). Percutaneous nephrostomy or ureteral stent placement may be necessary to divert urine and prevent urinoma formation. Obstruction from a ureteral or UPJ stone may result in significantly increased intraluminal pressures within the collecting system. Secondary findings include an identifiable cause of obstruction (stone or mass), renal enlargement, or a delayed nephrogram. The weakest portion of the collecting system that is prone to rupture is the forniceal region of the calyx. Spontaneous rupture of the collecting system with forniceal rupture may result in reduction or alleviation of the patient's flank pain.
- **Pyelonephritis/perinephric infection**. Perinephric infection and inflammatory changes are most commonly the result of pyelonephritis. Secondary findings to suggest pyelonephritis include renal enlargement and a striated nephrogram. Complications of pyelonephritis (such as renal abscess) may extend into the perinephric space or into the ipsilateral psoas muscle. The presence of urinary obstruction and secondary infection is a urologic emergency and is often treated with computed tomography (CT)-guided percutaneous nephrostomy. Additionally, infectious processes of adjacent structures, such as the colon or pancreas, can extend into the fat of the perinephric and pararenal spaces.

■ Diagnosis

Urinary leak (forniceal rupture from obstructed ureter)

✓ Pearls

- A renal laceration extending into the collecting system is best evaluated with delayed imaging.
- Perinephric hemorrhage without trauma requires follow-up imaging to exclude underlying malignancy.
- Urine extravasation may result from trauma or forniceal rupture from urinary obstruction.
- Perinephric infectious or inflammatory fat stranding is most often due to pyelonephritis.

Suggested Readings

Westphalen A, Yeh B, Qayyum A, Hari A, Coakley FV. Differential diagnosis of perinephric masses on CT and MRI. AJR Am J Roentgenol. 2004; 183(6):1697–1702

Case 73

Charles A. Tujo

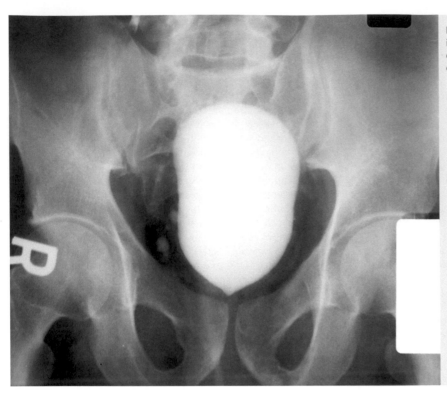

Fig. 73.1 Frontal view of the pelvis from an intravenous pyelogram (IVP) demonstrates elongation of the bladder with a "pear-shaped" configuration.

■ Clinical Presentation

A 45-year-old man with abdominal and pelvic fullness (▶Fig. 73.1).

■ Key Imaging Finding

Pear-shaped bladder

■ Top 3 Differential Diagnoses

- **Pelvic hematoma.** Bladder wall compression from hemorrhage within the pelvis usually results from blunt trauma, laceration of the internal iliac artery, or following surgery (i.e., prostatectomy). Mass effect usually is a bilateral, symmetric process on the bladder walls; the bladder base may be elevated. There may also be medial deviation of the ureters. In the setting of trauma, pelvic fractures and/or pubic diastasis are commonly associated findings.
- **Lymphadenopathy.** If massive, pelvic lymphadenopathy may compress the bladder and result in a pear-shape. The most common etiology in this setting would be non-Hodgkin lymphoma; however, metastatic disease from a local primary neoplasm, such as uterine, cervical, and carcinoma, is another consideration.
- **Pelvic lipomatosis.** A rare process primarily seen in overweight African American males, pelvic lipomatosis is the proliferation of nonencapsulated fat in the perivesical and perirectal space of the pelvis. Mass effect on the urinary bladder may result in an inverted pear-shaped bladder. The ureters may be symmetrically displaced medially, with up to 40% of patients developing urinary obstruction. Compression of the rectum occurs with elevation of the rectosigmoid junction on barium enema and can result in symptoms of constipation. Pelvic lipomatosis is associated with cystitis glandularis.

■ Additional Differential Diagnoses

- **Psoas hypertrophy.** Psoas muscle hypertrophy is a rare cause of symmetric bladder narrowing that could result in a pear-shaped bladder. It occurs more commonly in high-performance athletes and weightlifters with a narrow bony pelvis. Bilateral medial deviation of the ureters may also be seen. Enlarged psoas muscles are best appreciated on cross-sectional imaging. The renal axis may also be altered and the midureters may demonstrate an abrupt transition over the psoas muscle.
- **Iliac artery aneurysms.** Commonly found in patients with underlying atherosclerotic vascular disease and abdominal aortic aneurysms, large bilateral iliac artery aneurysms may result in a pear-shaped bladder. Ectasia and minimal aneurismal dilation are fairly common; however, the size necessary to produce compression of the bladder walls makes this a relatively rare etiology.

■ Diagnosis

Pelvic lipomatosis

✓ Pearls

- Pelvic hematomas may result from blunt trauma (look for pelvic fractures) or surgical complications.
- Pelvic lymphadenopathy is most often due to non-Hodgkin lymphoma; metastatic disease is less common.
- Pelvic lipomatosis is a benign proliferation of fat in the pelvis that compresses the bladder and rectum.

Suggested Readings

Dyer RB, Chen MY, Zagoria RJ. Intravenous urography: technique and interpretation. Radiographics. 2001; 21(4):799–821, discussion 822–824

Dyer RB, Chen MY, Zagoria RJ. Classic signs in uroradiology. Radiographics. 2004; 24(Suppl 1):S247–S280

Torigian DA, Siegelman ES. CT findings of pelvic lipomatosis of nerve. AJR Am J Roentgenol. 2005; 184(3, Suppl):S94–S96

Case 74

Todd M. Johnson

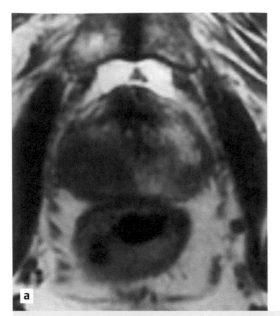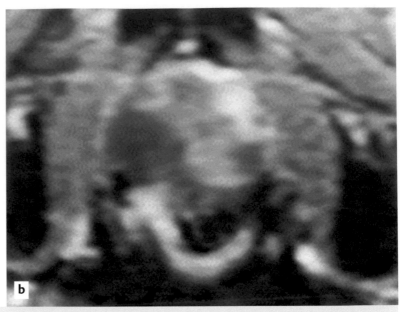

Fig. 74.1 (a) Axial T2 MR image through the prostate gland demonstrates large right and small left regions of hypointensity within the peripheral zone of the prostate gland. The lesion on the right has broad contact and bulges the prostate margin, consistent with extraprostatic extension. (b) Apparent diffusion coefficient (ADC) map demonstrates corresponding low values within the lesions. *Images courtesy of Dell Dunn, MD.*

■ Clinical Presentation

A 67-year-old man with elevated prostate-specific antigen (PSA) (▶ Fig. 74.1).

■ Key Imaging Finding

Prostate enlargement

■ Top 3 Differential Diagnoses

- **Prostate adenocarcinoma.** Prostate adenocarcinoma is second only to lung cancer as a cause of cancer-related death in males. It most frequently occurs in the peripheral zone of the prostate. On T2 magnetic resonance imaging (MRI) sequences, prostate cancer is hypointense to the typically hyperintense peripheral zone. Important MRI findings include invasion of the neurovascular bundle or seminal vesicles. Computed tomography (CT) cannot differentiate prostate cancer from normal peripheral zone tissue, but may detect gross extracapsular spread. Signs of extracapsular spread include obliteration of the periprostatic fat plane, lymphadenopathy, and invasion of adjacent structures, such as the urinary bladder or rectum. Microinvasion of the capsule is beyond the resolution of both MRI and CT. Many centers utilized advanced imaging with diffusion-weighted (restricted diffusion commonly seen in prostate cancer) and dynamic contrast-enhanced sequences, as well as spectroscopy, in the evaluation for prostate cancer. Hematogenous spread via the internal iliac veins and vertebral venous plexus results in osteoblastic metastases, readily detectable by bone scan.

- **Benign prostatic hypertrophy (BPH).** BPH is benign hypertrophy of the transitional zone of the prostate gland. Beyond the age of 50 years, nearly half of men will be affected by some degree of hypertrophy. Cross-sectional imaging can demonstrate prostate size. With intravenous urography (IVU), the effects of prostate enlargement on the bladder can be demonstrated. Bladder base elevation and a characteristic J-shaped appearance of the distal ureters may occur. With increasing outlet obstruction, poor bladder emptying with increased postvoid residual volume and bladder wall trabeculation with or without diverticula may be evident.
- **Prostatitis.** Prostatitis is an inflammatory condition of the prostate, which in the acute setting is most commonly a retrograde bacterial infection due to *Escherichia coli*. Enlargement of the prostate can occur, although this is not a specific finding. Chronic prostatitis also has nonspecific findings that may be indistinguishable from BPH and prostate carcinoma. Contrast-enhanced CT can be useful in the detection of prostatic abscess. Transrectal ultrasound-guided aspiration of a suspected prostatic abscess can help confirm the diagnosis.

■ Diagnosis

Prostate adenocarcinoma

✓ Pearls

- Prostate adenocarcinoma occurs in the peripheral zone and is hypointense on T2 sequences.
- An important prognostic factor in prostate adenocarcinoma is the presence of extracapsular spread.

- BPH is very common in older men and involves the transitional zone.
- Prostatitis is often secondary to a retrograde bacterial infection, most commonly *E. coli*.

Suggested Readings

de Rooij M, Hamoen EH, Fütterer JJ, Barentsz JO, Rovers MM. Accuracy of multiparametric MRI for prostate cancer detection: a meta-analysis. AJR Am J Roentgenol. 2014; 202(2):343–351

Oto A, Kayhan A, Jiang Y, et al. Prostate cancer: differentiation of central gland cancer from benign prostatic hyperplasia by using diffusion-weighted and dynamic contrast-enhanced MR imaging. Radiology. 2010; 257(3):715–723

Tan N, Margolis DJ, Lu DY, et al. Characteristics of detected and missed prostate cancer foci on 3-T multiparametric MRI using an endorectal coil correlated with whole-mount thin-section histopathology. AJR Am J Roentgenol. 2015; 205(1):W87–92

Case 75

Charles A. Tujo

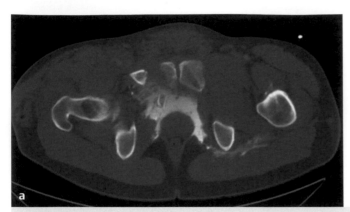 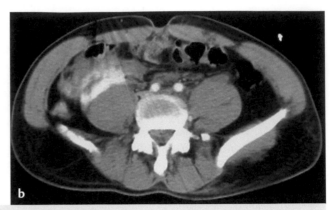

Fig. 75.1 **(a)** Axial CT image through the pelvis in bone window after retrograde filling of the bladder with contrast reveals extraperitoneal contrast within both the prevesical space and tracking along the left posterior thigh. There are multiple associated pelvic fractures. **(b)** Contrast-enhanced axial CT image through the upper pelvis in soft-tissue window demonstrates intraperitoneal contrast interposed between bowel loops in the right lower quadrant and layering along the paracolic gutter.

■ **Clinical Presentation**

Motor vehicle accident (▸Fig. 75.1).

■ Key Imaging Finding

Bladder rupture

■ Top 3 Differential Diagnoses

- **Extraperitoneal bladder rupture.** Extraperitoneal bladder rupture is more common than intraperitoneal (80–90% of cases) and is usually associated with pelvic fractures. Contrast from retrograde bladder filling (cystography) will accumulate in the perivesical and prevesical space, as well as the scrotum and thigh. A "Christmas tree" or "molar tooth" appearance of contrast can be seen with sharp or irregular margins. Management is typically nonsurgical with catheter placement and bladder decompression
- **Intraperitoneal bladder rupture.** Intraperitoneal bladder rupture is commonly associated with blunt trauma, typically with a full bladder. It can also occur spontaneously, which is more common with an underlying bladder process such as tumor, cystitis, and neurogenic bladder. Extravasated contrast

may be seen in the paracolic gutters, rectovesical/rectouterine pouch, or outlining bowel loops. This is readily seen on a computed tomography (CT) cystogram, where bowel loops are surrounded with contrast. Since the extravasated urine layers in larger spaces than the bladder and in smaller amounts, it can appear less dense since it is relatively more diluted. It is important to make the distinction between intraperitoneal and extraperitoneal bladder rupture, as intraperitoneal rupture is typically managed surgically.
- **Intra- and extraperitoneal bladder rupture.** Combined intraperitoneal and extraperitoneal bladder rupture occurs in 5 to 12% of cases of bladder injuries. Both patterns of injury listed above may be seen.

■ Additional Differential Diagnoses

- **Urethral injury.** More commonly seen in males, urethral injuries are classified by anatomic location, posterior versus anterior. Posterior urethral injuries can result in extravasation of contrast in the retropubic extraperitoneal space or perineum, which may mimic bladder rupture. If the bladder cannot be

filled retrograde, the injury to the urethra is complete. Anterior urethral injuries should not be confused with extraperitoneal bladder rupture, as extravasation during retrograde filling collects in the corpus spongiosum.

■ Diagnosis

Intra- and extraperitoneal bladder rupture

✓ Pearls

- Extraperitoneal bladder rupture is the most common type and is associated with pelvic fractures.
- Intraperitoneal bladder rupture is usually due to blunt trauma with a full bladder and treated surgically.

- Bladder rupture may also be spontaneous or iatrogenic.
- Despite a negative CT, cystography (CT or conventional) must be performed to exclude a suspected injury.

Suggested Readings

Gross JS, Rotenberg S, Horrow MM. Resident and fellow education feature. Bladder injury: types, mechanisms, and diagnostic imaging. Radiographics. 2014; 34(3):802–803

Morgan DE, Nallamala LK, Kenney PJ, Mayo MS, Rue LW, III. CT cystography: radiographic and clinical predictors of bladder rupture. AJR Am J Roentgenol. 2000; 174(1):89–95

Case 76

Michael Kuo

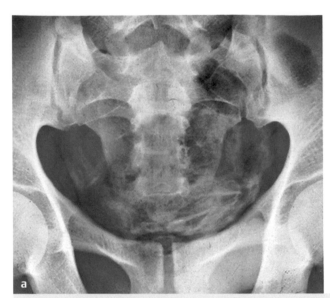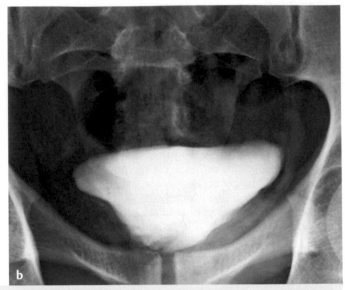

Fig. 76.1 **(a)** Frontal radiograph of the pelvis shows curvilinear calcifications within the pelvis. **(b)** Delayed intravenous urogram (IVU) centered over the pelvis shows portions of the calcification to be just superficial to the contrast-filled urinary bladder lumen.

■ **Clinical Presentation**

A 21-year-old man with history of dysuria (▶ Fig. 76.1).

■ Key Imaging Finding

Bladder wall calcifications

■ Top 3 Differential Diagnoses

- **Transitional cell carcinoma (TCC)**. TCC comprises 90 to 95% of epithelial bladder carcinomas and may show punctate, linear, or central calcifications. The most common presenting sign is painless hematuria, typically occurring in patients 50 to 60 years of age with a 4:1 male predominance. The bladder is the most common site of involvement, involved in 90% of cases of TCC. The renal pelvis, ureters, and proximal two-thirds of the urethra make up the remaining cases. The entire urothelium must be examined with follow-up imaging because of increased risk for synchronous or metachronous TCC.
- **Schistosomiasis**. Schistosomiasis is an infectious cause of cystitis and is the most common cause of bladder wall calcifica-tion worldwide. The parasite deposits ova within the bladder submucosa, which causes an inflammatory response. Mural calcifications may develop afterwards. Complications of schistosomiasis include bladder carcinoma, especially squamous cell carcinoma.
- **Cystitis**. Noninfectious causes of cystitis include cyclophosphamide-induced hemorrhagic cystitis and radiation-induced cystitis, both of which may also cause bladder wall calcification. Complications of chronic cystitis include hyperplastic uroepithelial cell clusters, which may led to cystitis cystica and cystitis glandularis.

■ Additional Differential Diagnoses

- **Tuberculosis (TB)**. TB of the urinary bladder is almost always secondary to TB infection of the kidney. End-stage disease causes bladder fibrosis, diminishing the capacity of the urinary bladder. Bladder wall calcifications are relatively uncommon. Complications include fistulae or sinus tract formation but are rare findings.
- **Urachal carcinoma**. Urachal carcinomas are adenocarcinomas (90%) that commonly calcify (70%). Fine punctuate calci-fications within a tumor on computed tomography (CT) may suggest mucinous adenocarcinoma. These arise from urachal remnants and are clinically silent until the bladder dome is invaded. Patients are typically between 40 and 70 years of age with a 3:1 male predominance, presenting with hematuria and/or mucoid discharge. Five-year survival is poor.

■ Diagnosis

Schistosomiasis

✓ Pearls

- TCC most often involves the bladder (90% of cases) and may have calcifications.
- Schistosomiasis is the most common cause of bladder wall calcification worldwide.
- Cystitis from infectious etiologies (TB), chemotherapy, or radiation may cause bladder wall calcifications.
- Urachal carcinomas are usually adenocarcinoma, which commonly calcify.

Suggested Readings

Dyer RB, Chen MYM, Zagoria RJ. Abnormal calcifications in the urinary tract. Radiographics. 1998; 18(6):1405–1424

Case 77

Todd M. Johnson

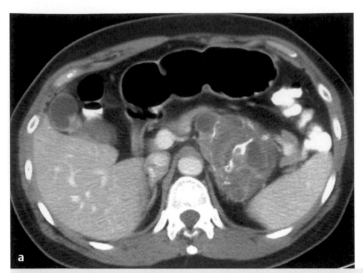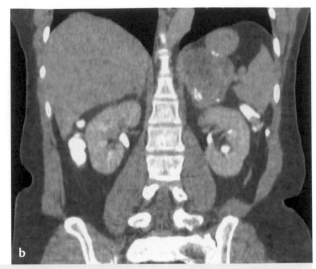

Fig. 77.1 Contrast-enhanced **(a)** axial and **(b)** coronal CT images demonstrate a large heterogeneously enhancing left adrenal mass with central cystic regions and irregular eccentric calcifications.

■ Clinical Presentation

History withheld (▶Fig. 77.1).

■ Key Imaging Finding

Adrenal mass

■ Top 3 Differential Diagnoses

- **Adrenal adenoma.** Adrenal adenomas are the most common adrenal tumors, occurring in nearly 10% of the population. The majority are small (<2 cm), circumscribed, and have low attenuation (<10 HU). Up to one-third can be lipid poor, requiring additional imaging such as enhancement washout (>40% relative or >60% absolute) or magnetic resonance (MR) noncontrast chemical shift imaging (signal loss in adenomas on opposed phase).
- **Metastases.** The adrenal glands are a common site for metastatic disease. Metastases may present as unilateral or bilateral, small or large, adrenal masses of soft-tissue density. MR appearance is usually hypointense on T1 and relatively hyperintense on T2. If complicated by hemorrhage or necrosis, they may have a heterogeneous appearance and irregular enhancement.
- **Hemorrhage.** Adrenal hemorrhage may be traumatic or nontraumatic. Nontraumatic etiologies include coagulopathy, stress (neonatal, surgery, sepsis, hypotension), and underlying mass. Hemorrhage may be unilateral or bilateral. Enlargement of the gland initially occurs with increased density in the acute to subacute phase; over time, the lesions decrease in size and attenuation and may develop calcifications.

■ Additional Differential Diagnoses

- **Pheochromocytoma.** Pheochromocytomas are rare tumors derived from chromaffin cells in the adrenal medulla. Patients can present with hypertension because of excess catecholamine secretion. Lesions can have variable imaging features depending on the degree of hemorrhage and necrosis. Classic imaging findings include avid contrast enhancement and marked hyperintensity on T2-weighted imaging. They typically demonstrate increased activity on I-131 meta-iodobenzylguanidine (MIBG) or In-111 Octreoscan nuclear scintigraphy.
- **Adrenal myelolipoma.** Myelolipomas are uncommon benign neoplasms that contain both hematopoietic and fat tissue. The fatty component is low density on computed tomography (CT; -30 to -90 HU) and hyperintense on T1-weighted imaging with signal loss on fat-suppressed sequences. Larger lesions may spontaneously hemorrhage.
- **Adrenocortical carcinoma.** Adrenocortical carcinoma is a rare tumor that is usually unilateral, nonfunctioning, and large at presentation (5–20 cm). Imaging features can be heterogeneous because of hemorrhage and necrosis, with variable degrees of enhancement. Calcifications are seen in up to 30% of cases. Metastatic disease is found in 20% of patients at presentation.

■ Diagnosis

Adrenocortical carcinoma

✓ Pearls

- Adrenal adenomas are the most common adrenal tumor and are classically of low attenuation on CT (<10 HU).
- Metastases are the second most common adrenal tumor and appear as soft-tissue lesions.
- Adrenal hemorrhage is most common in children.
- Pheochromocytomas are classically "light-bulb" bright on T2-weighted MR sequences.

Suggested Readings

Elsayes KM, Mukundan G, Narra VR, et al. Adrenal masses: MR imaging features with pathologic correlation. Radiographics. 2004; 24(Suppl 1):S73–S86

Kim YK, Park BK, Kim CK, Park SY. Adenoma characterization: adrenal protocol with dual-energy CT. Radiology. 2013; 267(1):155–163

Case 78

Todd M. Johnson

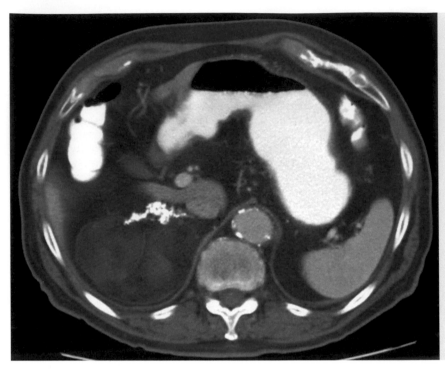

Fig. 78.1 Contrast-enhanced axial CT image through the upper abdomen demonstrates a large fat-containing retroperitoneal mass with soft-tissue elements and calcifications anteriorly.

■ Clinical Presentation

A 42-year-old man with vague right upper quadrant pain (▶Fig. 78.1).

■ Key Imaging Finding

Fatty retroperitoneal mass

■ Top 3 Differential Diagnoses

- **Renal angiomyolipoma (AML).** AML is a benign tumor of the kidney composed of vascular elements, smooth muscle, and adipose tissue. Gross fat (-30 to -90 HU) in a renal lesion is virtually diagnostic of AML, especially in the absence of calcification. Although there is no malignant potential, lesions composed predominately of vascular elements and smooth muscle can show significant enhancement, and are indistinguishable from renal cell carcinoma (RCC) by imaging. This slow-growing tumor is at risk for hemorrhage because of abnormal vessels and aneurysm formation, especially when the size is > 4 cm.
- **Adrenal myelolipoma.** Adrenal myelolipomas are rare benign tumors composed of variable amounts of adipose tissue and hematopoietic elements. On computed tomography (CT) imaging, a circumscribed heterogeneous lesion with fat density is characteristic. A small portion will have calcifications, especially if complicated by hemorrhage. Although patients are usually asymptomatic, spontaneous hemorrhage may occur in large lesions. When large, they may be difficult to distinguish from retroperitoneal liposarcomas.
- **Retroperitoneal liposarcoma.** Liposarcoma is the most common primary malignant lesion of the retroperitoneum. It originates from adipose tissue, usually located in the peri/paranephric space. CT imaging will reveal a fat and soft-tissue attenuation mass with heterogeneous enhancement. Lesions are usually large at the time of diagnosis, with displacement of adjacent structures.

■ Additional Differential Diagnoses

- **Renal cell carcinoma.** RCC has rarely been reported to contain macroscopic fat, which can represent engulfed fat. A de-differentiated RCC can have both calcification and fat. There should be a high suspicion for RCC if a fat density renal lesion contains calcifications.

■ Diagnosis

Adrenal myelolipoma (complicated by prior hemorrhage)

✓ Pearls

- Gross fat in a renal lesion is virtually diagnostic of AML in the absence of calcification.
- Adrenal myelolipomas consist of gross fat and hematopoietic elements; calcifications may be present.
- Liposarcoma is the most common retroperitoneal sarcoma; it contains gross fat and is typically large.
- Calcification within a fat-containing renal lesion should raise the suspicion for de-differentiated RCC.

Suggested Readings

Behranwala KA, Chettiar K, El-Bahrawy M, Stamp G, Kakkar AK. Retroperitoneal myolipoma. World J Surg Oncol. 2005; 3:72

Kim EY, Kim SJ, Choi D, et al. Recurrence of retroperitoneal liposarcoma: imaging findings and growth rates at follow-up CT. AJR Am J Roentgenol. 2008; 191(6):1841–1846

Case 79

Todd M. Johnson

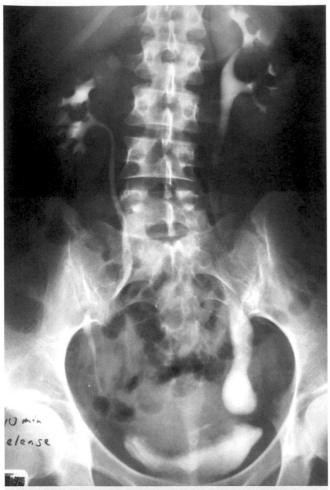

Fig. 79.1 Frontal projection from an IV urogram (IVU) demonstrates isolated dilatation of the distal left ureter with a normal-caliber proximal ureter, renal pelvis, and calyces.

■ Clinical Presentation

History withheld (▶Fig. 79.1).

■ Key Imaging Finding

Dilated ureter

■ Top 3 Differential Diagnoses

- **Ureteral obstruction**. Ureteral obstruction can result from stones, strictures, neoplasm, or extrinsic compression. Ureteral calculi may be radiopaque (most commonly calcium oxalate) or nonradiopaque (uric acid, xanthine, matrix, protease inhibitor). Strictures can result from prior infection/inflammation, instrumentation, or surgery. Transitional cell carcinoma, the most common primary neoplasm of the ureter, can present as a stricture on intravenous urogram (IVU). Pelvic neoplasms (ovarian, uterine, cervical, or colonic) can cause obstruction from mass effect and extrinsic compression, or from direct extension.
- **Reflux**. Vesicoureteral reflux is the abnormal flow of urine from the bladder into the upper urinary collecting system. Typically, it is the result of a short distal ureteral submucosal tunnel within the bladder wall, which normally serves as a valve mechanism. Reflux can be graded according to severity on voiding cystourethrogram (VCUG) (Grade I: ureter only; II: ureter, renal pelvis, and calyces; III: ureter and renal pelvis mildly dilated and calyces mildly blunted; IV: ureter and renal pelvis moderately dilated and calyces moderately blunted; and

V: gross dilatation and tortuosity of the ureter, severely dilated renal pelvis, and severely blunted calyces with loss of papillary impression). Nuclear cystography can be used for initial screening in females and as a follow-up study in both males and females with the benefit of lower patient radiation. VCUG is the initial study in males to evaluate the posterior urethra and exclude posterior urethral valves.
- **Primary megaureter**. Megaureter describes an enlarged ureter which may or may not have associated dilatation of the upper collecting system (megacalycosis). Primary megaureter can be classified into one of three categories: nonrefluxing and unobstructed (most common), obstructing, and refluxing. Nonrefluxing, unobstructed megaureter is idiopathic, and has neither reflux nor stenosis at the ureterovesical junction. The obstructing variant of primary megaureter has ureteral dilatation above a focal segment of normal caliber but aperistaltic juxtavesical ureter. It is thought that abnormal collagen deposition between muscle cells is a contributing cause of the aperistaltic segment. The refluxing variant of primary megaureter is a result of a short or absent intravesical ureter.

■ Additional Differential Diagnoses

- **Prune belly syndrome**. Prune belly syndrome is named after the appearance of the abdomen, which is wrinkled because of lack of the rectus muscles. It occurs almost exclusively in males. Urinary tract abnormalities include dilated tortuous ureters (with renal dysmorphism) and a megalocystic, dilated

prostatic urethra. The bladder is usually enlarged, and a majority of patients have vesicoureteral reflux. Additionally, the testicles are undescended and nonpalpable. Other abnormalities of the pulmonary, gastrointestinal, skeletal, and cardiac systems may be present.

■ Diagnosis

Primary megaureter

✓ Pearls

- Ureteral obstruction is most commonly due to renal calculi but may also be due to stricture or neoplasm.
- Fluoroscopic VCUG is used as the initial study to evaluate for reflux in males.

- Nuclear cystography minimizes patient dose for reflux studies in females or follow-up studies in males.
- Most cases of primary megaureter are of the nonrefluxing, unobstructed type.

Suggested Readings

Berrocal T, López-Pereira P, Arjonilla A, Gutiérrez J. Anomalies of the distal ureter, bladder, and urethra in children: embryologic, radiologic, and pathologic features. Radiographics. 2002; 22(5):1139–1164

Lebowitz RL, Olbing H, Parkkulainen KV, Smellie JM, Tamminen-Möbius TE; International Reflux Study in Children. International system of radiographic grading of vesicoureteric reflux. Pediatr Radiol. 1985; 15(2):105–109

Case 80

Todd M. Johnson

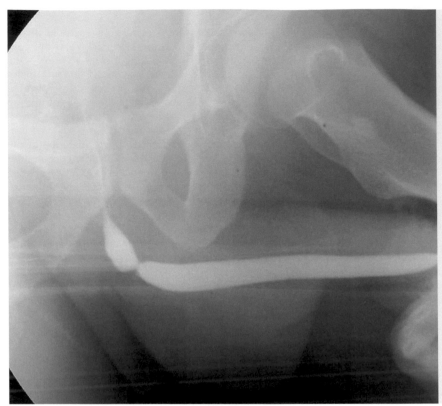

Fig. 80.1 Retrograde urethrogram demonstrates a focal stricture within the bulbous urethra.

■ Clinical Presentation

A 45-year-old man with history of urethritis (▶Fig. 80.1).

■ Key Imaging Finding

Urethral stricture

■ Top 3 Differential Diagnoses

- **Urethral trauma**. Straddle injury is one of the most common external causes of posttraumatic urethral stricture, usually involving the bulbous portion. Instrument-related iatrogenic strictures typically occur at the bulbomembranous urethra and penoscrotal junction. Posterior urethral strictures are usually a result of disruption from trauma (high-speed MVA with pelvic fractures) or surgery (transurethral prostate resection, radical prostatectomy). Retrograde urethrography is primarily used to diagnose anterior strictures, while simultaneous retrograde urethrography and antegrade cystourethrography help depict the length of posterior urethral strictures.
- **Postinfectious/postinflammatory stricture**. Gonococcal urethritis is one of the leading reportable sexually transmittable diseases in the United States. Nongonococcal urethritis is attributable to *Chlamydia trachomatis* in 30 to 50% of cases. Up to 15% of males with gonococcal urethritis will develop a stricture, typically in the distal bulbous urethra. It is thought that scars in this region occur because of the preponderance of Littré's glands; dilation of Littré's glands may also be seen

at urethrography. If urethrography demonstrates a narrowed, elongated, irregular, or asymmetric proximal bulbous urethra, there is a high association with stricture extension into the membranous urethra. Involvement of the membranous urethra is important for the urologist because of the location of the distal urethral sphincter; transection of this sphincter can result in iatrogenic urinary incontinence.
- **Urethral carcinoma**. Malignant tumors of the urethra are uncommon, and usually occur in individuals older than 50 years. Squamous cell carcinoma comprises the majority (>80%) of malignant tumors, involving the bulbomembranous urethra in 60% and the penile urethra in 30% of cases. Strictures from urethral carcinoma can be demonstrated on urethrography as a focal irregular narrowing; urethral fistulas and periurethral abscess may also develop. On magnetic resonance imaging (MRI), urethral carcinomas are typically low signal intensity masses relative to the normal corporal tissue on T1- and T2-weighted sequences.

■ Diagnosis

Postinfectious stricture (gonococcal urethritis)

✓ Pearls

- Posttraumatic strictures commonly occur at the bulbomembranous urethra or penoscrotal junction.
- Postinfectious/inflammatory urethral strictures typically involve the bulbous urethra.

- Strictures of the membranous urethra have surgical implications because of the location of the distal sphincter.
- Squamous cell carcinoma is the most common urethral neoplasm; it typically occurs in older males.

Suggested Readings

Kawashima A, Sandler CM, Wasserman NF, LeRoy AJ, King BF, Jr, Goldman SM. Imaging of urethral disease: a pictorial review. Radiographics. 2004; 24(Suppl 1):S195–S216

Part 4

Musculoskeletal Imaging

4

Case 81

Eva Escobedo

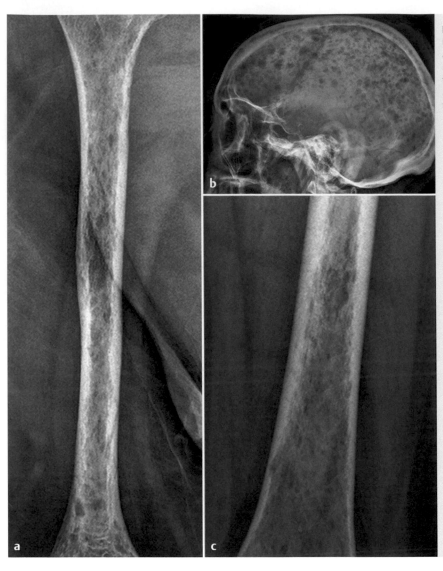

Fig. 81.1 **(a)** Anteroposterior (AP) view of the right humerus shows punched-out lytic lesions of shaft and endosteal scalloping. **(b)** Lateral view of skull reveals similar multiple lytic lesions. **(c)** AP view of the left distal femur shows punched-out lesions and focal erosion of the endosteal surface, which is typical of an intramedullary process.

■ Clinical Presentation

A 68-year-old woman with diffuse bone pain (▶Fig. 81.1).

■ Key Imaging Finding

Multiple lytic bony lesions

■ Top 3 Differential Diagnoses in an Adult

- **Metastases**. Bone metastases can be either well or poorly defined, and may be difficult to distinguish from multiple myeloma. Purely osteolytic lesions originate from primary thyroid, renal, uterine, head and neck, and gastrointestinal sources. Metastases arising from thyroid and renal primaries may produce bone expansion. Mixed osteolytic/osteosclerotic lesions may arise from lung, breast, cervix, ovarian, and testicular malignancies.
- **Multiple myeloma**. Multiple myeloma, a plasma cell dyscrasia, is the most common primary bone malignancy in adults. The predominant pattern of bone involvement is osteolysis and most commonly occurs at multiple sites, but can be solitary (plasmacytoma). The axial skeleton is the typical site of involvement, but extensive disease will affect the extremities as well. The classic pattern of bone involvement is multiple discrete "punched-out" lesions. Subcortical erosions of the endosteum may cause a characteristic "scalloped" appearance. The mandible is more commonly involved than with metastasis.
- **Lymphoma**. Skeletal involvement can be seen in both Hodgkin and non-Hodgkin lymphoma. The most common manifestation of non-Hodgkin lymphoma is multiple osteolytic lesions with a moth-eaten or permeative pattern of bone destruction, sometimes with endosteal scalloping and cortical destruction. Osteosclerosis is more commonly seen in Hodgkin lymphoma. Soft-tissue masses are common and may be seen in the absence of significant cortical disruption.

■ Top 3 Differential Diagnoses in a Child

- **Langerhans cell histiocytosis (LCH)**. Bone lesions may be seen in any of the LCHs, but eosinophilic granuloma is the most common subtype and manifests as single or multiple bone lesions in children or young adults. In tubular bones, eosinophilic granuloma usually presents as a well-defined lucent lesion. As it enlarges, there may be associated periosteal reaction and cortical erosion. Characteristic imaging appearances include "beveled edges" (greater involvement of inner than outer table) and "button sequestrum" (lucency with central devascularized bone) in the skull and "vertebra plana" of the spine.
- **Fibrous dysplasia (FD)**. FD is a sporadic disease of bone-forming mesenchyme with abnormal osteoblastic differentiation. Normal bone is replaced by immature woven bone and fibrous stroma. Lesions may be solitary or multiple, are typically well defined, and may have a lucent or hazy ("ground-glass") matrix with sclerotic borders. They may be expansile and contain internal calcifications. Deformities may occur due to abnormal weakened bone or fractures. There is no associated periosteal reaction.
- **Chronic recurrent multifocal osteomyelitis (CRMO)**. CRMO is a self-limiting inflammatory disorder of children of unknown etiology. It affects predominately long bone metaphyses but can occur at any skeletal site. Although initially osteolytic, the hallmark is reactive sclerosis.

■ Diagnosis

Multiple myeloma

✓ Pearls

- Common osteolytic metastases include thyroid and renal malignancy; lung and breast may be mixed.
- The classic appearance of multiple myeloma is multiple discrete "punched-out" lytic lesions.
- Non-Hodgkin lymphoma commonly demonstrates a moth-eaten or permeative pattern of bone destruction.
- LCH results in calvarial lesions with "beveled edges" and "button sequestrum," as well as vertebra plana.

Suggested Readings

Angtuaco EJ, Fassas AB, Walker R, Sethi R, Barlogie B. Multiple myeloma: clinical review and diagnostic imaging. Radiology. 2004; 231(1):11–23

Resnick D. Diagnosis of Bone and Joint Disorders. 4th ed. Philadelphia, PA: WB Saunders; 2002

Case 82

Michael A. Tall

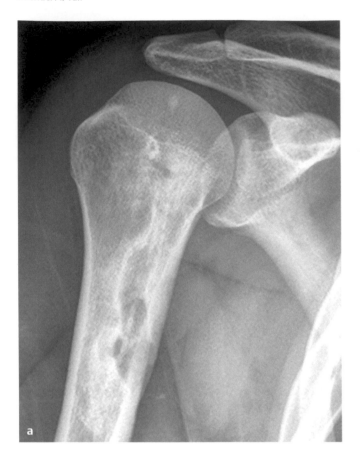
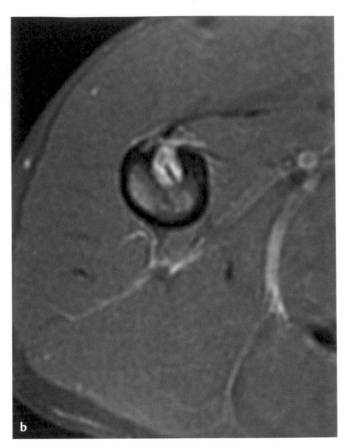
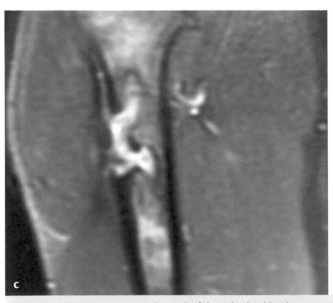

Fig. 82.1 **(a)** Anteroposterior radiograph of the right shoulder demonstrates an irregular lucency in the proximal humerus with a linear sclerotic density. **(b)** Axial and **(c)** sagittal contrast-enhanced fat-suppressed MR images through the proximal humerus show a centrally located, nonenhancing bony sequestrum surrounded by enhancing granulation tissue (involucrum). A cloaca is present, extending from the involucrum to the overlying cortex.

■ Clinical Presentation

A 23-year-old man with arm pain, swelling, and fevers (▶Fig. 82.1).

■ Key Imaging Finding

Sequestrum

■ Top 3 Differential Diagnoses

- **Osteomyelitis.** A sequestrum in the setting of osteomyelitis refers to a segment of dead, sclerotic bone that is separated from living bone by granulation tissue. The sequestrum may reside within the marrow and becomes a source of focal infection that can cause repeated flare-ups of acute osteomyelitis. A rim of living bone that surrounds the sequestrum is referred to as an involucrum. The involucrum may be permeated by a cloaca through which pus and the sequestrum itself may be expelled to the skin surface through a draining sinus tract.
- **Langerhans cell histiocytosis (LCH).** Eosinophilic granuloma is a subset of LCH that is characterized by multiple, predominantly lytic lesions throughout the axial and appendicular skeleton of children and young adults (<30 years of age). It accounts for approximately 70% of cases of LCH. Lesions within the long bones are characterized as lytic lesions with endosteal scalloping and occasionally periosteal reaction. Cranial involvement classically consists of a lytic lesion with beveled edges because of asymmetric involvement of the inner and outer tables. Lytic lesions of cranial vault sometimes contain a central radiodense fragment of bone, referred to as "button sequestrum."
- **Osteoid osteoma.** The classic radiographic findings in an osteoid osteoma include a centrally located oval or round radiolucent nidus surrounded by a uniform region of sclerotic bone. The central lucency is highly vascularized and is the target of surgical debridement or radiofrequency ablation. In 80% of cases, the nidus contains variable amounts of calcification. Common sites include the long bones of the lower extremities and spine. Adolescents and young adults often present with nighttime pain relieved by nonsteroidal anti-inflammatory drugs.

■ Additional Differential Diagnoses

- **Lymphoma.** Hodgkin and non-Hodgkin lymphoma can affect the bones in both primary and widespread multifocal disease. Primary non-Hodgkin lymphoma most commonly presents in the appendicular skeleton as an aggressive osteolytic lesion with poorly defined margins. Osteosclerosis, when evident, is more commonly found in Hodgkin disease, which can present with osteolytic lesions, osteosclerotic lesions, or a mixture of both. Sequestrum is more commonly seen in the Hodgkin variant.
- **Fibrosarcoma.** Fibrosarcomas are characterized by osteolytic foci with a geographic, moth-eaten, or permeative pattern of bone destruction. There is little osteosclerosis and a striking absence of a significant osseous reaction despite the underlying bone destruction. Occasionally, a sequestrum may be evident.

■ Diagnosis

Osteomyelitis

✓ Pearls

- Osteomyelitis may demonstrate a sequestrum surrounded by an involucrum and permeated by a cloaca.
- LCH results in lytic calvarial lesions with beveled edges and button sequestrum.

- Osteoid osteomas typically demonstrate a round or oval radiolucent nidus surrounded by sclerotic bone.
- The central nidus in osteoid osteoma is highly vascularized and is the target of radiofrequency ablation.

Suggested Readings

Jennin F, Bousson V, Parlier C, Jomaah N, Khanine V, Laredo JD. Bony sequestrum: a radiologic review. Skeletal Radiol. 2011; 40(8):963–975

Krasnokutsky MV. The button sequestrum sign. Radiology. 2005; 236:1026–1027

Helms CA. Fundamentals of Skeletal Radiology. 4th ed. Philadelphia, PA: Elsevier Saunders; 2014

Resnick D, Kransdorf MJ. Bone and Joint Imaging. 3rd ed. Philadelphia, PA: Elsevier Saunders; 2005

Case 83

Philip Granchi

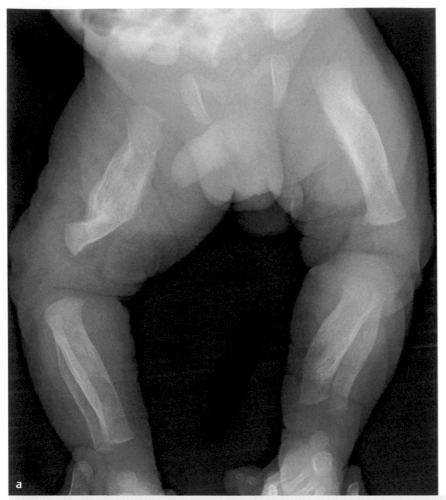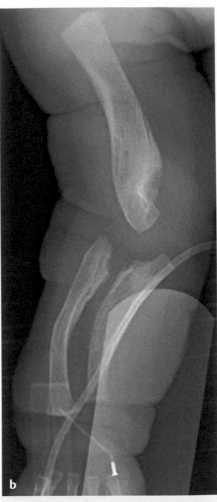

Fig. 83.1 (a) Frontal view of both lower extremities and (b) frontal view of right upper extremity show asymmetric, coarse periosteal reaction along long bones in this 4-week-old boy with irritability.

■ Clinical Presentation

Newborn with hyperirritability (▶Fig. 83.1).

■ Key Imaging Finding

Periosteal reaction in a newborn/infant

■ Top 3 Differential Diagnoses

- **Physiologic periosteal reaction.** Between 1 and 6 months of age, periosteal new bone formation occurs as thin lines parallel to the cortices of long bones with sparing of the metaphyses in about one-third of all infants. The key finding in recognizing this benign process is its symmetry. It commonly affects the humerus, femur, and tibia bilaterally. Follow-up films will show confluence of the periosteal reaction with the existing cortex. Physiologic periosteal bone formation is limited to the 1- to 6-month age group
- **Trauma.** Periosteal reaction occurs at sites of fracture from both accidental and nonaccidental trauma. In particular, nonaccidental trauma must be considered when periosteal reaction is identified in pediatric patients without an appropriate history of trauma to explain the underlying findings. Factors favoring nonaccidental trauma include multiple fractures of differing ages, as well as fractures with a high specificity for child abuse. The more common high specificity fractures include posterior rib and long bone metaphyseal corner fractures.
- **Infection.** Skeletal findings secondary to bony infection are diverse, but a common element is the presence of lucency, ranging from vertical or longitudinal bands in the setting of TORCH infections to poorly defined areas in osteomyelitis. The metaphyses are most commonly involved, which is a differentiating feature from normal physiologic periosteal bone formation.

■ Additional Differential Diagnoses

- **Prostaglandin therapy.** Patients with congenital heart disease may require patency of the ductus arteriosus to provide oxygenated blood to the systemic circulation. Prostaglandin therapy is used to keep the ductus open prior to corrective surgery. Although the periosteal reaction in this patient population is diffuse, patients will have clear history of cardiac anomaly and long-term treatment (4–6 weeks) with prostaglandins.
- **Infantile cortical hyperostosis (Caffey disease).** Occurring in the first few months of life, Caffey disease presents with fever, irritability, and periosteal reaction primarily involving the mandible, long bones, ribs, and scapulae. Key features that allow differentiation of Caffey disease include its coarse, irregular, and asymmetric periosteal reaction, as well as the presence of soft-tissue swelling over the affected areas.

■ Diagnosis

Caffey disease

✓ Pearls

- Physiologic periosteal reaction occurs between 1 and 6 months of age and does not involve the metaphyses.
- Trauma (accidental and nonaccidental) and infection result in localized periosteal reaction.
- Prostaglandin therapy may result in a diffuse periosteal reaction with long term (4–6 weeks) treatment.
- Caffey disease results in a coarse, irregular, asymmetric periosteal reaction with soft-tissue swelling.

Suggested Readings

Kirks D, Griscom NT. Practical Pediatric Imaging: Diagnostic Radiology of Infants and Children. 3rd ed. Philadelphia , PA: Lippincott-Raven; 1998:335–336

Nistala H, Mäkitie O, Jüppner H. Caffey disease: new perspectives on old questions. Bone. 2014; 60:246–251

Swischuk LE, ed. Imaging of the Newborn, Infant and Young Child. 5th ed. Philadelphia, PA: Lippincott Williams and Wilkins; 2004:733

Velaphi S, Cilliers A, Beckh-Arnold E, Mokhachane M, Mphahlele R, Pettifor J. Cortical hyperostosis in an infant on prolonged prostaglandin infusion: case report and literature review. J Perinatol. 2004; 24(4):263–265

Case 84

M. Jason Akers

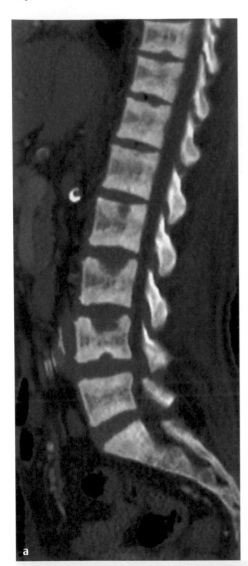
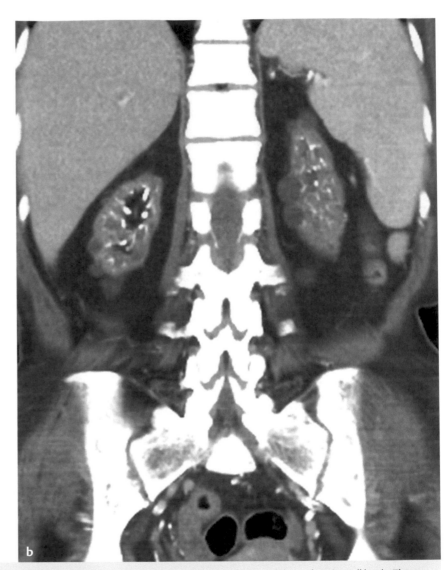

Fig. 84.1 (a) Sagittal reformation computed tomography (CT) image of lumbar spine shows superior and inferior endplate sclerosis at all levels. There is relative lucency within the central vertebral bodies between the areas of endplate sclerosis with an indistinct transition between the areas of sclerosis and the central areas of lucency. (b) Coronal reformation CT image of the abdomen in the same patient shows bilateral atrophic kidneys with multiple calcifications.

■ Clinical Presentation

A 43-year-old woman with back pain (▶ Fig. 84.1).

■ Key Imaging Finding

"Rugger-jersey" appearance of the spine

■ Top 3 Differential Diagnoses

- **Renal osteodystrophy**. Renal osteodystrophy represents a constellation of musculoskeletal abnormalities that occur in chronic renal failure, including secondary hyperparathyroidism, osteoporosis, osteosclerosis, osteomalacia, and soft-tissue and vascular calcifications. Osteosclerosis is common and results from an increased amount of abnormal osteoid. A classic site for osteosclerosis is the vertebral body endplates. The "rugger-jersey" appearance of the spine is created by the relative lucency of the central aspect of the vertebral bodies between the sclerotic endplates. The striate pattern is reminiscent of rugby players' alternating color horizontally striped shirts. The margins between the sclerotic and lucent portions of the vertebral body are smudgy, rather than sharp. Look for extraskeletal evidence of chronic renal failure to include atrophic native kidneys, surgical clips in the abdomen from nephrectomy or renal transplant, and dialysis catheters in the chest.

- **Osteopetrosis**. Osteopetrosis represents a group of hereditary disorders characterized by abnormal osteoclastic activity, resulting in dense bones. The "sandwich" appearance of the vertebral bodies is classic for osteopetrosis. The appearance is similar to the "rugger jersey" spine of renal osteodystrophy with the difference being a sharp margin between the sclerotic endplates and more lucent bone centrally. The classic "bone-in-bone" appearance occurs within the pelvis and long bones.

- **Paget disease**. Paget disease occurs in middle-aged and elderly patients and is characterized by excessive and abnormal bone remodeling. Most cases are polyostotic and the majority of cases involve the pelvis, spine, skull, femur, or tibia. The more common appearance of Paget disease in the spine is the "picture frame" vertebral body caused by overall increased density with sclerosis most marked at the periphery and a relatively lucent center. As in other bones, the classic features of Paget disease in the spine are bony (vertebral) enlargement, coarsened trabeculae, and overall increased bone density.

■ Diagnosis

Renal osteodystrophy

✓ Pearls

- The "rugger-jersey" appearance of the vertebral bodies in renal osteodystrophy has smudgy margins.
- The "sandwich" vertebrae in osteopetrosis have sharp interfaces between sclerotic and lucent bone.

- Paget disease is characterized by bony enlargement, coarsened trabeculae, and increased bone density.

Suggested Readings

Chew F. Musculoskeletal Imaging: A Teaching File. 3rd ed. Philadelphia, PA: Elsevier Saunders; 2005

Kirkland JD, O'Brien WT. Osteopetrosis – classic imaging findings in the spine. J Clin Diagn Res. 2015; 9(8):TJ01–TJ02

Lim CY, Ong KO. Various musculoskeletal manifestations of chronic renal insufficiency. Clin Radiol. 2013; 68(7):e397–e411

Martell BS, Dyer RB. The rugger jersey spine. Abdom Imaging. 2015; 40(8):3342–3343

Wittenberg A. The rugger jersey spine sign. Radiology. 2004; 230(2):491–492

Case 85

Michael A. Tall

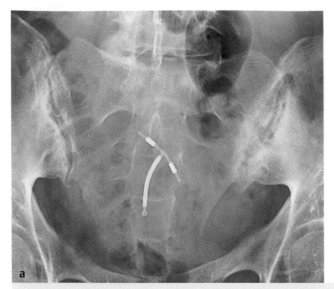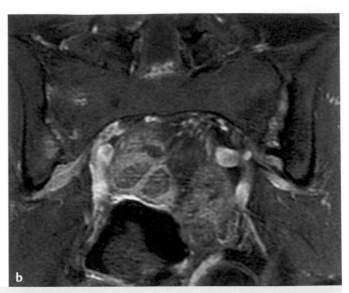

Fig. 85.1 **(a)** Anteroposterior radiograph of the pelvis demonstrates bilateral sclerosis and possible erosions involving the sacroiliac joints. **(b)** Coronal fat-suppressed postcontrast T1-weighted image of the posterior pelvis shows enhancing synovitis at both SI joints with erosions on the right.

■ Clinical Presentation

A 41-year-old woman with a 3-year history of worsening back and hip pain with morning stiffness (▶Fig. 85.1).

■ Key Imaging Finding

Sacroiliitis

■ Top 3 Differential Diagnoses if Bilateral & Symmetric

- **Ankylosing spondylitis (AS).** AS is a seronegative spondyloarthropathy. The earliest radiographic manifestations of AS involve the sacroiliac joints. The sacroiliac joints are typically involved in a bilateral symmetric fashion with sclerosis on both sides of the joint, along with small erosions. Eventually, ankylosis or fusion across the joint occurs. Magnetic resonance imaging (MRI) can facilitate early diagnosis and assessment of treatment response. Characteristic findings in the spine include erosions along the corners of the vertebral bodies (shiny corners), squaring of vertebral bodies, ossification and ankylosis along the annulus (bamboo spine), and interspinous ligament ossification (dagger sign).

- **Inflammatory bowel disease.** Between 5 and 15% of patients with Crohn disease develop sacroiliac and spinal changes. The radiographic manifestations of Crohn disease are identical to AS, including bilateral symmetric SI sclerosis on both sides of the joint, small erosions, and ankylosis.
- **Rheumatoid arthritis (RA).** Rheumatoid arthritis may result in bilateral, symmetric narrowing of the sacroiliac joints. Erosive changes occur, but usually to a lesser extent than what is seen with the spondyloarthropathies. Ankylosis, when present, involves the synovial portion of the joint only.

■ Top 3 Differential Diagnoses if Unilateral or Asymmetric

- **Psoriatic arthritis.** Psoriatic arthritis involves the sacroiliac joints in a bilateral but asymmetric fashion. Radiographic manifestations include erosions that are more prominent than AS or RA, along with sclerosis. Ankylosis, when present, occurs later in the disease process.
- **Reactive arthritis.** Reactive arthritis cannot be distinguished from psoriatic arthritis in radiographic changes of the SI joints, to include erosions along with sclerosis.

- **Septic arthritis.** Septic arthritis is almost always a unilateral process. Early in the disease process, abnormal widening, erosions, and bone destruction are present. This typically extends beyond the synovial portion of the joint. Bony ankylosis may eventually occur. Septic arthritis should be at least considered in any case of unilateral sacroiliitis. Failure to properly diagnose and treat this condition will result in significant joint destruction.

■ Diagnosis

Ankylosing spondylitis

✓ Pearls

- The earliest radiographic manifestation of AS involves the sacroiliac joints.
- The sacroiliac radiographic manifestations of Crohn disease are identical to AS.

- Psoriatic and reactive arthropathy involve the sacroiliac joints in a bilateral, asymmetric distribution.
- Septic arthritis should be suspected with unilateral sacroiliitis.

Suggested Readings

Bennett DL, Ohashi K, El-Khoury GY. Spondyloarthropathies: ankylosing spondylitis and psoriatic arthritis. Radiol Clin North Am. 2004; 42(1):121–134

Brower AC, Flemming DJ. Arthritis: In Black and White. 3rd ed. Philadelphia, PA: Saunders Elsevier; 2012

Navallas M, Ares J, Beltrán B, Lisbona MP, Maymó J, Solano A. Sacroiliitis associated with axial spondyloarthropathy: new concepts and latest trends. Radiographics. 2013; 33(4):933–956

Case 86

Michael A. Tall

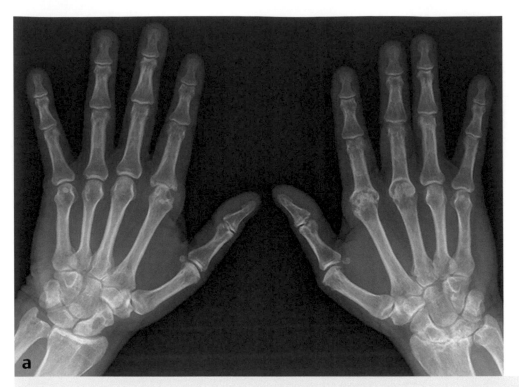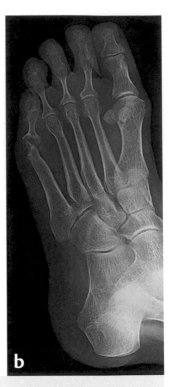

Fig. 86.1 (a) Dorsovolar radiograph of bilateral hands shows erosive changes and joint space narrowing at some of the MCP joints with severe joint space loss at right radiocarpal joint and cystic lucencies scattered at both wrists. **(b)** Oblique radiograph of the left foot reveals marked erosive changes at the fifth metatarsophalangeal joint.

■ Clinical Presentation

A 54-year-old woman with stiffness and pain in her hands and feet (▶Fig. 86.1).

■ Key Imaging Finding

Proximal arthropathy affecting primarily the metacarpophalangeal joints

■ Top 3 Differential Diagnoses

- **Rheumatoid arthritis (RA)**. The common radiographic manifestations of RA consist of periarticular osteopenia, uniform joint space loss, marginal erosions, subchondral cyst formation, and subluxations. Unlike psoriatic and reactive arthritis, there is a lack of bone formation. In the hand, the distribution primarily involves the metacarpophalangeal joints (MCPs), proximal interphalangeal joints (PIPs), and carpal bones in a bilateral fairly symmetric fashion. In the feet, often the earliest erosive changes are seen along the lateral aspect of the fifth metatarsal heads. Additional target sites of RA in the feet include metatarsophalangeal (MTP), PIP, and intertarsal joints. As the disease progresses, joint subluxations occur predominantly at the MCPs. Hand involvement precedes involvement of the feet in the vast majority of patients.
- **Crystalline arthropathy**. **Calcium pyrophosphate deposition disease (CPPD)** arthropathy is the most common crystalline arthropathy. The radiographic appearance resembles osteoarthropathy. Symmetric joint space narrowing, subchondral cysts, and osteophytes may be present. Unlike rheumatoid arthritis, erosions are absent. In the hand, the arthropathy is usually confined to the MCP joints. Chondrocalcinosis is often present, most frequently in the triangular fibrocartilage of the wrist. **Gout** is a crystalline arthropathy that primarily involves the hands and feet. The distribution is sporadic and bilateral involvement, when present, is asymmetric. Unlike rheumatoid arthritis, the erosions in gout demonstrate sclerotic borders with characteristic overhanging edges. Soft-tissue tophi occur in chronic disease. Bony mineralization is usually normal.
- **Collagen vascular disease (SLE)**. Systemic lupus erythematous is the most common of the collagen vascular diseases. Radiographic findings of SLE include juxta-articular osteopenia, joint subluxations and dislocations. Unlike RA, erosions are not typically present.

■ Additional Differential Diagnoses

- **Hemochromatosis**. In hemochromatosis, there is a predilection for the second and third MCP joints in the hands with subchondral cysts and characteristic hooked osteophytes. Bony mineralization is preserved, and there are no erosions. As in CPPD arthropathy, chondrocalcinosis may be present.

■ Diagnosis

Rheumatoid arthritis

✓ Pearls

- Rheumatoid arthritis demonstrates uniform joint space loss, marginal erosions, and subchondral cysts.
- Erosions in gout demonstrate sclerotic borders, often with overhanging edges; tophi may also be present.

- SLE demonstrates periarticular osteopenia, and subluxations without erosions.
- Hemochromatosis results in joint space narrowing, hooked osteophytes, and chondrocalcinosis.

Suggested Readings

Brower AC, Flemming DJ. Arthritis: In Black and White. 3rd ed. Philadelphia, PA: Saunders Elsevier; 2012

Gupta KB, Duryea J, Weissman BN. Radiographic evaluation of osteoarthritis. Radiol Clin North Am. 2004; 42(1):11–41, v

Jacobson JA, Girish G, Jiang Y, Resnick D. Radiographic evaluation of arthritis: inflammatory conditions. Radiology. 2008; 248(2):378–389

Case 87

Michael A. Tall

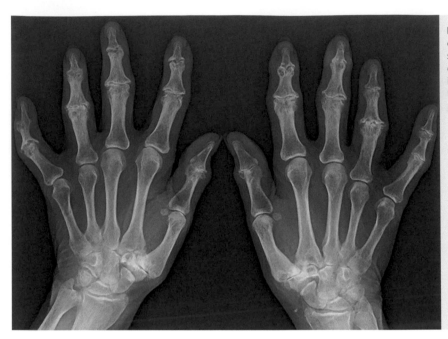

Fig. 87.1 Dorsovolar radiograph of the hands demonstrates joint space narrowing, irregularity, subchondral sclerosis, osteophytosis, and central erosions involving several proximal (PIP) and distal interphalangeal (DIP) joints of both hands. A few DIP joints show bony fusion. Bone mineralization is preserved.

■ Clinical Presentation

A 71-year-old woman with a history of longstanding bilateral hand and finger pain (▶ Fig. 87.1).

■ Key Imaging Finding

Distal arthropathy affecting primarily the interphalangeal joints

■ Top 3 Differential Diagnoses

- **Osteoarthritis**. Primary osteoarthritis in the hand involves the distal interphalangeal (DIP) and proximal interphalangeal (PIP) joints with relative sparing of the metacarpophalangeal (MCP) joints. There is nonuniform joint space loss with subchondral sclerosis and osteophyte formation in areas of greatest cartilage loss. Soft-tissue swelling around the DIP joint associated with osteophyte formation is called Heberden node, while that around the PIP joint is called Bouchard node. Erosions and ankylosis are not present
- **Erosive osteoarthritis**. Erosive osteoarthritis is seen primarily in postmenopausal women. It has the same distribution in the hand as primary osteoarthritis with involvement of the DIP and PIP joints in the fingers and the first carpometacarpal joint. In addition to osteophytes, however, central erosions are characteristic and produce two convexities at the joint surface likened to the wings of a seagull. Ankylosis of the joints may also occur.

- **Psoriatic arthritis**. The hands are most commonly involved in psoriatic arthritis with three different patterns of distribution. The first pattern is primarily DIP and PIP involvement. The second pattern is ray involvement wherein all joints in one to three digits will be involved, while the remaining digits are spared. The third pattern is similar to rheumatoid arthritis (RA) but there is usually DIP involvement and/or evidence of bone proliferation in contradistinction to RA. Erosions occur initially at the margins of the joint but eventually progress to involve the entire joint. The ends of the bones may become pointed and saucerized and give the classic "pencil-in-cup" appearance. Bone mineralization is usually preserved, even with severe erosive disease. Bone proliferation is one of the most important features of psoriatic arthritis and is almost always present in some form.

■ Additional Differential Diagnoses

- **Reactive arthritis**. Lower extremity involvement is more common with reactive arthritis. Upper extremity involvement, when present, typically occurs in the hands. The specific radiographic changes are essentially identical to psoriatic arthritis with erosive changes and new bone formation. This is often limited to just one digit. The PIP joints are more frequently involved to a greater extent than the DIPs or MTPs/MCPs.

- **Rheumatoid arthritis (RA)**. The common radiographic manifestations of RA consist of periarticular osteopenia progressing to generalized osteoporosis, uniform joint space loss, marginal erosions, subchondral cyst formation, and subluxations. Unlike psoriatic and reactive arthritis, there is a lack of bone formation. The distribution primarily involves the PIPs, MCPs, and carpal bones in a symmetric fashion.

■ Diagnosis

Erosive osteoarthritis

✓ Pearls

- The hallmarks of osteoarthritis include joint space narrowing, sclerosis, and osteophyte formation.
- Central erosions in the interphalangeal joints are characteristic of erosive osteoarthropathy.

- Marginal erosions and new bone formation are characteristic of reactive and psoriatic arthropathy.
- Advanced psoriatic arthritis may result in the classic "pencil-in-cup" deformity in the phalanges.

Suggested Readings

Brower AC, Flemming DJ. Arthritis: In Black and White. 3rd ed. Philadelphia, PA: Saunders Elsevier; 2012

Gupta KB, Duryea J, Weissman BN. Radiographic evaluation of osteoarthritis. Radiol Clin North Am. 2004; 42(1):11–41, v

Jacobson JA, Girish G, Jiang Y, Sabb BJ. Radiographic evaluation of arthritis: degenerative joint disease and variations. Radiology. 2008; 248(3):737–747

Case 88

Michael A. Tall

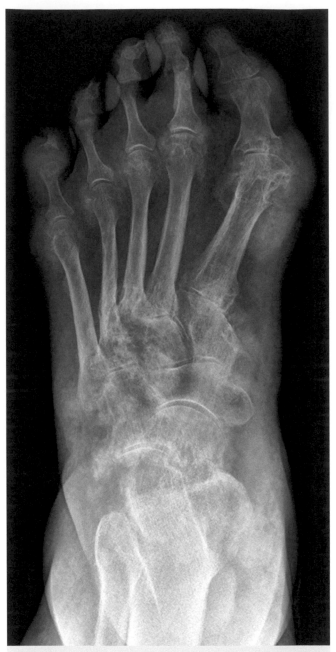

Fig. 88.1 Frontal radiograph of the foot demonstrates multiple erosions at all metatarsophalangeal (MTP) joints. The more prominent erosions at first and second MTP joints have sclerotic borders and overhanging edges. There are multiple soft-tissue masslike lesions with faintly increased density along the joints.

■ Clinical Presentation

A 72-year-old man with several year history of foot pain that is most pronounced at the great toe (▶ Fig. 88.1).

■ Key Imaging Finding

Erosive arthropathy involving the foot

■ Top 3 Differential Diagnoses

- **Rheumatoid arthritis (RA)**. RA is characterized by bilateral fairly symmetric distribution, uniform joint space narrowing, periarticular osteopenia, marginal erosions, and joint subluxations. The feet are involved in 80 to 90% of cases and usually lag behind the findings in the hands. The lateral aspect of the fifth metatarsal head is often the earliest site of involvement. Metatarsophalangeal (MTP), proximal interphalangeal (PIP), and intertarsal joint involvement can commonly be seen with sparing of distal interphalangeal (DIP) joints. Retrocalcaneal bursitis with erosions and Achilles tendonitis are also common findings with RA.
- **Gout**. Gouty arthritis is caused by the accumulation of monosodium urate crystals. It most commonly affects older men. Characteristic radiographic findings include well-defined, punched-out erosions often with a sclerotic border and overhanging edges, along with soft-tissue tophi. Bone mineralization is usually normal and joint spaces are preserved until late in the disease. The distribution is typically polyarticular and asymmetric. The first MTP joint is the most common joint involved and is referred to as podagra.
- **Reactive arthritis**. Early in the disease process, juxta-articular osteopenia, which may only affect a single joint, predominates in cases of reactive arthritis. Regions of osteopenia may normalize. Later in the disease process, uniform joint space narrowing, marginal erosions, and adjacent bone proliferation occur. Eventually, there may be ankylosis across the joint; however, it does not occur as frequently as in psoriatic arthritis. Small joints of the foot and the calcaneus are the most frequently involved joints with preferential involvement of the MTP and first IP joints.

■ Additional Differential Diagnoses

- **Psoriatic arthritis**. The hands are most commonly involved in psoriatic arthritis, but the feet may be involved as well. Marginal erosions coupled with bony proliferation are the hallmarks of the disease. Erosive changes may become so severe that they result in "pencil-in-cup" deformity. Diffuse soft-tissue swelling of an entire digit may also occur, which is referred to as a "sausage digit" deformity. Ankylosis is common. Characteristic distribution in feet involves IP joints, MTPs, and posterior margin of the calcaneus. DIP involvement tends to be seen early and more severe than PIP or MTP joints.

■ Diagnosis

Tophaceous gout

✓ Pearls

- The first MTP joint is the most commonly affected joint in gout and is referred to as podagra.
- Bony mineralization is normal and joint spaces are generally preserved until late in the course of gout.
- RA has symmetric joint space narrowing, marginal erosions, and periarticular osteopenia.
- Reactive arthritis involves the feet with joint space narrowing, marginal erosions, and bony proliferation.

Suggested Readings

Brower AC, Flemming DJ. Arthritis: In Black and White. 3rd ed. Philadelphia, PA: Saunders Elsevier; 2012

Girish G, Glazebrook KN, Jacobson JA. Advanced imaging in gout. AJR Am J Roentgenol. 2013; 201(3):515–525

Monu JU, Pope TL, Jr. Gout: a clinical and radiologic review. Radiol Clin North Am. 2004; 42(1):169–184

Case 89

Jasjeet Bindra

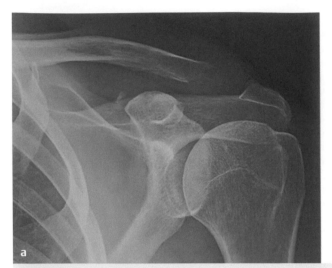 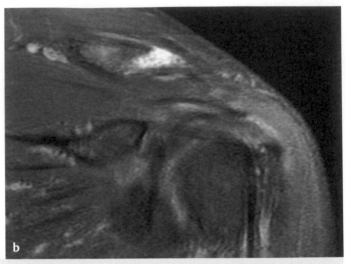

Fig. 89.1 **(a)** Frontal radiograph of the shoulder shows distal clavicular erosion/resorption. **(b)** Corresponding coronal oblique fat-saturated proton density MR image of the shoulder demonstrates osteolysis of distal clavicle with adjacent fluid signal.

■ Clinical Presentation

A 23-year-old man with shoulder pain (▶Fig. 89.1).

■ **Key Imaging Finding**

Distal clavicular erosion/resorption

■ **Top 3 Differential Diagnoses**

- **Traumatic**. Stress osteolysis of distal clavicle can occur when repeated forces are applied to the acromioclavicular (AC) joint. This is classically seen in weightlifters. Symptoms begin with aching pain in the AC region that is exacerbated by weight training (e.g., bench presses, push-ups, dips on the parallel bars, overhead activities, horizontal adduction). The most widely accepted etiology is that repetitive microtrauma causes subchondral stress fractures and remodeling in distal clavicle.
- **Rheumatoid arthritis (RA)**. RA can cause distal clavicular resorption that appears identical to other etiologies. Periarticular osteopenia, glenohumeral joint space narrowing, and

erosion of the humeral head on shoulder radiographs are suggestive of RA and can help in pinpointing the diagnosis.
- **Hyperparathyroidism**. Besides distal clavicular erosion, an additional finding that can be seen on shoulder or clavicular radiographs in cases of hyperparathyroidism is subligamentous resorption at the site of coracoclavicular ligament attachment on the clavicle. Generalized bone demineralization is a uniform feature of all types of hyperparathyroidism. Subchondral bone loss can also be seen at the sacroiliac, sternoclavicular, and temporomandibular joints and at the symphysis pubis, in addition to AC joint.

■ **Additional Differential Diagnoses**

- **Scleroderma**. Scleroderma is a multisystem connective tissue disease characterized as a systemic sclerosis. Radiographically, acro-osteolysis and soft-tissue calcifications are commonly seen involving the digits and distal clavicle. Erosions can occur; however, arthritis is not a prominent feature.
- **Infection**. Septic arthritis is a rare entity but should be entertained as a possibility in cases of distal clavicular erosion. Patients are often immunosuppressed and present with pain and elevated inflammatory markers. Early treatment with appropriate antibiotic coverage is essential.

■ **Diagnosis**

Posttraumatic osteolysis

✓ **Pearls**

- Posttraumatic distal clavicular osteolysis is most commonly associated with weight training.
- RA may cause distal clavicle resorption with additional glenohumeral joint space narrowing, osteopenia, and erosions.

- Hyperparathyroidism demonstrates generalized osteopenia with subligamentous and subperiosteal resorption.

Suggested Readings

Currie JW, Davis KW, Lafita VS, et al. Musculoskeletal mnemonics: differentiating features. Curr Probl Diagn Radiol. 2011; 40(2):45–71

Manaster BJ, May DA, Disler DG. Musculoskeletal Imaging, The Requisites. 4th ed. Philadelphia, PA: Mosby Elsevier; 2013

Schwarzkopf R, Ishak C, Elman M, Gelber J, Strauss DN, Jazrawi LM. Distal clavicular osteolysis: a review of the literature. Bull NYU Hosp Jt Dis. 2008; 66(2):94–101

Case 90

Eva Escobedo

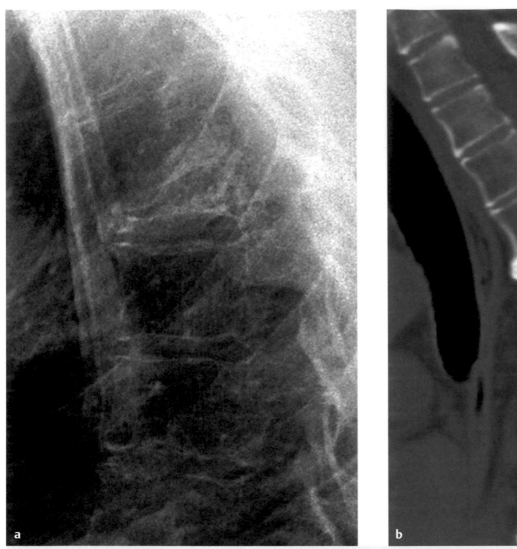
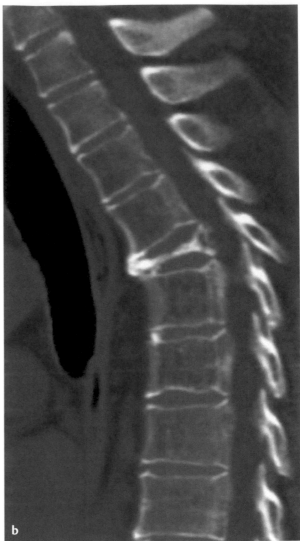

Fig. 90.1 (a) Lateral radiograph and (b) sagittal reformation CT image of thoracic spine show marked flattening of the T6 vertebral body with preservation of the disc spaces, consistent with vertebra plana.

■ Clinical Presentation

A 50-year-old man with back pain (►Fig. 90.1).

■ Key Imaging Finding

Vertebra plana

■ Top 3 Differential Diagnoses in an Adult

- **Multiple myeloma.** Multiple myeloma, a plasma cell dyscrasia, is the most common primary bone malignancy in adults. The predominant pattern is osteolysis that most commonly occurs at multiple sites, but can be solitary (plasmacytoma). The axial skeleton is the typical site of involvement, but extensive disease will affect the extremities as well. Osteopenia with compression fractures is a typical finding.
- **Metastases.** Bone metastases can be either well or poorly defined, and may be difficult to distinguish from multiple myeloma. Associated mass may be seen with metastasis or myeloma (especially plasmacytoma).
- **Trauma.** Compression fractures, and less commonly, vertebra plana, can be seen with relatively minor trauma in the setting of osteoporosis or steroids (endogenous or exogenous). Compression fracture from osteoporosis may be difficult to distinguish from myeloma, which often presents as diffuse osteoporosis.

■ Top 3 Differential Diagnoses in a Child

- **Langerhans cell histiocytosis (LCH).** LCH is by far the most common cause of vertebra plana in a child. In the spine, it most commonly occurs at a single site, but it may involve multiple levels as well. The compression deformity may be progressive and rapid. More often, however, LCH manifests as a lytic lesion rather than vertebra plana.
- **Leukemia/lymphoma.** Leukemia is the most common pediatric primary malignancy. Secondary lymphoma is much more common than primary lymphoma in the pediatric spine. Both entities may present with loss of vertebral height, with increased sclerosis being a common finding in the vertebral body. Constitutional symptoms and involvement of multiple levels are more commonly seen with these disease processes compared to LCH.
- **Osteomyelitis.** Both bacterial and granulomatous (TB) infection can present as vertebra plana. Bacterial infection commonly involves the intervertebral disc. TB spondylitis, on the other hand, more commonly results in predominant bone destruction with relative disc preservation, which can manifest as vertebra plana. However, some form of vertebral end plate irregularity, sclerosis, or destruction is usually present.

■ Diagnosis

Multiple myeloma

✓ Pearls

- Langerhans cell histiocytosis is by far the most common cause of vertebra plana in children.
- Leukemia or lymphoma may present with multiple levels of vertebral body collapse and sclerosis.
- Spinal involvement by multiple myeloma may be difficult to distinguish from osteoporosis or metastases.

Suggested Readings

Baghaie M, Gillet P, Dondelinger RF, Flandroy P. Vertebra plana: benign or malignant lesion? Pediatr Radiol. 1996; 26(6):431–433

Chang MC, Wu HT, Lee CH, Liu CL, Chen TH. Tuberculous spondylitis and pyogenic spondylitis: comparative magnetic resonance imaging features. Spine. 2006; 31(7):782–788

Greenlee JDW, Fenoy AJ, Donovan KA, Menezes AH. Eosinophilic granuloma in the pediatric spine. Pediatr Neurosurg. 2007; 43(4):285–292

Resnick D. Diagnosis of Bone and Joint Disorders. 4th ed. Philadelphia, PA: WB Saunders; 2002

Case 91

Philip Granchi

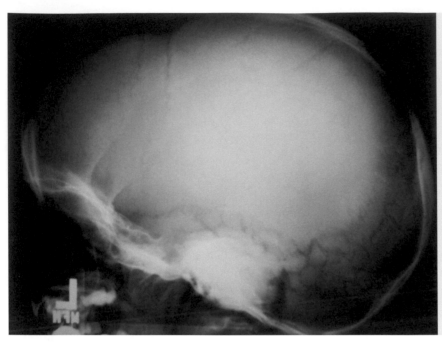

Fig. 91.1 Lateral skull radiograph reveals intrasutural ossification (wormian bones) involving the squamosal and lambdoid sutures.

■ Clinical Presentation

Child with facial abnormalities (►Fig. 91.1).

■ Key Imaging Finding

Wormian bones

■ Top 3 Differential Diagnoses

- **Idiopathic.** Wormian bones are a descriptive designation for irregular ossicles located within the sutures of calvarium (intrasutural bones). Idiopathic wormian bones are reported to be smaller and less numerous than those associated with an identifiable skeletal dysplasia, although no hard and fast criteria exist for this determination. Most commonly located within the lambdoid suture (50%), wormian bones may also occur in the coronal suture (25%) and have been identified in all cranial sutures and fontanelles.
- **Osteogenesis imperfecta (OI).** Wormian bones in OI may be numerous and demonstrate a mosaic ("crazy paving") pattern.

Besides wormian bones, other radiologic findings include osteoporosis, multiple fractures, gracile diaphysis, and scoliosis.
- **Cleidocranial dysostosis.** Cleidocranial dysostosis is a genetic disorder with abnormal membranous bone development that leads to findings of a small face, enlarged head, and hypertelorism. Wormian bones are one part of a radiographic constellation of findings that includes delayed closure of sutures and fontanelles, absence or hypoplasia of the clavicles, widened symphysis pubis, and coxa vara.

■ Additional Differential Diagnoses

- **Down syndrome.** Down syndrome (trisomy 21) is the most common genetic cause of mental impairment in children and has been associated with an increased incidence with advanced maternal age (>35 years of age). A host of radiographic findings are associated with Down syndrome, including wormian bones. Additional classic musculoskeletal findings include atlantoaxial instability, 11 rib pairs, short tubular bones of the hands, flared iliac wings, hip dysplasia, and patellar dislocation.

- **Metabolic disease (hypothyroidism, rickets).** Wormian bones may be found in patients with multiple metabolic deficiencies. In rickets, wormian bones are associated with the healing phase of the deficiency. Early extracranial findings include frayed physes and flaring (cupping) of the metaphyses. Hypothyroidism is characterized by markedly delayed skeletal maturity, "bullet" vertebrae at the thoracolumbar junction, and fragmentation of the epiphyses. Hypophosphatasia, a rare genetic defect of alkaline phosphatase, leads to rickets in the absence of dietary deficiency.

■ Diagnosis

Cleidocranial dysostosis

✓ Pearls

- Wormian bones may be idiopathic in etiology with the lambdoid suture most commonly involved.
- Wormian bones in OI may be numerous and demonstrate a mosaic pattern.

- Cleidocranial dysostosis presents with wormian bones and absence or hypoplasia of the clavicles.
- Wormian bones may be found with multiple metabolic disorders.

Suggested Readings

Jeanty P, Silva SR, Turner C. Prenatal diagnosis of wormian bones. J Ultrasound Med. 2000; 19(12):863–869

Manaster BJ, May DA, Disler DG. Musculoskeletal Imaging, The Requisites. 4th ed. Philadelphia: Mosby Elsevier; 2013

Marti B, Sirinelli D, Maurin L, Carpentier E. Wormian bones in a general paediatric population. Diagn Interv Imaging. 2013; 94(4):428–432

Paterson CR. Radiological features of the brittle bone diseases J Diagn Radiogr Imaging. 2003; 5(1):39–45

Case 92

Michael A. Tall

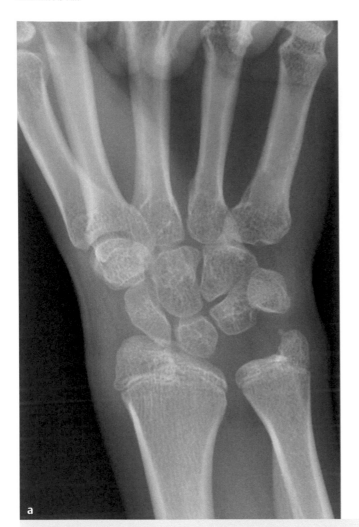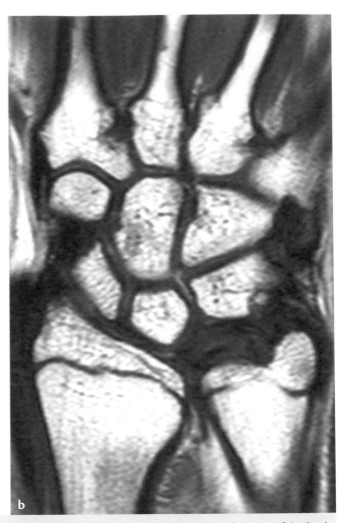

Fig. 92.1 **(a)** Frontal radiograph of the wrist and **(b)** corresponding coronal proton density MR image demonstrate a triangular configuration of the distal radius and ulna articulation with wedging of the proximal carpal bones between the distal radius and ulna, consistent with Madelung deformity.

■ Clinical Presentation

A 16-year-old girl with wrist pain and weakness (▶Fig. 92.1).

■ Key Imaging Finding

Madelung deformity

■ Top 3 Differential Diagnoses

- **Idiopathic Madelung deformity**. Idiopathic Madelung deformity often clinically manifests in young adulthood or adolescence and can present with visible deformity, pain, weakness, and limited range of motion. It results from premature closure of the medial volar aspect of the distal radial growth plate. Radiographic findings consist of increased inclination of the radial articular surface and volar tilt, proximal and volar migration of the lunate with triangulation of the carpus, relative ulnar lengthening, and dorsal subluxation of distal ulna. The isolated form of Madelung deformity is typically bilateral, asymmetric, and more common in women.
- **Posttraumatic**. Madelung-type deformity may be secondary to trauma or infection. It can result from single or repetitive axial loading trauma, an injury frequently seen in gymnasts. The Madelung-type of deformity results from premature closure along portions of the growth plate as a result of the injury and subsequent healing process.
- **Skeletal dysplasias**. Madelung deformity is frequently associated with Léri–Weill dyschondrosteosis, an autosomal dominant skeletal dysplasia. Patients with other osseous dysplasias, including Ollier disease, multiple epiphyseal dysplasia, and multiple hereditary exostoses, may present with Madelung-type deformity. It is also seen in <10% of patients with Turner syndrome. Involvement may be bilateral.

■ Diagnosis

Idiopathic Madelung deformity

✓ Pearls

- The isolated form of Madelung deformity is typically bilateral, asymmetric, and more common in women.
- Bilateral Madelung deformities may be present in several skeletal dysplasias.
- Trauma and infection are two common causes of a unilateral Madelung deformity.

Suggested Readings

Ali S, Kaplan S, Kaufman T, Fenerty S, Kozin S, Zlotolow DA. Madelung deformity and Madelung-type deformities: a review of the clinical and radiological characteristics. Pediatr Radiol. 2015; 45(12):1856–1863

Peh WC. Madelung deformity. Am J Orthop. 2001; 30(6):512

Resnick D, Kransforf MJ. Bone and Joint Imaging. 3rd ed. Philadelphia, PA: Elsevier Saunders; 2005

Schmidt-Rohlfing B, Schwöbel B, Pauschert R, Niethard FU. Madelung deformity: clinical features, therapy and results. J Pediatr Orthop B. 2001; 10(4):344–348

Case 93

Jasjeet Bindra

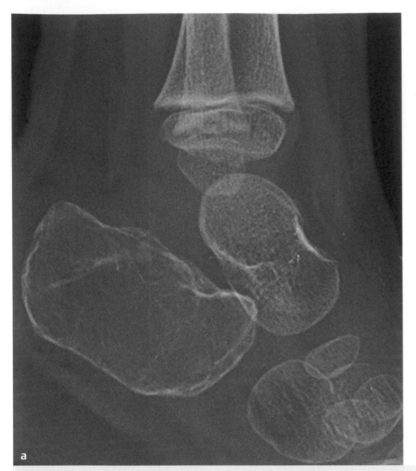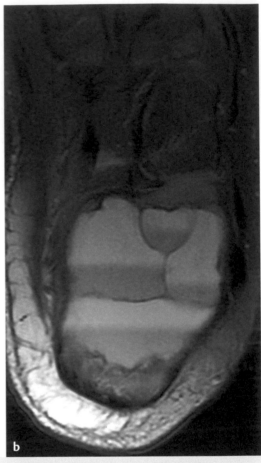

Fig. 93.1 **(a)** Lateral radiograph of the ankle shows a lucent expansile lesion involving the calcaneus. **(b)** Corresponding axial fat-saturated proton density MR image of the calcaneus shows the lesion with multiple fluid–fluid levels.

■ Clinical Presentation

A 5-year-old girl with heel pain (▶Fig. 93.1).

■ Key Imaging Finding

Osseous lesion with fluid–fluid levels

■ Top 3 Differential Diagnoses

- **Aneurysmal bone cyst (ABC)**. An ABC is an expansile lesion containing multiple thin-walled, blood-filled cystic cavities. Most of the ABCs are found in patients from 5 to 20 years of age, with a slight female preponderance. Typical sites include metaphyses of long bones and the posterior elements of the spine. Fluid–fluid levels occur whenever substances of different densities are layered within a cystic or compartmentalized structure. Fluid–fluid levels can be seen in ABCs on computed tomography (CT) or magnetic resonance imaging (MRI) and are believed to represent sedimentation of red blood cells within cystic cavities.
- **Unicameral (simple) bone cyst (SBC)**. A simple bone cyst is a fluid-containing lesion that usually arises in the metaphysis of long bones. The majority of these lesions are seen in patients younger than 20 years. Fluid–fluid levels have been reported in SBCs, usually in association with a pathologic fracture.
- **Telangiectatic osteosarcoma**. Telangiectatic osteosarcoma is a very aggressive type of osteosarcoma and is seen predominantly in patients in their second and third decades of life. The lesions are expansile and destructive, largely composed of cystic cavities containing necrosis and hemorrhage. Multiple aneurysmally dilated cystic cavities are separated by septations. Nodularity can be seen along septations, a key feature to differentiate from ABCs. Fluid–fluid levels are seen commonly.

■ Additional Differential Diagnoses

- **Fibrous dysplasia**. Fibrous dysplasia is a developmental dysplasia characterized by replacement of normal lamellar cancellous bone by abnormal fibrous tissue. It can be monostotic or polyostotic. The radiographic appearance varies with lesions containing greater fibrous tissue appearing more radiolucent with a characteristic "ground-glass" appearance. Lesions with greater osseous content are more sclerotic in appearance. Fluid–fluid levels have been reported in cases of cystic fibrous dysplasia.
- **Chondroblastoma**. Chondroblastoma is a solitary and benign cartilaginous neoplasm. A large percentage of cases are seen between the ages of 5 and 25 years. They usually arise in the epiphysis or apophysis of long bones. On imaging, chondroblastoma is frequently seen as a geographic, lytic lesion that may contain a chondroid matrix. They can show cystic features with fluid–fluid levels.

■ Diagnosis

Aneurysmal bone cyst

✓ Pearls

- ABCs commonly show fluid–fluid levels because of hemorrhagic blood products within the lesions.
- SBCs can show fluid–fluid levels in association with a pathologic fracture.
- Telangiectatic osteosarcomas can show septal or peripheral nodularity that can be a distinguishing feature.

Suggested Readings

Keenan S, Bui-Mansfield LT. Musculoskeletal lesions with fluid-fluid level: a pictorial essay. J Comput Assist Tomogr. 2006; 30(3):517–524

Van Dyck P, Vanhoenacker FM, Vogel J, et al. Prevalence, extension and characteristics of fluid-fluid levels in bone and soft tissue tumors. Eur Radiol. 2006; 16(12):2644–2651

Case 94

William T. O'Brien, Sr.

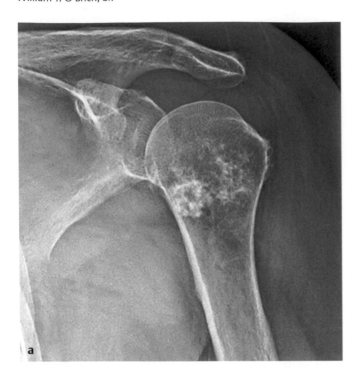

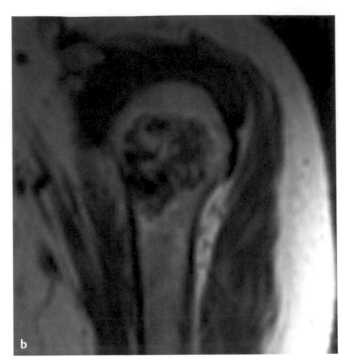

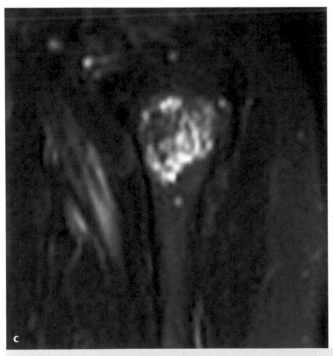

Fig. 94.1 (a) Frontal plain radiograph of the shoulder demonstrates a lucent lesion with internal chondroid/calcified matrix in an "arcs and swirls" pattern within the proximal humerus. (b) T1 coronal MR image through the proximal humerus reveals a lobulated, circumscribed, hypointense lesion centrally within the medullary cavity. (c) T2 coronal MR image through the same level shows high T2 signal lobules separated by thin low signal septations. More focal low signal intensities correspond to calcifications on plain radiograph.

■ **Clinical Presentation**

A 52-year-old woman with chronic shoulder pain (▶Fig. 94.1).

■ Key Imaging Finding

Medullary/chondroid lesion

■ Top 3 Differential Diagnoses

- **Enchondroma**. Enchondromas are benign chondroid lesions that contain a calcium matrix with a characteristic "arcs and swirls" pattern, except when they are located in the phalanges in which they will appear purely lucent. They are typically located centrally within the medullary cavity but may less commonly be eccentric. The proximal humerus, distal femur, proximal tibia, and phalanges are among the most common sites of involvement. On magnetic resonance imaging (MRI), enchondromas are composed of high T2 signal intensity lobules with thin intervening low T2 signal intensity septations. Internal calcifications are typically low signal on T2 and T1 sequences. On T1 sequences, enchondromas are characteristically low in signal intensity. Postgadolinium, the lesions will internally enhance in an "arcs and swirls" pattern.
- **Bone infarct**. Although some bone infarcts are idiopathic, the vast majority of patients have an underlying risk factor, including trauma, sickle cell disease, corticosteroid use, gly-cogen storage disease, alcoholism, or dyslipidemia. On plain radiographs, bone infarcts may simulate enchondromas with ill-defined patchy regions of sclerosis and lucency. More characteristically, bone infarcts will consist of a serpentine rim of calcification or demonstrate a "bone within bone" appearance. On MRI, bone infarcts present as geographic medullary lesions with central fat (bright on T1) and a margin that is hypointense on both T1- and T2-weighted sequences. Mixed internal signal intensity is due to fibrosis and calcification.
- **Chondrosarcoma**. Chondrosarcomas (especially low grade) have a similar imaging appearance to that of enchondromas, and it is often impossible to distinguish between the two based on imaging alone. Findings that would suggest chondrosarcoma include a size greater than 6 cm, rapid growth, cortical breakthrough, deep endosteal scalloping (more than two-thirds of the overlying cortex), and, most importantly, pain.

■ Additional Differential Diagnoses

- **Chronic osteomyelitis**. Chronic intramedullary infection typically presents on plain radiographs with sclerotic margins and endosteal thickening. A sclerotic sequestrum, which consists of isolated necrotic bone, is commonly seen. On MRI, these lesions will be internally hypointense on T1 and hyperintense on T2 sequences. The sequestrum will be low signal on both T1 and T2 sequences. Postcontrast images demonstrate rim enhancement, as well as regions of enhancing granulation tissue. Secondary findings to suggest infection include marrow edema, subperiosteal fluid, and a sinus tract.

■ Diagnosis

Enchondroma

✓ Pearls

- Enchondromas are benign chondroid lesions with calcifications in an "arcs and swirls pattern."
- Bone infarcts are geometric medullary lesions with a serpentine rim of calcification and fat centrally.
- Chondrosarcoma should be expected in the setting of pain or when malignant features are seen on imaging.
- Secondary findings to suggest chronic osteomyelitis include a sequestrum, marrow edema, and a sinus tract.

Suggested Readings

Flemming DJ, Murphey MD. Enchondroma and chondrosarcoma. Semin Musculo-skelet Radiol. 2000; 4(1):59–71

Murphey MD, Flemming DJ, Boyea SR, Bojescul JA, Sweet DE, Temple HT. Enchondroma versus chondrosarcoma in the appendicular skeleton: differentiating features. Radiographics. 1998; 18(5):1213–1237, quiz 1244–1245

Skaggs DL, Kim SK, Greene NW, Harris D, Miller JH. Differentiation between bone infarction and acute osteomyelitis in children with sickle-cell disease with use of sequential radionuclide bone-marrow and bone scans. J Bone Joint Surg Am. 2001; 83-A(12):1810–1813

Case 95

William T. O'Brien, Sr.

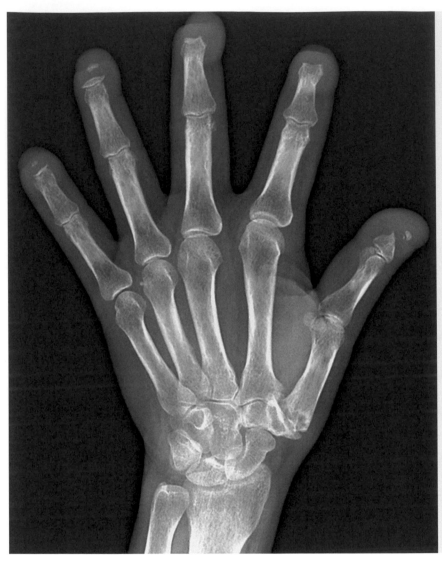

Fig. 95.1 Frontal plain radiograph of the left hand demonstrates resorption of all terminal phalangeal tufts (acro-osteolysis). There is complete resorption of terminal phalanges of second and third digits. Marked joint space narrowing and bony resorption are seen at the first carpometacarpal joint.

■ **Clinical Presentation**

A 49-year-old woman with chronic bilateral hand pain and ulcerations (▶Fig. 95.1).

■ Key Imaging Finding

Acro-osteolysis

■ Top 3 Differential Diagnoses

- **Hyperparathyroidism.** Hyperparathyroidism is a systemic abnormality of calcium homeostasis that can be primary (overproduction by the parathyroid glands), secondary (caused by renal failure or malabsorption), or tertiary (autonomous production by the parathyroid glands due to chronic renal failure or malabsorption). Subperiosteal resorption of bone, especially along the radial aspect of the second and third middle phalanges of the hands, is virtually diagnostic of hyperparathyroidism. Additional osseous abnormalities include resorption of the distal clavicles, bandlike osteosclerosis of the vertebral bodies referred to as "rugger-jersey" spine, brown tumors, and resorption of the terminal phalanges.
- **Scleroderma.** Scleroderma is a systemic connective tissue disorder that results in characteristic musculoskeletal abnormalities that are most prominent in the hands. The most common manifestations include bony erosions and soft-tissue resorption along the distal phalanges. Severe cases result in tapering

or complete destruction of the distal phalanges (acro-osteolysis). Soft-tissue calcifications are evident in approximately 10 to 30% of patients. CREST syndrome is a variant of scleroderma consisting of calcinosis, Raynaud phenomenon (distal extremity/phalangeal vasoconstriction due to cold temperatures or stress), esophageal dysmotility, sclerodactyly, and telangiectasias.
- **Trauma.** Thermal injury refers to either cold injury (frostbite) or burn injury. Both processes cause vascular occlusion and ischemia, resulting in soft-tissue and osseous abnormalities. Osseous manifestations include osteoporosis, periostitis, and resorption of the distal phalanges. In the setting of frostbite, the findings are typically bilateral with sparing of the thumbs secondary to clenched fists with the digits protecting the thumbs. Premature growth plate fusion is a complication in children.

■ Additional Differential Diagnoses

- **Psoriasis.** Psoriatic arthritis is a polyarticular arthritis with multiple variants. Although the distribution is variable, psoriasis has a predilection for the distal interphalangeal joints of the hands. Musculoskeletal involvement of the hand includes soft-tissue swelling, periarticular erosions, "fluffy" periostitis, and resorption of the distal phalanges. Bone mineralization is usually normal. Classic radiographic findings include the "sausage digit" (diffuse soft-tissue swelling) and the "pencil-in-cup" deformity from resorption and tapering of the distal aspect of the phalanges. Psoriasis may also involve the feet and sacroiliac joints.

- **Hajdu–Cheney syndrome.** Hajdu–Cheney is a rare syndrome that may occur sporadically or with an autosomal dominant familial inheritance. Patients have dysmorphic facies and cranial abnormalities, including an enlarged sella turcica, wormian bones, and basilar invagination. Hearing deficits and speech impediments are common. Osteolysis occurs within the distal phalanges of the hands and feet with classic bandlike lucencies that isolate proximal and distal osseous fragments in the terminal tufts.

■ Diagnosis

Scleroderma

✓ Pearls

- Hyperparathyroidism results in radial-sided subperiosteal resorption of the second and third middle phalanges.
- Scleroderma may result in soft-tissue resorption and calcifications with distal phalangeal acro-osteolysis.

- Thermal (burn and frost-bite) injuries may manifest as osteoporosis, periostitis, and acro-osteolysis.
- Hajdu–Cheney is a rare syndrome with dysmorphic facies and bandlike acro-osteolysis.

Suggested Readings

Avouac J, Guerini H, Wipff J, et al. Radiological hand involvement in systemic sclerosis. Ann Rheum Dis. 2006; 65(8):1088–1092

Resnick D, Kransdorf MJ. Bone and Joint Imaging. 3rd ed. Philadelphia, PA: Elsevier Saunders; 2005

Case 96

Jasjeet Bindra

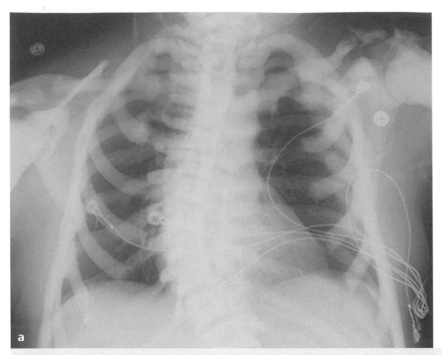
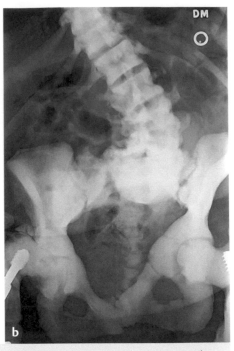

Fig. 96.1 (a) Frontal radiograph of the chest shows diffusely increased bone density. **(b)** Frontal image of lumbar spine and pelvis demonstrates similar diffuse osteosclerosis and transverse lucencies in both acetabula from fractures. Additional findings include scoliotic curvature of the spine, as well as postoperative changes and dislocation of the right hip.

■ Clinical Presentation

A 56-year-old woman with recurrent fractures (▶Fig. 96.1).

■ Key Imaging Finding

Diffusely increased bone density

■ Top 3 Differential Diagnoses

• **Metabolic disorders**. Renal osteodystrophy, primary hyperparathyroidism, hypervitaminosis D, and fluorosis are among the metabolic disorders that can cause increased bone density. Renal osteodystrophy is usually associated with soft-tissue calcifications, osteomalacia, and regions of osteosclerosis preferentially affecting the ribs, pelvis and spine. Osteosclerosis can produce the classic "rugger-jersey" spine radiographic appearance.

• **Osteoblastic metastases**. Several primary malignancies characteristically produce osteoblastic metastases, including carcinomas of the prostate, breast, and pancreas; mucinous adenocarcinoma of the gastrointestinal tract; transitional cell carcinoma; carcinoid tumor; lymphoma; medulloblastoma; and neuroblastoma. Differentiation from other causes of

increased bone density can often be made by correlation with medical history and the typically patchy nature of metastases.

• **Hematologic disorders**. Myelofibrosis, mastocytosis, and sickle cell anemia are some of the hematologic disorders that can show diffuse osteosclerosis. In myelofibrosis, bone marrow is replaced by fibrotic tissue, and osteosclerosis is most commonly found in the axial skeleton and proximal long bones, particularly the humerus and femur. In sickle cell disease, abnormal red blood cells result in bone infarcts that result in a markedly sclerotic appearance, especially in pelvis, spine, and ribs. Additional findings of spinal manifestations include "fish-mouth" vertebrae, avascular necrosis, and extramedullary hematopoiesis.

■ Additional Differential Diagnoses

• **Paget disease**. The incidence of Paget disease increases with age, with the majority cases occurring in elderly patients. In the blastic phase of Paget disease, there are areas of sclerosis with cortical thickening, coarsened trabeculae, and bony enlargement, especially in skull, spine, and pelvis.

• **Osteopetrosis**. Osteopetrosis is a rare inherited dysplasia characterized by increased bone density, especially in the long

bones, skull, and spine. Despite the increased density, involved bones are relatively fragile and prone to fractures. Classic radiographic findings include the "sandwich" appearance of the vertebral bodies with a sharp margin between the sclerotic endplates and more lucent bone centrally, as well as the "bone-in-bone" appearance occurs within the pelvis and long bones.

■ Diagnosis

Osteopetrosis

✓ Pearls

• Renal osteodystrophy results in the classic "rugger-jersey" spine, soft-tissue calcifications, and osteomalacia.

• Osteoblastic metastases most often present with patchy areas of increased density.

• Paget disease results in bony sclerosis, cortical thickening, coarsened trabeculae, and bony enlargement.

• Osteopetrosis is an inherited bony dysplasia with sclerotic but fragile bones.

Suggested Readings

Ejindu VC, Hine AL, Mashayekhi M, Shorvon PJ, Misra RR. Musculoskeletal manifestations of sickle cell disease. Radiographics. 2007; 27(4):1005–1021

Ihde LL, Forrester DM, Gottsegen CJ, et al. Sclerosing bone dysplasias: review and differentiation from other causes of osteosclerosis. Radiographics. 2011; 31(7):1865–1882

Murphey MD, Sartoris DJ, Quale JL, Pathria MN, Martin NL. Musculoskeletal manifestations of chronic renal insufficiency. Radiographics. 1993; 13(2):357–379

Case 97

M. Jason Akers

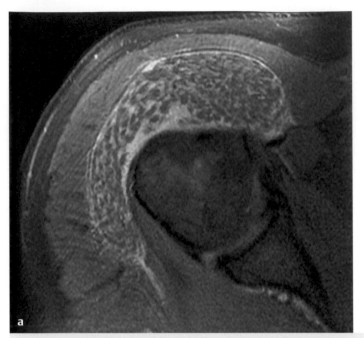
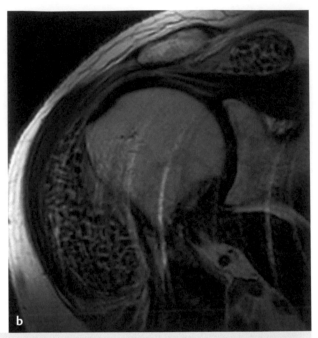

Fig. 97.1 **(a)** Axial fat-suppressed T2-weighted MRI of the shoulder and **(b)** coronal T2-weighted image of the same shoulder show marked distension of the subacromial-subdeltoid bursa with fluid containing multiple small iso- to hypointense nodules or bodies.

■ Clinical Presentation
....

A 71-year-old man with shoulder pain and swelling (▶ Fig. 97.1).

■ Key Imaging Finding

Loose bodies

■ Top 3 Differential Diagnoses

- **Synovial (osteo)chondromatosis.** Synovial (osteo)chondromatosis is a disease of the synovium resulting from synovial metaplasia, the cause of which is unknown. It is seen in men between the ages of 20 and 50 years and is most commonly intra-articular but may also occur in tendon sheaths and bursae. Occasionally, conglomerate masses may extend into the extracapsular soft tissues. The disease is typically monoarticular, with the knee, elbow, shoulder, and hip joints most commonly involved. Synovial metaplasia results in the formation of synovial villonodular projections that grow to form nodules. If the nodules remain attached to the synovium, they develop a blood supply and may become ossified. If the nodules break off, they are nourished by synovial fluid and become cartilaginous. Eighty-five percent have sufficient calcification to be detected on radiographs, appearing as multiple, round, similar-sized calcified bodies. The bodies are of variable magnetic resonance imaging (MRI) signal depending on the proportion of calcium, chondroid, and mature ossific tissue, ranging from low signal on all sequences to marrow signal on all sequences. Mechanical articular cartilage destruction results in well-marginated erosions. Malignant degeneration is rare. Treatment is resection of the bodies along with synovectomy. Recurrences after surgical debridement can occur.
- **Pigmented villonodular synovitis (PVNS).** PVNS is a benign neoplastic process of the synovium. It can occur intra-articularly and involve the joint diffusely or focally. It may also occur extra-articularly in a bursa or tendon sheath (giant cell tumor of the tendon sheath). The intra-articular form is characterized by villonodular proliferation of the synovium with associated hemorrhage. It is monoarticular with common locations including the knee and hip joints. On radiographs, PVNS manifests as a large joint effusion with or without associated erosions and subchondral cysts. Joint spaces are usually preserved. MRI shows a joint effusion and focal or diffuse synovial thickening that is low signal on T1 and T2 because of hemosiderin deposition. The hemosiderin causes susceptibility artifact and blooming on gradient-echo sequences. Treatment is synovectomy; incomplete resection is associated with high recurrence rates.
- **Rice bodies.** Multiple small loose bodies can occur within joints affected by rheumatoid arthritis and are termed "rice bodies" because of their resemblance to polished grains of rice. "Rice bodies" are small fragments of fibrous tissue that occur as a nonspecific response to synovial inflammation. The exact cause is unknown, but one theory postulates that "rice bodies" represent detached fragments of infarcted synovium. First described in association with tuberculous arthritis, "rice bodies" are now more frequently associated with rheumatoid arthritis. They can, however, also be seen in the absence of any underlying systemic disorder. On MRI, "rice bodies" are hypointense on T2 because of their fibrous nature and are associated with a joint effusion, synovial hypertrophy, and synovial enhancement after gadolinium administration.

■ Diagnosis

Rice bodies

✓ Pearls

- Synovial (osteo)chondromatosis is a synovial metaplasia that results in loose bodies; 85% are calcified.
- PVNS shows low-signal synovial thickening on T1 and T2 with blooming on gradient because of hemosiderin.

- "Rice bodies" are small loose bodies that are most frequently associated with rheumatoid arthritis.

Suggested Readings

Chung C, Coley BD, Martin LC. Rice bodies in juvenile rheumatoid arthritis. AJR Am J Roentgenol. 1998; 170(3):698–700

Cheung HS, Ryan LM, Kozin F, McCarty DJ. Synovial origins of Rice bodies in joint fluid. Arthritis Rheum. 1980; 23(1):72–76

Dürr HR, Stäbler A, Maier M, Refior HJ. Pigmented villonodular synovitis. Review of 20 cases. J Rheumatol. 2001; 28(7):1620–1630

Murphey MD, Vidal JA, Fanburg-Smith JC, Gajewski DA. Imaging of synovial chondromatosis with radiologic-pathologic correlation. Radiographics. 2007; 27(5):1465–1488

Stoller DW, Tirman PFJ, Bredella MA. Diagnostic Imaging: Orthopaedics. Salt Lake City, UT: Amirsys; 2004

Case 98

Philip Yen

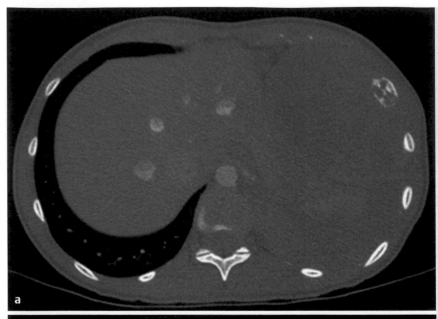

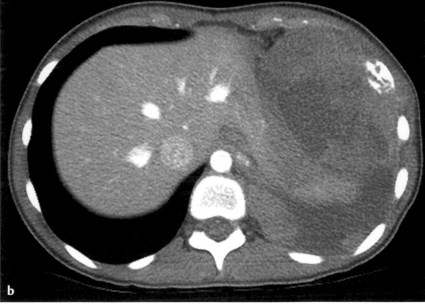

Fig. 98.1 (a, b) Axial CT images of the chest in bone and soft-tissue windows show an expansile, rib lesion of a left lower rib with a large heterogeneous soft-tissue component extending into the thoracic cavity.

■ **Clinical Presentation**

A 16-year-old girl with a chest wall mass (▶ Fig. 98.1).

■ Key Imaging Finding

Expansile rib lesion in a child

■ Top 3 Differential Diagnoses

- **Fibrous dysplasia**. Fibrous dysplasia is a benign skeletal disorder characterized by replacement of medullary bone with fibrous tissue. The ribs are the most common sites of involvement with monostotic disease. Polyostotic disease is termed McCune–Albright syndrome and is associated with endocrine dysfunction (most often precocious puberty) and café-au-lait spots. Bony lesions are expansile with variable internal matrix; the classic lesion has a characteristic ground-glass matrix.
- **Bone cyst**. Bone cysts are fluid-filled lesions that may be **unicameral** (**UBC**) or **aneurysmal** (**ABC**). They are expansile, lytic, and central in location. A pathognomonic finding in a UBC is the "fallen fragment" sign, which represents a bony fragment within the gravity-dependent area of the cyst and usually seen after a pathologic fracture. ABCs are multiloculated with fluid–fluid levels secondary to hemorrhage. Patients are typically younger than 30 years and asymptomatic unless complicated by fracture.
- **Enchondroma**. An enchondroma is a common benign cartilaginous bone tumor. When located in the phalanges, the lesions are expansile and purely lytic. In other locations, enchondromas are expansile with characteristic chondroid matrix and internal calcifications in an "arcs and swirls" patter. Multiple lesions are associated with Ollier (typically unilateral) and Maffucci syndromes (also has soft-tissue venous malformations/hemangiomas).

■ Additional Differential Diagnoses

- **Langerhans cell histiocytosis (LCH)**. Eosinophilic granuloma is the most benign form of LCH and is characterized by isolated osseous involvement. It is usually seen in children and young adults. Flat bones, including ribs, are involved more frequently than long bones. Although the imaging appearance is variable, they commonly present as expansile lytic lesions. Periosteal reaction may be seen.
- **Ewing sarcoma**. Ewing sarcoma is a malignant primary bone neoplasm that frequently affects the diaphysis or metaphysis of long bones in the first and second decades of life. Less commonly, it can involve flat bones and ribs. Radiographic findings include a permeative intramedullary destructive lesion with a "moth-eaten" appearance and aggressive periosteal reaction ("onion skin" or "sun burst" pattern). Computed tomography (CT) and magnetic resonance imaging (MRI) can better delineate associated soft-tissue components that can be very large.
- **Metastases**. Rib lesions may arise from any primary malignancy that metastasizes to bone, including Ewing sarcoma, osteosarcoma, lymphoma, rhabdomyosarcoma, neuroblastoma, and Wilms tumor. Radiographic findings vary based on the primary neoplasm; lesions are commonly multifocal.

■ Diagnosis

Ewing sarcoma

✓ Pearls

- Fibrous dysplasia classically has bony expansion with a "ground-glass" appearance to its matrix.
- "Fluid–fluid levels" can be seen in aneurysmal bone cysts.
- Ewing sarcoma tends to have a large associated soft-tissue mass with lytic appearance of the involved rib.

Suggested Readings

Glass RB, Norton KI, Mitre SA, Kang E. Pediatric ribs: a spectrum of abnormalities. Radiographics. 2002; 22(1):87–104

Helms CA. Fundamentals of Skeletal Radiology. 4th ed. Philadelphia, PA: Elsevier Saunders; 2014

Levine BD, Motamedi K, Chow K, Gold RH, Seeger LL. CT of rib lesions. AJR Am J Roentgenol. 2009; 193(1):5–13

Schulman H, Newman-Heinman N, Kurtzbart E, Maor E, Zirkin H, Laufer L. Thoracoabdominal peripheral primitive neuroectodermal tumors in childhood: radiological features. Eur Radiol. 2000; 10(10):1649–1652

Case 99

M. Jason Akers

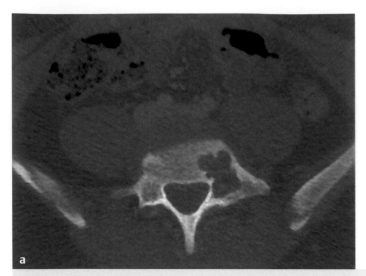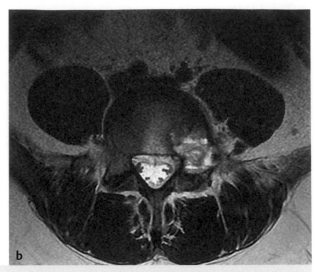

Fig. 99.1 **(a)** Axial CT image of lumbar spine shows a mildly expansile lytic lesion involving the left posterior L5 vertebral body and pedicle. **(b)** Axial T2-weighted magnetic resonance (MR) image at the same level shows fluid–fluid levels within the lesion.

▪ Clinical Presentation

Patient with chronic back pain (▶Fig. 99.1).

■ Key Imaging Finding

Posterior element lytic lesion

■ Top 3 Differential Diagnoses

- **Aneurysmal bone cyst (ABC).** ABC is a benign expansile lesion containing thin-walled blood-filled cavities thought to occur as a result of trauma. ABCs can be isolated or associated with other tumors. They are usually seen in children and young adults and commonly occur in long bone metaphyses and the posterior elements of the spine. In the spine, ABCs are classically centered in the pedicle and extend into the vertebral body. The pedicle appears absent on anteroposterior radiographs of the spine. Cortical thinning and focal cortical destruction are common. There may also be extension into the epidural space causing canal stenosis. Fluid–fluid levels result from hemorrhage within the lesion.
- **Osteoblastoma.** Osteoblastoma is a benign osteoid forming tumor thought to be a larger version (>1.5 cm) of osteoid osteoma. Forty percent occur in the spine and originate in the posterior elements, often extending into the vertebral body. They present as expansile lesions with narrow zones of transition and variable mineralization. The matrix is better visualized on computed tomography (CT) than radiographs. There may be an ABC component with fluid–fluid levels. Tumors can incite an inflammatory response with associated peritumoral edema that extends beyond the margins of the lesion.
- **Infection (tuberculosis [TB]).** TB causes granulomatous infection of the spine and adjacent soft tissues. Isolated posterior element involvement can occur particularly in the thoracic spine. Patients usually have prominent epidural and paraspinal disease with large paraspinal abscesses dissecting over multiple levels. Tuberculous spondylitis is more likely to spare intervertebral discs while causing prominent bony destruction.

■ Additional Differential Diagnoses

- **Metastases.** Metastases usually occur in older patients and involve the posterior vertebral body first with extension into the posterior elements. Metastases most commonly spread to the spine hematogenously. Lytic metastases tend to be less expansile and more permeative in appearance, occurring as a destructive lesion with an associated soft-tissue mass. Multiple vertebral levels are commonly involved.
- **Langerhans cell histiocytosis (LCH).** LCH is a disease occurring in children that is characterized by abnormal histiocyte proliferation producing granulomatous skeletal lesions. The classic presentation in the spine is vertebra plana with preservation of the disc space. LCH can also present as an aggressive lytic lesion with soft-tissue mass and extension into the spinal canal. Other sites of involvement include the skull with a beveled edge appearance, mandible, long bones, ribs, and pelvis.

■ Diagnosis

Aneurysmal bone cyst

✓ Pearls

- ABCs are benign expansile lytic lesions that contain fluid–fluid levels because of internal hemorrhage.
- Osteoblastoma has an osteoid matrix and typically has peritumoral edema that extends beyond the lesion.
- Posterior element involvement of the thoracic spine with paraspinal abscesses suggests TB spondylitis.
- Lytic metastases often occur in older patients, appear permeative/destructive, and may affect multiple levels.

Suggested Readings

DiCaprio MR, Murphy MJ, Camp RL. Aneurysmal bone cyst of the spine with familial incidence. Spine. 2000; 25(12):1589–1592

Long SS, Yablon CM, Eisenberg RL. Bone marrow signal alteration in the spine and sacrum. AJR Am J Roentgenol. 2010; 195(3):W178–200

Shaikh MI, Saifuddin A, Pringle J, Natali C, Sherazi Z. Spinal osteoblastoma: CT and MR imaging with pathological correlation. Skeletal Radiol. 1999; 28(1):33–40

Stoller DW, Tirman PFJ, Bredella MA. Diagnostic Imaging: Orthopaedics. Salt Lake City, UT: Amirsys; 2004

Case 100

Eva Escobedo

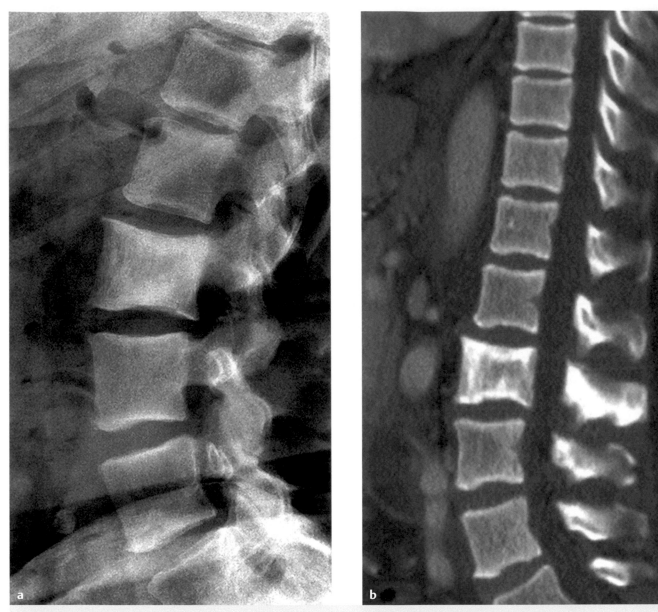

Fig. 100.1 **(a)** Lateral radiograph of lumbar spine shows diffusely dense and slightly enlarged L3 vertebral body. **(b)** Sagittal computed tomography (CT) reformation of lumbar spine shows similar appearance and involvement of posterior elements.

■ Clinical Presentation

A 60-year-old woman with back pain (▶Fig. 100.1).

■ Key Imaging Finding

Ivory vertebral body

■ Top 3 Differential Diagnoses

- **Osteoblastic metastasis**. Increased density in metastatic foci is due to abnormal stimulation of osteoblasts. Prostate and breast carcinoma are the most common sources of osteoblastic metastases. Less common sources include lymphoma (see below), bladder, colon, lung, and carcinoid. In most cases, there is involvement of multiple vertebral levels. In children, sclerotic vertebral metastasis can be seen with neuroblastoma and medulloblastoma.
- **Paget disease**. Paget disease, which is most common after 40 years of age, is characterized by excessive, abnormal remodeling of bone. The ivory vertebral body is seen in the inactive, sclerotic phase, and can either involve a single level or more than one level. The most common appearance with Paget disease in the vertebral body is trabecular thickening with enlargement of the vertebral body. Cortical thickening around the periphery of the body results in a "picture frame" appearance. Because of the common finding of expansion, Paget disease does not fully meet the original criteria of an ivory vertebral body, which is "increased density with retained size and shape," but is commonly included in the differential.
- **Lymphoma**. Skeletal involvement is common in both Hodgkin and non-Hodgkin lymphoma. Osteosclerosis is rare and more commonly seen with Hodgkin lymphoma. Spinal involvement in patients with Hodgkin disease may result in osteolysis, osteosclerosis, or a combination of the two. Destructive lytic lesions are more common than osteosclerosis. Lymphoma of the vertebral body is characteristically associated with a paraspinal soft-tissue mass. Margins of the vertebral body may show erosions caused by the surrounding mass.

■ Additional Differential Diagnoses

- **Mastocytosis**. A rare disorder of mast cell proliferation, mastocytosis may present with either osteopenia and lytic lesions or osteosclerosis, and may be focal or diffuse. In the spine, it commonly involves multiple levels. Multiple organ systems may be affected as well.
- **Myeloma**. Rarely, myeloma may present with osteosclerotic lesions. Sclerotic bone lesions may be seen with POEMS syndrome, a disease comprising multiple entities. POEMS is an acronym for the most common features of the syndrome: polyneuropathy, organomegaly, endocrinopathy, monoclonal gammopathy, and skin changes.

■ Diagnosis

Paget disease

✓ Pearls

- Enlargement of the vertebral body helps differentiate Paget from other causes of ivory vertebral body.
- The "picture frame" appearance is a characteristic sign in Paget disease.
- Prostate and breast carcinoma are the most common sources of osteoblastic metastases.
- Osteosclerosis is rare in lymphoma and more often seen with Hodgkin than with non-Hodgkin lymphoma.

Suggested Readings

Graham TS. The ivory vertebra sign. Radiology. 2005; 235(2):614–615
Mulligan ME. Myeloma and lymphoma. Semin Musculoskelet Radiol. 2000; 4(1):127–135

Resnick D. Diagnosis of bone and joint disorders. 4th ed. Philadelphia, PA: Saunders; 2002

Case 101

Sonia Kaur Ghei

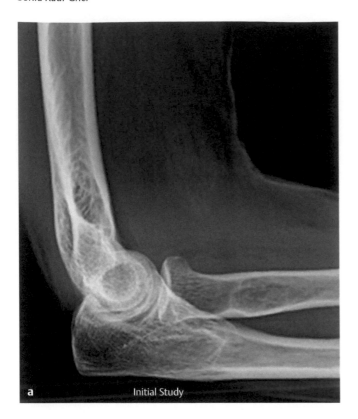

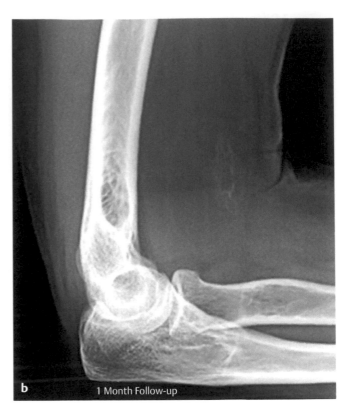

a — Initial Study

b — 1 Month Follow-up

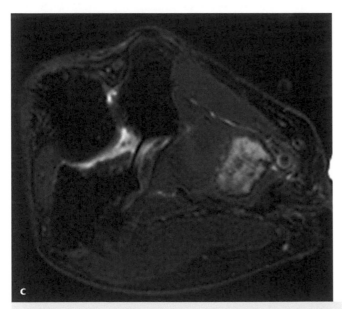

c

Fig. 101.1 (a) Initial and (b) 1 month follow-up lateral radiographs of the elbow show a mass with mineralization in the anterior soft tissues that demonstrates more mature appearance of mineralization on the 1 month follow-up radiograph. (c) Axial fat-suppressed T2 MR image of the elbow shows a corresponding hyperintense mass with a low signal intensity rim.

■ Clinical Presentation

A 60-year-old woman with palpable mass anterior to elbow (►Fig. 101.1).

■ **Key Imaging Finding**

Periarticular soft tissue calcifications

■ **Top 3 Differential Diagnoses**

- **Calcinosis of renal failure.** The most frequent cause of a calcified periarticular mass is chronic renal failure. These masses have amorphous, cloudlike calcifications and can become very large. They cannot be distinguished radiographically from tumoral calcinosis
- **Myositis ossificans.** Also known as heterotopic ossification, myositis ossificans occurs secondary to trauma or immobility and can present as an enlarging painful mass. Cloudlike calcification is seen 4 to 6 weeks after trauma with peripheral maturation to cortical bone. On radiographs, this so-called zonal phenomenon is seen with central lucency and a zone of mature ossification at the periphery (centripetal progression),

differentiating this entity from juxtacortical or extraskeletal osteosarcomas, which mature centrally or in centrifugal pattern.

- **Arthropathy with calcified soft tissue nodule.** If a soft tissue mass with calcification occurs near a joint, underlying arthropathy should be considered. For example, synovial osteochondromatosis can present as multiple calcified masses in a large joint such as the knee, hip, or shoulder and occurs secondary to metaplasia of synovial connective tissue. Gouty tophi, particularly involving the first metatarsophalangeal joint, can also calcify but are typically less dense than tumoral calcinosis.

■ **Additional Differential Diagnoses**

- **Scleroderma.** Scleroderma demonstrates characteristic findings in the hands with acro-osteolysis (resorption of the distal phalanges) and atrophy of the soft tissues at the distal fingers. Sharply marginated calcifications are seen in a subcutaneous and periarticular distribution. The calcifications associated with scleroderma are described as calcinosis circumscripta because of their well-defined margins.
- **Soft tissue sarcoma.** Soft tissue sarcomas include entities such as synovial sarcoma, extraskeletal osteosarcoma, and chondrosarcoma. Synovial sarcoma presents as a mass with amorphous calcifications in close proximity to a joint, particularly in the lower extremities. On T2 images, "triple signal intensity" is seen due to hemorrhage, fibrous tissue, and cystic

components that often contain fluid–fluid levels. Extraskeletal osteosarcomas demonstrate central ossification, which is referred to as "reverse zoning." Chondrosarcomas usually arise from underlying bone and contain annular or comma-shaped calcifications. Lesions are hyperintense on T2 magnetic resonance sequences, with hypointense calcifications.

- **Tumoral calcinosis.** Tumoral calcinosis is a rare idiopathic inherited disorder that predominantly occurs in people of African descent. It most often presents in the first or second decades of life with painless, enlarging periarticular calcifications. The hips, elbows, and shoulders are the most common sites of involvement.

■ **Diagnosis**

Heterotopic ossification or myositis ossificans

✓ **Pearls**

- Calcinosis of renal failure is the most frequent cause of a calcified periarticular mass.
- Myositis ossificans should eventually demonstrate a dense zone of mature ossification peripherally.

- Masses demonstrating central ossification or amorphous calcification may suggest a soft tissue sarcoma.

Suggested Readings

Greenspan A. Orthopedic Imaging - A Practical Approach. 5th ed. Philadelphia, PA: Lippincott Williams & Wilkins; 2011

Olsen KM, Chew FS. Tumoral calcinosis: Pearls, polemics, and alternative possibilities. Radiographics. 2006; 26(3):871–885

Case 102

Chirag V. Patel

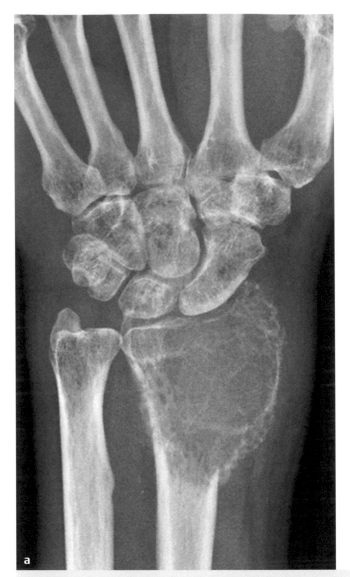 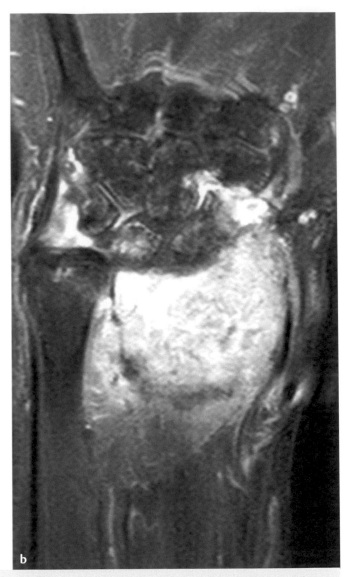

Fig. 102.1 **(a)** Frontal radiograph of wrist demonstrates an expansile lytic lesion involving the distal radius. There are subtle internal septations and adjacent soft-tissue swelling. The lesion has a narrow zone of transition. **(b)** Coronal postcontrast fat-suppressed T1 MR image of the same wrist shows diffuse enhancement of the mass.

▪ Clinical Presentation

A 40-year-old man with pain and swelling of the wrist (▶Fig. 102.1).

■ Key Imaging Finding

Benign expansile lytic lesion

■ Top 3 Differential Diagnoses

- **Fibrous dysplasia**. Fibrous dysplasia is a benign intramedullary fibro-osseous lesion with monostotic or less commonly polyostotic involvement. Common sites include long bones, ribs, craniofacial bones, and pelvis. Radiographically, it manifests as an intramedullary expansile lytic lesion, with metadiaphyseal localization, and, unlike other benign lytic bone lesions, demonstrates a thick "rind" of reactive bone. The tumor matrix has characteristic "ground-glass" appearance and may show internal calcification
- **Unicameral bone cyst**. Also known as simple bone cyst, unicameral bone cyst is a common bone lesion, following only nonossifying fibroma and osteochondroma in prevalence. It occurs in the 5- to 20-year age group, involving the metadiaphyses of long bones. Approximately 80% of the childhood cysts are located in the proximal humerus and proximal

femur, whereas in patients older than 17 years, about half of the lesions are located in the pelvis or calcaneus. Radiographic characteristics are a central location and cortical expansion, with a thin sclerotic rim.
- **Aneurysmal bone cyst (ABC)**. ABC is a benign bone lesion of unknown etiology, occurring in the 5- to 20-year age group. It most commonly occurs in the metadiaphyseal region of long bones and posterior elements of the spine. Radiographically, it presents as an expansile lytic lesion with thin septations, more commonly eccentric in location, giving a characteristic "soap-bubble" appearance. Computed tomography (CT) and magnetic resonance imaging (MRI) demonstrate fluid–fluid levels. The absence of ossification or calcification within the lesion and the absence of epiphyseal extension are other helpful distinguishing features.

■ Additional Differential Diagnoses

- **Giant cell tumor**. Giant cell tumor rarely occurs before closure of growth plate and is most commonly seen between 20 and 50 years of age. Epiphyseal extension is characteristic, and thin septations may be seen. The distal femur and proximal tibia account for more than 50% of giant cell tumors. Imaging characteristics include an eccentric location, extension to subcortical bone, and lack of a sclerotic rim. Approximately 5 to 10% of lesions may be malignant. Local recurrence after resection may occur in up to 25% of cases.
- **Eosinophilic granuloma**. Eosinophilic granuloma is the localized osseous form of Langerhans cell histiocytosis. The average age of onset is 10 to 14 years. Depending on the site of involvement and the stage of the disease, common manifestations include well-defined areas of cortical or medullary rarefaction; in the later stages, there may be a sclerotic margin, periosteal reaction, and bone expansion. Long bones are involved less commonly as compared to flat bones.

■ Diagnosis

Giant cell tumor

✓ Pearls

- Fibrous dysplasia classically has a ground-glass matrix with calcification and a thick rind of reactive bone.
- Approximately 80% of unicameral bones cysts in childhood involve the proximal humerus or femur.
- Fluid–fluid levels suggest an ABC but may be present in other lesions as well.
- Giant cell tumors occur after growth plate closure, extend to the subcortical bone, and lack a sclerotic rim.

Suggested Readings

Chakarun CJ, Forrester DM, Gottsegen CJ, Patel DB, White EA, Matcuk GR, Jr. Giant cell tumor of bone: review, mimics, and new developments in treatment. Radiographics. 2013; 33(1):197–211

Fitzpatrick KA, Taljanovic MS, Speer DP, et al. Imaging findings of fibrous dysplasia with histopathologic and intraoperative correlation. AJR Am J Roentgenol. 2004; 182(6):1389–1398

Mahnken AH, Nolte-Ernsting CC, Wildberger JE, et al. Aneurysmal bone cyst: value of MR imaging and conventional radiography. Eur Radiol. 2003; 13(5):1118–1124

Case 103

Adrianne K. Thompson

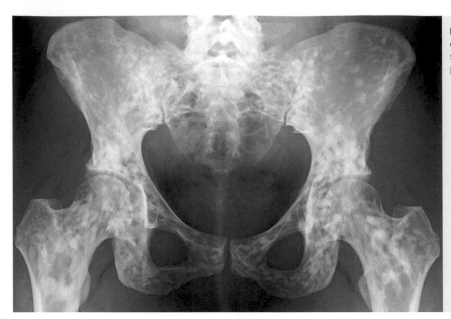

Fig. 103.1 Anteroposterior radiograph of the pelvis demonstrates multiple sclerotic lesions with a symmetric distribution throughout the pelvis and proximal femurs.

■ Clinical Presentation

A 40-year-old woman with hip pain (▶ Fig. 103.1).

■ Key Imaging Finding

Multiple sclerotic foci within the pelvis

■ Top 3 Differential Diagnoses

- **Osteopoikilosis**. Osteopoikilosis is an asymptomatic form of skeletal sclerotic dysplasia that occurs in both men and women. Cutaneous manifestations may be seen, such as keloids or fibrocollagenous infiltration of the skin. Imaging shows ovoid, well-defined, sclerotic foci, which are usually small and symmetrically distributed. Osteopoikilosis shows a predilection for long and short tubular bones, carpal and tarsal bones, pelvis, and scapulae. Usually, there is normal activity on bone scan. There may be an association with other osteosclerotic dysplasias such as osteopathia striata (Voorhoeve syndrome) and melorheostosis.
- **Metastatic disease**. Metastatic disease is a common cause of sclerotic foci within the pelvis, most often caused by prostate cancer in men and breast cancer in women. When presented with sclerotic foci within the pelvis, helpful features to suggest malignant disease include (1) lesion borders, which tend to be indistinct with a wide zone of transition, (2) presence of periosteal reaction, (3) soft tissue extension, (4) size, as metastatic lesions would be larger and less uniform than those seen in benign conditions, and (5) multiplicity, particularly when lesions are seen in bones outside of the pelvis.
- **Paget disease**. Paget disease is a disorder of bone metabolism seen in older patients with a slight male predilection and onset in the fifth and sixth decades of life. Numerous etiologies have been proposed, but the cause remains elusive. The disease shows increased bone remodeling, leading to an abnormal balance between bone resorption and replacement. Osteoblastic activity results in increased alkaline phosphatase, and increased osteoclastic activity leads to high levels of hydroxyproline in urine. Most commonly affected bones include the pelvis, femurs, skull, tibiae, and spine. Radiographic findings reflect the cellular activity taking place at that phase; there are three main phases: osteolytic, mixed, and osteoblastic. In the osteolytic phase, bone resorption occurs, causing radiolucent changes in bone. In the calvarium, this results in bone destruction termed *osteoporosis circumscripta*, whereas in the tibia, this results in a "blade-of-grass" appearance. The mixed phase shows both bone resorption and formation with prominent bony trabeculae and a "cotton-wool" appearance. Lastly, in the blastic phase, there is a drastic increase in bone density with cortical thickening and bony deformity. Specific changes within the pelvis include trabecular thickening of the iliopectineal/ilioischial lines, hemipelvic asymmetry, and bony enlargement. Complications include pathologic fractures, early degenerative joint disease, neurologic impingement, and malignant transformation.

■ Diagnosis

Osteopoikilosis

✓ Pearls

- Osteopoikilosis is asymptomatic and usually demonstrates normal activity on bone scan.
- Sclerotic metastatic disease to the pelvis most commonly originates from prostate and breast carcinoma.
- Paget disease in the pelvis may demonstrate thickening of the iliopectineal and ilioischial lines.

Suggested Readings

Greenspan A. Orthopedic Imaging: A Practical Approach. 5th ed. Philadelphia, PA: Lippincott Williams and Wilkins; 2011

Ihde LL, Forrester DM, Gottsegen CJ, et al. Sclerosing bone dysplasias: review and differentiation from other causes of osteosclerosis. Radiographics. 2011; 31(7):1865–1882

Resnick D, Kransdorf MJ. Bone and Joint Imaging. 3rd ed. Philadelphia, PA: Elsevier Saunders; 2005

Theodorou DJ, Theodorou SJ, Kakitsubata Y. Imaging of Paget disease of bone and its musculoskeletal complications: review. AJR Am J Roentgenol. 2011; 196(6, Suppl):S64–S75

Case 104

Sonia Kaur Ghei

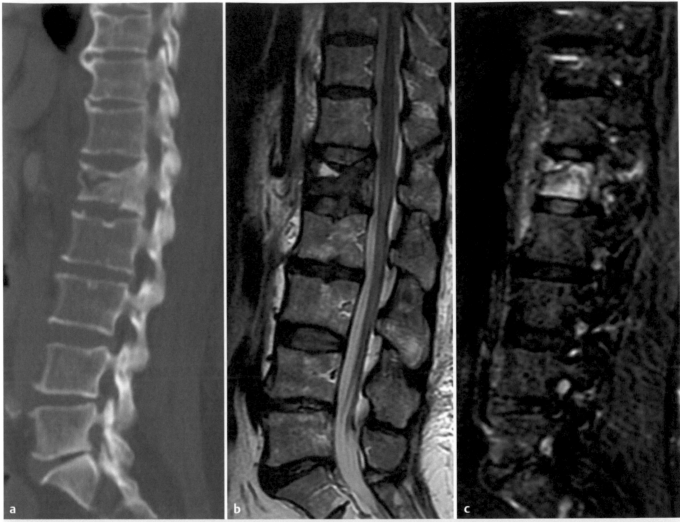

Fig. 104.1 **(a)** Sagittal reformatted CT image demonstrates an anterior wedge compression deformity of L1 in an elderly patient. There is sclerosis of the posterior vertebral body. **(b)** Sagittal T2-weighted MR image shows the L1 compression fracture with focal edema anteriorly and decreased signal intensity within the remainder of the vertebral body. **(c)** Sagittal short tau inversion recovery (STIR) image paramidline extending through the pedicle demonstrates extension of abnormal signal/marrow edema into the vertebral body pedicle with normal pedicle signal at other levels.

■ Clinical Presentation

A 72-year-old woman with acute back pain (►Fig. 104.1).

■ Key Imaging Finding

Vertebral body wedge fracture

■ Top 3 Differential Diagnoses

- **Traumatic fracture**. Traumatic vertebral fractures tend to occur in the upper lumbar spine, and a history of fall or significant trauma is usually present. These most often involve the superior endplate, and surrounding paravertebral soft tissue swelling or hematoma can often be seen. This soft tissue should be smooth and rim-shaped rather than irregular or nodular. If the fracture extends into the posterior elements, abnormal signal intensity may be seen in these regions
- **Insufficiency fracture**. Insufficiency fractures of the spine tend to occur in older osteoporotic patients. These tend to have similar imaging characteristics as a traumatic fracture but can occur at any level. In an older patient, the images should be carefully examined for signs of underlying malignancy because the spine is a common site of metastatic disease, and a fracture may be the presenting abnormality. Marrow edema in insufficiency fractures is limited to the vertebral body; extension of abnormal signal into the pedicles suggests an underlying lesion or traumatic event. In addition, the soft tissue component should be smooth and rim-shaped.

- **Pathological fracture**. A pathological fracture can occur anywhere in the spine where there is an underlying lesion. There are four magnetic resonance imaging (MRI) features that suggest an underlying malignant etiology: (1) abnormal marrow signal with ill-defined margins (all fractures will demonstrate increased T2 and inversion recovery signal secondary to marrow edema and hemorrhage, but it should be well-defined if benign), (2) abnormal marrow signal extending into the pedicles, (3) associated soft tissue lesion with irregular or nodular borders (smooth paravertebral soft tissue swelling is normally seen surrounding a fracture), and (4) marked enhancement (mild enhancement can normally be seen with benign fractures). Also, because traumatic fractures tend to occur in the upper lumbar spine, an underlying lesion should be considered in a younger patient with a lower lumbar spine fracture, particularly if there is no history of significant antecedent trauma.

■ Diagnosis

Pathological fracture (metastatic disease)

✓ Pearls

- Traumatic fractures commonly involve the superior endplates within the upper lumbar spine.
- Insufficiency fractures tend to occur in older, osteoporotic patients and spare the posterior elements.

- Atraumatic marrow edema within pedicles or marked enhancement is concerning for pathological fracture.
- Pathological fractures should be considered in a younger patient without significant trauma.

Suggested Readings

Griffith JF, Guglielmi G. Vertebral fracture. Radiol Clin North Am. 2010; 48(3):519–529

Haba H, Taneichi H, Kotani Y, et al. Diagnostic accuracy of magnetic resonance imaging for detecting posterior ligamentous complex injury associated with thoracic and lumbar fractures. J Neurosurg. 2003; 99(1, Suppl):20–26

Shih TT, Huang KM, Li YW. Solitary vertebral collapse: distinction between benign and malignant causes using MR patterns. J Magn Reson Imaging. 1999; 9(5):635–642

Wintermark M, Mouhsine E, Theumann N, et al. Thoracolumbar spine fractures in patients who have sustained severe trauma: depiction with multi-detector row CT. Radiology. 2003; 227(3):681–689

Case 105

Adrianne K. Thompson

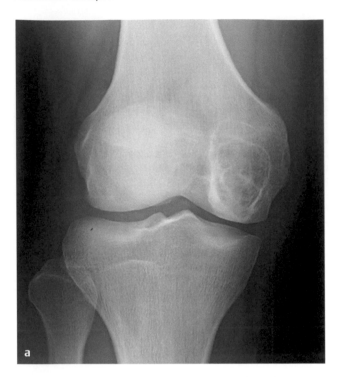

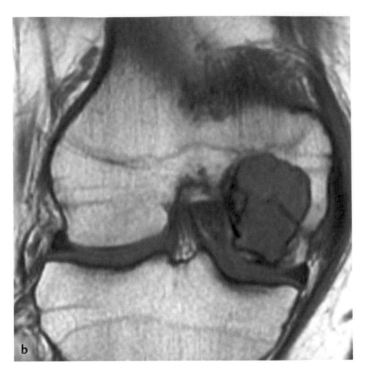

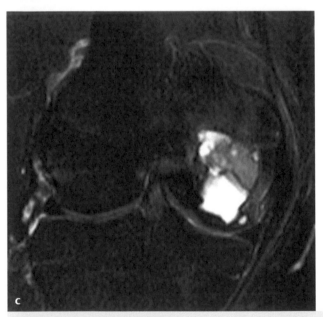

Fig. 105.1 **(a)** Frontal radiograph of the knee demonstrates a circumscribed eccentric lucent lesion with thin sclerotic margins and a narrow zone of transition within the epiphyseal region of the medial femoral condyle. **(b)** Coronal T1 and **(c)** fat-suppressed T2 images of the same knee reveal a benign appearing circumscribed T1 intermediate to hypointense and T2 mixed (intermediate to hyperintense) intensity epiphyseal lesion.

■ Clinical Presentation

A young man with knee pain (▶Fig. 105.1).

■ Key Imaging Finding

Epiphyseal/epiphyseal equivalent lucent lesion

■ Top 3 Differential Diagnoses

- **Chondroblastoma.** Chondroblastomas are rare lesions that occur in the epiphyses of long bones and are usually seen before skeletal maturity. The most common locations include the humerus, tibia, and femur, as well as within epiphyseal equivalents, such as the patella. On radiographs, chondroblastomas tend to be well-defined lucent lesions with a thin rim of sclerosis; calcifications can be seen in approximately 50% of cases. Periosteal reaction can occasionally be seen quite a distance away from the primary lesion. On MRI, they tend to show decreased signal intensity on T1 and variable signal intensity on T2 sequences, depending upon the amount of chondroid matrix and calcification. However, chondroblastomas are associated with significant surrounding marrow edema that may extend into the soft tissues. They demonstrate increased uptake on nuclear medicine bone scans
- **Giant cell tumor (GCT).** GCTs are locally aggressive bone tumors composed of giant cells, connective tissue, and stromal cells. They are most common in the third and fourth decades of life and more so in women than men. Its fundamental feature

is extensive epiphyseal involvement and is usually seen after growth plate closure. GCT favors long tubular bones, but can also be seen in the spine and flat bones, such as the clavicles, ribs, and sternum. Radiographic evaluation shows a lucent, expansile, eccentric lesion producing overlying cortical thinning. Margins can be well- or poorly defined. Approximately 5 to 10% of lesions may be malignant. They can also have recurrence after treatment.
- **Langerhans cell histiocytosis (LCH).** LCH typically occurs in children, adolescents, and young adults and has a 2:1 male predominance. Although LCH can be multiple, solitary lytic bone lesions predominate with a "punched-out" appearance; it commonly involves the skull ("punched-out" lesion with beveled edges), mandible (floating tooth), spine (flattened vertebral body or vertebra plana), ribs, and long bones. These lesions occur in the epiphyses and can cross an open growth plate. LCH can mimic more aggressive processes, such as infection or Ewing sarcoma, both clinically and radiographically.

■ Additional Differential Diagnoses

- **Intraosseous ganglion cyst.** Intraosseous ganglion cysts tend to occur within the subchondral/subarticular regions of the shoulder, knee, ankle, hip, and carpal joints after skeletal mat-

uration. On radiographs, they are well-defined lucent lesions with surrounding sclerotic margins. They demonstrate low T1 and high T2 signal intensity.

■ Diagnosis

Chondroblastoma

✓ Pearls

- Chondroblastomas usually occur in epiphyses or epiphyseal equivalents before skeletal maturity.
- Chondroblastomas tend to be associated with a significant amount of marrow and soft tissue edema.

- GCTs typically involve the epiphysis or epiphyseal equivalents after skeletal maturity.
- LCH can occur in the epiphysis and can cross an open growth plate.

Suggested Readings

Douis H, Saifuddin A. The imaging of cartilaginous bone tumours. I. Benign lesions. Skeletal Radiol. 2012; 41(10):1195–1212

Greenspan A, Jundt G, Remagen W. Differential Diagnosis in Orthopedic Oncology. 2nd ed. Philadelphia, PA: Lippincott Williams and Wilkins; 2007

Resnick D, Kransdorf MJ. Bone and joint imaging. 3rd ed. Philadelphia, PA: Elsevier Saunders; 2005

Part 5

Head and Neck Imaging

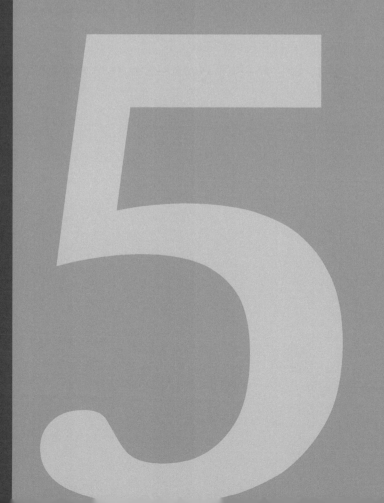

Case 106

William T. O'Brien, Sr.

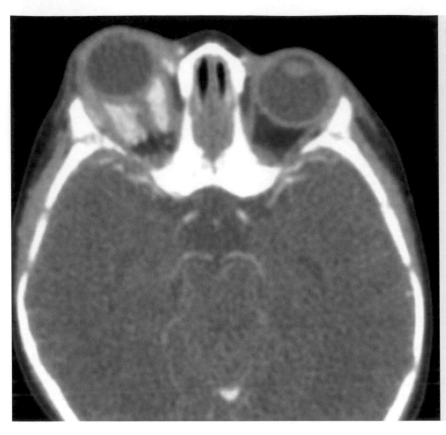

Fig. 106.1 Axial contrast-enhanced CT image demonstrates enhancing intraconal mass on both sides of the optic nerve sheath complex with associated proptosis. Restricted mobility of the globe is suggested by the disconjugate gaze during imaging despite the eyes being open.

■ Clinical Presentation

A young patient with proptosis and visual changes (▶Fig. 106.1).

■ Key Imaging Finding

Enhancing orbital mass

■ Top 3 Differential Diagnoses

- **Cavernous "hemangioma"**. Orbital cavernous "hemangiomas" are truly nonneoplastic, encapsulated venous vascular malformations. They represent the most common intraorbital masses and often present with proptosis or pain. Lesions are well-circumscribed a with round, oval, or lobulated configuration. Most commonly, they are intraconal and retrobulbar in location, although they may occur anywhere in the orbit. They are typically hyperdense on computed tomography (CT), T1 hypointense, and T2 hyperintense with intense enhancement. Calcifications are occasionally seen and are characteristic. Larger lesions may remodel adjacent bony structures
- **Lymphatic malformation**. Orbital lymphatic malformations are benign hamartomatous lesions that occur in children and young adults. Patients typically present with proptosis as the lesion enlarges. Although they most commonly involve the extraconal compartment, orbital lymphatic malformations may involve any and multiple compartments. They are typically multilocular, cystic, and prone to hemorrhage. Fluid–fluid levels are common and characteristic after episodes of hemorrhage. Enhancement of septations is typically seen.
- **Meningioma**. Orbital meningiomas most often occur in middle-aged women; there is also an increased incidence in children with neurofibromatosis type II (NF-2). Extraconal involvement is often due to intraorbital spread from a sphenoid wing or cavernous sinus meningioma. Optic nerve sheath meningiomas, on the other hand, are true intraconal lesions that typically do not extend intracranially, a differentiating feature from an optic nerve glioma. Meningiomas enhance avidly and may have calcifications. Enhancement pattern is characterized as "tram track" on axial images (bright nerve sheath/meningioma enhancement peripherally, and hypodense [CT] or hypointense [T1 magnetic resonance imaging, MRI] optic nerve centrally). Meningiomas cause bony hyperostosis.

■ Additional Differential Diagnoses

- **Metastases**. Metastases may involve any portion of the orbit to include the bony orbit, globe, and intraconal and extraconal spaces. Breast and lung cancer are the most common primary tumors in adults, followed by prostate, gastrointestinal, genitourinary, and soft tissue sarcomas. In children, neuroblastoma, leukemia, Wilms tumor, and Ewing sarcoma are most common. Larger lesions may result in proptosis and loss of visual acuity. Breast cancer metastases may result in enophthalmos due to a desmoplastic response.
- **Lymphoma**. Lymphoma usually involves the orbit secondarily and is of the non-Hodgkin variant. Patients are often elderly with proptosis or painless swelling. Less often, children and young adults may be affected. Lymphoma is commonly circumscribed and may be bilateral, a helpful distinguishing feature. CT may show increased density with enhancement. Lesions are low to intermediate on T1 and variable but typically T2 hyperintense. Common areas of involvement include the lacrimal gland and superior aspect of the orbit.
- **Nerve sheath tumor**. Both schwannomas and neurofibromas may occur within the orbit. Schwannomas are usually more heterogeneous and prone to cystic degeneration. They are often intermediate on T1 and hyperintense on T2 sequences with heterogeneous but avid solid enhancement. Neurofibromas are generally more homogeneous but less well-defined and typically occur in NF-1; they are commonly multiple and bilateral. MR reveals an intermediate T1 and hyperintense T2 mass with solid enhancement.

■ Diagnosis

Orbital "hemangioma" (cavernous venous malformation)

✓ Pearls

- Cavernous venous malformations are the most common orbital mass; they enhance intensely, and may have calcifications.
- Extraconal meningiomas involve the orbit secondarily; intraconal meningiomas occur along the optic nerve.
- Metastases and lymphoma involve the orbit secondarily and may be bilateral.

Suggested Readings

Tanak A, Mihara F, Yoshiura T. Differentiation of cavernous hemangioma from schwannoma of the orbit. AJR Am J Roentgenol. 2004; 183:1799–1804

Case 107

William T. O'Brien, Sr.

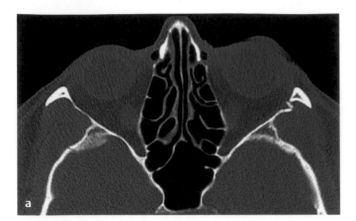

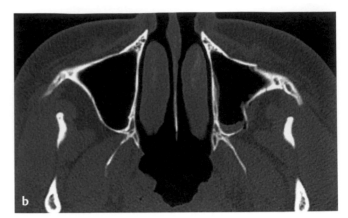

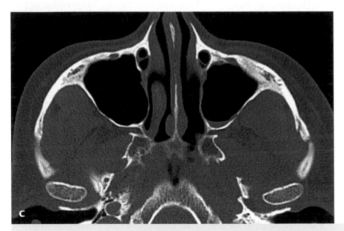

Fig. 107.1 Axial CT images demonstrate **(a)** a comminuted and mildly displaced fracture of the left lateral orbital wall, **(b)** comminuted fracture of the left lateral maxillary sinus wall with an additional fracture of the anterior maxillary sinus wall, **(b,c)** a small amount of hemorrhage within the maxillary sinus, and a mildly displaced comminuted fracture of the left zygomatic arch **(c)**.

■ Clinical Presentation

A young adult man with facial trauma (▶Fig. 107.1).

■ Key Imaging Finding

Orbital rim fracture

■ Top 3 Differential Diagnoses

- **Orbital wall blowout fracture**. An orbital wall blowout fracture results from a direct blow to the globe. Increased intraorbital pressure is transmitted to the thin orbital floor, resulting in a characteristic fracture pattern. A fracture fragment may protrude inferiorly into the maxillary sinus with a "trap-door" appearance; a "Bombay door" configuration occurs with two fragments along the orbital floor. Intraorbital fat is usually displaced inferiorly into the maxillary sinus, and there is often a hyperdense air–fluid level within the sinus due to hemorrhage. The inferior rectus muscle may extend into or through the site of fracture, resulting in muscle entrapment. Imaging findings suggestive of clinical entrapment include a focal change in course or contour of the rectus musculature in the region of fracture. It is important to evaluate for globe injury, as well as additional orbital and facial fractures. A fracture through the medial orbital wall (lamina papyracea) results in herniation of orbital fat into the ethmoid sinus with associated hemorrhage; entrapment of the medial rectus muscle may be seen

- **Zygomaticomaxillary complex fracture**. A zygomaticomaxillary complex fracture (also referred to as a tripod fracture) is a common facial fracture that is caused by a direct blow to the zygomatic bone. The fractures involve the zygomatic arch and the inferior and lateral orbital walls, resulting in disassociation of the anterior zygoma from the remainder of the facial bones.

Patients commonly present with facial swelling, a localized deformity, and, occasionally, the inability to open the jaw due to impingement upon the mandibular coronoid process from the fracture fragment.

- **Le Fort fracture**. Le Fort fractures are characterized by some form of facial disassociation as a result of bilateral fractures and are categorized into three major subtypes. All subtypes involve fractures of the pterygoid plates. *Le Fort I* fractures occur through the maxillary bone below the orbital floor. There may be extension into one or both maxillary sinuses. The inferior portion of the maxilla below the fracture site is disassociated from the remainder of the facial bones. In *Le Fort II* fractures, the fracture is pyramidal in shape, involving bilateral maxilla and converging superiorly and medially through the inferior and medial orbital walls and nasal bridge. The nasal bridge and maxilla below the fracture is disassociated from the remainder of the facial bones. The *Le Fort III* fracture is the most severe and is characterized by complete craniofacial disassociation. This complex set of fractures involves the bilateral zygomaticofrontal sutures, the nasofrontal suture, and the lateral, medial, and inferior orbital walls. Pure Le Fort type fractures are unusual; most fractures are complex with components of different subtypes.

■ Diagnosis

Zygomaticomaxillary complex (tripod) fracture

✓ Pearls

- Orbital wall blowout fractures are due to a direct blow to the globe; muscle entrapment may be seen.
- Zygomaticomaxillary complex fractures involve the zygoma, inferior orbital wall, and lateral orbital wall.

- Le Fort fractures are characterized by varying degrees of facial disassociation; type III is the most severe.

Suggested Readings

Dolan KD, Jacoby CG, Smoker WR. The radiology of facial fractures. Radiographics. 1984; 4:575–663

Case 108

Adam J. Zuckerman

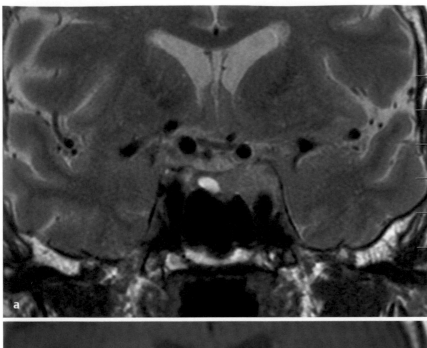

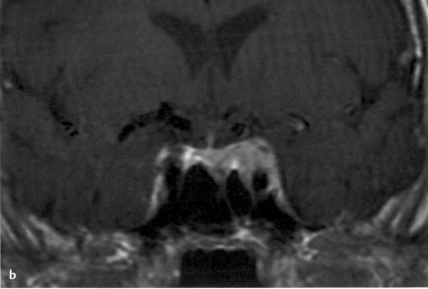

Fig. 108.1 (a) Axial T2 and (b) coronal T1 postcontrast MR images demonstrate left cavernous sinus mass, which is isointense to gray matter on T2 and avidly enhances. There is encasement and inferior displacement of the left cavernous internal carotid artery without luminal narrowing.

■ Clinical Presentation

A 31-year-old postpartum female complaining of facial numbness (▶Fig. 108.1).

■ Key Imaging Finding

Cavernous sinus mass/enhancement

■ Top 3 Differential Diagnoses

- **Meningioma**. Meningiomas are benign dural-based masses and represent the most common extra-axial masses. With cavernous sinus involvement, patients often present with oculomotor symptoms related to mass effect on cranial nerves (CNs). They characteristically encase and narrow the internal carotid artery (ICA). Meningiomas are iso- to hyperdense compared to gray matter with or without calcification. Overlying bony hyperostosis may be seen. Meningiomas are iso- to hypointense on T1 and iso- to hyperintense on T2 with avid enhancement and a dural tail
- **Schwannoma**. Schwannomas are nerve sheath tumors and represent the second most common extra-axial masses. Cavernous sinus schwannomas most often involve the trigeminal nerve. On computed tomography (CT), schwannomas are typically isodense compared to brain parenchyma with heterogeneous enhancement. Unlike meningiomas, calcification is rare.

When located near the skull base or exiting foramina, smooth bony remodeling and foraminal enlargement are commonly seen. On magnetic resonance imaging (MRI), schwannomas are iso- to hypointense on T1 and variably hyperintense on T2 and demonstrate heterogeneous but avid enhancement.
- **Pituitary macroadenoma**. Pituitary macroadenoma (>10 mm) is the most common suprasellar mass in adults. The best diagnostic clue is a sellar mass without a separate identifiable pituitary gland. The tumor is most commonly isodense on CT, isointense on T1, and iso- to hyperintense on T2 sequences compared to gray matter. Enhancement is usually heterogeneous. With cavernous sinus invasion, there may be carotid artery encasement (more than two-thirds is typically considered a sign of cavernous sinus invasion) without narrowing. Patients often present with visual field defects or CN palsy because of local mass effect.

■ Additional Differential Diagnoses

- **Tolosa–Hunt syndrome**. Tolosa–Hunt syndrome is an idiopathic, inflammatory process of the cavernous sinus, which is pathologically related to orbital pseudotumor. The syndrome is characterized by recurrent, painful ophthalmoplegia with involvement of the oculomotor nerve from the superior orbital fissure to the cavernous sinus. MRI features are similar to inflammatory orbital pseudotumor, demonstrating iso- to hypointense signal intensity on both T1 and T2 sequences. Enhancement may be ill-defined or masslike.
- **Carotid-cavernous fistula (CCF)**. A CCF is an abnormal shunt between the carotid artery and cavernous sinus venous spaces. They are most often direct fistulas involving the ICA from trauma; aneurysm rupture and indirect fistulas involving dural arterial branches are less common. Patients present with

headaches, bruit, exophthalmos, and ophthalmoplegia. Angiographically, CCFs demonstrate early venous filling of the cavernous sinus, superior ophthalmic vein, and/or inferior petrosal sinus. MRI shows cavernous sinus enlargement and enhancement with flow voids. Endovascular treatment options (glue or coils) are favored.
- **Perineural spread of tumor or infection**. Infiltrating sinonasal or head and neck carcinomas or invasive infections (e.g. fungal) may extend into the cavernous sinus via entry through the skull base foramina. Postcontrast fat-saturated MRI is most helpful in demonstrating intracranial extension, especially when asymmetric or unilateral. Oftentimes, the primary origin may be identified if not already known clinically.

■ Diagnosis

Pituitary macroadenoma

✓ Pearls

- Cavernous sinus meningiomas avidly enhance with a dural tail; they may encase and narrow the ICA.
- Cavernous sinus schwannomas most commonly involve CN V, and skull base remodelling may be seen.

- Pituitary macroadenomas present as sellar/suprasellar masses without a separate identifiable pituitary gland.
- Tolosa–Hunt is an inflammatory process of the cavernous sinus, which is related to orbital pseudotumor.

Suggested Readings

Lee JH, Lee HK, Park JK, Choi CG, Suh DC. Cavernous sinus syndrome: clinical features and differential diagnosis with MR imaging. AJR Am J Roentgenol. 2003; 181(2):583–590

Case 109

William T. O'Brien, Sr.

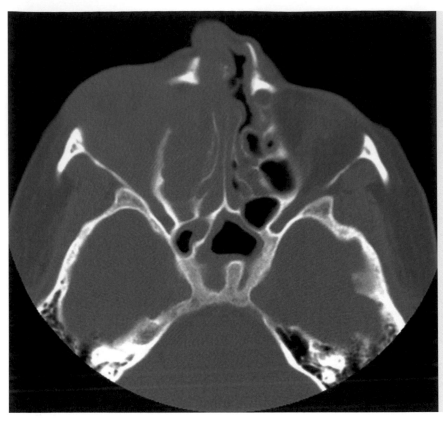

Fig. 109.1 Axial CT image through the paranasal sinuses in bone window reveals complete opacification of the right ethmoid sinus with bony erosion and overlying cartilage deformity. There is disruption of the right lamina papyracea with infiltration of the orbital fat. Mild mucosal thickening is noted involving the sphenoid and left ethmoid sinuses.

■ Clinical Presentation

A 32-year-old woman with chronic, progressive nasal congestion and cough (►Fig. 109.1).

■ Key Imaging Finding

Aggressive sinus disease with bony destruction

■ Top 3 Differential Diagnoses

- **Invasive fungal sinusitis (IFS)**. IFS most commonly occurs in immunosuppressed patients, especially elderly diabetics. Mucormycosis and Aspergillosis are the most common causative agents, with Aspergillus also occurring in otherwise healthy individuals. Mucormycosis has a tendency to spread through the cavernous sinus and orbits, resulting in a life-threatening infection. Aspergillus invades vasculature, which results in mycotic aneurysm formation and vessel spasm or thrombosis. Fungal secretions are often hyperdense on computed tomography (CT) scans; calcifications are common. Hypointensity on both T1 and T2 (more so on T2) is characteristic of fungal infection. Bony erosion and extension beyond sinus margins are suggestive of an aggressive infection
- **Granulomatous disease (Wegener/sarcoid)**. Wegner granulomatosis is a systemic vasculitis that primarily affects the kidneys and respiratory tract. Patients present with recurrent sinonasal "infections," respiratory symptoms, and renal insufficiency. The necrotizing vasculitis of small and medium size vessels results in sinus disease (usually within the maxillary sinus) with locally erosive features. Early in the disease, the nasal septum is most involved. As the disease progresses, there is formation of a sinus mass with extensive bony erosion and involvement of adjacent compartments, to include the orbits. The soft tissue mass is hypointense on T1- and T2-weighted sequences and enhances. Sarcoid has a similar appearance on imaging and nearly always has associated pulmonary disease, which manifests as hilar/mediastinal adenopathy and/or interstitial lung disease.
- **Sinonasal carcinoma**. Squamous cell carcinoma (SCC) accounts for approximately 90% of sinus malignancies. The maxillary sinus is most commonly involved, followed by the ethmoid sinus. Patients present relatively late in the disease process with obstructive sinus symptoms. On CT, SCC presents as a soft tissue mass with bony destruction; extension beyond the sinus margins may be seen. Involvement of the pterygopalatine fossa allows for communication with the orbit and middle cranial fossa, most commonly through perineural spread of tumor. The tumor is hypointense on T1 and intermediate to hypointense on T2 sequences, with heterogeneous enhancement. Less common sinonasal neoplasms include sinonasal undifferentiated carcinoma, adenocarcinoma (associated with wood working and chemical exposures), and rhabdomyosarcoma (most common in children).

■ Additional Differential Diagnoses

- **Lymphoma**. Lymphoma of the paranasal sinuses is of the non-Hodgkin variant. The imaging appearance is nearly identical to that of SCC, with typically a unilateral sinus mass that invades bone and is intermediate to hypointense on T2 sequences. A key distinguishing feature is the presence of lymphadenopathy within the neck and involvement of Waldeyer's tonsillar ring (a pharyngeal ring of lymphoid tissue composed of the adenoids, tubal tonsils, palatine tonsils, and lingual tonsils).
- **Cocaine nose**. Chronic use of cocaine results in a granulomatous response with a soft tissue mass and cartilaginous erosion. The local granulomatous response combined with the vasoconstrictive properties of cocaine results in necrosis of the nasal septum. Continued insults lead to expansion of the septal perforation.

■ Diagnosis

Wegener granulomatosis

✓ Pearls

- IFS most often occurs in immunosuppressed patients and may be hyperdense (CT) and hypointense (magnetic resonance imaging [MRI]).
- Wegner granulomatosis results in aggressive sinus disease, pulmonary symptoms, and renal insufficiency.
- SCC (by far the most common) and lymphoma commonly involve the sinuses.
- Chronic cocaine abuse can lead to ischemic necrosis with bony and cartilaginous destruction.

Suggested Readings

Allbery SM, Chaljub G, Cho NL, Rassekh CH, John SD, Guinto FC. MR imaging of nasal masses. Radiographics. 1995; 15(6):1311–1327

Valencia MP, Castillo M. Congenital and acquired lesions of the nasal septum: a practical guide for differential diagnosis. Radiographics. 2008; 28(1):205–224, quiz 326

Case 110

William T. O'Brien, Sr.

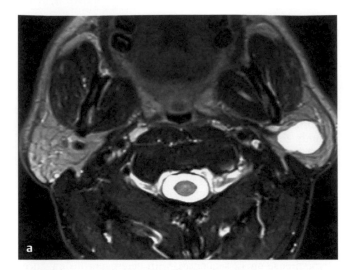

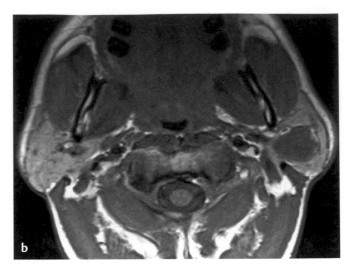

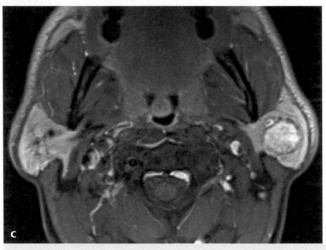

Fig. 110.1 **(a)** Axial T2, **(b)** T1, and **(c)** T1 fat-suppressed postcontrast MR images show a circumscribed, lobulated T2 hyperintense, T1 hypointense left parotid gland mass with homogeneous enhancement. The mass is centered in the superficial parotid lobe, with a small component extending medial to the retromandibular vein into the deep parotid lobe.

■ Clinical Presentation

A 43-year-old man with palpable abnormality (▶Fig. 110.1).

■ Key Imaging Finding

Unilateral parotid mass

■ Top 3 Differential Diagnoses

- **Pleomorphic adenoma**. Benign parotid neoplasms are far more common (80%) than malignant primary neoplasms. Of all benign parotid neoplasms, pleomorphic adenoma is the most common (80%). Patients are often middle-aged and may be asymptomatic or present with nonspecific symptoms or a palpable mass. On computed tomography (CT), pleomorphic adenomas appear as well-circumscribed heterogeneous round, oval, or lobulated masses. They may be located within the superficial and/or deep parotid lobe, an important distinction for surgical planning; the facial nerve/retromandibular vein is the demarcation between the superficial and deep parotid lobes. On magnetic resonance imaging (MRI), the lesions are iso- to hypointense on T1 and characteristically hyperintense on T2 sequences. Delayed enhancement is typical.
- **Warthin tumor**. Warthin tumors, also known as papillary cystadenoma lymphomatosum, are the second most common benign parotid neoplasm and most commonly occur in middle-aged or elderly men. The may be both multifocal and bilateral. On imaging, the lesions are well-circumscribed with mixed cystic and solid components. CT findings include a slightly heterogeneous mass with enhancement of solid components. On MRI, the enhancing solid portions are generally hypointense on T1 and intermediate in signal on T2 sequences, whereas the cystic components typically follow fluid signal intensity (T1 hypointense and T2 hyperintense).
- **Parotid carcinoma**. Malignant neoplasms are more common in salivary glands other than the parotid gland (e.g., sublingual and submandibular). Of the malignant subtypes, mucoepidermoid is the most common in the parotid gland. Imaging appearance and clinical presentation vary based on the aggressiveness of the lesion. In general, a well-circumscribed lesion is more characteristic of a low grade neoplasm, whereas an ill-defined infiltrative appearance with intermediate density and T1/T2 signal intensity suggests a more aggressive lesion. Adenoid cystic carcinoma (ACC) is the second most common parotid malignancy and is typically an aggressive, infiltrative mass. Perineural spread is common, which leads to neuropathy involving the facial nerve, especially when located within the deep parotid lobe.

■ Additional Differential Diagnoses

- **Lymphadenopathy**. Lymphadenopathy may occur within the parotid gland from inflammatory, infectious, or neoplastic processes. Infectious or inflammatory etiologies typically resolve with follow-up imaging. Lymphoma may involve intraparotid lymph nodes and present as solitary, multiple, or bilateral masses. Lymphoma may also involve the parotid parenchyma in a diffuse, infiltrative pattern. Metastases from head and neck cancer (squamous cell carcinoma [SCC]) or skin cancer (SCC or melanoma) may also involve intraparotid lymph nodes, as these nodes provide primary regional lymphatic drainage for portions of the scalp.
- **Branchial cleft cyst**. A developmental defect of the first branchial cleft may result in a type 1branchial cleft cyst occurring anywhere from the external auditory canal to the angle of the mandible, to include within the parotid gland parenchyma. The lesions are typically asymptomatic unless superinfected. Patients commonly present in adulthood with inflammation and/or a palpable mass. CT and MRI reveal a well-circumscribed cystic mass with varying degrees of peripheral enhancement.

■ Diagnosis

Pleomorphic adenoma

✓ Pearls

- Pleomorphic adenomas are benign, represent the most common parotid masses, and are bright on T2-weighted imaging.
- Warthin tumors are typically mixed cystic and solid, occur in middle-aged and elderly men, and may be bilateral.

- Malignant parotid tumors include mucoepidermoid and ACC (prone to perineural spread).
- Lymphadenopathy may result from inflammatory, infectious, or neoplastic processes.

Suggested Readings

Kinoshita T, Ishii K, Naganuma H, Okitsu T. MR imaging findings of parotid tumors with pathologic diagnostic clues: a pictorial essay. Clin Imaging. 2004; 28(2):93–101

Case 111

William T. O'Brien, Sr.

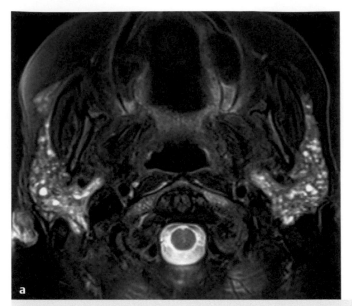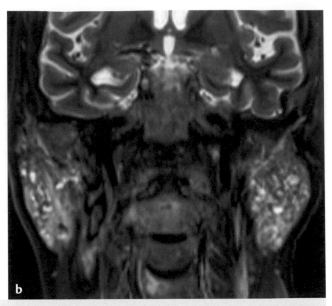

Fig. 111.1 **(a)** Axial and **(b)** coronal T2 fluid-sensitive images with fat suppression demonstrate numerous bilateral small hyperintense lesions within the parotid glands.

■ Clinical Presentation

An adult woman with facial "swelling" (▶Fig. 111.1).

■ Key Imaging Finding

Bilateral parotid masses

■ Top 3 Differential Diagnoses

• **Lymphadenopathy**. Lymphadenopathy may occur within the parotid gland from inflammatory, infectious, or neoplastic processes. Infectious or inflammatory etiologies typically resolve with follow-up imaging. Lymphoma may involve intraparotid lymph nodes and present as solitary, multiple, or bilateral masses. Lymphoma may also involve the parotid parenchyma in a diffuse, infiltrative pattern. Metastases from head and neck cancer (squamous cell carcinoma [SCC]) or skin cancer (SCC or melanoma) may also involve intraparotid lymph nodes, as intraparotid lymph nodes provide primary regional lymphatic drainage for portions of the scalp

• **Warthin tumors**. Warthin tumors, also known as papillary cystadenoma lymphomatosum, are the second most common benign parotid neoplasm and most commonly occur in middle-aged or elderly men. The may be both multifocal and bilateral. On imaging, the lesions are well-circumscribed with mixed cystic and solid components. Computed tomogra-

phy (CT) findings include a slightly heterogeneous mass with enhancement of solid components. On magnetic resonance imaging (MRI), the enhancing solid portions are generally hypointense on T1 and intermediate in signal on T2 sequences, whereas the cystic components typically follow fluid signal intensity (T1 hypointense and T2 hyperintense).

• **Sjögren syndrome**. Sjögren syndrome is an autoimmune disease that most commonly occurs in middle-aged to elderly women and results in lymphocytic infiltration of glandular tissue. The classic triad consists of parotid gland enlargement with keratoconjunctivitis sicca (dry eyes) and xerostomia (dry mouth). On CT and MRI, Sjögren syndrome presents as heterogeneous glandular enlargement with scattered enhancing nodules and fluid pockets. The appearance can mimic benign lymphoepithelial lesions or lymphoma. Patients with long-standing Sjögren syndrome are at increased risk of developing lymphoma.

■ Additional Differential Diagnoses

• **Lymphoepithelial lesions**. Benign lymphoepithelial lesions most often occur in acquired immunodeficiency syndrome (AIDS) patients who present with painless bilateral parotid gland enlargement. Pathologically, there is lymphocytic infiltration of the gland (similar to Sjögren syndrome) with lymphoepithelial cyst formation. CT and MRI reveal bilateral cystic and solid parotid lesions with diffuse gland enlargement. Associated cervical lymphadenopathy and tonsillar hypertrophy is commonly seen.

• **Sarcoidosis**. Sarcoidosis is a multisystem granulomatous disorder that most commonly occurs in adult African-Americans. Diffuse sarcoidosis can lead to granulomatous infiltration of glandular tissue, including the parotid and lacrimal glands. Patients typically have elevated angiotensin-converting enzyme levels and may also present with uveitis and cranial nerve deficits. On imaging, there is heterogeneous glandular enlargement, which is usually bilateral and symmetric. Gallium scan will reveal the classic "panda sign" with increased uptake in the parotid and lacrimal glands.

■ Diagnosis

Sjögren syndrome

✓ Pearls

• Warthin tumors are typically mixed cystic and solid, occur in middle-aged and elderly men, and may be bilateral.
• Sjögren syndrome is characterized by parotid enlargement/lesions, dry eyes, and dry mouth.

• Lymphoepithelial lesions occur in AIDS patients and present with bilateral cystic and solid parotid lesions.
• Sarcoidosis results in bilateral heterogeneous parotid enlargement; the "panda sign" is seen on gallium-67 scans.

Suggested Reading

Kinoshita T, Ishii K, Naganuma H, Okitsu T. MR imaging findings of parotid tumors with pathologic diagnostic clues: a pictorial essay. Clin Imaging. 2004; 28(2):93–101

Case 112

Matthew J. Moore

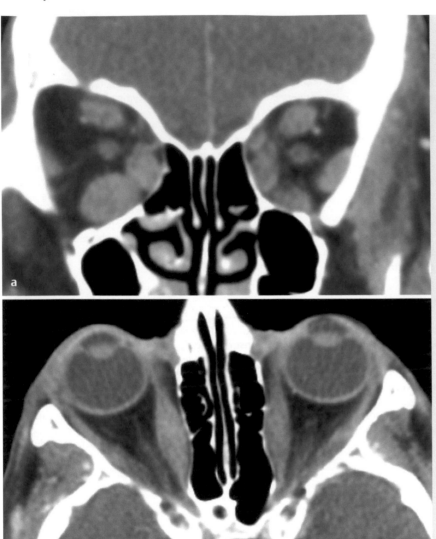

Fig. 112.1 **(a)** Coronal and **(b)** axial CT images demonstrate bilateral enlargement of the extraocular muscles, with sparing of the myotendinous junctions on the axial view **(b)**.

■ Clinical Presentation

A 35-year-old woman complaining of 3 months of "eye bulging" (▶Fig. 112.1)

■ Key Imaging Finding

Orbital extraocular muscle (EOM) enlargement

■ Top 3 Differential Diagnoses

- **Thyroid associated orbitopathy (TAO).** TAO, also known as Grave's ophthalmopathy, is the most common cause of proptosis in adults. TAO is an autoimmune inflammatory condition characterized by enlargement of multiple EOM bellies with sparing of myotendinous junctions. It is typically bilateral and preferentially affects the inferior > medial > superior > lateral > superior oblique muscles (*"I'M SLOW"* mnemonic). Increased orbital fat and lacrimal gland enlargement can also be seen. Look for stretching or compression of the optic nerve. TAO tends to affect young and middle aged adults, women more so than men. Corticosteroid treatment is effective; some will require surgical therapy for uncontrolled mass effect
- **Orbital pseudotumor.** Orbital pseudotumor, the most common cause of a painful orbital mass in adults, is an idiopathic inflammatory disease, causing infiltrative or masslike enhancement of any part of the orbit. EOM involvement, including the myotendinous junction, is the most common pattern. Multiple EOMs may be involved, but the findings are often unilateral. With isolated lateral rectus muscle enlargement, it is more likely orbital pseudotumor and essentially never thyroid orbitopathy. Other presentations include lacrimal gland enlargement and involvement of retrobulbar fat. Involvement of the cavernous sinus is known as Tolosa–Hunt.
- **Infectious myositis.** Infectious cellulitis–myositis may be a complication of sinonasal infection, most often involving the ethmoids. The most common finding is enlargement of the medial rectus muscle with associated ethmoid sinus disease. Secondary findings, in addition to adjacent sinus opacification, include subperiosteal abscess formation, osseous erosion or osteitis, and inflammatory intraorbital fat stranding.

■ Additional Differential Diagnoses

- **Neoplasm.** Lymphoma, leukemia, rhabdomyosarcoma, and metastases may involve the EOMs. Lymphoma has many orbital manifestations but most often presents as a homogenously enhancing, painless, orbital mass in an elderly patient (older than 60 years). It may also involve the lacrimal glands or occasionally the EOMs, simulating thyroid orbitopathy. Rhabdomyosarcoma is the most common soft tissue sarcoma in childhood. They vast majority occur within orbital soft tissues rather than within the EOMs. Lesions are isodense to muscle on computed tomography (CT), T1 hypointense, and T2 hyperintense with moderate enhancement.
- **Sarcoidosis.** Approximately 25% of sarcoid patients have ophthalmic disease. The most common imaging findings include masslike lacrimal gland enlargement with enhancement, EOM enlargement, optic nerve thickening and enhancement, and orbital pseudotumor-like intraorbital masses. The most common presenting signs/symptoms include acute uveitis, chronic dacryoadenitis, and lacrimal gland enlargement.
- **Vascular congestion.** High-flow arteriovenous shunting may result in increased intraorbital pressure and vascular congestion. Carotid–cavernous fistulas are most common and consist of abnormal shunts between the carotid artery and cavernous sinus. The vast majority are direct fistulas from trauma. Chemosis, pulsatile exophthalmos, and an orbital bruit are found clinically. Magnetic resonance imaging (MRI) shows a convex lateral cavernous sinus border, cavernous sinus flow voids, enlarged ipsilateral superior ophthalmic vein and EOMs, and proptosis.

■ Diagnosis

Thyroid associated orbitopathy

✓ Pearls

- Thyroid orbitopathy is the most common cause of EOM enlargement; it is most often bilateral.
- Pseudotumor presents as a painful orbital mass; myotendinous junction involvement is characteristic.
- Infectious myositis is most commonly secondary to intraorbital extension from ethmoid sinus disease.
- Orbital lymphoma most commonly presents as an indolent painless mass in an elderly patient.

Suggested Readings

LeBedis CA, Sakai O. Nontraumatic orbital conditions: diagnosis with CT and MR imaging in the emergent setting. Radiographics. 2008; 28(6):1741–1753

Case 113

William T. O'Brien, Sr.

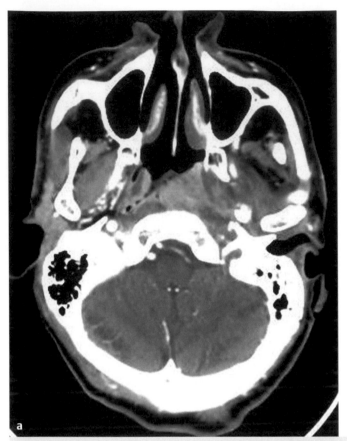 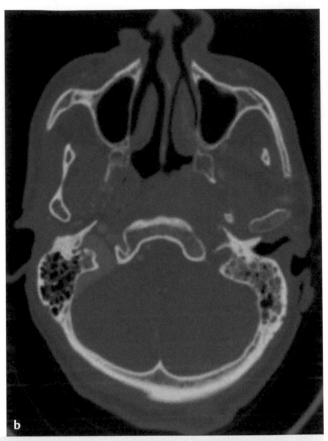

Fig. 113.1 **(a)** Axial CT image through the nasopharynx and posterior fossa in soft tissue window reveals a heterogeneous mass in the fossa of Rosenmüller on the left with mass effect on the Eustachian tube and nasopharyngeal airway. **(b)** Corresponding axial CT image in bone window demonstrates fluid within the left mastoid air cells as a result of Eustachian tube obstruction.

■ Clinical Presentation

A 58-year-old man with progressive nasal fullness and chronic ear "infections" (▶Fig. 113.1)

■ Key Imaging Finding

Pharyngeal mucosal mass

■ Top 3 Differential Diagnoses

- **Squamous cell carcinoma (SCC).** SCC is the most common primary malignancy of the head and neck. It commonly originates in the nasopharynx or oropharynx. The lesions are clinically occult until late in the disease process. Nasopharyngeal carcinoma arises from the fossa of Rosenmüller. Patients may be asymptomatic or present with nasal obstruction or hearing deficits due to obstruction of the Eustachian tube and subsequent accumulation of fluid within the middle ear and mastoid air cells. Oropharyngeal SCC commonly extends laterally to involve the parapharyngeal space. The imaging appearance is that of an ill-defined heterogeneously enhancing mass. There may be local spread and lymphatic spread to cervical lymph nodes, which characteristically demonstrate central necrosis. Treatment of nasopharyngeal and oropharyngeal carcinoma depends upon staging, which is determined by the local extent of the primary tumor, size and location of regional lymph node spread, and presence or absence of distant metastases
- **Infection/Abscess.** Pharyngeal mucosal infections/abscesses most often result from adenoidal/tonsillar infections. Patients often present with fever and sore throat. Tonsillitis often demonstrates striated enhancement in a "tigroid" pattern

without focal fluid collection. As the infection progresses and organizes, a rim-enhancing abscess may develop. With phlegmon, imaging often demonstrates ill-defined or partially organized inflammatory changes without complete rim enhancement. It is important to realize that the presence of complete rim enhancement is not 100% specific for an abscess since failed aspiration/drainage may occur in approximately 25% of cases of suspected abscesses by computed tomography (CT). Prompt treatment is necessary to prevent retropharyngeal spread, which may allow for further spread to the mediastinum.
- **Lymphoma.** Non-Hodgkin lymphoma may involve the pharyngeal mucosa and appear similar to SCC. Patients with systemic lymphoma commonly have constitutional symptoms, along with abdominal lymphadenopathy, which are helpful discriminators. In the absence of constitutional symptoms or widespread disease, the presence of multiple enlarged cervical lymph nodes without necrosis is also suggestive of lymphoma. In some cases, biopsy may ultimately be necessary to establish the diagnosis.

■ Additional Differential Diagnoses

- **Thornwaldt cyst.** Thornwaldt cysts are benign notochord remnants within the nasopharynx. They are cystic and midline and situated between the longus coli muscles. The amount of proteinaceous material determines the imaging appearance. They are T2 hyperintense and variable but often T1 hyperintense. Although incidental findings, they may cause halitosis and may become superinfected. These can usually be differentiated from mucous retention cysts, which are typically off midline and within adenoidal tissue or pharyngeal mucosa.
- **Minor salivary gland tumor.** Benign (e.g., pleomorphic adenoma) and malignant (e.g., mucoepidermoid) minor salivary gland tumors may rarely involve the pharyngeal mucosal space. Imaging appearance is determined by the histology of the lesion. In general, benign lesions tend to be well-circumscribed, whereas more aggressive lesions may be ill-defined and heterogeneous with an imaging appearance that mimics SSC. Metastases and associated lymphadenopathy are uncommon.

■ Diagnosis

Nasopharyngeal squamous cell carcinoma

✓ Pearls

- Nasopharyngeal SCC arises at the fossa of Rosenmüller and may obstruct the Eustachian tube.
- Striated tonsillar enhancement is seen with tonsillitis; abscesses show rim enhancement.

- The presence of constitutional symptoms or lymphadenopathy without necrosis suggests lymphoma.
- Thornwaldt cysts are midline notochord remnants and are often hyperintense on both T1 and T2 sequences.

Suggested Readings

Shin JH, Lee HK, Kim SY, Choi CG, Suh DC. Imaging of parapharyngeal space lesions: focus on the prestyloid compartment. AJR Am J Roentgenol. 2001; 177(6):1465–1470

Case 114

William T. O'Brien, Sr.

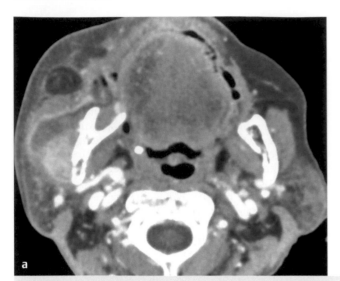 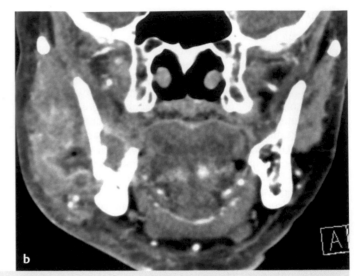

Fig. 114.1 **(a)** Axial and **(b)** reformatted coronal postcontrast CT images demonstrate a right masticator mass with regions of low attenuation and peripheral rim enhancement, heterogeneous increased enhancement, and surrounding fatty infiltration. A portion of the low attenuation extends into the right mandible **(a)** and contains a small focus of gas/air **(b)**.

■ Clinical Presentation

An adult woman with facial swelling and pain (▶Fig. 114.1).

■ Key Imaging Finding

Masticator space mass

■ Top 3 Differential Diagnoses

- **Infection/abscess**. Most infections of the masticator space evolve from a dental origin. Infections may present as osteomyelitis, cellulitis, or an organized abscess. Osteomyelitis has variable imaging appearances, including lucent, sclerotic, or mixed, and often mimics an aggressive, infiltrative process. Periosteal reaction may be seen. Care should be taken to evaluate the full extent of the infection since spread to other spaces and even the intracranial compartment can occur along nerve roots and fascial planes. Bony erosion and marrow infiltration are important findings, as are drainable fluid collections, since these may alter clinical management

- **Sarcoma**. Sarcomas most often arise from bone (chondrosarcoma, osteosarcoma, or Ewing sarcoma) or muscle (rhabdomyosarcoma). Occasionally, squamous cell carcinoma from a head and neck primary can secondarily involve the masticator space. Chondrosarcomas arise near the temporomandibular joint. There is typically a soft tissue mass; the presence of a chondroid matrix is a helpful distinguishing feature. Osteosarcoma occurs anywhere in the mandible and is aggressive with bone formation and periosteal reaction. Ewing sarcoma presents within the first two decades of life with permeative bone destruction and a soft tissue mass. The degree of periosteal reaction is variable. Rhabdomyosarcoma arises from the muscles of mastication and typically occurs in children. On magnetic resonance imaging (MRI), it may be difficult to distinguish between the types of sarcomas, as they all can be intermediate on T1 and variably hyperintense on T2 sequences and demonstrate heterogeneous enhancement.

- **Venolymphatic malformation**. Venolymphatic malformations represent a spectrum of venous and lymphatic developmental abnormalities. Pure venous malformations avidly enhance and may contain flow voids on T2 MRI; the presence of phleboliths is pathognomonic. Pure lymphatic malformations are fluid-filled and may be unilocular or multilocular. Fluid-fluid levels, most often due to hemorrhage, are characteristic. Many cases demonstrate characteristics of both. Lesions often cross fascial planes to involve multiple spaces of the neck.

■ Additional Differential Diagnoses

- **Nerve sheath tumor**. Both schwannomas and neurofibromas may occur within the masticator space, typically involving the mandibular division of the trigeminal nerve (V3) or peripheral nerves. Schwannomas are usually more heterogeneous and may have regions of cystic degeneration. They are often intermediate on T1 and hyperintense on T2 sequences with heterogeneous but avid enhancement. Neurofibromas are generally more homogeneous and occur in the setting of neurofibromatosis type 1; they are commonly multiple and bilateral. MRI reveals intermediate T1 and hyperintense T2 signal intensity with heterogeneous enhancement. The target sign, characterized by centrally decreased and peripherally increased T2 signal intensity, is more frequently seen with neurofibromas.

- **Hemangioma**. Hemangiomas are unencapsulated, proliferative vascular neoplasms and are the most common benign tumors of infancy. The proliferative growth phase typically occurs in the first year of life; infantile and rapidly involuting congenital variants (RICH) then undergo involution with fatty replacement; noninvoluting congenital variants (NICH) do not regress. Treatment is conservative unless there is mass effect on adjacent vital structures. Clinically, patients present with a superficial mass, which is bluish or scarlet in color. MRI reveals a lobulated hyperintense T2 and slightly hyperintense T1 mass with avid enhancement.

■ Diagnosis

Infection/abscess (odontogenic origin)

✓ Pearls

- Most masticator space infections arise from a dental origin; look for signs of osteomyelitis or abscess.
- Masticator space sarcomas typically arise from bone or muscle; imaging findings often overlap.

- Venolymphatic malformations occur within the masticator space and may involve multiple compartments.
- Nerve sheath tumors (neurofibromas and schwannomas) occur along the mandibular division of cranial nerve V3 or peripheral nerves.

Suggested Reading

Shin JH, Lee HK, Kim SY, Choi CG, Suh DC. Imaging of parapharyngeal space lesions: focus on the prestyloid compartment. AJR Am J Roentgenol. 2001; 177(6):1465–1470

Case 115

William T. O'Brien, Sr.

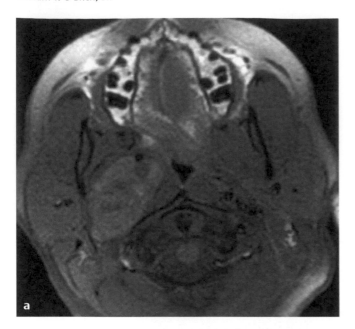
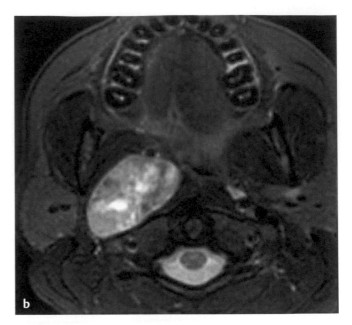
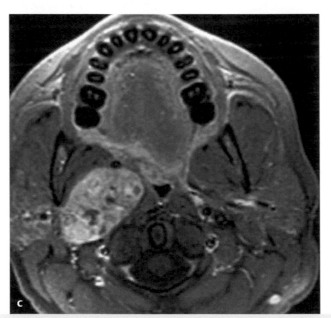
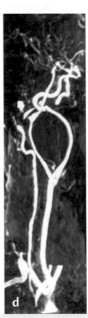

Fig. 115.1 **(a)** Axial T1 precontrast with fat suppression, **(b)** T2, and **(c)** T1 postcontrast with fat suppression images through the neck demonstrate a heterogeneous, well-circumscribed T1 intermediate to hyperintense and T2 hyperintense mass that avidly enhances. There are small cystic foci internally. **(d)** An oblique sagittal reformatted magnetic resonance angiography (MRA) image of the neck reveals that the mass results in splaying of the right internal and external carotid arteries without significant internal hypervascularity. (Images courtesy of Rebecca Cornelius, MD, University of Cincinnati)

■ **Clinical Presentation**

A 48-year-old woman with "fullness in throat" (▶Fig. 115.1)

■ Key Imaging Finding

Carotid space mass

■ Top 3 Differential Diagnoses

- **Paraganglioma**. Paragangliomas arise from neural crest cells and are most common in middle-aged women. Up to 10% are malignant and 10% may be bilateral. The two most common paragangliomas to present as carotid space masses are the carotid body tumor, which is the most common and occurs at the carotid bifurcation, and the glomus vagale, which occurs more superiorly along the course of the vagus nerve. The carotid body tumor splays the internal and external carotid arteries, which is characteristic but not pathognomonic, as other lesions may also occasionally splay the carotid arteries, including glomus vagale and nerve sheath tumors. Glomus vagale typically displaces the internal carotid artery anteriorly. Paragangliomas are highly vascular and commonly contain calcifications and flow voids, resulting in a "salt-and-pepper" appearance on magnetic resonance imaging (MRI). They are associated with multiple endocrine neoplasia syndromes but are typically hormonally inactive
- **Nerve sheath tumor**. Both schwannomas and neurofibromas may occur within the carotid space, most often involving the vagus nerve or cervical nerve roots. When located more superiorly within the carotid space near the nasopharynx, cranial nerves IX, XI, and XII may also be involved. Schwannomas are usually more heterogeneous with cystic and solid components when large. They are often intermediate in signal intensity on

T1 and hyperintense on T2 sequences. Avid but heterogeneous enhancement of the solid components is typically seen. Neurofibromas are generally more homogeneous and occur in the setting of neurofibromatosis type 1 (NF-1), in which case they are most often multiple and bilateral. On computed tomography (CT), the lesions are hypodense. MRI reveals intermediate signal intensity on T1 and heterogeneous signal on T2 sequences; enhancement is typical. Compared to schwannomas, neurofibromas more commonly demonstrate a target sign on T2 sequences with centrally decreased and peripherally increased signal intensity.

- **Vascular abnormality**. Vascular abnormalities and asymmetries are common causes of palpable abnormalities. The most important role of the radiologist is to identify the vascular origin of the abnormality so that inadvertent biopsy is avoided. Normal variants, such as a dominant jugular vein, are commonly seen. In the setting of hypertension or trauma, aneurysms and pseudoaneurysms can present as carotid space masses. Venous thrombosis as a result of recent line placement, surrounding inflammation or neoplasm, or hypercoagulable state, can present a diagnostic dilemma; often, the wall and surrounding soft tissues enhance, mimicking a mass. The key is to identify the vascular origin of the abnormality.

■ Additional Differential Diagnoses

- **Lymphadenopathy**. Lymph node enlargement may be reactive, inflammatory, or neoplastic in nature. Reactive and inflammatory etiologies demonstrate nonspecific lymph node enlargement, which is often self-limiting. Squamous cell carcinoma from a head and neck origin is the most common cause of nodal metastases and often demonstrates abnormal nodal architecture and central necrosis. Papillary thyroid carcinoma and atypical infections (e.g. *Mycobacterium* and *Bartonella*

subspecies) are additional causes of centrally necrotic lymph nodes. Lymphoma presents with prominent lymph node enlargement and may be of the Hodgkin or non-Hodgkin variant. Hodgkin lymphoma spreads in a contiguous fashion from the mediastinum and is most often unilateral. Non-Hodgkin lymphoma is typically bilateral with associated abdominal lymphadenopathy.

■ Diagnosis

Nerve sheath tumor (vagal schwannoma)

✓ Pearls

- Paragangliomas arise from neural crest cells, may have a "salt-and-pepper" appearance, and avidly enhance.
- Schwannomas and neurofibromas may occur along the course of the vagus nerve within the carotid space.

- Vascular abnormalities and asymmetries within the carotid space may mimic enhancing masses.
- Neoplastic lymphadenopathy is most commonly due to squamous cell carcinoma, followed by lymphoma.

Suggested Readings

Fruin ME, Smoker WR, Harnsberger HR. The carotid space in the suprahyoid neck. Semin Ultrasound CT MR. 1990; 11(6):504–519

Case 116

William T. O'Brien, Sr.

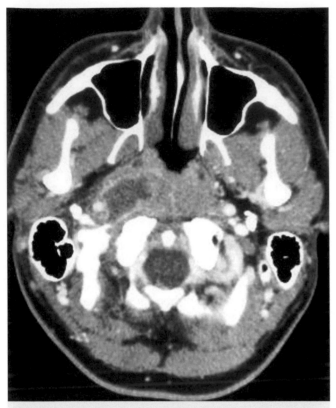

Fig. 116.1 Contrast-enhanced axial CT image through the suprahyoid neck demonstrates a rim-enhancing fluid collection within the retropharyngeal space on the right. The adjacent distal cervical right internal carotid artery is slightly smaller in caliber compared to the contralateral side.

■ Clinical Presentation

An adult man with sore throat (▶Fig. 116.1).

■ Key Imaging Finding

Retropharyngeal mass

■ Top 3 Differential Diagnoses

• **Infection/abscess**. Patients with a retropharyngeal infection or abscess commonly present with fever, sore throat, and elevated white blood cell count. Involvement of the retropharyngeal space most often occurs secondary to spread of infection from tonsillar tissue. Lateral radiographs will show prevertebral soft tissue swelling, prompting cross-section imaging. Contrast-enhanced computed tomography (CT) demonstrates soft tissue swelling within the retropharyngeal space with associated inflammatory changes. Adenitis refers to inflammatory changes within retropharyngeal lymph nodes, which typically demonstrate enlargement and abnormal central hypoattenuation. Suppurative retropharyngeal adenitis may appear identical to an extralymphatic retropharyngeal abscess. If left untreated, suppurative adenitis may extend beyond the nodal capsule and result in a true retropharyngeal abscess. Phlegmon presents with ill-defined hypodensity and variable enhancement. As the infectious process becomes more organized, an abscess develops, demonstrating central fluid density with complete, peripheral rim enhancement. Prompt treatment is necessary since the retropharyngeal space allows for contiguous spread of infection into the mediastinum and within the danger space.

• **Nodal metastases**. The vast majority of nodal metastases within the retropharyngeal space result from spread of squamous cell carcinoma (SCC), which is the most common neoplasm of the pharyngeal mucosa. Involvement of the lateral retropharyngeal nodes of Rouvière is characteristic, and central necrosis is common. Extracapsular spread appears as disruption of the peripheral lymph node margin with ill-defined hypoattenuation extending into the surrounding soft tissues and portends a worse prognosis. Thyroid carcinoma (papillary variant) may also metastasize to the retropharyngeal lymph nodes, commonly resulting in central necrosis. Imaging of the remainder of the head and neck will help identify the primary lesion as originating from the pharyngeal mucosa (SCC) or thyroid gland.

• **Lymphoma**. Non-Hodgkin lymphoma commonly presents with lymphadenopathy within the neck. Patients with systemic lymphoma often have constitutional symptoms, along with abdominal lymphadenopathy, which are helpful discriminators. In the absence of constitutional symptoms or widespread disease, the presence of multiple enlarged cervical lymph nodes without necrosis is suggestive of lymphoma. However, unlike other nodal chains within the neck, isolated retropharyngeal lymph node enlargement may rarely be the initial presentation of lymphoma.

■ Additional Differential Diagnoses

• **Venolymphatic malformation**. Venolymphatic malformations represent a spectrum of venous and lymphatic developmental abnormalities. Pure venous malformations avidly enhance and may contain flow voids on T2 magnetic resonance imaging (MRI); the presence of phleboliths is pathognomonic. Pure lymphatic malformations may be unilocular or multilocular and demonstrate fluid attenuation and signal intensity. Fluid–fluid levels, most often due to hemorrhage, are characteristic. Many cases demonstrate characteristics of both. Venolymphatic malformations often cross fascial planes to involve multiple spaces of the neck.

■ Diagnosis

Retropharyngeal abscess (with adjacent carotid vasospasm)

✓ Pearls

• Retropharyngeal infections cause soft tissue swelling and inflammation; abscesses reveal rim enhancement.
• SCC is the most common cause of retropharyngeal nodal metastases, followed by papillary thyroid cancer.

• Non-Hodgkin lymphoma commonly presents with constitutional symptoms and diffuse lymphadenopathy.
• Venolymphatic malformations have varying degrees of cystic/vascular components and cross fascial planes.

Suggested Readings

Shin JH, Lee HK, Kim SY, Choi CG, Suh DC. Imaging of parapharyngeal space lesions: focus on the prestyloid compartment. AJR Am J Roentgenol. 2001; 177(6):1465–1470

Case 117

William T. O'Brien, Sr.

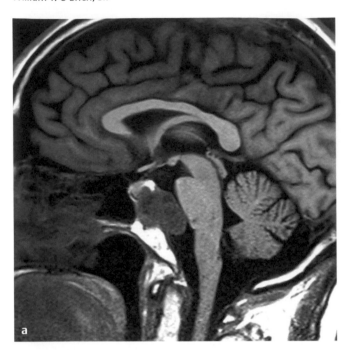

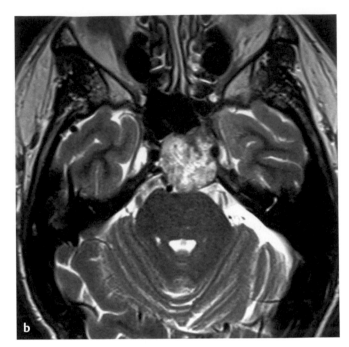

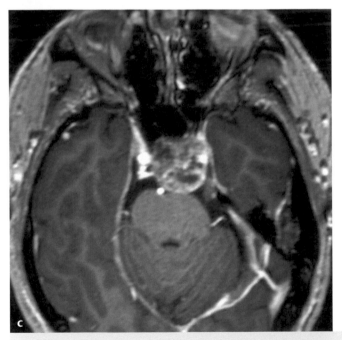

Fig. 117.1 (a) Sagittal T1 image demonstrates a lobulated hypointense mass centered within the clivus with extension superiorly along the inferior sella and posteriorly into the prepontine cistern. (b) The mass is T2 hyperintense with regions of intermediate signal intensity and demonstrates heterogeneous enhancement on axial fat-suppressed postcontrast image (c). The mass partially encases the left internal carotid artery without frank cavernous sinus extension.

■ Clinical Presentation

A 63-year-old man with headaches (▶Fig. 117.1).

■ Key Imaging Finding

Clival mass

■ Top 3 Differential Diagnoses

- **Metastases**. Metastatic disease commonly involves the skull base. Common primary neoplasms include breast, lung, and prostate carcinoma; lymphoma may be primary or secondary. Breast and lung carcinoma are most often lytic, along with renal and thyroid carcinomas. Prostate (and occasionally breast) carcinoma produces sclerotic metastases. Computed tomography (CT) demonstrates bony evolvement in better detail than magnetic resonance imaging (MRI), especially along the skull base. MRI is superior in evaluating the soft tissue component as well as intracranial involvement. Metastases are hypointense on T1 and hyperintense on T2 with avid enhancement; lymphoma may be T2 hypointense.
- **Chordoma**. Chordoma is a malignant tumor that arises from notochordal remnants. It most commonly affects the clivus and sacrum in young to middle-aged adults and is more common in men; vertebral body involvement is less common.

Patients with clival involvement often present with headache and ophthalmoplegia due to cranial nerve involvement. CT reveals a midline, expansile, lytic mass with hyperdense foci centrally. Chordomas are classically hyperintense on T2 sequences with hypointense fibrous septations. They are typically hypo- to isointense on T1 sequences with heterogeneous but avid enhancement.
- **Chondrosarcoma**. Chondrosarcoma is a malignant primary bone lesion that may involve the skull base where it is typically off midline. They may occur at any age but are most common in middle-aged patients who present with cranial nerve deficits. CT demonstrates an expansile lesion with internal chondroid matrix in an "arcs and swirls" pattern. The soft tissue component is commonly hyperdense. On MRI, the chondroid matrix is hyperintense on T2 sequences; internal calcifications are hypointense. Heterogeneous enhancement is typical.

■ Additional Differential Diagnoses

- **Invasive pituitary macroadenoma**. Pituitary adenomas are common benign neoplasms of the pituitary gland. They are characterized as microadenomas (<10 mm) or macroadenomas (≥10 mm). As a general rule, microadenomas are hormonally active, whereas macroadenomas are inactive but exert local mass effect. Occasionally, a macroadenoma can display infiltrative characteristics, invading the cavernous sinus, paranasal sinuses, clivus/skull base, and brain parenchyma. Imaging findings include a large, expansile soft tissue mass with decreased T1 and increased T2 signal; avid enhancement is typical. The normal pituitary gland is obliterated by the mass, which is a key differentiating feature.
- **Plasmacytoma**. Plasmacytoma is the result of abnormal proliferation of plasma cells; it is the solitary form of multiple myeloma. Patients are often ≥40 years of age. Presentation

depends upon the location of the mass; pain, headache, and cranial neuropathies are common. CT demonstrates a poorly defined, expansile lytic lesion. On MRI, they are typically isointense to gray matter on T1 and T2 sequences; homogeneous enhancement is typical. Flow voids may be present. Patients must be followed to exclude multiple myeloma.
- **Meningioma**. Extradural meningiomas are relatively rare, accounting for fewer than 2% of cases. Intraosseous meningiomas are a subset of extradural meningiomas, most often involve the calvarium, skull base, or facial bones, and are centered in the diploic space. They typically present in adults. CT reveals bony expansion and sclerosis; they may mimic fibrous dysplasia or malignancies. There may be a soft tissue component. Sclerotic components are hypointense on both T1 and T2 MRI sequences; avid enhancement is typical.

■ Diagnosis

Chordoma

✓ Pearls

- Chordomas arise from notochord remnants; they are midline and characteristically bright on T2 sequences.
- Chondrosarcoma demonstrates a chondroid matrix with "arcs and swirls" calcifications and bright T2 signal.

- Invasive macroadenomas may involve the clivus, cavernous and paranasal sinuses, and brain parenchyma.

Suggested Reading

Kimura F, Kim KS, Friedman H, Russell EJ, Breit R. MR imaging of the normal and abnormal clivus. AJR Am J Roentgenol. 1990; 155(6):1285–1291

Case 118

Adam J. Zuckerman

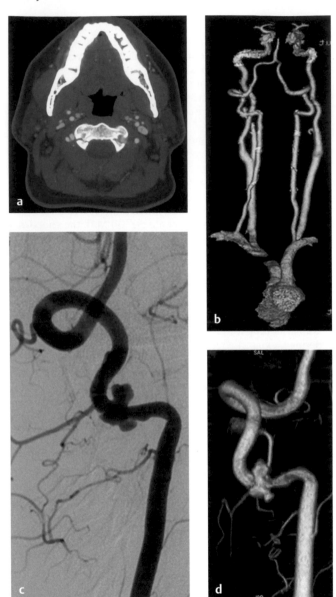

Fig. 118.1 **(a)** Contrast-enhanced axial CT image from a neck CT angiography demonstrates a vertebral fracture through the foramen transversarium with an ovoid area of opacification adjacent to the right vertebral artery. **(b)** CT angiographic, **(c)** conventional angiographic, and **(d)** three-dimensional rotational angiographic images depict a multilobular outpouching along the distal cervical right vertebral artery.

■ Clinical Presentation

A 36-year-old cyclist with neck pain following a collision (▶Fig. 118.1).

■ Key Imaging Finding

Vascular neck injury

■ Top 3 Differential Diagnoses

- **Dissection**. Arterial dissections are the result of intimal injury. They most commonly involve the cervical internal carotid and vertebral arteries; vertebral injury is most common in the V3 segment near the skull base where the vessel is most mobile. Early dissection can often present with complete occlusion of the vessel lumen preceded by a segment of tapered narrowing. Classic angiographic findings include the presence of an intimal flap or irregular segmental luminal narrowing. Computed tomography (CT) angiography reveals eccentric luminal narrowing with relative enlargement of the cross-sectional area of the affected artery compared to contralateral side secondary to thickening from mural hematoma. Axial fat-suppressed T1 magnetic resonance (MR) images demonstrate an eccentric, crescentic periarterial rim of hyperintense signal abnormality along the margin of a flow void. Dissections can be complicated by pseudoaneurysm, thromboembolic, or occlusive phenomena. First-line treatment involves anticoagulation with refractory cases necessitating endovascular or surgical intervention.

- **Pseudoaneurysm**. Pseudoaneurysms are typically due to penetrating or blunt trauma and are frequently associated with arterial dissection. They can also be due to infectious or iatrogenic causes. Pseudoaneurysms are commonly ovoid in appearance and located at the distal aspect of a stenotic segment. Doppler ultrasound of a pseudoaneurysm may demonstrate the classic "to-and-fro" appearance. Management is dependent upon size, location, and etiology. Patients are at risk for expansion of the lesion with compression of adjacent structures and possible rupture. They are also prone to thrombus formation with distant emboli. Treatment options include surgical resection/reconstruction or endovascular stent placement with or without coil embolization of the pseudoaneurysm.

- **Vascular occlusion**. Complete or partial vascular occlusion commonly occurs in association with blunt or penetrating neck injuries. Vascular imaging with CT or conventional angiography demonstrates decreased or absent opacification of the involved vascular structures with or without other associated vascular injuries, including an underlying dissection or intramural hematoma.

■ Additional Differential Diagnoses

- **Arteriovenous fistula (AVF)**. AVFs are usually the result of a penetrating neck injury with partial transection of an artery and adjacent vein. AVFs may also occur spontaneously or be the result of blunt trauma with cervical spine fracture, infection, or iatrogenia. Patients often present with a neck bruit or ischemic symptoms; however, up to 30% of cases may be asymptomatic. AVFs can be diagnosed angiographically with early venous filling during the arterial phase. CT and magnetic resonance imaging (MRI) provide additional detail on the relationship of an AVF to surrounding structures. Endovascular treatment aims to close the fistula while preserving flow in the parent artery.

■ Diagnosis

Pseudoaneurysm of the right vertebral artery

✓ Pearls

- Dissections result from intimal injury; common findings include an intramural hematoma and intimal flap.
- Pseudoaneurysms commonly result from penetrating injuries; they are at risk of expansion and rupture.

- Complete or partial vascular occlusion commonly occurs in association with blunt or penetrating neck injuries.
- AVFs are direct communications between an artery and vein, typically because of penetrating injuries.

Suggested Readings

Herrera DA, Vargas SA, Dublin AB. Endovascular treatment of traumatic injuries of the vertebral artery. AJNR Am J Neuroradiol. 2008; 29(8):1585–1589

Núñez DB, Jr, Torres-León M, Múnera F. Vascular injuries of the neck and thoracic inlet: helical CT-angiographic correlation. Radiographics. 2004; 24(4):1087–1098, discussion 1099–1100

Provenzale JM. Dissection of the internal carotid and vertebral arteries: imaging features. AJR Am J Roentgenol. 1995; 165(5):1099–1104

Case 119

William T. O'Brien, Sr.

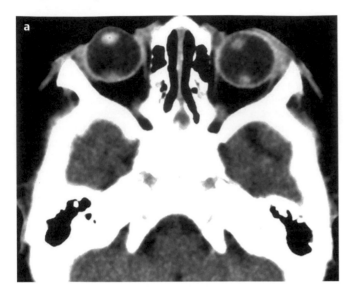

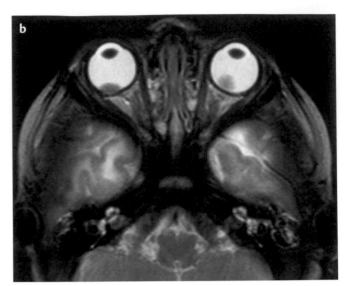

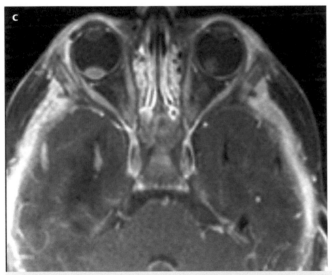

Fig. 119.1 **(a)** Unenhanced axial CT image of the orbits demonstrates abnormal hyperdense soft tissue density along the posterior aspect of the globes, which are normal in size and morphology. The lesions are hypointense on axial T2 sequences **(b)** and demonstrate enhancement **(c)**. The increased T2 signal intensity within the subcortical temporal lobe white matter represents normal myelination pattern (unmyelinated) for age.

■ Clinical Presentation

An infant boy with abnormal screening examination (▶ Fig. 119.1).

■ Key Imaging Finding

Globe lesion in a child

■ Top 3 Differential Diagnoses

- **Retinoblastoma**. Retinoblastoma is a malignant neoplasm of the retina and represents the most common globe tumor in children. Nearly all cases present prior to 5 years of age, with leukocoria (white pupillary reflex) being the most common presenting sign. Approximately 75% are unilateral, whereas the remaining are bilateral. Trilateral (bilateral globe plus pineal gland involvement) and quadrilateral (trilateral plus suprasellar involvement) disease is seen in familial cases. Unenhanced computed tomography (CT) demonstrates a hyperdense globe mass with calcifications (95%). Globe size is normal. The mass is hyperintense on T1 and hypointense on T2 sequences, with avid enhancement. Treatment options include chemotherapy, radiation, and enucleation. Distinguishing features include a normal globe size and presence of calcification
- **Persistent hyperplastic primary vitreous (PHPV)**. PHPV results from persistence of the embryonic vascularity within the vitreous, which may result in vitreous hemorrhage, cataracts, and retinal detachment. In severe disease, phthisis bulbi may occur with globe deformity. Characteristic imaging findings include microphthalmia and increased density in the vitreous. The density may change location with repositioning of the patient. Magnetic resonance imaging (MRI) findings consist of increased T1 and T2 signal within the vitreous. Calcifications are not a feature of PHPV. This may be difficult to distinguish from other entities, especially noncalcified retinoblastoma. Key distinguishing features are microphthalmia in a full-term infant.
- **Coats disease**. Coats disease occurs primarily in young male children and is characterized by subretinal exudates, retinal detachment, and vascular anomalies of the retina. The primary imaging findings are exudates in the region of the retina and retinal detachment. CT reveals increased density within the affected globe without calcification. Subretinal exudates are better visualized on MRI as regions of increased T1 and T2 signal. Distinguishing features include normal globe size and lack of calcification.

■ Additional Differential Diagnoses

- **Retinopathy of prematurity (ROP)**. ROP, also referred to as retrolental fibroplasia, occurs as a sequela of prolonged oxygen therapy in premature infants, resulting in abnormal vascular development and hemorrhage. Imaging features include bilateral (usually) microphthalmia. Resultant hemorrhage leads to increased density within the globe and retinal detachment. Calcification may occur in advanced cases. Bilateral involvement and a history of prematurity help distinguish this entity from the other differentials.
- **Toxocariasis**. Ocular toxocariasis results from a hypersensitivity reaction to the larval form of *Toxocara*. The infection is transmitted through contact with dogs and cats. Patients present with unilateral visual disturbances. On CT, imaging findings include hyperdensity within the globe often without a focal mass. The lesion is isointense on T1- and hyperintense on T2-weighted sequences. Distinguishing features include normal globe size, lack of calcification, and history of contact with dogs or cats.

■ Diagnosis

Retinoblastoma (bilateral)

✓ Pearls

- Retinoblastoma is the most common globe tumor in children and presents with leukocoria and calcification.
- PHPV is due to persistent embryonic vascularity and presents as microphthalmia in a full-term infant.
- Coats disease is characterized by retinal detachment and lack of calcification with a normal globe size.
- ROP is caused by prolonged oxygenation; bilateral microphthalmia without calcification is characteristic.

Suggested Reading

Chung EM, Specht CS, Schroeder JW. From the archives of the AFIP: Pediatric orbit tumors and tumorlike lesions: neuroepithelial lesions of the ocular globe and optic nerve. Radiographics. 2007; 27(4):1159–1186

Case 120

William T. O'Brien Sr.

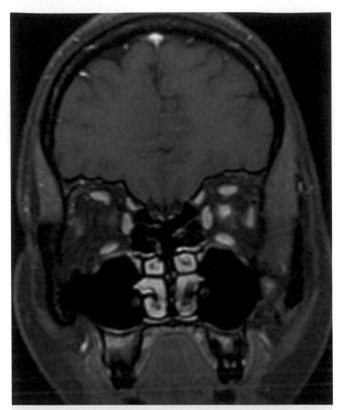

Fig. 120.1 Coronal T1 postcontrast image with fat suppression demonstrates diffuse enlargement and abnormal enhancement involving the left optic nerve with some mild adjacent inflammatory changes. There is normal enhancement of the extraocular muscles.

■ Clinical Presentation

A young adult woman with pain and visual changes (▶ Fig. 120.1).

■ Key Imaging Finding

Optic nerve enlargement and enhancement

■ Top 3 Differential Diagnoses

- **Optic neuritis**. Optic neuritis is most often due to demyelination secondary to an autoimmune or viral process. Other etiologies include ocular infection, toxic or metabolic degeneration, ischemia, and meningitis/encephalitis. Multiple sclerosis (MS) involves the optic nerve in roughly one-third of cases. Approximately one-half to three-fourths of patients who present with their first episode of optic neuritis will develop MS within 15 years. Patients present with ipsilateral orbital pain with eye movement and vision loss which occurs over hours to days. MR demonstrates abnormal increased T2/FLAIR signal intensity within the affected optic nerve, best visualized on coronal sequences. Postcontrast studies may reveal abnormal optic nerve enlargement and enhancement. In chronic stages, the optic nerve may become atrophic.

- **Optic nerve glioma**. Optic nerve gliomas are low-grade neoplasms (typically juvenile pilocytic astrocytomas) that most often occur between 5 and 15 years of age. Patients present with vision loss with or without proptosis. Optic nerve gliomas may occur sporadically or be associated with neurofibromatosis type 1 (NF-1); bilateral optic nerve involvement is pathognomonic for NF-1. Tumors cause enlargement, elongation, and "buckling" of the optic nerve, resulting in the "dotted i" sign on axial images. Enlargement and benign bony remod-

eling of the optic canal may also be seen. The enhancement pattern is variable. Optic nerve gliomas may extend along the optic pathways (optic chiasm, tracts, and radiations). NF-1 predominantly involves the optic nerve with preservation of nerve morphology. Non-NF-1 cases most often involve the optic chiasm or hypothalamus, are larger and more masslike, commonly have cystic degeneration, and may extend beyond the optic pathways.

- **Optic nerve sheath meningioma**. Meningiomas arise from arachnoid rests in the meninges covering the optic nerve. Eighty percent of the cases occur in women and typically present in the fourth decade of life with progressive loss of vision (optic nerve atrophy). They may occur as tubular (most common), fusiform, or eccentric masses associated with the optic nerve. The lesions may be hyperdense on computed tomography; calcification is common (20–25%). On magnetic resonance, they are typically isointense to gray matter on T1 and variable in signal on T2 sequences. Enhancement is intense and relatively homogeneous. The "tram track" sign on postcontrast imaging represents linear bands of enhancement surrounding the central nonenhancing optic nerve. Sphenoid bone and/or optic canal hyperostosis may be seen.

■ Additional Differential Diagnoses

- **Leukemia/lymphoma**. Leukemia (acute myeloid leukemia) and non-Hodgkin lymphoma may involve the orbit in a variety of presentations. Involvement of the optic nerve sheath complex with regions of enhancement is the least common manifestation. When present, lesions are often (but not exclusively) bilateral.

- **Sarcoidosis**. Sarcoidosis is a systemic process characterized by noncaseating granulomas. Symptomatic central

nervous system involvement (neurosarcoidosis) occurs in approximately 5% of patients with sarcoidosis. Isolated optic nerve involvement is rare but should be considered in the differential diagnosis of an optic nerve lesion in a patient with sarcoidosis. Varying degrees and patterns of enhancement are seen, but nodular enhancement is most common.

■ Diagnosis

Optic neuritis

✓ Pearls

- Optic nerve gliomas are the most common cause of optic nerve enlargement in kids and are associated with NF-1.
- Optic neuritis is commonly due to demyelination; the majority of patients will develop MS within 15 years.

- Optic nerve sheath meningiomas demonstrate "tram track" enhancement on axial imaging.

Suggested Readings

Kornreich L, Blaser S, Schwarz M, et al. Optic pathway glioma: correlation of imaging findings with the presence of neurofibromatosis. AJNR Am J Neuroradiol. 2001; 22(10):1963–1969

LeBedis CA, Sakai O. Nontraumatic orbital conditions: diagnosis with CT and MR imaging in the emergent setting. Radiographics. 2008; 28(6):1741–1753

Case 121

Adam J. Zuckerman

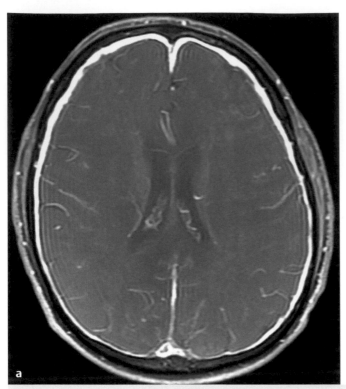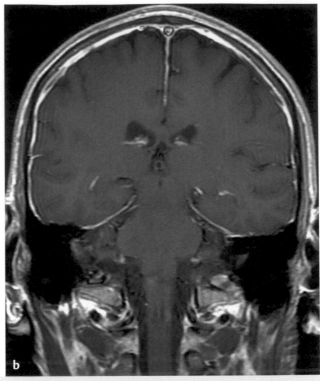

Fig. 121.1 **(a)** Postcontrast axial fat-suppressed and **(b)** coronal T1 images demonstrate diffuse abnormal pachymeningeal (dural) enhancement.

■ Clinical Presentation

An adult man with weakness, fatigue, and failure to thrive
(▶Fig. 121.1).

■ Key Imaging Finding

Pachymeningeal (dural) enhancement

■ Top 3 Differential Diagnoses

• **Intracranial hypotension**. Intracranial hypotension results from decreased intracranial pressure due to cerebrospinal fluid (CSF) leak. Common etiologies include trauma, iatrogenia (lumbar puncture or postoperative), and idiopathic or spontaneous CSF leaks. Patients present clinically with orthostatic headaches. Classic imaging findings include diffuse pachymeningeal (dural) enhancement and caudal displacement of the cerebellar tonsils ("sagging brain" appearance). The presence of dural thickening, subdural fluid collections, venous engorgement/distention, and pituitary hyperemia may also be seen. If the site of the CSF leak is unknown, computed tomography (CT), magnetic resonance imaging (MRI), or radionuclide cisternography may be useful in determining the origin of the leak. Conservative therapies (bed rest, hydration, and caffeine) and epidural blood patches are the most common first-line treatments.

• **Metastases**. Metastatic disease commonly affects the dura either from hematogenous spread or direct extension from calvarial lesions. Breast, lung, and prostate carcinomas are the most common primary neoplasms; hematologic malignancies, such as lymphoma and leukemia, may also demonstrate abnormal dural enhancement. The regions of abnormal enhancement may be smooth or nodular and focal or diffuse. Although dural lesions are often asymptomatic, cranial neuropathies are common with skull base involvement.

• **Pachymeningitis**. Meningeal infection may be due to bacterial, viral, or fungal etiology. The diagnosis is made clinically with CSF sampling; imaging is useful for the evaluation of suspected complications. Meningeal enhancement is evident only in approximately 50% of patients with meningitis and commonly involves both the leptomeninges and pachymeninges. *Mycobacterium tuberculosis* classically results in meningeal disease involving the skull base, cerebritis, and intracranial abscess formation (tuberculoma); isolated tuberculosis pachymeningitis with associated enhancement has been described in immunocompromised patients.

■ Additional Differential Diagnoses

• **Sarcoidosis**. Approximately 5% of sarcoid patients develop symptomatic CNS involvement. Neurosarcoidosis most often presents with smooth or nodular dural and/or leptomeningeal enhancement, especially along the basal cisterns. There is often involvement of the optic chiasm, hypothalamus, infundibulum, internal auditory canals, and cranial nerves at the skull base. Brain parenchyma can also be involved in one-third of patients.

• **Subdural hemorrhage**. Subdural hemorrhage typically results from tearing of bridging veins and is most often due to trauma. In contrast to epidural hemorrhage, subdural collections may cross sutures but cannot cross midline. The blood products within the hemorrhage vary in attenuation (CT) and signal intensity (MR) based on the age of hemorrhage, as well as additional factors. Hyperdense or T1-hyperintense blood products may mimic dural enhancement. In addition, blood products are a source of meningeal irritation, which may manifest as true meningeal enhancement on CT or MRI. Patients often have an antecedent history of trauma.

■ Diagnosis

Metastases/Pachymeningeal carcinomatosis

✓ Pearls

• Intracranial hypotension results from a CSF leak; findings include dural enhancement and tonsillar ectopia.

• Dural-based metastases may result from hematogenous spread or direct spread from a skull-based lesion.

• Common imaging findings of meningitis include both leptomeningeal and pachymeningeal enhancement.

• Neurosarcoidosis often results in nodular meningeal enhancement; cranial neuropathies are common.

Suggested Readings

Castillo M. Imaging of meningitis. Semin Roentgenol. 2004; 39(4):458–464

Schievink WI, Maya MM, Louy C, Moser FG, Tourje J. Diagnostic criteria for spontaneous spinal CSF leaks and intracranial hypotension. AJNR Am J Neuroradiol. 2008; 29(5):853–856

Smirniotopoulos JG, Murphy FM, Rushing EJ, Rees JH, Schroeder JW. Patterns of contrast enhancement in the brain and meninges. Radiographics. 2007; 27(2):525–551

Case 122

William T. O'Brien Sr.

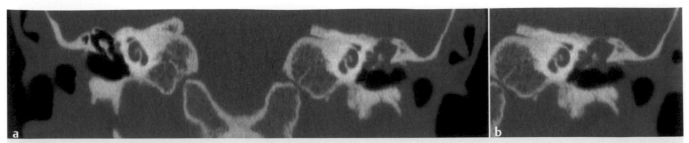

Fig. 122.1 **(a)** Coronal CT image from an unenhanced temporal bone CT with **(b)** a magnified view of the left temporal bone demonstrates lobulated soft-tissue density within the left middle ear, involving the epitympanum, including the lateral attic or Prussak space, and the mesotympanum. There is mild blunting of the scutum, as well as demineralization and erosion of the ossicles and tegmen tympani (roof of the middle ear cavity).

■ Clinical Presentation

Chronic ear pain and conductive hearing loss (▶ Fig. 122.1).

■ Key Imaging Finding

Middle ear mass

■ Top 3 Differential Diagnoses

- **Acquired cholesteatoma.** Cholesteatomas are epidermoid cysts composed of keratinized squamous epithelium. Within the middle ear, the vast majority result from chronic otitis media. Patients suffer from multiple ear infections with perforation of a retracted tympanic membrane and conductive hearing loss. On imaging, cholesteatomas appear as soft-tissue masses in Prussak space within the lateral attic. There is often blunting of the scutum (lateral wall of the attic) and erosion of the ossicles. When large, cholesteatomas may extend into the mastoid air cells. It is important to identify the bony margin of the facial nerve and integrity of the tegmen tympani (roof of tympanic cavity) for presurgical planning, as well as to define the full extent of the mass for the surgeon. On magnetic resonance imaging (MRI), cholesteatomas commonly show increased signal on diffusion weighted imaging. Complications include coalescent mastoiditis, meningitis, epidural abscesses, and venous sinus thrombosis.

- **Facial nerve schwannoma.** Facial nerve schwannomas may occur anywhere along the course of the facial nerve. When involving the tympanic segment in the middle ear, there is often enlargement of the bony facial nerve canal. Postcontrast images demonstrate tubular enlargement and enhancement of the involved segment; involvement of the labyrinthine segment is a helpful finding to distinguish this entity from other middle ear masses. As small lesions can be subtle, it is important to look for asymmetry with the contralateral side.
- **Glomus tympanicum.** Glomus tympanicum is a paraganglioma which occurs within the middle ear along the cochlear promontory. It arises from neural crest origin and is highly vascular with avid enhancement. As the mass grows, it may fill the middle ear and encroach on the ossicles. Bony erosion may be seen. When large, glomus tumors may contain calcifications and flow voids, resulting in a "salt and pepper" appearance on MRI. Clinically, patients present with conductive hearing loss and pulsatile tinnitus.

■ Additional Differential Diagnoses

- **Normal variant vasculature.** An aberrant internal carotid artery (ICA) is a developmental abnormality which likely results from regression of the cervical and proximal petrous ICA and the development of alternate anastomoses. Imaging findings include deviation and narrowing of the ICA within the temporal bone (extending into the middle ear), along with absence of the cervical and proximal portion of the petrous ICA. A dehiscent jugular bulb occurs when the sigmoid plate of the jugular bulb is absent, allowing for extension of the jugular bulb into the middle ear cavity. Imaging findings are diagnostic and typically straightforward.

- **Cholesterol granuloma.** Cholesterol granulomas occur secondary to nonspecific chronic inflammatory changes and are seen most commonly in the temporal bone (middle ear and petrous apex). Computed tomography reveals a soft-tissue mass within the middle ear without osseous erosion. On physical examination, there is a bluish or purplish coloration of the tympanic membrane. The lesions are hyperintense on both T1- and T2-weighted MR sequences due to hemorrhage within the lesions. There may be peripheral rim enhancement.

■ Diagnosis

Acquired cholesteatoma

✓ Pearls

- Acquired cholesteatomas occur in Prussak space and cause blunting of the scutum and ossicular erosion.
- Facial nerve schwannoma presents as an enhancing mass within an expanded facial nerve canal.

- Glomus tympanicum is a highly vascular paraganglioma and occurs along the cochlear promontory.
- Normal variant vasculature (aberrant ICA and dehiscent jugular bulb) may present as a middle ear mass.

Suggested Readings

Betts A, Esquivel C, O'Biren WT. Vascular retrotympanic mass. J Am Osteopath Coll Radiol. 2012; 1(1):31–33

Swartz JD, Harnsberger HR, Mukherji SK. The temporal bone. Contemporary diagnostic dilemmas. Radiol Clin North Am. 1998; 36(5):819–853, vi

Remley KB, Coit WE, Harnsberger HR, Smoker WR, Jacobs JM, McIff EB. Pulsatile tinnitus and the vascular tympanic membrane: CT, MR, and angiographic findings. Radiology. 1990; 174(2):383–389

Case 123

William T. O'Brien Sr.

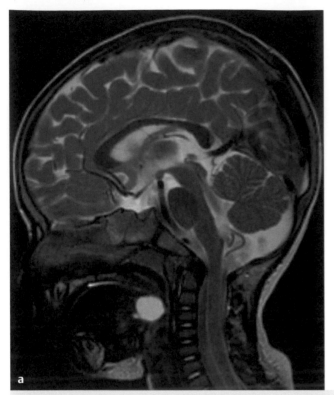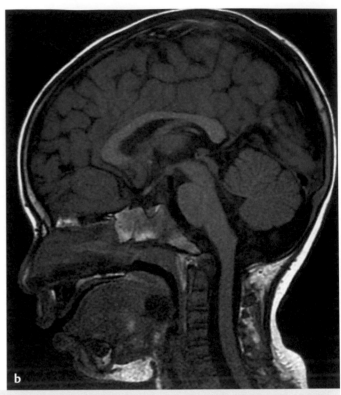

Fig. 123.1 (a) Sagittal T2 and **(b)** T1 MR images reveal a circumscribed cystic mass involving the root and base of the tongue. There is incidental note of a mega cisterna magna with hyperdynamic CSF flow both intracranially and within the cervical spinal canal **(a)**. The sphenoid sinus has yet to pneumatize in this child (open synchondroses).

■ Clinical Presentation

A young child with globus sensation (▶Fig. 123.1).

■ Key Imaging Finding

Base of tongue mass in a child

■ Top 3 Differential Diagnoses

- **Thyroglossal duct cyst**. Thyroglossal duct cysts represent the most common congenital neck lesions. The vast majority (≈85%) are midline. Approximately 25% of the cysts are suprahyoid in location with the remaining 75% being infrahyoid. Suprahyoid lesions occur anywhere from the foramen cecum at the tongue base to the hyoid bone; infrahyoid lesions may be midline or paramedian and are characteristically embedded within the strap muscles. Thyroglossal duct cysts are most often well circumscribed and may have lobulations or septations. They typically follow fluid attenuation (computed tomography [CT]) or signal intensity (magnetic resonance imaging [MRI]). Increased protein content may result in increased attenuation and T1 signal intensity. Superimposed infection or hemorrhage results in a heterogeneous imaging appearance, which may include peripheral enhancement.
- **Lingual thyroid**. Lingual thyroid refers to ectopic thyroid tissue located at the foramen cecum, involving the base and root of the tongue; 90% of ectopic thyroid cases occur in this location. It is important to evaluate the thyroid bed in the lower neck for the presence of additional thyroid tissue; in ≈75% of cases, the lingual thyroid represents the only functioning thyroid tissue. Most patients are hypothyroid with the remainder of patients being euthyroid. On cross-sectional imaging, ectopic thyroid tissue follows thyroid attenuation and signal intensity. It is hyperdense on CT with moderate enhancement. On MR, it is hyperintense on T1 and T2 sequences and demonstrates avid enhancement. Nuclear medicine thyroid imaging is also a useful adjunct in identifying functioning thyroid tissue. Rarely, thyroid cancer may occur in ≈1 to 3% of cases; concerning imaging characteristics include soft-tissue nodular components or calcification.
- **Epidermoid/dermoid cyst**. Epidermoid and dermoid cysts are developmental abnormalities that may involve the oral cavity, oropharynx, or floor of mouth. Epidermoids contain epithelial elements, while dermoids contain epithelial elements along with dermal elements. Both appear cystic on imaging with low attenuation on CT and T2 hyperintensity on MR. There may be thin peripheral enhancement, if any. Dermoids may contain macroscopic fat which is a key discriminator, when present. Epidermoids show restricted diffusion.

■ Additional Differential Diagnoses

- **Hemangioma**. Hemangiomas are benign vascular tumors which may involve the oral cavity or oropharynx. Capillary hemangiomas are common in infancy but naturally regress after a proliferative phase. CT and MR demonstrate a well-circumscribed, lobulated, hyperdense, and T2 hyperintense mass with avid enhancement.
- **Tonsillar hypertrophy**. The lingual tonsils are a component of Waldeyer ring and are located within the oropharynx along the base of the tongue. Tonsillar hypertrophy refers to enlargement of the tonsils which may occur in isolation or secondary to a local infectious or inflammatory process. It is most often symmetric; if asymmetric, it may mimic a mass. Contrast-enhanced CT demonstrates homogeneous hyperattenuation of tonsillar tissue. On MR, tonsillar tissue is T2 hyperintense with enhancement similar to mucosal tissue.
- **Venolymphatic malformation**. Venolymphatic malformations represent a spectrum of venous and lymphatic developmental abnormalities. Pure venous malformations avidly enhance and contain flow voids on T2 MR; the presence of phleboliths is pathognomonic. Pure lymphatic malformations may be unilocular or multilocular and demonstrate fluid attenuation and signal intensity. Fluid–fluid levels, most often due to hemorrhage, are characteristic. Venolymphatic malformations often cross fascial planes to involve multiple spaces of the neck.

■ Diagnosis

Thyroglossal duct cyst

✓ Pearls

- Thyroglossal duct cysts are common congenital lesions which present as circumscribed, midline cystic masses.
- Lingual thyroid is the most common form of ectopic thyroid; it is typically the only functioning thyroid tissue.
- Dermoid cysts often contain macroscopic fat; epidermoids show restricted diffusion.

Suggested Reading

Fang WS, Wiggins RH, III, Illner A, et al. Primary lesions of the root of the tongue. Radiographics. 2011; 31(7):1907–1922

Case 124

William T. O'Brien Sr.

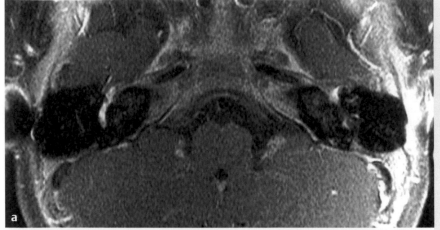
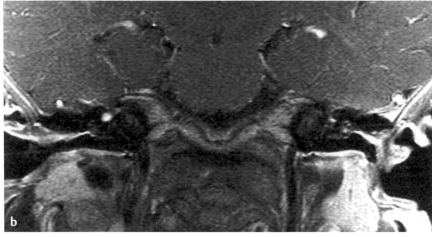

Fig. 124.1 (a) Axial and (b) coronal T1 postcontrast MR images with fat suppression reveal abnormal asymmetric enhancement and enlargement of the tympanic segment of the right facial nerve. The coronal image (b) shows the normal nonenhancing labyrinthine segments bilaterally (medially above the cochlea) and normal size and enhancement of the tympanic segment (just lateral to the labyrinthine segment) of the left facial nerve.

■ Clinical Presentation

A young adult man with facial asymmetry (▶ Fig. 124.1).

■ **Key Imaging Finding**

Facial nerve enhancement

■ **Top 3 Differential Diagnoses**

- **Normal facial nerve enhancement**. The proximal portions of the facial nerve which are surrounded by CSF—cisternal, canalicular, and labyrinthine segments—should not enhance; enhancement of these segments is considered abnormal. Beginning at the geniculate ganglion and extending distally into the horizontal (tympanic) and vertical (mastoid) segments, the facial nerve may enhance normally. Normal enhancement is typically symmetric but may be mildly asymmetric.
- **Bell palsy**. Bell palsy refers to acute onset infectious or postinfectious ipsilateral facial nerve palsy. Most cases are self-limiting and thought to result from herpes simplex virus type 1, the same virus which causes cold sores. On magnetic resonance (MR), the geniculate ganglion, tympanic segment, and mastoid segment of the facial nerve may enhance in normal patients. With Bell palsy, there is often smooth asymmetric enhancement of the involved tympanic and/or mastoid seg-

ments, as well as abnormal enhancement of the portions of the facial nerve that are usually protected by the blood–nerve barrier, to include the intracanalicular and labyrinthine segments. The distal intracanalicular and labyrinthine segments are most commonly involved.
- **Nerve sheath tumor**. Schwannomas arise from perineural Schwann cells. They are composed of two tissue types: Antoni A (densely packed) and B (loosely packed, T2 hyperintense). Patients present with hearing loss or facial neuropathy. Temporal bone computed tomography (CT) reveals smooth enlargement of the involved segments of the facial nerve canal. The geniculate ganglion is the most common site with extension into adjacent facial nerve segments. MR demonstrates abnormal signal, enlargement, and enhancement of the involved segments.

■ **Additional Differential Diagnoses**

- **Facial nerve hemangioma**. Facial nerve hemangioma is a vascular tumor, which occurs along the course of the facial nerve. It most often occurs in the region of the geniculate ganglion, followed by the distal IAC and junction of the horizontal (tympanic) and vertical (mastoid) segments of the facial nerve. CT reveals a characteristic honeycomb bony matrix. On MR, lesions are T2 hyperintense with avid enhancement, corresponding to the vascular nature of the tumor.
- **Perineural spread of tumor**. Perineural spread along the facial nerve most often results from parotid tumors, specifically adenoid cystic carcinoma. Facial nerve involvement from primary head and neck or skin neoplasms is much less common. On CT, perineural spread most often manifests as abnormal enlargement of the bony facial nerve canal within the involved segments, typically extending proximally from the stylomas-

toid foramen. MR demonstrates abnormal enlargement, signal intensity, and enhancement of the involved portions of the facial nerve. Imaging should extend through the neck to evaluate for a primary origin.
- **Ramsey Hunt**. Ramsey Hunt syndrome is caused by reactivation of the varicella zoster virus, which lies dormant in the geniculate ganglion. Patients are often elderly or immunocompromised and present with ipsilateral otalgia, a vesicular rash involving the external auditory canal and auricle, and facial neuropathy. MR reveals abnormal enhancement within the involved segments of the facial nerve; abnormal enhancement of the vestibulocochlear nerve and labyrinthine structures is also commonly seen. Patients are typically treated with steroids and antiviral medications (e.g. acyclovir). There is a good prognosis/recovery in approximately 50 to 70% of cases.

■ **Diagnosis**

Facial nerve schwannoma

✓ **Pearls**

- Bell palsy most often involves the distal intracanalicular and labyrinthine segments; it is usually self-limiting.
- Tumors (schwannoma and perineural spread) result in abnormal signal, enhancement, and nerve enlargement.

- Hemangiomas are vascular tumors that result in a honeycomb matrix on CT and avid enhancement on MR.

Suggested Reading

Saremi F, Helmy M, Farzin S, Zee CS, Go JL. MRI of cranial nerve enhancement. AJR Am J Roentgenol. 2005; 185(6):1487–1497

Case 125

William T. O'Brien Sr.

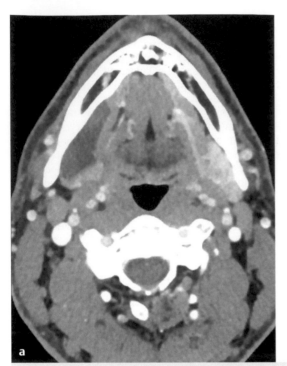
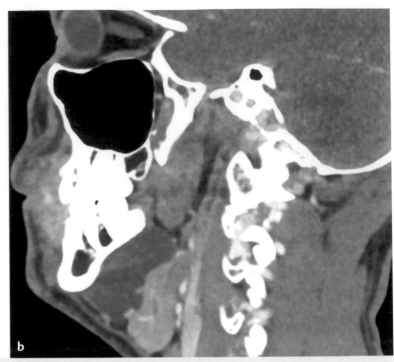

Fig. 125.1 **(a)** Axial contrast-enhanced CT image demonstrates a hypodense mass within the floor of the mouth along the inner margin of the right mandible. **(b)** Reformatted sagittal CT image confirms extension of the mass into the submandibular space with inferior and posterior displacement of the right submandibular gland.

■ Clinical Presentation

A 27-year-old man with facial asymmetry and palpable mass (►Fig. 125.1).

■ Key Imaging Finding

Floor of the mouth mass

■ Top 3 Differential Diagnoses

- **Squamous cell carcinoma (SCC)**. SCC is the most common neoplasm of the aerodigestive tract and is highly associated with tobacco usage. Common locations include the base of tongue, palate, and floor of the mouth. Patients are often asymptomatic until late in the disease process. The mylohyoid muscle divides floor of the mouth carcinomas into sublingual (above) and submandibular (below) compartments. SCC often presents as an ill-defined enhancing mass. Lymphadenopathy, which may be centrally necrotic, is commonly seen.
- **Infection/abscess**. Cellulitis and abscesses within the floor of the mouth are commonly due to dental infections or procedures. Cellulitis presents with inflammatory changes which are typically ill defined, while abscesses are organized fluid collections with rim enhancement. The term *Ludwig angina*

refers to a severe, potentially life-threatening infection with abscess formation involving the sublingual, submental, and submandibular spaces. The life-threatening nature of the infection results from airway compression.
- **Ranula**. Ranulas are mucous retention cysts of the salivary glands in the floor of the mouth. When confined to the sublingual space, they are referred to as simple ranulas; when they extend below the mylohyoid muscle into the submandibular space, they are referred to as diving or plunging ranulas. The plunging ranulas lack true cyst walls. Ranulas typically follow fluid attenuation and signal intensity and are most often unilocular. Peripheral enhancement may be seen, especially with superimposed infection.

■ Additional Differential Diagnoses

- **Venolymphatic malformation**. Venolymphatic malformations represent a spectrum of venous and lymphatic developmental abnormalities. Pure venous malformations avidly enhance and may contain flow voids on T2 MR; the presence of phleboliths is pathognomonic. Pure lymphatic malformations may be unilocular or multilocular and demonstrate fluid attenuation and signal intensity. Fluid–fluid levels, most often due to hemorrhage, are characteristic. Many cases demonstrate characteristics of both. Venolymphatic malformations often cross fascial planes to involve multiple compartments and spaces of the neck.
- **Epidermoid/dermoid cyst**. Epidermoid and dermoid cysts are developmental abnormalities which may involve the oral cavity, oropharynx, or floor of the mouth. Epidermoids contain ep-

ithelial elements, while dermoids contain epithelial elements along with dermal elements. Both appear cystic on imaging with low attenuation on CT and T2 hyperintensity on MR. There may be thin peripheral enhancement, if any. Dermoids may contain macroscopic fat which is a key discriminator, when present. Epidermoids demonstrate restricted diffusion.
- **Hemangioma**. Hemangiomas are benign vascular tumors which may involve the oral cavity or oropharynx; rarely, they may present as a submucosal floor of the mouth mass. Capillary hemangiomas are common in infancy but naturally regress following a proliferative phase. CT and MR demonstrate a well-circumscribed, lobulated, hyperdense, and T2 hyperintense mass with avid enhancement.

■ Diagnosis

Ranula (diving/plunging)

✓ Pearls

- SCC is the most common malignancy of the aerodigestive tract and may have associated necrotic adenopathy.
- Cellulitis and abscesses are typically of dental origin; Ludwig angina is severe and potentially life threatening.

- Ranulas are mucous retention cysts and characterized based on their relation to the mylohyoid muscle.
- Venolymphatic malformations, epidermoid/dermoid cysts, and hemangiomas may involve the floor of the mouth.

Suggested Reading

Coit WE, Harnsberger HR, Osborn AG, Smoker WR, Stevens MH, Lufkin RB. Ranulas and their mimics: CT evaluation. Radiology. 1987; 163(1):211–216

Case 126

William T. O'Brien Sr.

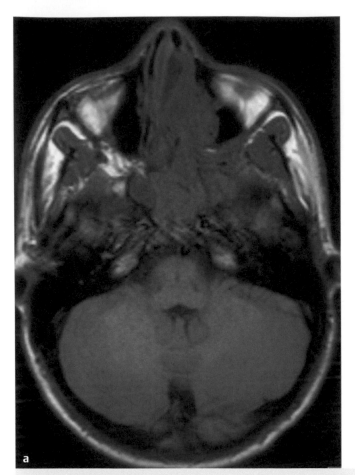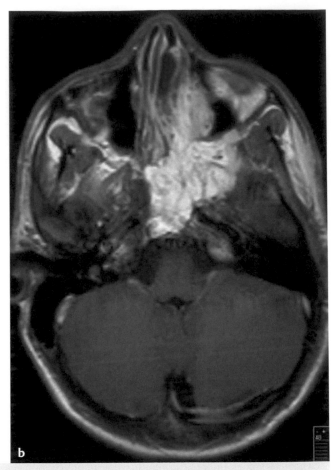

Fig. 126.1 **(a)** Pre- and **(b)** postcontrast T1-weighted MR images demonstrate a large T1 hypointense mass which demonstrates intense homogeneous enhancement. The mass involves the left nasopharynx, nasal cavity, and pterygopalatine fossa and extends laterally through the sphenopalatine foramen. The maxillary sinus is also involved. There was no intracranial or intraorbital extension (images not shown).

■ Clinical Presentation

A child with chronic stuffy nose, facial asymmetry, and visual disturbances (▶Fig. 126.1).

■ Key Imaging Finding

Aggressive nasal mass in a child/adolescent

■ Top 3 Differential Diagnoses

- **Juvenile nasopharyngeal angiofibroma (JNA)**. JNAs are benign but locally aggressive lesions that occur in adolescent boys. They originate in the nasopharynx adjacent to the sphenopalatine foramen and pterygopalatine fossa. The lesions commonly extend into multiple compartments, including infratemporal, intracranial, and intraorbital, as well as into the paranasal sinuses. Anterior bowing of the posterior maxillary sinus wall is commonly seen. Patients present with nasal obstruction and epistaxis. JNAs are hypointense to intermediate on T1 and intermediate to hyperintense on T2 sequences. They avidly enhance; flow voids are commonly seen. Lesions are resected with preoperative embolization to minimize intraoperative bleeding.
- **Esthesioneuroblastoma (ENB)**: ENB is a malignant neuroendocrine tumor which arises from olfactory endothelium within the superior nasal cavity. It most commonly occurs in adolescents and middle-aged patients who present with nasal obstruction and epistaxis. Imaging findings include an enhancing mass which is hypointense to intermediate on T1 and hyperintense on T2 sequences. Intracranial extension through the cribriform plate is common. The classic finding is a "dumbbell-shaped" mass in the nasal cavity/nasopharynx and anterior cranial fossa with a narrowed waist at the level of the cribriform plate. Intracranial portions of the tumor often demonstrate cystic components.
- **Rhabdomyosarcoma**. Rhabdomyosarcoma represents a malignant tumor composed of striated musculature and is the most common nasal sarcoma in adolescents. It may involve the sinuses, nasal cavity, and nasopharynx with bony destruction. Intracranial extension is common. The mass is relatively homogeneous, iso- to hypointense on T1 and hyperintense on T2 compared to musculature, and avidly enhances.

■ Additional Differential Diagnoses

- **Hemangioma**. Hemangiomas are benign tumors which may occur within the nasal cavity at any age but most often present in the pediatric population or during pregnancy. These may be capillary (more common) or cavernous and typically occur along the nasal septum or turbinates. Presenting symptoms include nasal obstruction and epistaxis. Imaging findings include well-circumscribed, lobulated avidly enhancing nasal soft-tissue mass which is hypointense to intermediate on T1 and hyperintense on T2 sequences.
- **Sinonasal lymphoma**. Non-Hodgkin lymphoma (NHL) commonly involves the head and neck, most often with cervical lymphadenopathy. Paranasal sinus involvement is less common and may present as a well-defined or infiltrative soft-tissue mass. On MR imaging, NHL is most often iso- to hyperintense on T1 and hyperintense on T2 sequences compared to musculature. T2 signal intensity may be more variable with aggressive variants. Homogeneous enhancement is typically seen.
- **Inverted papilloma (IP)**. IPs are benign, locally aggressive neoplasms which may occur in adolescents but are most common in adult men who present with nasal obstruction. They originate along the middle meatus and extend into the paranasal sinuses. Calcifications may be seen on CT. They are isointense on T1 and hyperintense on T2 MR sequences with characteristic linear striations. There is heterogeneous enhancement.

■ Diagnosis

Juvenile nasopharyngeal angiofibroma

✓ Pearls

- JAFs occur in adolescent boys, avidly enhance, and commonly extend into multiple compartments.
- ENBs are malignant neuroendocrine tumors which may extend intracranially through the cribriform plate.
- Hemangiomas most commonly occur along the septum and turbinates in children and during pregnancy.
- IPs are locally aggressive, may have calcifications, and have a characteristic striated appearance on MRI.

Suggested Reading

Valencia MP, Castillo M. Congenital and acquired lesions of the nasal septum: a practical guide for differential diagnosis. Radiographics. 2008; 28(1):205–224, quiz 326

Case 127

William T. O'Brien Sr.

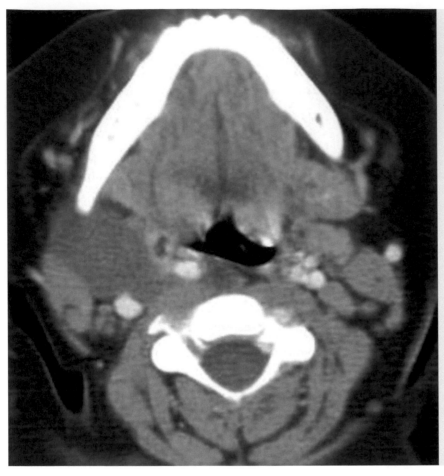

Fig. 127.1 Contrast-enhanced axial CT image through the neck demonstrates an ovoid fluid attenuation mass located at the angle of the mandible on the right. There is extension into the parapharyngeal space, as well as the carotid space with splaying of the carotid artery and internal jugular vein.

■ Clinical Presentation

A young patient with a palpable neck mass (▶Fig. 127.1).

■ Key Imaging Finding

Cystic neck mass

■ Top 3 Differential Diagnoses

- **Congenital cyst**. *Thyroglossal duct cysts* (TDCs) represent the most common congenital cystic neck masses. They are typically midline (85%) or slightly off-midline and ≈75% are infrahyoid in location. *Branchial cleft cysts* result from developmental abnormalities of the branchial apparatus. There are four types with the second being the most common, followed by the first. Type 1 branchial cleft cysts may occur anywhere from the external auditory canal to the angle of the mandible, including within the parotid gland. Type 2 branchial cleft cysts most commonly occur near the angle of the mandible anterior and medial to the sternocleidomastoid (SCM) muscle. Third and fourth branchial cleft cysts are rare and frequently result in sinus formation. Type 3 branchial cleft cysts occur deep to the SCM muscle or posteriorly, while type 4 branchial cleft cysts occur near the larynx or thyroid gland. *Thymic cysts* are the least common congenital cystic neck masses. They may occur anywhere along the tract of thymus descent from the angle of the mandible into the mediastinum. They are lateral in location, either deep or superficial to the SCM muscle, and may be unilocular or multilocular. All congenital cysts demonstrate fluid attenuation (CT) or signal intensity (MR); internal debris and peripheral enhancement may be appreciated with superimposed infection or hemorrhage.

- **Abscess**. Abscesses may occur anywhere in the neck but are typically found within the peritonsillar, retropharyngeal, or perioral regions. Less common etiologies include penetrating trauma or postoperative complications. Clinical signs and symptoms include pain, fever, and elevated white blood cell count. Imaging characteristics include a rim-enhancing fluid collection with variable wall thickness and surrounding inflammatory changes. Percutaneous or surgical drainage with antibiotic therapy is commonly warranted.

- **Lymphatic malformation**. Lymphatic malformations are common in the head and neck region. They are fluid-filled and may be unilocular or multilocular. Fluid–fluid levels, most often due to hemorrhage, are characteristic. Peripheral enhancement may be seen with superimposed inflammation or infection; internal regions of enhancement, when present, correspond to venous components of a venolymphatic malformation. Lesions may grow quite large and insinuate between and cross fascial plains. Lymphatic malformations previously characterized as "cystic hygromas" are a common subtype which typically occur posteriorly and may be associated with chromosomal abnormalities, such as Turner or Down syndrome.

■ Additional Differential Diagnoses

- **Cystic lymph node**. Cystic lymph nodes may result from local or regional spread of infectious or malignant processes. Squamous cell carcinoma (SCC) and papillary thyroid cancer are the two most common primary neoplasms that demonstrate cystic metastases within cervical lymph nodes. Atypical infections, such as *Mycobacterium* and *Bartonella* subspecies, are the common infectious etiologies for cystic lymph nodes.

- **Cystic nerve sheath tumor**. Cystic nerve sheath tumors, such as schwannomas, may occur within the neck and are typically oriented along the course of the traversing nerve; communication with the neural foramina may be seen with more central lesions and is characteristic. The presence of enhancing soft-tissue components is a useful discriminator to exclude a congenital cyst or pure lymphatic malformation.

■ Diagnosis

Congenital thymic cyst

✓ Pearls

- The most common congenital cystic neck masses are TDCs (midline) and branchial cleft cysts (lateral).
- Abscesses commonly occur within the neck, are rim enhancing, and typically require drainage.

- Lymphatic malformations may be unilocular or multilocular, have fluid–fluid levels, and cross fascial planes.
- Cystic lymphadenopathy may occur from infectious or neoplastic (SCC and papillary thyroid) processes.

Suggested Reading

Lev S, Lev MH. Imaging of cystic lesions. Radiol Clin North Am. 2000; 38(5):1013–1027

Case 128

Adam J. Zuckerman

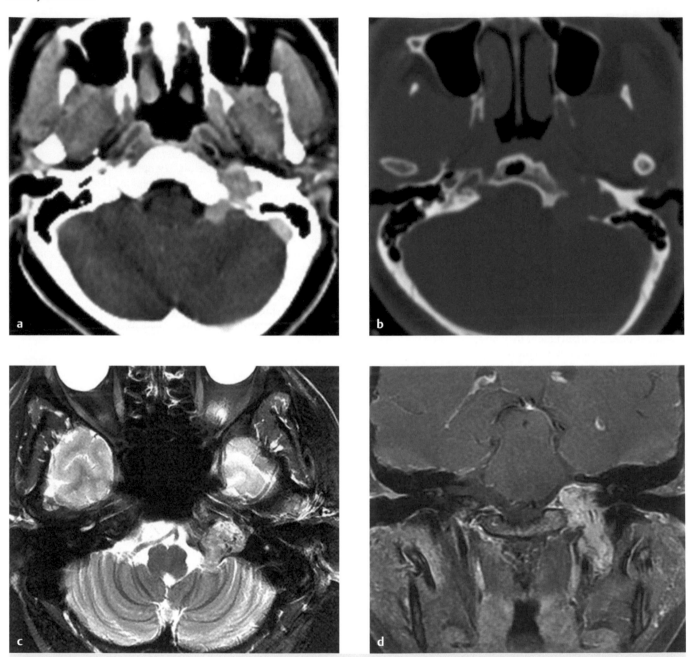

Fig. 128.1 (a) Contrast-enhanced axial CT images in soft tissue and (b) bone windows demonstrate an enhancing soft-tissue mass with expansion and erosion of the jugular foramen. (c) T2-weighted axial image reveals the presence of multiple flow voids within an intermediate signal intensity left jugular foramen mass. (d) Coronal T1 postcontrast MR image shows the extent of the avidly enhancing lesion originating from the jugular foramen.

■ Clinical Presentation

An adult woman with tinnitus and cranial neuropathies
(▶Fig. 128.1).

■ Key Imaging Finding

Jugular foramen mass

■ Top 3 Differential Diagnoses

- **Paraganglioma**. Jugular foramen paragangliomas (glomus jugulare) are highly vascular lesions that enlarge the jugular foramen, often with associated irregular, permeative bone destruction. The infiltrative osseous pattern is best appreciated on computed tomography (CT) bone windows. These aggressive lesions are associated with jugular vein invasion and intraluminal growth. On magnetic resonance (MR), glomus jugulare tumors often demonstrate the classic "salt and pepper" appearance, characterized by multiple T2-hypointense flow voids and occasional intralesional calcifications. The solid components of the mass are isointense on T1, iso- to hyperintense on T2, and avidly enhance. The tumors commonly extend intracranially, as well as inferiorly into the cervical region. Tumors which also involve the middle ear cavity are termed *glomus jugulotympanicum*.
- **Schwannoma**. Schwannomas of the jugular foramen are fairly uncommon and most often arise along the glossopharyngeal nerve. Clinical symptoms are related to local mass effect; unilateral hearing loss and dysphagia are the most common presenting symptoms. The benign, slow-growing nature of schwannomas causes smooth osseous expansion/remodeling of the jugular foramen. Larger lesions may compress the ipsilateral jugular vein and/or sigmoid sinus. On CT, schwannomas tend to be isodense to brain parenchyma and avidly enhance. On MR, they most often appear hypointense on T1 and hyperintense on T2 sequences with marked enhancement; cystic degeneration may occasionally occur.
- **Meningioma**. Meningiomas are the most common extra-axial tumors and may occasionally arise within or adjacent to the jugular foramen. On CT, meningiomas typically appear iso- to slightly hyperdense relative to brain parenchyma and may contain internal calcifications. The presence of adjacent bony hyperostosis is a useful discriminator, when present. On MR, lesions appear relatively isointense with respect to gray matter on T1- and T2-weighted sequences with diffuse homogeneous enhancement, a broad dural base, and a dural tail.

■ Additional Differential Diagnoses

- **Metastases**. Metastatic involvement of the jugular foramen may have a variety of appearances, ranging from a nonaggressive pattern with osseous remodeling to an aggressive pattern with erosive, destructive osseous changes. Breast, lung, and prostate carcinoma are the most common primary tumors associated with skull base metastases. The lesions have variable soft-tissue attenuation (CT) and signal intensity (MR), as well as variable enhancement patterns based on the origin and cell type of the primary tumor. Metastatic foci may be multifocal; therefore, it is important to search for additional osseous, meningeal, or parenchymal lesions.
- **Jugular bulb variants**. The most common jugular bulb variant is asymmetric prominence, which is seen on most brain MRIs.

The increased prominence may cause variable signal intensity at the junction of the sigmoid sinus and internal jugular vein, resulting in a pseudolesion. When in doubt, a pseudolesion can be confirmed on CT or MR venography. A dehiscent or high-riding (far more common) jugular bulb has a prevalence of ≈6% in the general population and may occasionally be a cause of tinnitus. When the jugular bulb is seen above the inferior margin of the round window, it is considered high riding. High-resolution CT can evaluate for the presence of bony dehiscence of the petrous septum between the middle ear and jugular bulb. CT venography may also be helpful in confirming the diagnosis.

■ Diagnosis

Paraganglioma (glomus jugulare)

✓ Pearls

- Paragangliomas are highly vascular tumors which may demonstrate a "salt and pepper" appearance on MR.
- Jugular foramen schwannomas are sharply demarcated and result in smooth osseous expansion/remodeling.
- Jugular foramen meningiomas may be hyperdense on CT with calcification and avid enhancement.

Suggested Reading

Caldemeyer KS, Mathews VP, Azzarelli B, Smith RR. The jugular foramen: a review of anatomy, masses, and imaging characteristics. Radiographics. 1997; 17(5):1123–1139

Case 129

William T. O'Brien Sr.

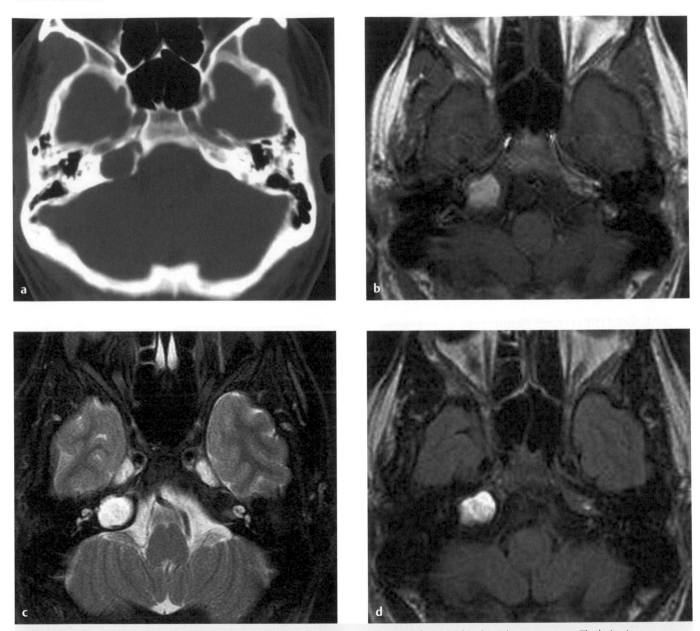

Fig. 129.1 (a) Axial CT image through the brain in bone window demonstrates an expansile lesion within the right petrous apex. The lesion is hyperintense on (b) T1, (c) T2 with fat suppression, and (d) FLAIR weighted images. The lesion did not enhance on postcontrast sequences (not shown).

■ **Clinical Presentation**

An adult man with headaches and mild hearing loss (▶ Fig. 129.1).

■ Key Imaging Finding

Petrous apex mass

■ Top 3 Differential Diagnoses

• **Cholesterol granuloma.** Cholesterol granulomas occur secondary to nonspecific chronic inflammatory changes and are seen most commonly in the temporal bone (petrous apex and middle ear cavity). They represent the most common primary lesion of the petrous apex. Computed tomography (CT) reveals a hypodense mass, which is often expansile with benign bony remodeling; bony erosion is less commonly seen. On magnetic resonance (MR), the lesions are characteristically hyperintense on both unenhanced T1 and T2 sequences due to hemorrhage within the lesions. Occasionally, a T2 hypointense hemosiderin ring is seen. There may be peripheral rim enhancement, but the lesions themselves will not enhance.

• **Mucous retention cyst or mucocele.** Mucous retention cysts and mucoceles are typically seen in the paranasal sinuses but may also occur within a pneumatized petrous apex. They result from entrapped secretions in an aerated petrous apex. They are hypodense and often expansile (more common with mucoceles) on CT. On MR, lesions are typically T1 hypointense and T2 hyperintense. With inspissated, proteinaceous secretions, they may be slightly hyperintense on T1, however, not to the same degree as cholesterol granulomas. The lesions do not enhance, although peripheral inflammatory enhancement may be seen.

• **Congenital cholesteatoma.** Congenital cholesteatomas are epidermoids which most commonly occur within the middle ear and petrous apex, similar to cholesterol granulomas. On CT, the lesions are hypodense and expansile. MR demonstrates increased T2 signal intensity secondary to internal cystic components. The lesions are commonly hypointense to slightly hyperintense on T1-weighted sequences. As with other epidermoids, there is typically increased signal on diffusion weighted imaged, which is fairly characteristic. Thin peripheral enhancement may be seen, but the lesions themselves do not enhance.

■ Additional Differential Diagnoses

• **Apical petrositis.** Serous or reactive fluid within a pneumatized petrous apex is a common finding in asymptomatic patients and is of little clinical significance. Apical petrositis, however, refers to superimposed infection of a pneumatized petrous apex, often in association with otomastoiditis. CT reveals fluid within the petrous apex, as well as possible adjacent bony erosion. The fluid is T1 hypointense and T2 hyperintense. Inflammatory changes result in enhancement, which often extends along the overlying dura. Gradenigo syndrome refers to retro-orbital pain and diplopia secondary to cranial nerve VI (abducens) deficits as a result of petrous apicitis; the infectious process compresses the nerve as it extends through the dural reflection of Dorello canal. Prompt diagnosis and treatment is necessary to reduce morbidity associated with this entity.

• **Neoplasm.** Metastases commonly involve the skull base secondary to direct or hematogenous spread. Direct spread may result from nasopharyngeal or sinonasal primary neoplasms. Lung, breast, renal cell, and prostate cancers disseminate via hematogenous spread. Primary involvement can be seen with chondrosarcoma, multiple myeloma, or plasmacytoma. Chondrosarcomas are expansile, off-midline, and characteristically T2 bright due to a chondroid matrix; CT shows internal calcifications in an "arcs and swirls" pattern. Bony destruction is often irregular and aggressive with tumors. Enhancement is prominent and best seen with fat suppression.

■ Diagnosis

Cholesterol granuloma

✓ Pearls

• Cholesterol granuloma is the most common primary petrous apex lesion and is bright on T1- and T2-weighted images.

• Mucous retention cysts and mucoceles may occur within a pneumatized petrous apex with entrapped secretions.

• Apical petrositis may lead to Gradenigo syndrome (apical petrositis, retro-orbital pain, and cranial nerve VI deficits).

• Chondrosarcomas may arise from the petrous bone, are T2 bright, and contain "arcs and swirls" calcifications.

Suggested Readings

Chapman PR, Shah R, Curé JK, Bag AK. Petrous apex lesions: pictorial review. AJR Am J Roentgenol. 2011; 196(3, Suppl):WS26–WS37, Quiz S40–S43

Connor SE, Leung R, Natas S. Imaging of the petrous apex: a pictorial review. Br J Radiol. 2008; 81(965):427–435

Case 130

Matthew J. Moore

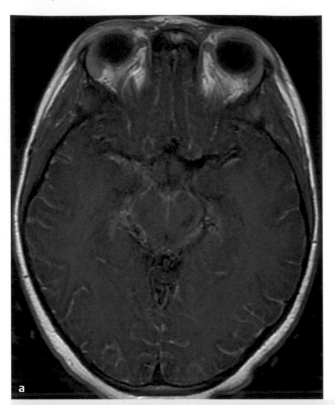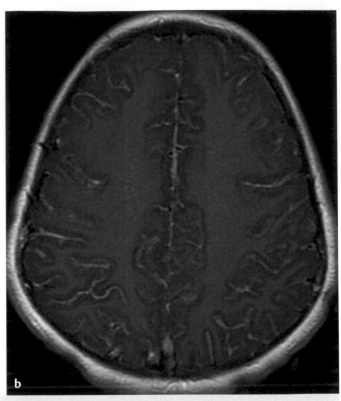

Fig. 130.1 **(a)** Axial T1 postcontrast images through the basal cisterns and **(b)** centrum semiovale reveal diffuse, symmetric abnormal leptomeningeal enhancement throughout the visualized sulci and along the surface of the brainstem.

■ Clinical Presentation

A patient with chronic headaches and long-standing medical issues (▶Fig. 130.1).

■ Key Imaging Finding

Leptomeningeal enhancement

■ Top 3 Differential Diagnoses

- **Meningitis**. Meningitis is an inflammatory infiltration of the pia, arachnoid, and cerebrospinal fluid (CSF) most often due to hematogenous dissemination of a distant infection. Lumbar puncture is the most sensitive test, revealing increased white blood cells and protein with decreased glucose. The exact values vary based on the etiology of infection (most often viral or bacterial). MRI may show hyperintense fluid-attenuated inversion recovery (FLAIR) signal and enhancement of the subarachnoid space from the exudative inflammatory process. Potential complications include hydrocephalus, ventriculitis, cerebral abscesses, empyema, infarction, and venous thrombosis.

- **Leptomeningeal carcinomatosis**. Leptomeningeal carcinomatosis may be caused by hematogenous spread of malignancy (most commonly lung and breast), CSF dissemination or direct extension of a central nervous system (CNS) primary tumor, or secondary lymphoma. MRI is the most sensitive imaging modality; lumbar puncture demonstrates tumor cells on cytologic examination. Overall sensitivity is increased when both procedures are performed. MR images show smooth or nodular leptomeningeal enhancement, which may be focal or diffuse. The ependymal surfaces of the ventricles and cranial nerves may be coated. Hyperintense FLAIR signal within the subarachnoid space may be seen. Communicating hydrocephalous is a potential complication from interference with CSF absorption. CT is relatively insensitive for leptomeningeal disease, but will show hydrocephalus. The presence of additional parenchymal or calvarial metastatic foci is a useful discriminator.

- **Neurosarcoidosis**. Sarcoidosis is a systemic inflammatory granulomatous (noncaseating) disease with a peak onset in the third and fourth decades of life. Symptomatic CNS involvement is uncommon (~5 of cases) and presents with smooth or nodular meningeal enhancement, especially along the basal cisterns. There is often involvement of the optic chiasm, hypothalamus, infundibulum, and cranial nerves at the skull base. Perivascular and ependymal enhancement may be seen. Brain parenchyma can also be involved in one-third of patients with the hypothalamus most often involved, followed by the brainstem and cerebral or cerebellar hemispheres. If not already obtained, look for a lymphadenopathy with or without interstitial lung disease on chest X-ray or CT.

■ Additional Differential Diagnoses

- **Collateral vascular flow**. Leptomeningeal vasculature is an important source of collateral flow in the setting of proximal arterial stenosis or occlusion. Given the relatively slow flow seen in collateral vessels, leptomeningeal enhancement is noted on postcontrast imaging. Common etiologies of proximal stenoses include atherosclerosis, primary or secondary moyamoya, and vasculitis. On imaging, the appearance of leptomeningeal vascular enhancement has been referred to as the "climbing ivy" sign.

- **Subacute infarction**. Contrast-enhanced CT or MRI of a subacute infarction can show gyriform parenchymal enhancement and swelling of cerebral or cerebellar cortex within a vascular distribution. In addition, there is often overlying leptomeningeal enhancement, representing collateral flow. Remember the "2–2–2" rule: gyriform enhancement begins as early as 2 days, peaks at 2 weeks, and typically resolves by 2 months.

■ Diagnosis

Collateral vascular flow (Moyamoya)

✓ Pearls

- Meningitis results from hematogenous spread of infection; leptomeningeal enhancement is commonly seen.
- Leptomeningeal carcinomatosis may be due to distant metastases, direct extension, or CSF dissemination.

- Neurosarcoidosis presents with leptomeningeal enhancement, most often along the basal cisterns.

Suggested Readings

Phillips ME, Ryals TJ, Kambhu SA, Yuh WT. Neoplastic vs inflammatory meningeal enhancement with Gd-DTPA. J Comput Assist Tomogr. 1990; 14(4):536–541

Smirniotopoulos JG, Murphy FM, Rushing EJ, Rees JH, Schroeder JW. Patterns of contrast enhancement in the brain and meninges. Radiographics. 2007; 27(2):525–551

Part 6

Brain and Spine Imaging

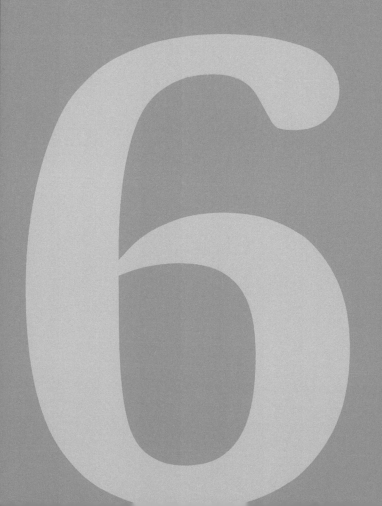

Case 131

William T. O'Brien Sr.

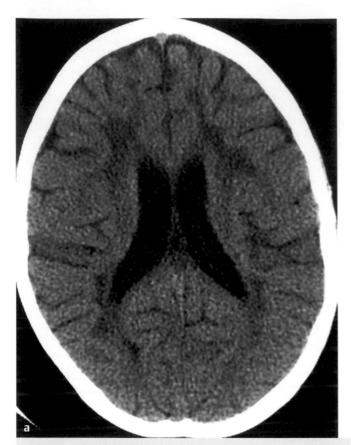
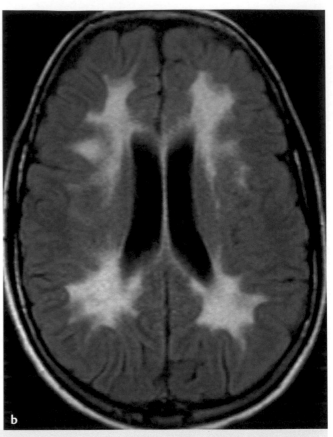

Fig. 131.1 (a) Axial CT image demonstrates bilateral, symmetric, confluent regions of hypoattenuation involving the superficial and deep white matter. (b) Axial fluid-attenuated inversion recovery (FLAIR) image shows corresponding increased signal abnormality throughout the white matter with sparing of the subcortical U-fibers.

■ Clinical Presentation

A young child with developmental delay (▶ Fig. 131.1).

■ **Key Imaging Finding**

Confluent white matter lesions in a child

■ **Top 3 Differential Diagnoses**

- **Acute disseminated encephalomyelitis (ADEM).** ADEM is a monophasic demyelinating disease which occurs in children following an antecedent viral infection or vaccination. The demyelination is thought to be secondary to an autoimmune response against myelin due to cross-reaction with a viral protein. Patients present with neurologic deficits that mimic multiple sclerosis (MS). Disease course varies from self-limiting to fulminant, hemorrhagic encephalitis. Computed tomography (CT) and magnetic resonance imaging (MRI) reveal large, usually bilateral, white matter lesions that are high signal on T2. Postcontrast images may demonstrate open-ring or nodular enhancement, corresponding to active regions of demyelination. Compared to MS, ADEM is more likely to be confluent and involve gray matter.
- **Multiple sclerosis (MS).** MS is the most common demyelinating disease overall. It occurs preferentially in young to middle-aged women, but also affects men and children. Patients present with optic neuritis, cranial neuropathies, and/or sensorimotor deficits. Most patients have a relapsing and remitting course. MR findings include increased T2 signal intensity within the periventricular white matter, optic pathways, corpus callosum, cerebellum, cerebellar peduncles, and brainstem/cord. Periventricular lesions are ovoid and perpendicular to the ventricles, resulting in characteristic Dawson fingers. Active demyelination may enhance in a nodular or ring pattern

with the open ring toward the overlying cortex. Compared to adults, children with MS tend to have fewer but larger lesions with less enhancement. The Marburg variant is a fulminant, aggressive form which leads to rapid death. Schilder disease is a rare progressive form which begins in childhood. Devic's disease (neuromyelitis optica) affects the optic nerves and spinal cord with relative sparing of the brain; it is considered a separate entity from MS, as it responds differently to therapy.
- **Dysmyelinating disease.** Leukodystrophies are a group of rare metabolic disorders characterized by dysmyelination secondary to accumulation of toxic metabolites as a result of enzyme deficiencies (lysosomal, peroxisomal, or mitochondrial disorders). Patients present most commonly at an early age with visual or behavioral disturbances. MRI demonstrates bilateral symmetric increased T2 signal intensity along white matter tracts. Metachromatic leukodystrophy has a predilection for the occipital lobes and splenium of the corpus callosum with sparing of subcortical U-fibers. Adrenoleukodystrophy has a similar pattern, commonly affects males (x-linked), also affects the adrenal glands, and involves subcortical U-fibers in late stages of the disease. Alexander disease has frontal lobe predominance and Canavan disease is associated with increased levels of N-acetylaspartate (NAA) on spectroscopy. Both Alexander and Canavan diseases often result in macrocephaly in addition to the white matter manifestations.

■ **Additional Differential Diagnoses**

- **Treatment-related leukoencephalopathy.** Both chemotherapy and radiation therapy may result in confluent regions of signal abnormality, predominantly involving the white matter. The corpus callosum, cerebellum, and brainstem may be involved as well. Chemotherapy changes are typically bilateral and symmetric; radiation changes correspond to a treatment field.

■ **Diagnosis**

Dysmyelinating disease (metachromatic leukodystrophy)

✓ **Pearls**

- ADEM is a monophasic demyelinating process which follows an antecedent viral infection or vaccination.
- MS is the most common demyelinating process; multiple forms exist with varying presentations.

- Leukodystrophies are rare metabolic disorders which result in diffuse dysmyelination.

Suggested Readings

Banwell B, Shroff M, Ness JM, Jeffery D, Schwid S, Weinstock-Guttman B; International Pediatric MS Study Group. MRI features of pediatric multiple sclerosis. Neurology. 2007; 68(16, Suppl 2):S46–S53

Cheon JE, Kim IO, Hwang YS, et al. Leukodystrophy in children: a pictorial review of MR imaging features. Radiographics. 2002; 22(3):461–476

Case 132

Paul M. Sherman

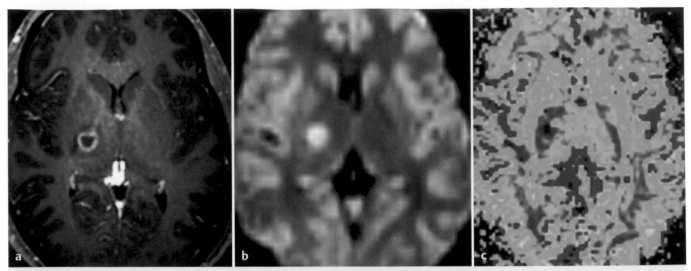

Fig. 132.1 **(a)** Axial T1 postcontrast image with fat suppression reveals a ring-enhancing mass centered within the posterior limb of the right internal capsule with surrounding edema. **(b)** Diffusion-weighted image demonstrates central restricted diffusion (was dark on apparent diffusion coefficient map). **(c)** Perfusion imaging shows corresponding decreased perfusion (blue-black) relative to the surrounding and contralateral deep white matter.

■ Clinical Presentation

A young man with mental status changes (▶Fig. 132.1).

■ Key Imaging Finding

Ring-enhancing lesion

■ Top 3 Differential Diagnoses

• **Neoplasm**. High-grade gliomas, lymphoma, and metastases represent the majority of ring-enhancing tumors. Glioblastoma multiforme (GBM) is the most common primary brain tumor in adults and is highly aggressive (World Health Organization [WHO] grade IV). There is rapid growth with neovascularity. Lesions are typically solitary with marked mass effect, surrounding vasogenic edema, thick irregular peripheral enhancement, and central necrosis. The tumor is predominantly T2 hyperintense; regions of hemorrhage and restricted diffusion (due to high cellularity) are common. Involvement of the corpus callosum is often seen. Primary CNS lymphoma typically involves the deep gray/white matter. Corpus callosal and ependymal involvement is common. Lesions may be T2 hypointense due to high cellularity. There is solid enhancement in immunocompetent patients; ring enhancement is seen following treatment or in immunosuppressed patients. Positron emission tomography (PET) or thallium imaging demonstrates increased metabolic activity, distinguishing lymphoma from Toxoplasmosis. As with other tumors, there is increased perfusion. Metastatic lesions may be solitary (~45%) or multiple, involving the gray–white matter junction, deep gray–white matter, and posterior fossa. There is often pronounced edema,

except for cortical metastases which show little edema. Ring enhancement occurs with cystic or necrotic metastases.

• **Abscess**. Abscesses result from hematogenous spread; direct spread from sinonasal or otomastoid infections, trauma, or surgery; or as a complication of meningitis. They may be solitary or multiple. Abscesses have a T2 hypointense capsule which is thinner toward the ventricles (prone to intraventricular rupture) with smooth rim enhancement and surrounding vasogenic edema. Pyogenic abscesses demonstrate central restricted diffusion. Toxoplasmosis, a parasitic infection in immunosuppressed patients, does not typically show restricted diffusion. Abscesses have decreased perfusion. MR spectroscopy shows an elevated lipid-lactate doublet.

• **Subacute infarct**. Cortically based infarcts are typically located in a vascular distribution; deep infarcts may be more difficult to characterize. The presence of edema, mass effect, hemorrhagic transformation, and subacute enhancement may mimic a mass lesion, especially if ring enhancing. Infarcts show restricted diffusion acutely, which may persist into the subacute phase. This is helpful but nonspecific, as abscesses and cellular neoplasms may also show restricted diffusion. Enhancement begins as early as 2 days and peaks at 2 weeks.

■ Additional Differential Diagnoses

• **Demyelinating disease**. Multiple sclerosis is the most common primary demyelinating disease; ADEM is monophasic and more common in children. Characteristic features include ovoid T2/FLAIR hyperintense lesions oriented perpendicular to the ventricles (Dawson fingers). High specificity locations include the corpus callosum, optic pathways, and posterior fossa. Enhancement suggests active demyelination. The enhancement pattern may be nodular or "open-ring" with the open portion facing the cortex. Tumefactive lesions mimic neoplasms.

• **Resolving contusion**. A history of trauma is important in differentiating a contusion from other ring-enhancing lesions. Blood products are present in varying stages, depending on the age of the hematoma. Rim enhancement occurs within a few days in a vascularized capsule. Acute blood products are isointense on T1 and hypointense on T2. Subacute blood products (intra- or extracellular methemoglobin [MetHb]) are T1 hyperintense. Intracellular MetHb is T2 hypointense; extracellular MetHb is T2 hyperintense.

■ Diagnosis

Subacute infarct

✓ Pearls

• GBM, lymphoma, and metastases are the most common tumors to present as ring-enhancing lesions.
• Abscesses characteristically have a T2 hypointense capsule with smooth enhancement and restricted diffusion.

• Enhancement pattern of demyelinating plaques may be "open-ring" with the open portion facing the cortex.

Suggested Reading

Smirniotopoulos JG, Murphy FM, Rushing EJ, Rees JH, Schroeder JW. Patterns of contrast enhancement in the brain and meninges. Radiographics. 2007; 27(2):525–551

Case 133

William T. O'Brien Sr.

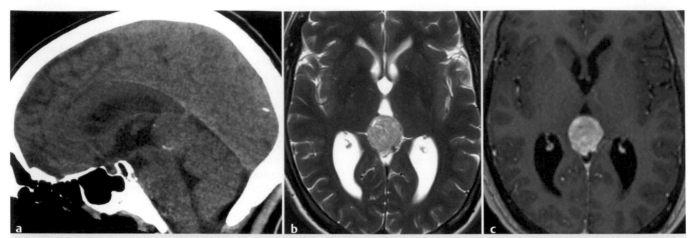

Fig. 133.1 **(a)** Sagittal reformatted CT image demonstrates a large, circumscribed, isodense pineal region mass with mass effect on the brainstem and cerebral aqueduct. Linear calcification is seen along the inferior periphery of the mass. The mass is **(b)** T2 hyperintense with **(c)** avid enhancement on T1 postcontrast image with fat suppression.

■ Clinical Presentation

An adult man with occasional headaches and ocular dysmotility (►Fig. 133.1).

■ Key Imaging Finding

Pineal region mass

■ Top 3 Differential Diagnoses

- **Pineal cyst**. Pineal cysts are common and usually incidental. Rarely, large cysts (>15 mm) may produce symptoms secondary to local mass effect with headaches or visual disturbances. Simple cysts follow fluid signal intensity and lack central, solid enhancement; surrounding enhancement involving the cyst wall and within the pineal substance is commonly seen. The cysts may demonstrate increased signal intensity on T1 sequences due to proteinaceous content or occasionally hemorrhage with trauma. Cysts greater than 10 mm are often followed with serial imaging to ensure stability, especially if atypical features are identified.
- **Germ cell tumor (GCT)**. GCTs are the most common malignant neoplasms of the pineal gland with germinomas representing more than 60% of cases. Most occur in adolescent and young adult males. Presenting symptoms are often secondary to mass effect resulting in obstructive hydrocephalus, Parinaud syndrome (paralysis of upward gaze), or endocrine dysfunction. Germinomas are hyperdense on computed tomography (CT) due to a high nuclear-to-cytoplasmic ratio and may contain calcifications centrally. On MRI, germinomas are intermediate signal intensity on T1 and T2 sequences with avid enhancement. On occasion, germinomas may appear cystic. As cerebrospinal fluid (CSF) dissemination is common, the entire spine must be imaged to evaluate for drop metastases. Other GCTs include teratomas, yolk sac tumors, and choriocarcinomas. Teratomas will typically have macroscopic fat and calcification. Yolk sac tumors may be cystic and associated with elevated levels of alpha-fetoprotein. Choriocarcinomas have a propensity to bleed and are associated with elevated levels of human chorionic gonadotropin.
- **Pineal cell tumor**. Pineal cell origin tumors consist of pineoblastomas, pineocytomas, and pineal parenchymal tumors of intermediate differentiation (PPTID). Pineoblastomas are more malignant with a peak incidence in the first decade of life. Seeding of the CSF is common. Pineocytomas (World Health Organization [WHO] grade I) have a peak incidence in the third and fourth decades of life and are less aggressive. PPTIDs are intermediate tumors (WHO grade II or III) which occur most commonly in young adults. On imaging, the tumors may closely resemble one another. On average, pineoblastomas are larger at presentation. All are iso- to hyperdense on CT due to high cellularity. When calcifications occur, they are typically along the periphery in an "exploded" pattern. On MRI, pineal cell tumors are of intermediate signal intensity on T1 and intermediate to hyperintense on T2 sequences with avid enhancement. As with GCTs, the spine must be imaged to evaluate for drop metastases.

■ Additional Differential Diagnoses

- **Tectal plate glioma**. Tectal gliomas are slow growing, low-grade astrocytomas which occur primarily in children. Patients present with symptoms related to increased intracranial pressure. Imaging reveals bulbous enlargement of the tectal plate with narrowing or obstruction of the cerebral aqueduct. There is increased T2 signal intensity and typically no or minimal enhancement. Treatment is geared toward CSF diversion.
- **Meningioma**. Meningiomas are the most common extra-axial intracranial tumors. They may occur along the margin of the tentorium, mimicking a pineal gland mass. The pineal gland and internal cerebral veins are often displaced superiorly. On noncontrast CT, meningiomas may be hyperdense; calcification is common. Enhancement pattern is typically avid and homogenous with a dural tail.

■ Diagnosis

Pineal cell tumor (pineocytoma)

✓ Pearls

- GCTs are the most common pineal neoplasms and commonly result in CSF dissemination.
- Pineal origin tumors are the second most common pineal neoplasms and may also result in CSF dissemination.
- Tectal plate gliomas are low-grade T2 hyperintense astrocytomas which obstruct the cerebral aqueduct.

Suggested Reading

Smith AB, Rushing EJ, Smirniotopoulos JG. From the archives of the AFIP: lesions of the pineal region: radiologic-pathologic correlation. Radiographics. 2010; 30(7):2001–2020

Case 134

William T. O'Brien Sr.

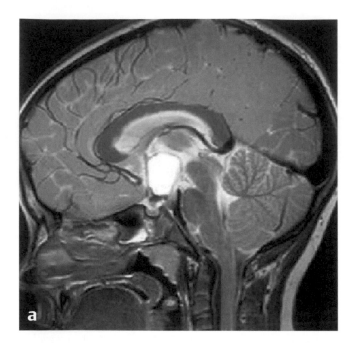

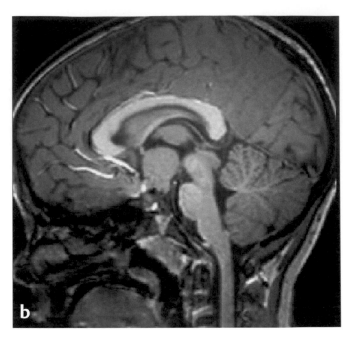

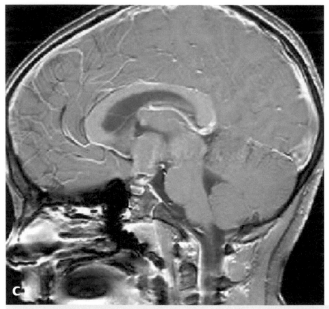

Fig. 134.1 (a-c) Sagittal MR images demonstrate a large mixed cystic and solid suprasellar mass with extension into the superior aspect of the sellar. The cystic component along the superior aspect of the mass is T2 (a) and mildly T1 (b) hyperintense. The smaller solid component of the mass inferiorly demonstrates regions of enhancement on the T1 postcontrast image with fat suppression (c).

■ Clinical Presentation

A 6-year-old girl with headache (►Fig. 134.1).

■ Key Imaging Finding

Sellar/Suprasellar mass in a child

■ Top 3 Differential Diagnoses

• **Craniopharyngioma**. Craniopharyngiomas represent the most common suprasellar masses in children. They are benign tumors which arise from Rathke pouch epithelium. There are two subtypes, each with varying age peaks and imaging features: adamantinomatous (peak age: 5–15 years) and papillary (peak age: >50 years). Pediatric adamantinomatous craniopharyngiomas present as multicystic suprasellar masses which may extend into the sella, anterior and middle cranial fossae, and retroclival regions. Computed tomography (CT) demonstrates amorphous calcifications in more than 90% of cases. There is often sellar expansion and clival remodeling or erosion. Both CT and MRI reveal a mixed cystic and solid suprasellar mass with enhancement of the solid components and cyst walls. The cystic content may be hyperdense on CT, hyperintense on T1, and variable on T2 sequences due to increased protein content, which is described as "crank case oil" on gross pathologic examination. In contrast, the adult variant (papillary) most commonly presents as a solid enhancing suprasellar mass without calcifications.

• **Germ cell tumor (GCT)**. GCTs are most common in the pediatric population. They occur most often in the pineal region, followed by the suprasellar region and are typically midline. Germinomas are the most common subtype and present as infiltrating sellar and/or suprasellar masses which typically follow gray matter signal and homogeneously enhance. With sellar involvement, there is often absence of the posterior pituitary bright spot on precontrast T1 images. Teratomas are more heterogeneous and usually have regions of macroscopic fat and calcification. Dermoid cysts may follow cerebrospinal fluid (CSF) signal on T2-weighted sequences but are often slightly hyperintense to CSF on T1 and may have wall calcification. When present, fat–fluid levels are characteristic. GCTs may seed the CSF due to direct extension (germinomas) or rupture (dermoid cysts).

• **Rathke cleft cyst**. Rathke cleft cysts are nonneoplastic lesions which arise from remnants of Rathke cleft. The lesions are often intrasellar; many will have suprasellar extension. Lesions may occasionally be purely suprasellar. Roughly 10 to 15% will have curvilinear wall calcification. On magnetic resonance imaging (MRI), the cystic fluid may have variable signal intensity based on mucinous content. Lesions with high mucin content will be hyperintense on T1 sequences. An intracystic nodule is commonly seen, which is a useful discriminator. There is no internal enhancement, but a rim of enhancing pituitary gland is often seen.

■ Additional Differential Diagnoses

• **Optic nerve/hypothalamic glioma**. Optic nerve gliomas are low-grade tumors that often occur between 5 and 15 years of age. They may be sporadic or associated with NF-1; bilateral optic nerve gliomas are pathognomonic for NF-1. Tumors cause enlargement, elongation, and "buckling" of the optic nerve. Enhancement is variable. The tumor may extend along the optic pathway. Non-NF-1 cases tend to involve the optic chiasm and/or hypothalamus, are typically larger and more masslike, commonly have cystic degeneration, and often extend beyond the optic pathways. Hypothalamic gliomas are similar in appearance but centered in the hypothalamus.

• **Hypothalamic hamartoma**. Hypothalamic hamartomas are benign lesions that occur in children with gelastic seizures or precocious puberty. The hamartomas are isointense to gray matter on T1 and iso- to hyperintense on T2 sequences. No enhancement should be seen; the presence of enhancement suggests a hypothalamic glioma rather than hamartoma. Clinical features combined with imaging findings are key to making the diagnosis.

■ Diagnosis

Craniopharyngioma

✓ Pearls

• Pediatric craniopharyngiomas present as multilobulated, multicystic masses with regions of calcification.
• GCTs occur in the midline and may seed the CSF; germinoma is the most common subtype.

• Optic nerve and hypothalamic gliomas may occur sporadically or be associated with NF-1.
• Patients with hypothalamic hamartomas may present with precocious puberty and gelastic seizures.

Suggested Reading

Hershey BL. Suprasellar masses: diagnosis and differential diagnosis. Semin Ultrasound CT MR. 1993; 14(3):215–231

Case 135

Paul M. Sherman

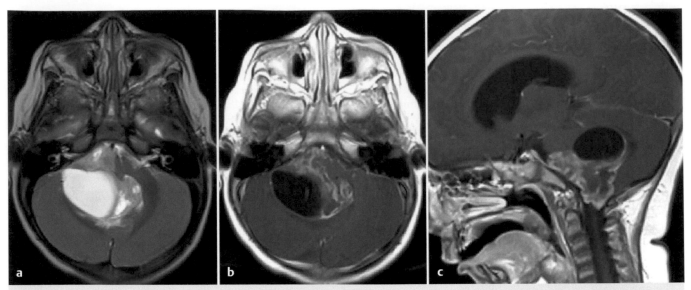

Fig. 135.1 **(a)** Axial T2 and **(b)** T1 postcontrast images demonstrate a mixed cystic and solid posterior fossa mass, which is slightly eccentric to the right. There is enhancement of the solid components. The mass extends into the right cerebellopontine angle and prepontine cistern with leftward displacement and compression of the brainstem. **(c)** Sagittal T1 postcontrast image shows the extraventricular extension, as well as inferior extension below the plane of the foramen magnum. There is obstructive hydrocephalus with enlargement of the lateral ventricle.

■ Clinical Presentation

A young girl with headaches and loss of balance (▶Fig. 135.1).

■ Key Imaging Finding

Posterior fossa mass in a child

■ Top 3 Differential Diagnoses

- **Medulloblastoma.** Medulloblastoma is an aggressive (World Health Organization [WHO] grade IV) primitive neuroectodermal tumor (PNET) and is the most common posterior fossa tumor in children. Peak incidence is within the first decade of life. As with all posterior fossa tumors, patients often present with headache or symptoms related to obstructive hydrocephalus. The tumor typically arises from the superior medullary velum or roof of fourth ventricle. Although characteristically midline, lateral (cerebellar hemisphere) origin may be seen in older children and young adults. Lesions are hyperdense on computed tomography (CT; ~90%) and demonstrate regions of restricted diffusion on magnetic resonance (MR) due to high cellular content. They are T1 hypointense and T2 iso- to hyperintense with heterogeneous enhancement. Cystic changes occur in half of the cases; calcification occurs in approximately 20%. Subarachnoid seeding is noted in up to one-third of the cases at presentation; therefore, evaluation of the neuroaxis is required prior to surgical resection.
- **Juvenile pilocytic astrocytoma (JPA).** JPA (WHO grade I astrocytoma) is the second most common primary posterior fossa tumor in children with an incidence slightly below medulloblastoma. They may be sporadic or associated with NF1.

Peak incidence is 5 to 15 years of age. The tumor arises from the cerebellar hemisphere; therefore, it is typically off-midline. The most common presentation is a cystic mass with an enhancing mural nodule. The cystic component is T1 iso- to hypointense and T2/FLAIR hyperintense. The solid component is T2 and FLAIR hyperintense and enhances avidly. Enhancement of the cyst wall suggests the presence of tumor cells. A less common imaging appearance includes a solid mass with a cystic/necrotic center.
- **Ependymoma.** Ependymoma is a slow-growing, midline posterior fossa tumor that originates along the floor of the fourth ventricle. It characteristically squeezes through the fourth ventricle foramina into the foramen magnum, cerebellopontine angle, or cisterna magna. Mean age of presentation is 6 years of age. On CT, calcification is seen in approximately 50% of cases; cystic change and hemorrhage occur in approximately 20%. Two-thirds arise from the fourth ventricle; one-third of the cases are supratentorial and centered in the brain parenchyma. The tumor is iso- to hypointense on T1 and hyperintense on T2 sequences. There is mild to moderate heterogeneous enhancement of solid components. CSF dissemination occurs but is less common than with medulloblastoma.

■ Additional Differential Diagnoses

- **Brainstem glioma.** Brainstem glioma represents approximately 10 to 20% of pediatric brain tumors and commonly presents within the first and second decades of life. It typically presents as a diffuse, infiltrating pontine mass (WHO grade II–III) with exophytic components which may engulf the basilar artery or project into the fourth ventricle. It is typically T1 hypointense and T2 hyperintense with variable enhancement. Higher grade regions demonstrate restricted diffusion, increased enhancement, and increased perfusion. Prognosis is poor.

- **Atypical teratoid rhabdoid tumor (ATRT).** ATRT is a rare, aggressive embryonal tumor composed of rhabdoid cells and PNET components. It often presents in the first few years of life with most located in the posterior fossa and the remainder occurring supratentorially. Its appearance on gross examination and imaging is nearly identical to medulloblastoma. Key distinction is patient's age at presentation. Subarachnoid seeding is common. Prognosis is dismal; mean survival is less than 6 months if younger than 3 years at the time of presentation.

■ Diagnosis

Ependymoma

✓ Pearls

- Medulloblastoma is the most common posterior fossa mass in a child, is midline, and often seeds the CSF.
- JPA most commonly presents as an off-midline cystic mass with enhancing mural nodule.

- Ependymoma is a midline tumor which extends through the ventricular foramina.

Suggested Readings

O'Brien WT. Imaging of posterior fossa brain tumors in children. J Am Osteopath Coll Radiol. 2013; 2(3):2–12

Poretti A, Meoded A, Huisman TA. Neuroimaging of pediatric posterior fossa tumors including review of the literature. J Magn Reson Imaging. 2012; 35(1):32–47

Case 136

Paul M. Sherman

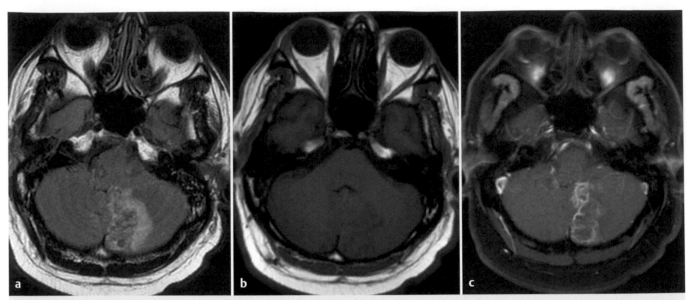

Fig. 136.1 (a) Axial fluid attenuation inversion recovery (FLAIR) image through the brain demonstrates a heterogeneous increased signal intensity lesion along the medial, inferior left cerebellum with local mass effect and surrounding edema. **(b)** Axial T1 pre- and **(c)** postcontrast images demonstrate gyral enhancement in a vascular territory distribution (posterior inferior cerebellar artery).

■ Clinical Presentation

A 52-year-old man with headache and gait disturbances (►Fig. 136.1).

■ Key Image Finding

Posterior fossa mass in an adult

■ Top 3 Differential Diagnoses

- **Infarction**. Ischemic changes commonly affect the posterior fossa and may have a masslike appearance. The morphology of an infarct is often wedge-shaped and corresponds to a vascular territory (posterior inferior, anterior inferior, and superior cerebellar arteries). Other differentiating features include restricted diffusion in the acute and early subacute stages and occasionally vascular occlusion demonstrated on computed tomography angiography (CTA) or magnetic resonance angiography (MRA). Edema, mass effect, hemorrhagic transformation, and subacute enhancement may mimic a mass.
- **Metastatic disease**. Metastatic disease represents the most common posterior fossa parenchymal neoplasm in middle-aged and older adults. Lung, breast, and gastrointestinal malignancies are among the most common. Metastases are more often multiple, although solitary lesions are not uncommon. Tumors are typically solid; cystic change and calcification occasionally occur with mucinous adenocarcinomas. Hemorrhagic metastases, which may occur with breast, lung, renal cell, thyroid, melanoma, and choriocarcinoma, tend to have strong enhancement and a hemosiderin rim. Renal cell carcinoma metastases may mimic hemangioblastoma, as they are very vascular.

- **Hemangioblastoma**. Hemangioblastomas are low-grade (WHO grade I) meningeal neoplasms and are the most common primary posterior fossa neoplasms in adults. Ninety to 95% occur within the posterior fossa, typically within the cerebellar hemispheres, while 5 to 10% are supratentorial. Supratentorial lesions commonly occur in the setting of von Hippel Lindau (VHL) disease (autosomal dominant, chromosome 3). Larger lesions present as cystic masses with enhancing mural nodules (similar to juvenile pilocytic astrocytoma) which abut the pial surface; smaller lesions commonly present as solid enhancing masses. The cyst and nodule are T2 hyperintense. Solid components avidly enhance, abut the pial surface, and may demonstrate flow voids. When identified, the entire neuroaxis should be imaged to look for additional cord lesions. Approximately one-fourth to one-half of patients with posterior fossa hemangioblastomas will have VHL. Patients with VHL may also have retinal hemangioblastomas, endolymphatic sac tumors, renal cell carcinoma, pheochromocytoma, islet cell tumors, and visceral cysts.

■ Additional Differential Diagnoses

- **Vascular malformation**. Arteriovenous malformations (AVMs) consist of a nidus of abnormal connections between arteries and veins without intervening capillaries. CT may demonstrate regions of increased density or calcification. MRI reveals a tangle of enlarged vessels; perinidal aneurysms are a common source of hemorrhage. Cavernous malformations (CMs) consist of blood-filled sinusoids and cavernous spaces without intervening parenchyma. CT may be normal or show subtle regions of calcification or hemorrhage. Lesions have foci of increased and decreased T1 and T2 signal centrally with a T2 dark (hemosiderin) capsule on MRI.

- **Hypertensive hemorrhage**. Hypertensive hemorrhage commonly involves the posterior fossa, to include the pons and cerebellar hemispheres. Hemorrhagic foci are typically round or oval. Acute hemorrhage is hyperdense on CT with mass effect and surrounding edema. MR appearance varies based on the age of blood products and composition of the hemoglobin moiety. Gradient echo and susceptibility weighted imaging often identify additional foci of microhemorrhage associated with hypertension in the lentiform nuclei and thalami.

■ Diagnosis

Subacute posterior inferior cerebellar artery territory infarct

✓ Pearls

- Ischemia commonly affects the posterior fossa, follows a vascular distribution, and has restricted diffusion.
- Metastases are the most common posterior fossa parenchymal tumors in adults and may be multiple.

- Hemangioblastomas present as cystic masses with mural nodules; they may be sporadic or inherited (VHL).

Suggested Readings

Cormier PJ, Long ER, Russell EJ. MR imaging of posterior fossa infarctions: vascular territories and clinical correlates. Radiographics. 1992; 12(6):1079–1096

Poretti A, Meoded A, Huisman TA. Neuroimaging of pediatric posterior fossa tumors including review of the literature. J Magn Reson Imaging. 2012; 35(1):32–47

Case 137

William T. O'Brien Sr.

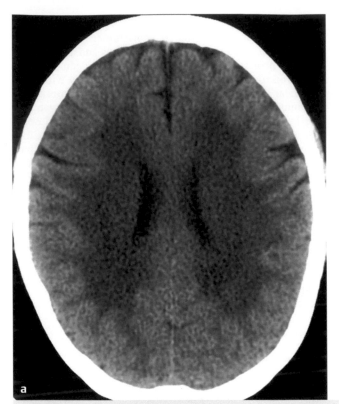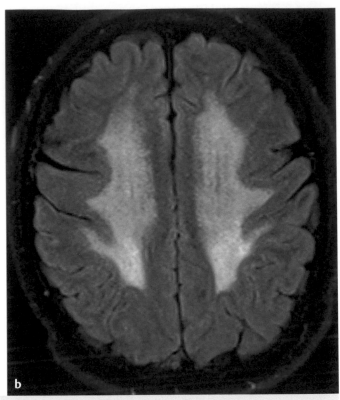

Fig. 137.1 **(a)** Unenhanced axial CT image demonstrates symmetric, confluent hypoattenuation throughout the superficial and deep white matter of the bilateral cerebral hemispheres. **(b)** Axial fluid attenuation inversion recovery (FLAIR) image reveals corresponding increased signal intensity within the involved white matter.

■ Clinical Presentation

A 59-year-old woman with lymphoma undergoing treatment with mental status changes (▶Fig. 137.1).

■ Key Imaging Finding

Confluent white matter lesions in an adult

■ Top 3 Differential Diagnoses

- **Vasculopathy.** Microvascular ischemic disease is common in the elderly and can be advanced for age. Imaging reveals subcortical and periventricular white matter hypodensity (computed tomography [CT]) and increased T2 signal (magnetic resonance imaging [MRI]) without enhancement. Lesions may be confluent and extensive with associated volume loss. Vasculitis most often presents as multifocal gray and white matter lesions which are bilateral, usually cortical or subcortical and often involve the basal ganglia and thalami. Lesions may enhance and often have regions of microhemorrhage. Digital subtraction angiography reveals alternating stenoses and dilatation.
- **Demyelinating disease.** Multiple sclerosis (MS) demonstrates multiple perpendicular periventricular T2 hyperintensities with perivenular extension (Dawson fingers). Lesions are bilateral and asymmetric, often involving the optic pathways, corpus callosum, cerebellum, cerebellar peduncles (brachium pontis), and brainstem/cord. There may be transient nodular or "open ring" enhancement during active demyelination. Plaques may also be confluent or masslike (tumefactive). "Black holes" are hypointense on T1 and represent burnt-out plaques. MS most commonly has a relapsing, remitting course,

unlike acute disseminated encephalomyelitis (ADEM) which is monophasic. Both processes may involve the spinal cord. Lyme disease is a tick-borne illness caused by the spirochete *Borrelia burgdorferi*. White matter lesions simulate MS, but there may be an associated viral-like illness or skin rash. Cranial nerve VII, leptomeningeal, and cauda equina involvement may be seen.

- **Neoplasm.** Gliomatosis cerebri is an infiltrating glial tumor which involves three or more lobes and may be bilateral. Although centered within the hemispheric white matter, the cortex may also be involved. There is relative preservation of the underlying brain architecture and no or minimal enhancement. Anaplastic astrocytoma may be more discrete, with enhancement ranging from none to focal or patchy. Primary central nervous system (CNS) lymphoma characteristically involves the deep gray matter or periventricular white matter and classically involves the corpus callosum. There is often T2 hypointensity and CT hyperdensity due to its high cellularity (small, round, blue cell tumor). Enhancement is typically homogeneous unless the patient is immunocompromised or steroids have been administered; then there may be ring enhancement.

■ Additional Differential Diagnoses

- **Atypical infection.** HIV may primarily affect the CNS, resulting in confluent, symmetric periventricular signal abnormality, along with increased atrophy for age. Progressive multifocal leukoencephalopathy (PML) is an atypical virus (JC virus) which affects oligodendrocytes. The vast majority of cases are seen in patients with AIDS. MRI demonstrates confluent white matter T2 hyperintensities without mass effect and with characteristic involvement of subcortical U-fibers. White matter involvement may be bilateral but is typically asymmet-

ric. There is usually no enhancement; if present, it is faint and peripheral.
- **Treatment-related leukoencephalopathy.** Both chemotherapy and radiation therapy may result in confluent regions of signal abnormality, predominantly involving the white matter. Chemotherapy changes are typically bilateral and symmetric, while radiation changes most often correspond to a treatment field.

■ Diagnosis

Treatment-related leukoencephalopathy (chemotherapy)

✓ Pearls

- Demyelinating processes are a common cause of white matter lesions and may be confluent when severe.
- Gliomatosis cerebri and lymphoma may present as infiltrating masses involving white matter tracts.

- HIV results in symmetric periventricular signal abnormality; PML is usually bilateral but asymmetric.
- Treatment-related leukoencephalopathy is confluent and may be diffuse or localized to a treatment field.

Suggested Readings

Bag AK, Curé JK, Chapman PR, Roberson GH, Shah R. JC virus infection of the brain. AJNR Am J Neuroradiol. 2010; 31(9):1564–1576

Filippi M, Rocca MA. MR imaging of multiple sclerosis. Radiology. 2011; 259(3):659–681

Case 138

William T. O'Brien Sr.

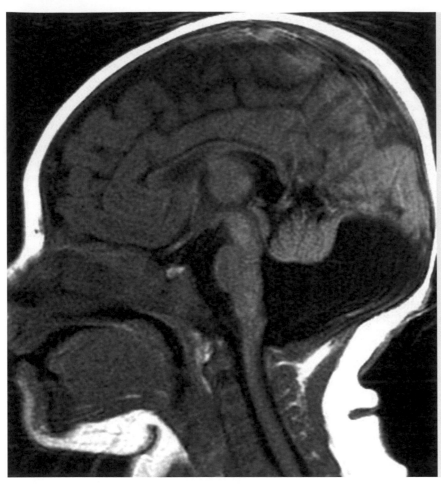

Fig. 138.1 Sagittal T1 MR image demonstrates a posterior fossa cerebrospinal fluid collection that communicates with an enlarged fourth ventricle. There is hypoplasia of the cerebellar vermis inferiorly, as well as an enlarged posterior fossa with elevation of the torcula (confluence of sinuses) above the lambdoid suture (torcular-lambdoid inversion). The corpus callosum appears thin but completely formed.

■ Clinical Presentation

A young child with developmental delay (▶Fig. 138.1).

■ Key Imaging Finding

Posterior fossa cerebrospinal fluid (CSF) collection/cyst

■ Top 3 Differential Diagnoses

• **Mega cisterna magna.** Mega cistern magna is a common normal variant in which the CSF-filled cisterna magna posterior to the cerebellum is prominent. It can usually be differentiated from an arachnoid cyst or Dandy-Walker malformation by the normal appearance and size of the posterior fossa, normal cerebellar vermis and fourth ventricle, minimal to no mass effect, and the presence of internal vessels and the falx cerebelli.

• **Arachnoid cyst.** Arachnoid cysts are developmental CSF-filled spaces within the arachnoid. Although typically asymptomatic and discovered incidentally, they may exert local mass effect. The majority are supratentorial within the middle cranial fossa or along the convexities. Common infratentorial locations include the cerebellopontine angle and cistern magna. When located within the posterior fossa, they may be large enough to compress the fourth ventricle or cerebral aqueduct, resulting in obstructive hydrocephalus. Arachnoid cysts follow CSF fluid signal on all magnetic resonance imaging pulse sequences; occasionally, they may have slight increased signal intensity on proton density due to stasis of CSF. Mass effect is evident

by displacement of vessels and the falx cerebelli around the arachnoid cyst and scalloping of overlying cortex.

• **Dandy-Walker continuum.** Dandy-Walker malformation is a developmental abnormality which results from a defect in the cerebellar vermis and fourth ventricle during embryogenesis. The malformation consists of an enlarged posterior fossa, partial or complete absence of the cerebellar vermis, hypoplasia of the cerebellar hemispheres, and a dilated fourth ventricle which is in direct communication with a posterior CSF-filled fluid collection. The enlarged posterior fossa results in superior displacement of the torcula above the lambdoid sutures (torcular-lambdoid inversion). Dandy-Walker malformation is associated with additional central nervous system anomalies, to include corpus callosal agenesis or hypogenesis and neuronal migration abnormalities. The Dandy-Walker variant is characterized by vermian hypoplasia and an enlarged fourth ventricle which communicates with a prominent cistern magna posteriorly; the posterior fossa is typically normal in size.

■ Additional Differential Diagnoses

• **Blake pouch cyst.** Blake pouch is an embryological structure that is located at the foramen of Magendie and normally regresses; its regression allows for flow of CSF from the fourth ventricle through foramen Magendie. Persistence of a Blake pouch cyst may result in an infravermian cyst that may be an incidental finding or cause obstructive hydrocephalus. As the lesion is essentially a fourth ventricle diverticulum, choroid plexus may be seen extending into the superior portion of the cyst. MRI best characterizes the infravermian cyst, its mass effect, and resultant hydrocephalus, if present.

• **Joubert syndrome (vermian hypoplasia).** Joubert syndrome is an uncommon posterior fossa malformation characterized

by a dysplastic and hypoplastic cerebellar vermis, as well as malformations of various nuclei and tracts. Patients present with neonatal hyperpnea, apnea, and mental retardation. Imaging findings include a dysplastic and hypoplastic cerebellar vermis (more pronounced superiorly); a bulbous fourth ventricle which has a characteristic "bat wing" configuration; and a "molar tooth" appearance of the midbrain secondary to a narrow, deep interpeduncular cistern and elongated superior cerebellar peduncles that are parallel with each other. Prominence of the cisterna magna in association with vermian hypoplasia may be seen.

■ Diagnosis

Dandy-Walker malformation

✓ Pearls

• Mega cisterna magna is a normal variant with a normal sized posterior fossa and normal cerebellar vermis.

• Arachnoid cysts follow CSF signal on all pulse sequences and exert local mass effect.

• Dandy-Walker continuum results from vermian aplasia or hypoplasia.

• Joubert syndrome results in a "bat wing" configuration of the fourth ventricle and "molar tooth" midbrain.

Suggested Readings

Barkovich AJ, Kjos BO, Norman D, Edwards MS. Revised classification of posterior fossa cysts and cystlike malformations based on the results of multiplanar MR imaging. AJR Am J Roentgenol. 1989; 153(6):1289–1300

Bosemani T, Orman G, Boltshauser E, et al. Congenital abnormalities of the posterior fossa. RadioGraphics. 2015; 35:200–220

Ten Donkelaar HJ, Lammens M. Development of the human cerebellum and its disorders. Clin Perinatol. 2009; 36(3):513–530

Case 139

Jeffrey P. Tan

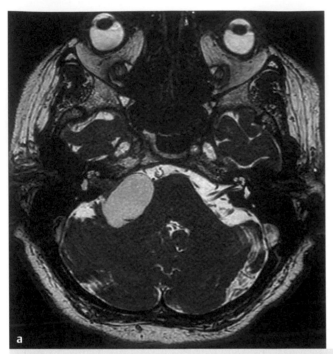
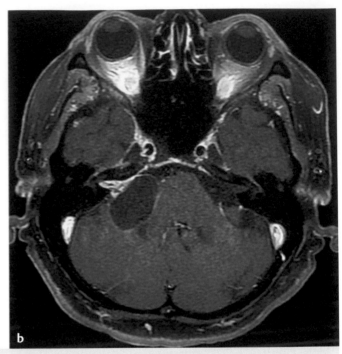

Fig. 139.1 **(a)** High-resolution axial FIESTA image reveals a cystic mass in the right cerebellopontine angle with soft-tissue signal within the right internal auditory canal (IAC). **(b)** Postcontrast axial T1 image with fat suppression shows avid enhancement of the solid component within the IAC and extending through the porous acousticus.

■ Clinical Presentation

A 32-year-old man with sensorineural hearing loss (▶ Fig. 139.1).

■ Key Imaging Finding

Cerebellopontine angle (CPA) mass

■ Top 3 Differential Diagnoses

- **Vestibular schwannoma.** Vestibular schwannomas arise from perineural Schwann cells. They are composed of two tissue types: Antoni A and Antoni B. Antoni A tissue is densely packed, which results in darker signal on T2 sequences; Antoni B tissue is loosely packed and T2 hyperintense. Vestibular schwannomas may involve the superior or inferior divisions of the vestibular nerve within the posterior internal auditory canal (IAC). There is typically expansion of the IAC and flaring of the porus acousticus. The border of a schwannoma typically makes an acute angle with the petrous temporal bone. Lesions are variable in signal but typically hyperintense on T2 sequences. Cystic change and hemorrhage may occur; calcification is uncommon. Enhancement is heterogeneous but avid. Bilateral vestibular schwannomas are diagnostic of neurofibromatosis type 2.
- **Meningioma.** Meningiomas arise from meningothelial arachnoid cells and are the most common extra-axial tumors. They typically occur in adult women; they may also be seen in children with NF-2 or a history of prior cranial radiation.

CPA meningiomas may be circumscribed or plaquelike. They often have a broad dural base along the petrous temporal bone and avidly enhance with a dural tail. An isolated intracanalicular meningioma is rare. On unenhanced computed tomography (CT), meningiomas are iso- to hyperdense compared to brain parenchyma with adjacent bony remodeling or hyperostosis. Calcification is common.

- **Arachnoid cyst.** Arachnoid cysts are cerebrospinal fluid (CSF) collections contained within arachnoid. The vast majority are developmental due to embryonic failure of meningeal fusion; acquired cases have also been described. The most common locations include the middle cranial fossa, followed by the posterior fossa. Cysts are hypodense on CT and follow CSF signal on MR. Slight increased signal may be seen on T2 sequences due to lack of normal CSF pulsations. There is no restricted diffusion, which is a key discriminator from epidermoid cysts, and no enhancement. Larger cysts exert mass effect on the adjacent parenchyma.

■ Additional Differential Diagnoses

- **Epidermoid.** Epidermoid cysts are lesions of ectodermal origin, composed of keratinaceous debris, and lined by stratified squamous epithelium. The most common intracranial location is the CPA. Epidermoids are hypointense on T1 and hyperintense on T2 sequences. There is typically heterogeneous hypointensity on FLAIR imaging. The key distinction between arachnoid cysts is the presence of restricted diffusion, which is characteristic of epidermoid cysts. In addition, epidermoid cysts have irregular margins and engulf vessels and nerves rather than displace them, in contradistinction to arachnoid cysts.

- **Lipoma.** Intracranial lipomas result from persistence of the meninx primitiva, which is a precursor to the pia and arachnoid. They are typically midline and supratentorial; however, the CPA is the most common posterior fossa location. Lipomas are hypodense on CT and follow fat signal intensity on all pulse sequences. Chemical shift artifact and fat suppression are key to making the diagnosis. Lesions are considered incidental; however, cranial neuropathies may rarely occur. Resection is reserved for symptomatic lesions.

■ Diagnosis

Vestibular schwannoma

✓ Pearls

- Vestibular schwannomas are the most common CPA masses; bilateral lesions are diagnostic of NF-2.
- Meningiomas are hyperdense on CT, may have calcification, intensely enhance, and have a dural tail.

- Arachnoid cysts follow CSF signal on all pulse sequences and may exert local mass effect.
- Epidermoids mimic arachnoid cysts with the exception of restricted diffusion, which is characteristic.

Suggested Readings

Bonneville F, Savatovsky J, Chiras J. Imaging of cerebellopontine angle lesions: an update. Part 1: enhancing extra-axial lesions. Eur Radiol. 2007; 17(10):2472–2482

Bonneville F, Savatovsky J, Chiras J. Imaging of cerebellopontine angle lesions: an update. Part 2: intra-axial lesions, skull base lesions that may invade the CPA region, and non-enhancing extra-axial lesions. Eur Radiol. 2007; 17(11):2908–2920

Case 140

Paul M. Sherman

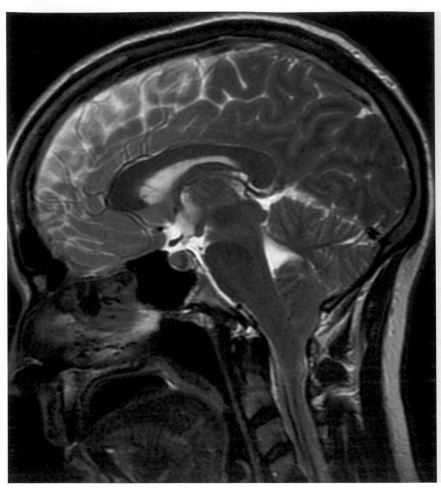

Fig. 140.1 Sagittal T2 image demonstrates inferior displacement of the cerebellar tonsils below the foramen magnum to the level of the midposterior arch of C1 with effacement of cerebrospinal fluid at the craniocervical junction. Heterogeneous T2 signal intensity is noted within the ventral epidural space of the upper cervical spine with posterior displacement of the T2 hypointense dura.

■ Clinical Presentation

A 42-year-old woman with positional headaches (▶ Fig. 140.1).

■ Key Imaging Finding

Cerebellar tonsillar herniation

■ Top 3 Differential Diagnoses

• **Chiari malformations.** Both type I and II Chiari malformations, while distinct entities, demonstrate a small posterior fossa with caudal extension of peg-shaped cerebellar tonsils below the foramen magnum ≥5 mm. The degree of tonsillar ectopia and crowding at the craniocervical junction is often greater with Chiari II. Chiari I is associated with bony abnormalities of the skull base and cervical spine (e.g., Klippel Feil syndrome) and syringohydromyelia of the cord. Patients with Chiari I typically do not have additional central nervous system (CNS) malformations and often present with headaches or symptoms related to brainstem compression or syringohydromyelia. Chiari II malformations are associated with a lumbosacral myelomeningocele (open neural tube defect) and additional intracranial anomalies. Imaging findings include tonsillar ectopia, cervicomedullary kinking, compressed and elongated fourth ventricle, beaked tectum, "towering" cerebellum protruding cranially through the incisura, enlarged massa intermedia, low lying torcula, and a Luckenschadel skull (bony dysplasia which lasts up until 6 months of age). Dysgenesis of the corpus callosum is seen in approximately 90% of cases. Hydrocephalus is present in nearly all cases. Chiari III malformations are exceedingly rare and consist of low occipital and/or high cervical cephaloceles with intracranial findings of Chiari II malformations and upper cervical spine dysraphism.

• **Intracranial hypotension.** Intracranial hypotension results in "sagging" of the brain and inferior tonsillar displacement. Etiologies include iatrogenia (postsurgical or procedural, such as lumbar puncture), trauma, violent coughing or strenuous exercise, spontaneous dural tear, ruptured arachnoid diverticulum, severe dehydration, and, rarely, disc protrusion with dural injury. Reduced intracranial pressure results in brain descent. Tonsillar ectopia is seen in approximately 75% of cases. Additional findings include diffuse thickened, fluid attenuation inversion recovery (FLAIR) hyperintense, enhancing dura and subdural fluid collections, typically hygromas. There is a "sagging" midbrain (below dorsum sella) and "fat midbrain sign" (elongated midbrain and pons). Radionuclide cisternography or computed tomography myelography can be used to search for the site of cerebrospinal fluid (CSF) leak if blood patch therapy fails.

• **Ependymoma.** Ependymoma is the third most common posterior fossa tumor in children (after medulloblastoma and juvenile pilocytic astrocytoma) and arises from the ependymal cells of the fourth ventricle. It is a soft, pliable tumor which may extend through the fourth ventricular outlet foramina into the cerebellopontine angle or foramen magnum. Extension through the foramen magnum may mimic cerebellar tonsillar ectopia. Calcification is seen in approximately 50% of cases; cysts and hemorrhage are less common. The mass is heterogeneous and typically iso- or hyperintense on T2 images with heterogeneous enhancement. Patients often present with headache, vomiting, and/or ataxia. Peak incidence is in the first decade of life.

■ Additional Differential Diagnoses

• **Posterior fossa mass.** Any primary or secondary posterior fossa mass may cause tonsillar herniation secondary to local mass effect. Common causes in children include medulloblastoma and juvenile pilocytic astrocytomas; common lesions in adults include infarction, metastases, hemangioblastoma, vascular malformations, and hypertensive hemorrhage.

■ Diagnosis

Intracranial hypotension (secondary to CSF leak)

✓ Pearls

• Chiari I is characterized by tonsillar ectopia, skull base/cervical spine malformations, and syrinx.
• Chiari II is characterized by tonsillar ectopia, myelomeningocele, and multiple intracranial abnormalities.

• A posterior fossa mass or "sagging" from intracranial hypotension may result in tonsillar ectopia.

Suggested Readings

Fishman RA, Dillon WP. Dural enhancement and cerebral displacement secondary to intracranial hypotension. Neurology. 1993; 43(3, Pt 1):609–611
Koeller KK, Sandberg GD; Armed Forces Institute of Pathology. From the archives of the AFIP. Cerebral intraventricular neoplasms: radiologic-pathologic correlation. Radiographics. 2002; 22(6):1473–1505

Milhorat TH, Chou MW, Trinidad EM, et al. Chiari I malformation redefined: clinical and radiographic findings for 364 symptomatic patients. Neurosurgery. 1999; 44(5):1005–1017

Case 141

Paul M. Sherman

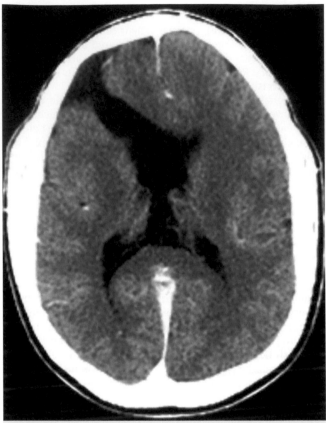

Fig. 141.1 Contrast-enhanced axial CT image through the lateral ventricles demonstrates a gray matter–lined CSF cleft which communicates with the frontal horn of the right lateral ventricle. There is also absence of the septum pellucidum.

■ Clinical Presentation

An adolescent boy with seizures (▶ Fig. 141.1).

■ Key Imaging Finding

Cerebrospinal fluid (CSF)-lined cortical cleft

■ Top 3 Differential Diagnoses

- **Schizencephaly**. Schizencephaly is a congenital malformation characterized by parenchymal clefts which extend from the pial surface to the lateral ventricles. The clefts are lined by dysplastic (usually polymicrogyric) gray matter and often parasylvian in location. In type I or "closed lip" schizencephaly, the gray matter linings are apposed, making the malformation less conspicuous. Along the ventricular aspect of the cleft, there is often a "dimple" with CSF extending from the ventricle into the opening of the cleft. Type II or "open lip" schizencephaly is characterized by a large CSF-filled cleft lined by dysplastic gray matter. Approximately 50% of cases of schizencephaly are bilateral; when bilateral, the "open lip" variant is more common. Clinical manifestations depend on the severity of the defect, as well as the presence of additional malformations. Patients with type I schizencephaly are often almost normal in terms of development, but may have seizures and hemiparesis. Patients with type II schizencephaly usually have significant neurological deficits, especially if bilateral, including mental retardation, seizures, paresis, mutism, and/or blindness. Both variants may be associated with septo-optic dysplasia. Heterotopia or cortical dysplasia may be associated findings.
- **Porencephalic cyst**. Porencephalic cysts are CSF-filled cavities that are lined by gliotic white matter and typically communicate with the ventricles and/or subarachnoid space. In many cases, the communication with the ventricles or subarachnoid space may be occult. Porencephalic cysts may be congenital secondary to a perinatal insult after brain development or acquired from a postnatal insult in childhood or young adulthood. Common acquired causes include infarct, infection, and trauma. Familial porencephaly has been described but is rare. The cysts vary significantly in size from relatively small to quite large and may be unilateral or bilateral. In general, congenital cysts are smooth with little surrounding gliosis, while acquired cysts tend to have irregular walls and more pronounced gliosis. The adjacent ventricle is typically enlarged due to volume loss. Occasionally, the cysts may enlarge due to a ball-valve–type communication with the ventricle or adhesions. Superficial cysts may remodel the overlying calvarium, similar to arachnoid cysts. When symptomatic, treatment includes resection or fenestration of the cysts. Patients with porencephaly often present with spastic hemiplegia and seizures. Severe neurological deficits may be seen with large or multiple regions of porencephaly. Porencephaly has been described in association with various syndromes, as well as amygdala-hippocampal atrophy, which may be related to seizure activity.
- **Encephalomalacia**. Parenchymal injury results in volume loss with encephalomalacia and compensatory dilatation of the ventricles and adjacent sulci. Common causes of encephalomalacia include arterial infarct, primary intracranial hemorrhage, and hemorrhagic venous infarct. The region of encephalomalacia approaches CSF attenuation (computed tomography) and signal (magnetic resonance) and is lined by gliotic white matter, similar to porencephalic cysts. The morphology depends on the location, size, and type of parenchymal injury. Occasionally, it may appear cystic. Arterial infarcts are typically wedge-shaped. On magnetic resonance imaging, the gliotic parenchyma along the border of encephalomalacia is increased in T2 and fluid attenuation inversion recovery (FLAIR) signal intensity. Hemosiderin staining may be seen along the margin of encephalomalacia on gradient echo or susceptibility-weighted imaging.

■ Diagnosis

Schizencephaly (type II, open lip)

✓ Pearls

- Schizencephaly results in CSF clefts lined by dysplastic gray matter; it is caused by an intrauterine insult.
- Schizencephaly is associated with neural migration abnormalities and septo-optic dysplasia.
- Porencephalic cysts are often caused by a perinatal insult and are lined by dysplastic white matter.
- Encephalomalacia results in volume loss from prior parenchymal injury; arterial infarct is the most common cause.

Suggested Readings

Denis D, Chateil JF, Brun M, et al. Schizencephaly: clinical and imaging features in 30 infantile cases. Brain Dev. 2000; 22(8):475–483

Van Tassel P, Curé JK. Nonneoplastic intracranial cysts and cystic lesions. Semin Ultrasound CT MR. 1995; 16(3):186–211

Case 142

Paul M. Sherman

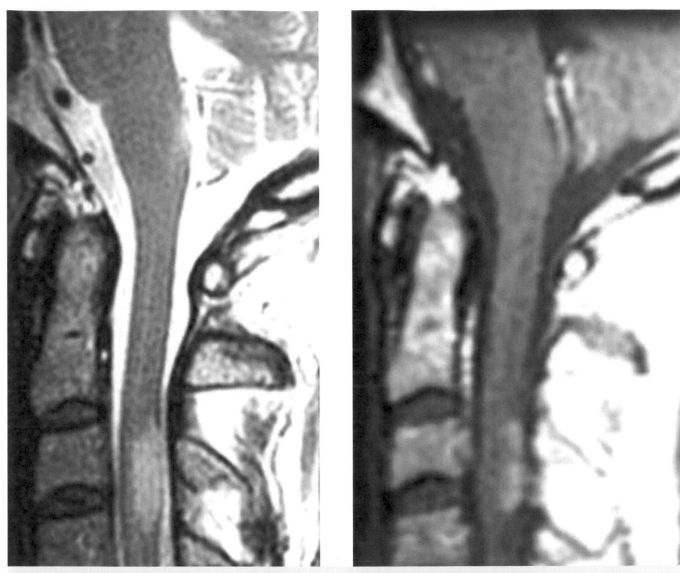

Fig. 142.1 **(a)** Sagittal T2 image demonstrates a region of cord signal abnormality along the midposterior aspect of the cord at the C3–C4 level, extending approximately 1.5 vertebral levels in craniocaudal dimension. **(b)** Sagittal T1 postcontrast image shows focal regions of enhancement. There is minimal to no cord expansion.

■ **Clinical Presentation**

An adult woman with neck pain and paresthesias (▶ Fig. 142.1).

■ Key Imaging Finding

Enhancing intramedullary spinal lesion/mass

■ Top 3 Differential Diagnoses

- **Ependymoma**. Ependymoma is the most common spinal cord tumor in adults. They may occur at any age but have a peak incidence in the fourth and fifth decades of life. The cellular variant originates from the ependymal lining of the central canal and most commonly occurs within the cervical followed by thoracic spine. It is a circumscribed, central lesion which often has symmetric cord expansion but may have exophytic components. It usually spans three to four vertebral segments with surrounding cord edema. Intratumoral cysts are present in the majority of cases, and adjacent cord syrinx is common. Enhancement may be intense and homogenous or nodular and heterogeneous. Hemorrhage is seen more often than with astrocytoma and presents as a T2 hypointense hemosiderin cap along the cranial and/or caudal end of the tumor. The myxopapillary variant occurs in the conus medullaris, filum terminale, or cauda equina. When located along the filum or cauda equina, it may mimic an extramedullary mass. It is a circumscribed ovoid or lobular mass, which commonly spans two to four vertebral segments. Mucin may cause T1 hyperintensity. The solid components intensely enhance. Both subtypes may cause widening of the interpediculate distance and scalloping of the vertebral bodies. The cellular variant may also cause scoliosis, while the myxopapillary variant may extend through neural foramina.

- **Astrocytoma**. Astrocytomas are the most common intramedullary spinal cord tumor in children and young adults. They are most common in the cervical followed by thoracic spine but may also be holocord. Common imaging presentation includes an infiltrating, expansile mass spanning up to four vertebral segments. Fusiform but eccentric expansion of cord is typical with occasional exophytic components. Syrinx and cystic components are less common compared to ependymoma. Solid components are T1 hypo- or isointense and T2 hyperintense with heterogeneous enhancement. They are typically low grade with an 80% 5-year survival.

- **Demyelinating disease**. Demyelinating disease may affect any portion of the cord but preferentially involves the posterolateral cervical cord. The lesions are often flame-shaped and T2 hyperintense with little or no cord swelling or edema. Enhancement may be seen during active demyelination. Concomitant brain lesions are usually present, although isolated cord disease is seen in 10 to 20% of cases. Lesions typically span less than two vertebral segments and involve less than half the cross-sectional area of the cord. Acute disseminated encephalomyelitis, however, may be more extensive, involving multiple segments and a larger cross-sectional area of the cord.

■ Additional Differential Diagnoses

- **Hemangioblastoma**: Hemangioblastomas are low-grade neoplasms of the cord and cerebellum. In the cord, 75% are sporadic and 25% are associated with von Hippel-Lindau (VHL) syndrome in which case they are often multiple. They are subpial and most often dorsal in location. Hemangioblastomas are typically T1 isointense T2 hyperintense with cord edema. Signal is more heterogeneous with hemorrhage. Smaller lesions show solid enhancement, while larger lesions demonstrate the characteristic cystic mass with enhancing mural nodule.

Prominent flow voids may be seen. The brain and entire spine should be imaged if VHL is suspected.

- **Metastatic disease**: Intramedullary metastases are relatively uncommon. The most common primary neoplasms include lung carcinoma (especially small cell), breast carcinoma, melanoma, lymphoma, and renal cell carcinoma. There is typically a nidus of enhancement and extensive edema. Pial metastatic lesions can mimic hemangioblastomas.

■ Diagnosis

Demyelinating disease (multiple sclerosis)

✓ Pearls

- Ependymomas are the most common cord tumor in adults; a characteristic hemosiderin cap may be seen.
- Astrocytomas are the most common cord tumors in children and present as infiltrating, expansile masses.

- Demyelinating disease preferentially involves the posterolateral cord; enhancement suggests active disease.

Suggested Reading

Carra BJ, Sherman PM. Intradural spinal neoplasms: a case based review. J Am Osteopath Coll Radiol. 2013; 2(3):13–21

Case 143

Paul M. Sherman

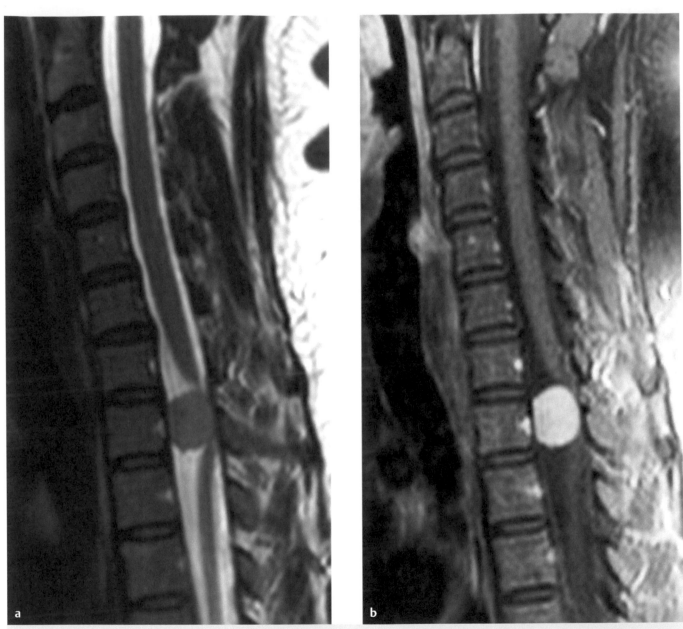

Fig. 143.1 **(a)** Sagittal T2 image demonstrates a circumscribed, iso- to hyperintense intradural extramedullary mass within the upper thoracic spine, resulting in posterior displacement and severe compression of the cord. **(b)** T1 postcontrast image with fat suppression reveals avid and homogeneous enhancement, along with a dural base anteriorly.

■ Clinical Presentation

A young adult woman with pain and radiculopathy (▶ Fig. 143.1).

■ Key Imaging Finding

Intradural extramedullary spinal mass

■ Top 3 Differential Diagnoses

- **Nerve sheath tumor**. Schwannomas are the most common intradural extramedullary masses. They may be purely intradural (most common), intra- and extradural with a classic dumbbell configuration, or rarely extradural. They may cause bony remodeling with foraminal enlargement or posterior vertebral body scalloping. Schwannomas are circumscribed, iso- to hypointense to cord on T1, variably hyperintense on T2, and intensely enhance. Cystic change and hemorrhage may be seen with larger lesions. Most cases are solitary and sporadic; they may be multiple in the setting of NF-2. Neurofibromas (NFs) are often indistinguishable from schwannomas on imaging, especially when solitary and sporadic (90%). However, they are more likely to demonstrate the "target" sign with centrally decreased and peripherally increased T2 signal intensity. Multiple NFs are seen in patients with NF-1. Plexiform NFs are a specific subtype which demonstrate T2 hypointense septations and may undergo malignant degeneration in 5% of cases (suggested by rapid growth). Other spinal stigmata of NF-1 include thoracic scoliosis/kyphosis, vertebral anomalies, meningocele, and dural ectasia.
- **Meningioma**. Meningiomas are the second most common intradural extramedullary masses and are more common in women and patients with NF-2. The vast majority (90%) are intradural; the remainder present as intra- and extradural, or rarely paraspinal or intraosseous. They are most common in the thoracic spine (80%), followed by the cervical and lumbar spine. They are typically round in shape and may have a broad dural base. Meningiomas are isointense to cord on T1 and iso- to hyperintense on T2 images. Up to 5% may calcify. Flow voids may occasionally be present. The lesions intensely enhance; the presence of a dural tail is a useful discriminator but is less common than with intracranial meningiomas.
- **Metastatic disease**. Cerebrospinal fluid (CSF) metastases may result from hematogenous spread of a distant primary tumor or dissemination from a primary central nervous system (CNS) tumor. Common extra-CNS tumors with hematogenous spread include lung, breast, and melanoma; CNS tumors prone to CSF dissemination include high-grade astrocytomas, medulloblastomas, germ cell tumors, choroid plexus neoplasm, and ependymomas. Metastases may present as a solitary intradural extramedullary mass, multiple enhancing masses, or smooth or nodular leptomeningeal infiltration with "sugar coating" of the cord/ nerve roots. Extensive disease may fill the thecal sac, resulting in increased precontrast T1 signal of the CSF (dirty appearance of the CSF). Rarely, metastases may present as an intramedullary mass. Bony lesions of the spine may be seen in association with hematogenous metastases.

■ Additional Differential Diagnoses

- **Lymphoma/leukemia**. Lymphoma and leukemia have a variety of imaging appearances within the spine, including leptomeningeal infiltration, intradural extramedullary spinal masses, epidural masses, and vertebral masses; leptomeningeal involvement is the most common and presents with smooth or nodular enhancement. Intradural extramedullary masses typically occur in the setting of diffuse CSF involvement; a focal, solitary mass is rare. Intradural extramedullary lesions are often well circumscribed with homogeneous enhancement.
- **Paraganglioma**. Paragangliomas are neural crest tumors that most often occur in the adrenal gland, followed by the head and neck region; they may rarely present as intradural, extramedullary masses, often occurring along the filum/cauda equina. Magnetic resonance imaging reveals a circumscribed T2 hyperintense avidly enhancing mass. Hemosiderin cap and vascular flow voids may be seen. Increased activity is noted on metaiodobenzylguanidine (MIBG) scans.

■ Diagnosis

Meningioma

✓ Pearls

- Nerve sheath tumors (specifically schwannoma) are the most common intradural extramedullary spinal masses.
- Meningiomas are more common in women and patients with NF-2; they may have a broad dural base.

- CSF malignancies may result from hematogenous spread, drop metastases, or lymphoma/leukemic infiltration.

Suggested Reading

Carra BJ, Sherman PM. Intradural spinal neoplasms: a case based review. J Am Osteopath Coll Radiol. 2013; 2(3):13–21

Case 144

Paul M. Sherman

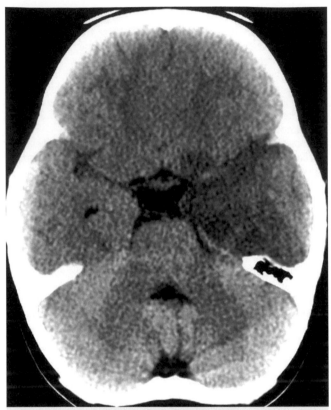

Fig. 144.1 Axial unenhanced CT image demonstrates diffuse hypoattenuation throughout the left temporal lobe and posteroinferior frontal lobe with loss of gray-white matter differentiation and sulcal effacement. There is mild medial displacement of the uncus on the left.

■ Clinical Presentation

A 64-year-old man with headache and seizures (▶ Fig. 144.1).

■ Key Imaging Finding

Diffuse, infiltrating temporal lobe mass/edema

■ Top 3 Differential Diagnoses

- **Herpes encephalitis**. Brain parenchymal infection secondary to herpes simplex virus type 1 (HSV-1) in adults characteristically involves the limbic system, including the temporal lobes, insula, inferior frontal lobes, and cingulate gyri. Patients present with acute onset of fever, headaches, seizures, and/or focal neurological deficits. Imaging typically reveals bilateral, asymmetric involvement of the cortex and subcortical white matter with sparing of the basal ganglia. There is edema with loss of gray-white differentiation and local mass effect, typically in a nonvascular distribution. Foci of hemorrhage and restricted diffusion are commonly seen. Mild, patchy enhancement may be seen acutely, developing into gyriform enhancement usually within 1 week. Mortality is 50 to 70% if not recognized and treated promptly.
- **Ischemia/Infarction**. Infarcts result from vascular occlusion. Patients present acutely with focal neurological deficits, altered mental status, and/or aphasia. Arterial etiologies include thromboembolic disease (most common), dissection, vasculitis, and hypoperfusion. Imaging reveals cytotoxic edema with loss of gray-white matter differentiation and sulcal effacement in a vascular distribution. Occlusion of the proximal middle cerebral artery (MCA) may show a characteristic "dense MCA" sign on computed tomography with hypoattenuation involv-

ing the basal ganglia and insula. Both computed tomography angiography and magnetic resonance angiography may demonstrate the site of vascular occlusion. Acute infarcts show restricted diffusion. Perfusion imaging evaluates for a penumbra, or potentially viable parenchyma. Hemorrhagic transformation occurs in 15 to 20% of cases. Venous infarcts occur in patients with one of many hypercoagulable states. Temporal lobe involvement is common due to occlusion of the vein of Labbe. Imaging shows cytotoxic edema in a nonvascular distribution. Hemorrhage is common, especially with thrombus extending into cortical veins.
- **Gliomatosis cerebri**. Gliomatosis cerebri is a WHO grade III infiltrating astrocytoma with a peak incidence in the fifth and sixth decades of life. Patients often present with headaches, seizures, or focal neurological deficits. Imaging reveals diffuse, confluent regions of T2/FLAIR hyperintensity with mass effect, often centered within the centrum semiovale. There is involvement of three or more lobes, and there may be extension across white matter tracts to involve the contralateral hemisphere. There is typically no or minimal patchy enhancement. Involvement of the cortex, deep gray matter, cerebellum, brainstem, and spinal cord may be seen.

■ Additional Differential Diagnoses

- **Limbic encephalitis**. Limbic encephalitis is a paraneoplastic syndrome associated with a primary malignancy, typically lung or breast cancer. Imaging findings may be indistinguishable from herpes encephalitis with unilateral or bilateral regions of signal abnormality with a predilection for limbic system; however, hemorrhage does not occur. Clinically, the onset of symptoms is usually more insidious (weeks to months) rather than acute. Treatment of the primary malignancy may result in stabilization or improvement of symptoms.

- **Status epilepticus**. Seizures result in focal increased cerebral perfusion and disruption of the blood–brain barrier. There is associated ill-defined edema involving the cortex and subcortical white matter; the temporal lobe is commonly involved. Enhancement may occasionally be seen. Follow-up imaging after cessation of seizures demonstrates improvement or resolution. It is important to remember that the region of edema may be remote from the actual seizure focus.

■ Diagnosis

Herpes encephalitis

✓ Pearls

- Herpes encephalitis is a life-threatening infection which preferentially involves the limbic system.
- Ischemia results in cortical edema, sulcal effacement, and restricted diffusion in a vascular distribution.

- Gliomatosis cerebri is an infiltrating neoplasm involving three or more lobes.
- Limbic encephalitis is a paraneoplastic syndrome with insidious rather than acute onset of symptoms.

Suggested Reading

Peerauly T, Landolfi JC. Herpes encephalitis masquerading as tumor. ISRN Neurol. 2011; 2011:474672

Case 145

William T. O'Brien Sr.

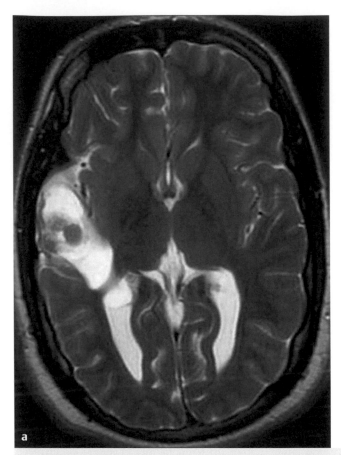 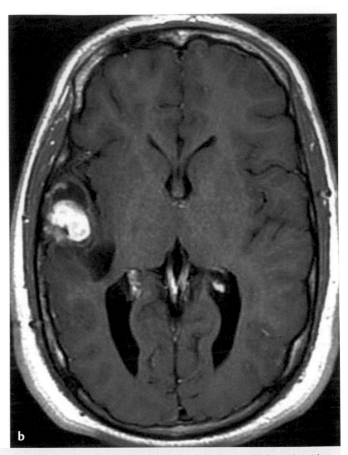

Fig. 145.1 **(a)** Axial T2 and **(b)** T1 postcontrast images demonstrate a cortically based mixed cystic and solid mass in the right temporal lobe with avid enhancement of the solid, nodular component. There is no significant surrounding edema.

■ Clinical Presentation

A 15-year-old boy with seizures (▶Fig. 145.1).

■ Key Imaging Finding

Cortically based cystic temporal lobe mass in a patient with seizures

■ Top 3 Differential Diagnoses

- **Ganglioglioma**. Ganglioglioma is a low-grade (typically WHO grade 1), cortically based neuroepithelial tumor, which is composed of neoplastic ganglion and glial cells. It most often occurs in the temporal lobes and is the most common neoplastic cause of temporal lobe seizures in adolescents and young adults. Additional symptoms include headache and focal neurological deficits. Although its imaging appearance varies, the most common presentation is a superficial mixed cystic and solid mass; the solid components often present as a mural nodule and are hyperintense on T2 sequences. As the lesion is cortically based, cortical expansion and overlying bony remodeling is often seen. Calcifications and enhancement of solid components are noted in approximately half of cases. Meningeal enhancement and surrounding edema is mild, when present.
- **Dysembryoplastic neuroepithelial tumor (DNET)**. DNET is a benign tumor which is composed of both glial and neuronal elements. A unique feature is its association with adjacent regions of cortical dysplasia. It typically occurs in adolescents and young adults; the most common presentation is seizures. Surgical resection must include the foci of cortical dysplasia to ensure resolution of seizures. DNET most often occurs in the temporal lobes. On magnetic resonance (MR), DNET presents as a circumscribed, wedge-shaped, cortically based mass. It is T2 hyperintense with a characteristic "bubbly" or multicystic appearance. Calcification and enhancement are fairly uncommon, occurring in approximately one-fifth to one-third of cases. There is often no significant edema. As the mass is cortically based, expansion of the cortex and calvarial remodeling are commonly seen.
- **Pleomorphic xanthoastrocytoma (PXA)**. PXA is a low-grade, cortically based astrocytoma which most often occurs during childhood and early adulthood. Patients commonly present with seizures, headache, and occasionally focal neurological deficits. The majority of cases involve the temporal lobe, resulting in temporal lobe epilepsy. On MR, PXA presents as a T2-hyperintense cortically based cystic and solid mass with a solid mural nodule. The solid nodular component extends along the pial surface. Prominent enhancement and surrounding vasogenic edema may be seen. The majority of cases demonstrate overlying meningeal enhancement, which is a useful discriminator. Computed tomography may show calcification, as well as bony remodeling.

■ Additional Differential Diagnoses

- **Balloon cell (Taylor) cortical dysplasia**. Focal cortical dysplasia (FCD) is a neuronal migration disorder characterized by abnormal cortical development secondary to some form of insult. There are two subtypes: Type 1 in which there is abnormal cortical development without abnormal neurons and Type 2 in which there is both abnormal cortical development and dysmorphic neurons. Taylor dysplasia is a subset of type 2 that contains characteristic balloon cells on pathologic examination. On MR, cortical dysplasia presents with increased T2/FLAIR signal intensity involving the cortex and subcortical white matter with blurring of the gray-white matter junction. The signal abnormality is commonly wedge-shaped with tapered signal pointing toward the ventricles. The overlying cortex may be thickened. Regions of increased cortical signal intensity on heavily T1-weighted sequences are fairly characteristic and helpful in distinguishing from neoplasms. There is no enhancement or surrounding edema. Patients present with seizures or focal neurological deficits.

■ Diagnosis

Ganglioglioma

✓ Pearls

- Ganglioglioma is a common cause of temporal lobe epilepsy in young adults; it is mixed cystic and solid.
- DNET presents as a nonenhancing, "bubbly," multicystic mass with adjacent regions of cortical dysplasia.

- PXA presents as a cystic mass with enhancing mural nodule; meningeal enhancement is often seen.
- Taylor dysplasia presents as wedge-shaped cortical/subcortical signal abnormality tapering toward ventricles.

Suggested Readings

Colombo N, Tassi L, Galli C, et al. Focal cortical dysplasias: MR imaging, histopathologic, and clinical correlations in surgically treated patients with epilepsy. AJNR Am J Neuroradiol. 2003; 24(4):724–733

Koeller KK, Henry JM; Armed Forces Institute of Pathology. From the archives of the AFIP: superficial gliomas: radiologic-pathologic correlation. Radiographics. 2001; 21(6):1533–1556

Case 146

Paul M. Sherman

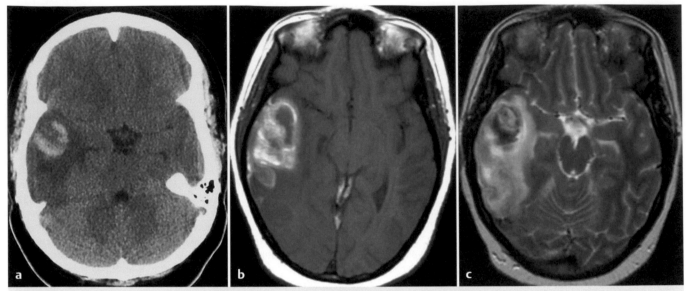

Fig. 146.1 (a) Axial unenhanced CT image demonstrates an intraparenchymal hemorrhage within the right temporal lobe with surrounding vasogenic edema. There is mass effect with sulcal effacement and medial deviation of the right uncus. Axial (b) T1 and (c) T2 images reveal similar findings. The hemorrhage is predominantly T1 hyperintense with regions of both T2 hyperintense and hypointense signal intensity, consistent with subacute hemorrhage.

■ Clinical Presentation

An adult woman with headache and altered mental status (▶Fig. 146.1).

■ Key Imaging Finding

Intraparenchymal hemorrhage

■ Top 3 Differential Diagnoses

• **Hemorrhagic infarct.** Hypertensive infarcts occur in adults or in younger patients with malignant hypertension or illicit drug use. They most often involve the basal ganglia/external capsule, thalamus, and posterior fossa. Hemorrhage is typically round or elliptical with surrounding edema. There may be extension into the ventricles. There is often no enhancement. Hemorrhagic transformation of an arterial infarct usually occurs in the subacute phase when gyral enhancement is seen or more acutely with use of thrombolytics. Arterial infarcts are characteristically wedge-shaped and follow a vascular distribution. Restricted diffusion is seen in the acute setting. Hemorrhagic venous infarcts occur in patients with hypercoagulable states and associated dural venous sinus or cortical vein (more commonly associated with parenchymal hemorrhage) thrombosis. Clot is hyperdense on unenhanced computed tomography (CT) ("cord sign" for cortical veins); the "empty delta" sign on contrast studies corresponds to enhancement of the sinus surrounding the nonenhancing thrombus. Computed tomography or magnetic resonance venography demonstrates the region of venous thrombosis. Gradient recalled echo (GRE) and susceptibility-weighted imaging (SWI) sequences are sensitive for hemorrhage.

• **Vascular malformation.** Arteriovenous malformations (AVMs) are abnormal networks of arteries and veins with no intervening capillary bed. The vast majority are solitary and supratentorial. CT demonstrates iso- to hyperdense serpentine vessels; calcifications are common. MR reveals flow voids in a "bag of worms" pattern with avid enhancement. Associated aneurysms (arterial, venous, or intranidal) are a primary source of hemorrhage. AVMs are classified based on size, location (eloquent or noneloquent brain), and venous drainage (superficial or deep). They may be treated endovascularly or surgically. Cavernous malformations (CMs) consist of blood-filled sinusoids and cavernous spaces without intervening parenchyma. The majority of lesions are solitary. CT may be normal or show subtle increased density. A "popcorn" appearance on MR is secondary to mixed T1 and T2 hyper- and hypointense blood products. There is blooming on GRE and SWI sequences.

• **Hemorrhagic neoplasm.** Glioblastoma multiforme (GBM) is the most common primary brain neoplasm in adults. It is highly aggressive (WHO grade IV) with vasogenic edema and regions of central necrosis, tumoral enhancement, and neovascularity, which makes it prone to hemorrhage. Hemorrhagic metastases may be solitary or multiple. Primary neoplasms prone to hemorrhage include lung, breast, renal cell carcinoma, thyroid, and melanoma. Metastases may involve the gray-white matter junction or end arterioles within the deep brain parenchyma.

■ Additional Differential Diagnoses

• **Contusion.** Contusions present as patchy, superficial parenchymal hemorrhages with surrounding edema. They involve characteristic locations where parenchyma contacts the adjacent calvarium, including the anterior temporal, inferior frontal, and parasagittal parenchyma. Within the first few days following trauma, contusions may expand and then subsequently regress. Calvarial fractures and foci of extra-axial hemorrhage are associated findings. GRE and SWI (more sensitive) demonstrate blooming associated with hemorrhage.

• **Cerebral amyloid disease.** Amyloid angiopathy typically presents as spontaneous, lobar parenchymal hemorrhages in elderly patients. There is an association with underlying white matter disease and dementia. The parietal and occipital lobes are most common, although any lobe may be involved. Roughly one-third of patients will have MR findings of old lobar or petechial hemorrhages, best seen on GRE and SWI sequences.

■ Diagnosis

Hemorrhagic infarct (venous infarct secondary to vein of Labbe thrombosis)

✓ Pearls

• AVMs are most commonly solitary and supratentorial, have flow voids, and avidly enhance.
• Hemorrhagic infarcts include hypertensive hemorrhages, hemorrhagic conversion, and venous infarcts.

• GBM and hypervascular metastases may present as hemorrhagic intraparenchymal masses.
• Cerebral amyloid angiopathy presents as spontaneous, lobar parenchymal hemorrhages in elderly patients.

Suggested Reading

Linn J, Brückmann H. Differential diagnosis of nontraumatic intracerebral hemorrhage. Klin Neuroradiol. 2009; 19(1):45–61

Case 147

Paul M. Sherman

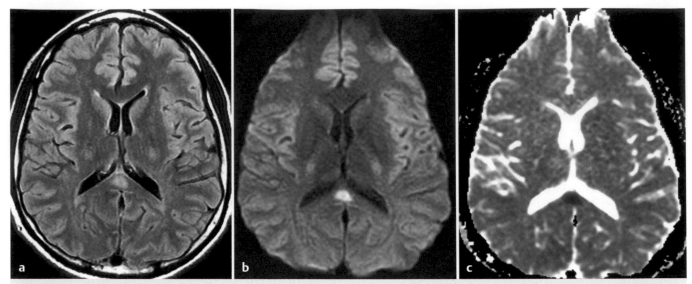

Fig. 147.1 **(a)** Axial fluid attenuation inversion recovery (FLAIR) image demonstrates a focal region of signal abnormality within the splenium of the corpus callosum. Restricted diffusion is confirmed with **(b)** increased signal on diffusion-weighted imaging and **(c)** corresponding decreased signal on the apparent diffusion coefficient map.

■ Clinical Presentation

An adult man with headaches and altered mental status (▶Fig. 147.1).

■ Key Imaging Finding

Corpus callosal lesion

■ Top 3 Differential Diagnoses

- **Demyelinating disease**. Multiple sclerosis (MS) and acute disseminated encephalomyelitis (ADEM) are the most common demyelinating diseases. MS is more common in adults and ADEM primarily affects children. Imaging features include ovoid T2 hyperintense periventricular white matter lesions perpendicular to the ventricles (Dawson fingers). High specificity locations include the optic tracts, corpus callosum, cerebellum, brainstem, and cord. Enhancement (nodular or ring enhancing) and restricted diffusion may be seen during active demyelination. Tumefactive MS (large masslike enhancing lesions) is rare but may mimic neoplasm.
- **Neoplasm (GBM and lymphoma)**. Glioblastoma multiforme (GBM) and lymphoma present as masses. GBM is an aggressive WHO grade IV astrocytoma and is the most common primary malignant brain tumor in adults. It extends across white matter tracts to involve the contralateral hemisphere, hence the term "butterfly glioma" of corpus callosum. It rapidly enlarges with central necrosis and neovascularity. There is marked mass effect; thick, irregular enhancement; and adjacent T2 hyperintensity which represents edema and tumor invasion. The tumor is primarily T2 hyperintense with necrosis and hemorrhage. Flow voids may be seen. Foci of restricted diffusion correspond to high cellularity or hemorrhage. GBM most commonly occurs in middle-aged and elderly adults. Primary central nervous system lymphoma is of the non-Hodgkin variant. It occurs within the deep gray and white matter and commonly involves the corpus callosum and ependymal surfaces of the ventricles. Lymphoma may be solitary or multiple and circumscribed or infiltrative. Lesions are often hyperdense on CT, T1 and T2 iso- to hypointense, and demonstrate increased signal on diffusion-weighted imaging due to high cellularity. Enhancement is homogenous in immunocompetent patients and peripheral or ring enhancing in immunocompromised patients. Unlike toxoplasmosis, lymphoma is hypermetabolic on thallium and positron emission tomography imaging.
- **Ischemia/edema**. The corpus callosum is less prone to ischemic change due to the compact nature of white matter tracts; however, ischemic injury and edema are increasingly more common. Ischemic change may occur anywhere within the corpus callosum but is most common in the posterior body and splenium. Restricted diffusion may be seen acutely. Seizure-related edema has a propensity for the splenium, especially in kids. The edema typically resolves after the seizure activity subsides, unless there are superimposed ischemic changes.

■ Additional Differential Diagnoses

- **Diffuse axonal injury (DAI)**. DAI results from white matter shear injury and presents as multifocal hemorrhagic or nonhemorrhagic lesions involving the gray-white matter junction (grade 1), corpus callosum (grade 2), deep gray matter, and dorsolateral brainstem (grade 3). Gradient echo (T2*GRE) and susceptibility-weighted imaging are sensitive for hemorrhagic shear injury due to susceptibility from blood products. Associated traumatic brain injury (contusions and extra-axial hemorrhage) is commonly seen.

- **Toxic demyelination**. Chronic alcoholism (classically Italian red wine) and poor nutrition may result in focal demyelination, involving predominantly the splenium of the corpus callosum, termed *Marchiafava-Bignami*. Imaging findings of Wernicke encephalopathy are often absent. Other causes of toxic demyelination include medication toxicity secondary to chemotherapy, antiepileptic drugs, some antibiotics, and illicit drug abuse.

■ Diagnosis

Ischemia (heat stroke)

✓ Pearls

- Characteristic MS lesions include Dawson fingers and involvement of the corpus callosum and posterior fossa.
- GBM and lymphoma are the most common neoplasms to involve and cross the corpus callosum.

- DAI is due to shear injury and may involve the corpus callosum; GRE is sensitive for hemorrhagic lesions.

Suggested Reading

Bourekas EC, Varakis K, Bruns D, et al. Lesions of the corpus callosum: MR imaging and differential considerations in adults and children. AJR Am J Roentgenol. 2002; 179(1):251–257

Case 148

Paul M. Sherman

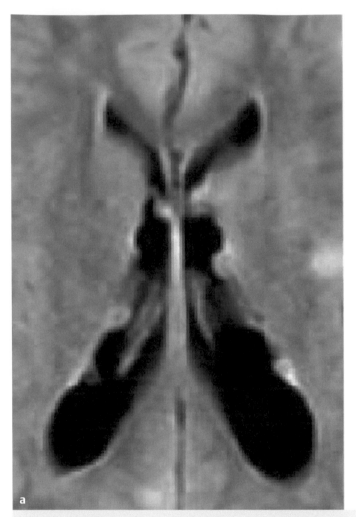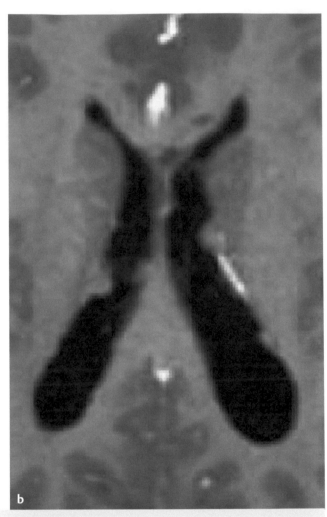

Fig. 148.1 **(a)** Axial fluid attenuation inversion recovery (FLAIR) image demonstrates multiple hyperintense subependymal nodular lesions. Regions of cortical and subcortical hyperintense signal abnormality are partially noted. **(b)** Axial T1 postcontrast image shows no discernible enhancement within the visualized lesions.

■ Clinical Presentation

A 19-year-old man with seizures (▶Fig. 148.1).

■ Key Imaging Finding

Subependymal nodules

■ Top 3 Differential Diagnoses

- **Tuberous sclerosis (TS).** TS is a neurocutaneous syndrome that results from gene mutations affecting chromosomes 9q34.3 (hamartin) and 16p13.3 (tuberin). Two-thirds of cases occur sporadically, while the remaining cases occur in an autosomal dominant fashion with variable penetrance. The classic triad consists of facial angiofibromas, mental retardation, and seizures but is seen only in approximately one-third of cases. Central nervous system (CNS) manifestations include cortical/subcortical tubers, white matter lesions that occur in a radial pattern along paths of neuronal migration, subependymal nodules, and subependymal giant cell astrocytomas (SEGAs). The cortical/subcortical tubers are composed of disorganized glial tissue and heterotopic neuronal elements. They present as triangular regions of cortical and subcortical signal abnormality which may calcify and occasionally demonstrate enhancement. Subependymal nodules have variable T1 and T2 signal intensity and commonly enhance. They demonstrate gradient echo susceptibility (hypointensity) when calcified; the majority are calcified by 20 years of age. SEGAs are low-grade tumors which occur in approximately 10 to 15% of cases. They are located at foramen of Monro, enlarge over time, and enhance. Interval growth is the best sign to distinguish SEGAs from dominant subependymal nodules. Treatment is typically geared toward cerebrospinal fluid diversion. Common abnormalities associated with TS include retinal hamartomas, cardiac rhabdomyomas, renal cysts and angiomyolipomas, pulmonary lymphangioleiomyomatosis, subungual fibromas, and skin lesions, such as ash-leaf spots and shagreen patches.

- **Heterotopic gray matter.** Heterotopic gray matter results from arrest or disruption of normal neuronal migration from the subependymal region to the overlying cortex. It is thought to occur secondary to some form of fetal insult during development. Heterotopia may be nodular or bandlike. Subependymal heterotopic gray matter is isointense to gray matter on all magnetic resonance (MR) sequences, does not enhance, and does not calcify. Patients often present with seizures and developmental delay. Mild cases, however, may be asymptomatic.

- **TORCH infection.** The primary TORCH infections consist of toxoplasmosis, rubella, cytomegalovirus (CMV), and herpes simplex virus. CMV is the most common TORCH infection to result in subependymal and periventricular calcifications, mimicking tuberous sclerosis on computed tomography. Toxoplasmosis also causes intracranial calcifications; however, the distribution is more random with less propensity for the periventricular region. Common associated findings include microcephaly and neuronal migration abnormalities, including polymicrogyria and pachygyria. Patients commonly suffer from mental retardation, seizures, and hearing loss.

■ Additional Differential Diagnoses

- **Metastatic disease.** Subependymal metastatic disease may result from primary CNS neoplasms or hematogenous spread from extracranial malignancies. Primary CNS neoplasms prone to subependymal spread include glioblastoma multiforme, medulloblastoma, ependymoma, primary CNS lymphoma, germ cell neoplasms, pineal cell neoplasms, and choroid plexus tumors. Extracranial metastases from multiple primary sites may involve the subependymal surfaces and choroid plexus, particularly breast carcinoma.

■ Diagnosis

Tuberous sclerosis

✓ Pearls

- Tuberous sclerosis results in subependymal nodules, which calcify and demonstrate enhancement.
- Heterotopic gray matter is due to an insult in utero and follows gray matter signal on all MR sequences.

- CMV is the most common TORCH infection to cause subependymal/periventricular calcifications.

Suggested Readings

Barkovich AJ, Chuang SH, Norman D. MR of neuronal migration anomalies. AJR Am J Roentgenol. 1988; 150(1):179–187

Braffman BH, Bilaniuk LT, Naidich TP, et al. MR imaging of tuberous sclerosis: pathogenesis of this phakomatosis, use of gadopentetate dimeglumine, and literature review. Radiology. 1992; 183(1):227–238

Fink KR, Thapa MM, Ishak GE, Pruthi S. Neuroimaging of pediatric central nervous system cytomegalovirus infection. Radiographics. 2010; 30(7):1779–1796

Case 149

William T. O'Brien Sr.

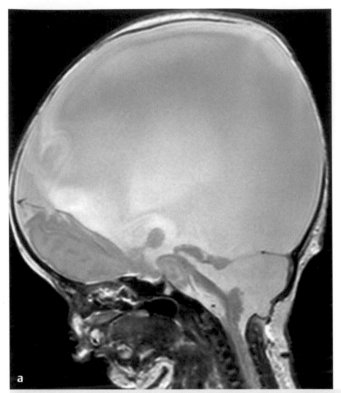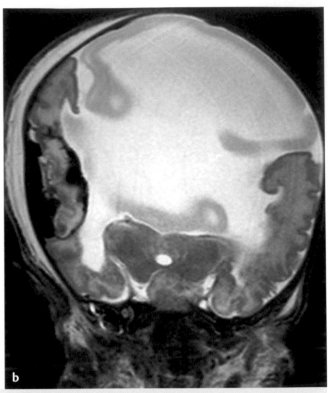

Fig. 149.1 **(a)** Sagittal T2 image demonstrates a massive supratentorial cerebrospinal fluid collection and macrocrania. There is focal narrowing at the cerebral aqueduct. Brain parenchyma is compressed anteriorly and superiorly with volume loss throughout, including the posterior fossa. **(b)** Coronal T2 image shows peripheral displacement of the brain parenchyma along the inner calvarium. The falx and septum pellucidum are not seen due to pressure erosion. The thalami were noted to be separate.

■ Clinical Presentation

A neonate with enlarged head size and lethargy (▶Fig. 149.1).

■ Key Imaging Finding

Massive supratentorial cerebrospinal fluid (CSF) collection in a newborn

■ Top 3 Differential Diagnoses

- **Massive hydrocephalus.** Hydrocephalus refers to ventriculomegaly due to obstruction, overproduction, or decreased absorption. In the newborn, this results in macrocephaly because the sutures are open. Massive hydrocephalus compresses the brain parenchyma along the peripheral calvarial margin, mimicking hydranencephaly or holoprosencephaly. Key distinguishing features include a thin mantle of cortex along the inner calvarium and the presence of the falx, respectively. Aqueductal stenosis is a common cause of massive hydrocephalus. Other causes include obstructing posterior fossa, pineal gland, tectal plate, and intraventricular masses. Transependymal edema is seen with acute uncompensated hydrocephalus. Nonobstructive communicating hydrocephalus may be seen with prior meningitis, ventriculitis, or hemorrhage.

- **Hydranencephaly.** Hydranencephaly is characterized by liquefactive necrosis of the supratentorial brain parenchyma in the anterior (internal carotid artery) circulation secondary to some form of in utero insult. There is sparing of parenchyma in the posterior (posterior cerebral artery and cerebellar branch vessels) circulation. Most cases are thought to result from an ischemic, traumatic, or toxic insult between approximately 20 and 27 weeks of gestation. Key distinguishing features include the presence of the falx cerebri; intact thalami, brainstem, cerebellum, and typically portions of the posterior occipital and parietal lobes; and absence of a cortical mantle around a large supratentorial CSF-filled cavity. Neonates commonly present with neurologic function limited to the brainstem; death typically occurs in infancy or early childhood.

- **Alobar holoprosencephaly.** Holoprosencephaly is a spectrum of congenital forebrain malformations characterized as alobar, semilobar, and lobar. The alobar form is the most severe and is characterized by a large dorsal interhemispheric cyst and fusion of the thalami and remaining brain parenchyma, which is flattened anteriorly. The corpus callosum, anterior falx, interhemispheric fissure, and Sylvian fissures are absent. Craniofacial abnormalities include hypotelorism, fused metopic suture, and cleft palate. Semilobar and lobar variants are less severe forms with varying degrees of defective separation of the anterior and central brain structures and complete or partial absence of the falx. An azygous anterior cerebral artery is commonly seen.

■ Additional Differential Diagnoses

- **Agenesis of the corpus callosum (ACC) with midline interhemispheric cyst.** ACC may be associated with midline interhemispheric cysts in addition to elevation of the third ventricle. The cysts may represent a diverticulum of the lateral ventricle (type I) or multiple interhemispheric cysts (type II). Ventriculomegaly is commonly seen. The interhemispheric cysts result in lateral displacement of the brain parenchyma. One-half to three-fourths of cases of ACC have additional central nervous system malformations.

- **Bilateral open-lip schizencephaly.** Type II (open lip) schizencephaly consists of a large CSF-filled cleft which is lined by polymicrogyric gray matter. The abnormality may be bilateral in up to half of cases and may be associated with septo-optic dysplasia. Differentiating features include gray matter–lined clefts and an intact falx. Heterotopia or cortical dysplasia may be associated findings. Patients often present with seizures and varying degrees of developmental delay and/or motor deficits.

■ Diagnosis

Massive hydrocephalus (aqueductal stenosis)

✓ Pearls

- Massive hydrocephalus in a neonate is commonly due to obstruction; a thin peripheral cortical mantle is seen.
- Hydranencephaly is liquefactive necrosis in the anterior circulation; falx is present with no cortical mantle.

- Alobar holoprosencephaly results in a large dorsal monoventricle with fused parenchyma anteriorly.

Suggested Readings

Dublin AB, French BN. Diagnostic image evaluation of hydranencephaly and pictorially similar entities, with emphasis on computed tomography. Radiology. 1980; 137(1, Pt 1):81–91

Case 150

Paul M. Sherman

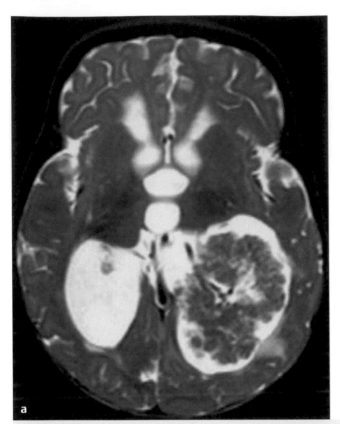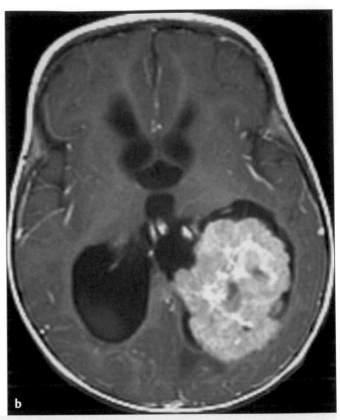

Fig. 150.1 (a) Axial T2-weighted sequence through the level of the lateral ventricles demonstrates a lobulated hypointense mass within the left lateral ventricle with frondlike margins. (b) Axial T1 postcontrast image through the same level reveals intense homogeneous enhancement (precontrast image not shown). There is associated hydrocephalus with transependymal interstitial edema. There is no brain parenchymal invasion.

■ Clinical Presentation

A young patient with persistent vomiting (▶Fig. 150.1).

■ Key Imaging Finding

Intraventricular mass

■ Top 3 Differential Diagnoses

- **Meningioma**. Meningiomas are the most common primary adult intracranial tumor and occur more frequently in women. Although intraventricular meningiomas are uncommon, they still represent the most common atrial masses in adults. They may also be seen in children, especially in the setting of NF-2. Meningiomas arise from arachnoid cap cells within the choroid plexus or velum interpositum. On computed tomography (CT), they are circumscribed and often hyperdense compared to brain parenchyma; calcification is common. On magnetic resonance (MR), meningiomas are T1 iso- to hypointense and variably hyperintense on T2 sequences; regions of calcification are T2 hypointense. Mass effect may result in ventricular dilatation and parenchymal edema. Lesions intensely enhance.
- **Choroid plexus tumor**. Choroid plexus tumors consist of benign choroid plexus papilloma (CPP) and malignant choroid plexus carcinoma (CPC). They occur most often in children within the atria of the lateral ventricles and less commonly in adults within the fourth ventricle. Infants and toddlers present with enlarging head size, vomiting, and ataxia secondary

to hydrocephalus due to overproduction of cerebrospinal fluid (CSF). They are well circumscribed with frondlike projections and a vascular pedicle. Calcifications are seen in 25% of cases. The lesions are hypointense on T1 and hyperintense on T2 sequences. CPP enhances intensely and homogeneously. Heterogeneous enhancement and brain parenchymal invasion suggests a CPC rather than benign CPP.
- **Central neurocytoma**. Central neurocytomas are histologically distinct but similar to oligodendrogliomas. They arise from and have a broad attachment to the septum pellucidum or ventricular wall. Nearly half of cases occur near the foramina of Monro. Peak incidence is between 20 and 40 years of age. Patients may present with ventricular obstruction, visual disturbances, or hormonal changes. Lesions appear as circumscribed, lobulated masses with numerous cysts, often with a "soap bubble" appearance. Solid components are iso- to hyperdense on CT, variable on T1, and heterogeneously hyperintense on T2. There is moderate enhancement. Calcifications are seen in approximately 50% of cases. Surrounding parenchymal edema may be seen with larger lesions.

■ Additional Differential Diagnoses

- **Ependymoma/Subependymoma**. In addition to being common posterior fossa tumors in kids, ependymomas may also be supratentorial, within the ventricles or brain parenchyma (more common). Ependymomas are T1 isointense and T2 hyperintense with heterogeneous enhancement. Cystic change, calcification, and hemorrhage may be seen. Subependymomas occur more often in adults within the fourth and lateral ventricles. In the lateral ventricles, they may mimic central neurocytomas with a "bubbly" appearance. On MR, lesions are T1 iso- to hypointense and T2 hyperintense with faint enhancement. They commonly have regions of calcification.
- **Subependymal giant cell astrocytomas (SEGAs)**. SEGAs are WHO grade I mixed glioneuronal tumors that occur at the foramina of Monro in approximately 15% of tuberous sclerosis patients. Most present in the first and second decades of life. Lesions are identified based on interval growth of a subependymal nodule in the characteristic location; enhancement pattern is not a distinguishing feature. Lesions may result in hydrocephalus. Treatment options include CSF diversion or tumor resection; newer medical therapies are promising. On CT, SEGAs are iso- to hypodense and may have calcification. On MR, lesions are T1 hypointense and T2 hyperintense; calcifications are T2 hypointense. Enhancement pattern is variable.

■ Diagnosis

Choroid plexus tumor (papilloma)

✓ Pearls

- Meningiomas are the most common primary intracranial and intraventricular/atrial tumors in adults.
- Choroid plexus tumors most often occur in the atria of the lateral ventricles (children) and fourth ventricle (adults).

- Central neurocytoma occurs along the septum pellucidum or ventricular wall with a "soap bubble" appearance.

Suggested Reading

Koeller KK, Sandberg GD; Armed Forces Institute of Pathology. From the archives of the AFIP. Cerebral intraventricular neoplasms: radiologic-pathologic correlation. Radiographics. 2002; 22(6):1473–1505

Case 151

Paul M. Sherman

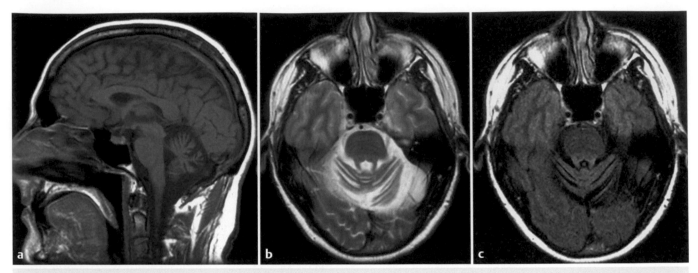

Fig. 151.1 (a) Sagittal T1-, (b) axial T2-, and (c) axial FLAIR-weighted MR sequences through the brain demonstrate diffuse cerebellar atrophy, which is markedly disproportionate to the supratentorial compartment.

■ Clinical Presentation

A 53-year-old man with history of seizures (▶Fig. 151.1).

■ Key Imaging Finding

Cerebellar atrophy

■ Top 3 Acquired Differential Diagnoses

- **Alcohol abuse.** Alcohol abuse results in progressive cerebellar degeneration. Alcohol is neurotoxic, causing cerebellar and cortical (frontal lobe predominant) degeneration, as well as peripheral polyneuropathies. There is disproportionate involvement of the superior vermis and cerebellum compared to the cerebral hemispheres. Associated findings include Wernicke encephalopathy, which presents as abnormal T2 hyperintensity within the periaqueductal gray matter, mammillary bodies, medial thalamus, and hypothalamus, and less commonly Marchiafava–Bignami disease, which results in abnormal signal intensity within the corpus callosum.
- **Anticonvulsant therapy.** Both seizures and long-term anticonvulsant therapy may produce irreversible cerebellar degeneration with disproportionate cerebellar atrophy. Patients present with ataxia, nystagmus, and peripheral neuropathies. Phenytoin is the most common and may also result in diffuse calvarial thickening.
- **Paraneoplastic syndrome.** Cerebellar degeneration may occur as a result of a paraneoplastic syndrome. Breast and lung cancer are by far the most common primary neoplasms. Less common associated malignancies include gastrointestinal and genitourinary neoplasms, Hodgkin lymphoma, and neuroblastoma. The cerebellar degeneration is thought to result from autoantibodies to Purkinje fibers or a cytotoxic process associated with T-cells. The paraneoplastic cerebellar degeneration often precedes the diagnosis of a primary tumor.

■ Top 3 Sporadic or Inherited Differential Diagnoses

- **Sporadic olivopontocerebellar atrophy (sOPCA).** sOPCA, also referred to as multisystem atrophy, is a neurodegenerative disorder that typically presents in adulthood. Imaging reveals atrophy of the ventral pons and midbrain with enlargement of the fourth ventricle and widening of the superior and middle cerebellar peduncles. There is hemispheric greater than vermian cerebellar atrophy. Less pronounced cerebral atrophy preferentially involves the frontal and parietal lobes. Cruciformlike T2 hyperintensity in the pons gives the classic "hot cross bun" sign. Signal abnormality is also seen in the middle cerebellar peduncles and dorsolateral putamen. Patients present with parkinsonian features, ataxia, dysarthria, and autonomic dysfunction.
- **Ataxia telangiectasia (AT).** AT is an autosomal recessive complex which results in spinocerebellar degeneration, ocular and cutaneous telangiectasias, radiation sensitivity, immunodeficiencies, and increased risk of neoplasms. Patients often present as toddlers with signs of ataxia. The neurological decline is progressive. Cross-sectional imaging demonstrates cerebellar atrophy with enlargement of the cerebellar sulci and compensatory enlargement of the fourth ventricle. There is also atrophy of the dentate nuclei. Intracranial telangiectasias may result in scattered foci of gradient echo susceptibility secondary to microhemorrhages. Occasionally, associated supratentorial white matter demyelination or dysmyelination may be seen.
- **Friedreich ataxia.** Also known as spinocerebellar ataxia, Friedreich ataxia typically presents in the second decade of life and has both autosomal dominant and recessive forms. Cross-sectional imaging demonstrates mild atrophy of the vermis and paravermian structures, a small medulla, and significant atrophy of the spinal cord. The dorsal cord has a flattened appearance. Clinically, patients often present with lower extremity ataxia, upper extremity tremors, and kyphoscoliosis.

■ Diagnosis

Anticonvulsant therapy (long-term phenytoin use)

✓ Pearls

- Alcohol, anticonvulsant therapy, and paraneoplastic syndromes are secondary causes of cerebellar atrophy.
- OPCA results in cerebellar and brain stem atrophy; pontine hyperintensity is referred to as "hot cross bun" sign.
- AT presents with spinocerebellar degeneration, telangiectasias, immunodeficiencies, and risk of neoplasms.

Suggested Readings

Fischbein NJ, Dillon WP, Barkovich AJ. Teaching Atlas of Brain Imaging. New York, NY: Thieme; 1999

Huang YP, Tuason MY, Wu T, Plaitakis A. MRI and CT features of cerebellar degeneration. J Formos Med Assoc. 1993; 92(6):494–508

Case 152

Paul M. Sherman

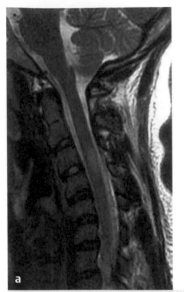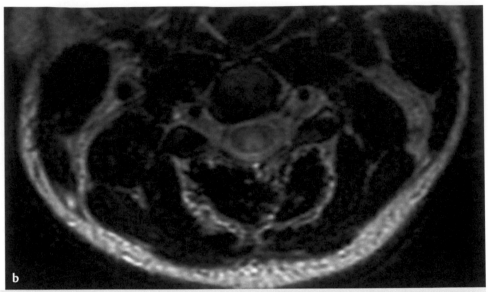

Fig. 152.1 (a) Sagittal and (b) axial T2-weighted images through the cervical spine demonstrate a large hyperintense lesion involving the midposterior aspect of the cord at the C3–C4 level. There is no cord expansion.

■ Clinical Presentation

Young adult with cervical myelopathy (▶ Fig. 152.1).

■ Key Imaging Finding

Spinal cord signal abnormality

■ Top 3 Differential Diagnoses

- **Demyelinating disease**. Demyelinating processes, such as multiple sclerosis (MS) and acute disseminated encephalomyelitis (ADEM), may affect the spinal cord in addition to the brain. Isolated cord disease is seen in approximately 10 to 20% of cases. Lesions are hyperintense on T2 sequences and most commonly located along the posterolateral aspect of the cord. There is little edema, if any; enhancement may be seen during periods of active demyelination. The plaques are typically small, usually spanning less than two vertebral bodies in length. Patients commonly present with neurologic deficits. MS demonstrates relapsing and remitting symptoms, while ADEM is characteristically monophasic after an antecedent viral infection or vaccination.
- **Transverse myelitis (TM)**. TM refers to abnormalities involving the ventral and dorsal cord at a particular level. It may be caused by a variety of factors, including infectious, ischemic, autoimmune (collagen vascular diseases), demyelinating, and paraneoplastic processes. When no cause is identified, it is termed idiopathic TM. Patients with TM present with pain and sensorimotor deficits corresponding to the affected level. Imaging shows abnormal cord signal, which may affect the whole cord at that level; enhancement is variable.
- **Intramedullary neoplasm**. The most common intramedullary neoplasms include ependymomas, which are most common in adults, and astrocytomas, which are more common in children. Ependymomas may be either myxopapillary at the caudal end of the cord or cellular within the central portion of the cord. Both neoplasms may extend up to 4 vertebral bodies in length, although astrocytomas may rarely be holocord. In general, ependymomas are more circumscribed and heterogeneous; intratumoral cysts and cord edema are commonly seen. Astrocytomas are typically more ill-defined and diffuse, causing fusiform cord expansion.

■ Additional Differential Diagnoses

- **Cord contusion**. Cord contusions occur with trauma and present with acute-onset neurologic deficits. There is increased T2 signal intensity and edema within the involved segment of the cord. Foci of hemorrhage and cord expansion may be seen. Secondary findings of trauma include spinal fractures, marrow edema, ligamentous injury, and soft-tissue injuries. The cervical spine is the most common portion of the spine involved.
- **Cord ischemia**. The spinal cord arterial supply consists of a single anterior spinal artery and paired posterior spinal arteries. Cord infarcts are multifactorial and may be caused by arterial occlusion, usually the anterior spinal artery, or venous hypertension. Imaging findings of arterial infarcts include central increased T2 signal intensity involving the cord gray matter, as well as cord edema and swelling. Venous edema and infarcts are less specific in their imaging pattern and are often due to spinal dural arteriovenous fistulas or underlying causes of impaired venous drainage.
- **Subacute combined degeneration (SCD)**. SCD results from a vitamin B12 deficiency and is often due to pernicious anemia or malabsorption (e.g., Crohn disease). Patients present with weakness, spasticity, ataxia, and loss of proprioception. Imaging demonstrates signal abnormality involving the posterior columns with a characteristic "inverted V" appearance on axial sequences. Treatment consists of B12 replacement therapy.

■ Diagnosis

Demyelinating disease (ADEM)

✓ Pearls

- Demyelinating disease commonly affects the posterolateral aspect of the cord; active lesions may enhance.
- The most common intramedullary neoplasms include ependymomas (adults) and astrocytomas (children).
- Cord contusions occur in the setting of trauma; hemorrhage, edema, and cord expansion may be seen.
- Cord ischemia is usually due to arterial occlusion; signal abnormality preferentially affects central gray matter.

Suggested Readings

Bourgouin PM, Lesage J, Fontaine S, et al. A pattern approach to the differential diagnosis of intramedullary spinal cord lesions on MR imaging. AJR Am J Roentgenol. 1998; 170(6):1645–1649

Case 153

Paul M. Sherman

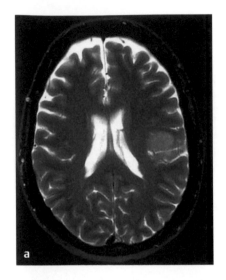

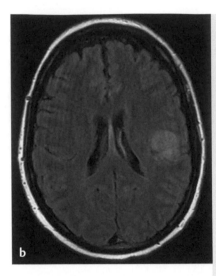

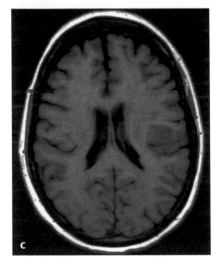

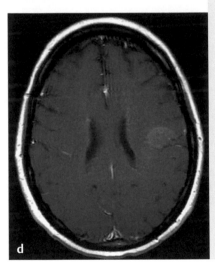

Fig. 153.1 (a) Axial T2 and (b) FLAIR images of the brain demonstrate a cortically based hyperintense lesion within the left frontal lobe with no significant vasogenic edema. The mass (c) is hypointense on T1-weighted sequences and (d) demonstrates mild homogeneous enhancement after contrast administration.

■ Clinical Presentation

Adult woman with seizures and focal neurologic deficits (▶Fig. 153.1).

■ Key Imaging Finding

Solitary region of cortical and subcortical signal abnormality in an adult

■ Top 3 Differential Diagnoses

- **Ischemia/infarct.** Cerebrovascular disease is common in adults and most often results from thromboembolic disease. In younger patients, vasculitis and dissection are prevalent. Arterial infarcts result in wedge-shaped cortical and subcortical hypoattenuation (computed tomography [CT]) and T2 hyperintensity (magnetic resonance imaging [MRI]). Cytotoxic edema results in cortical swelling with effacement of sulci. Acute infarcts demonstrate restricted diffusion. Gyral or patchy enhancement may be seen in the subacute phase, beginning as early as 2 days and peaking around 10 to 14 days. CT angiography and MR angiography may show vascular occlusion. Perfusion imaging is useful in identifying the penumbra, which represents viable parenchyma at risk of infarct. Hemorrhagic transformation occurs in 15 to 20% of cases. Venous infarcts do not follow a vascular territory and are prone to hemorrhage. CT venography or MR venography reveals the region of thrombosis.
- **Neoplasm.** Astrocytomas are the most common primary brain tumors in adults. Variants that present with cortical signal abnormality include fibrillary (WHO grade II) and anaplastic (WHO grade III). Fibrillary astrocytoma often presents with indistinct or less commonly well-defined signal abnormality centered in the white matter with or without cortical involvement. Enhancement, if present, is mild. Anaplastic astrocytoma is more aggressive with regions of increased perfusion, edema, and enhancement. MR spectroscopy reveals increased choline and decreased *N*-acetylaspartate (NAA). Restricted diffusion is not seen, unless there is focal progression to a high-grade tumor. Oligodendrogliomas occur in middle-aged adults who present with seizures. They are centered within the subcortical white matter and commonly extend to the cortex. The frontal lobe is the most common location. Lesions are well defined with little edema and mild enhancement. Calcification is typically seen.
- **Cerebritis.** Cerebritis refers to focal infection of the brain parenchyma and may result from hematogenous spread, direct spread, or as a complication of meningitis. Patients present with fever, headache, seizures, or focal neurologic deficits. On imaging, cerebritis presents as ill-defined cortical and subcortical hypoattenuation (CT) and increased T2/FLAIR signal intensity (MRI). Restricted diffusion may be seen, which may mimic an infarct acutely. Enhancement, if present, is ill-defined or thin and linear. Meningeal enhancement is a useful discriminator.

■ Additional Differential Diagnoses

- **Contusion.** Cerebral contusions result from trauma as the brain contacts the skull base or dural reflections. Common locations include the inferior frontal lobes, anterior temporal lobes, and parasagittal locations. Contusions beneath the site of impact are referred to as coup injuries, while those on the opposite side of injury are referred to as contrecoup injuries. Acutely, there is cortical and subcortical edema and swelling. Foci of parenchymal or extra-axial hemorrhage are hyperdense on CT and variable in signal on MRI depending on the timing of imaging. MRI is more sensitive than CT and typically demonstrates additional foci of parenchymal injury. Within the first 2 to 3 days, contusions may enlarge. Encephalomalacia is often seen chronically.
- **Seizure edema.** Seizure edema results in cortical and subcortical edema which is transient. It typically occurs with status epilepticus where seizure activity lasts for ≥30 minutes. Acutely, there is gyral swelling and sulcal effacement. Restricted diffusion and patchy enhancement may be seen. The edema decreases or resolves if the patient remains seizure-free. The regions of edema may or may not correspond to area of seizure focus.

■ Diagnosis

Neoplasm (astrocytoma)

✓ Pearls

- Infarcts often result from thromboembolic disease; vasculitis and dissection are common in younger patients.
- Astrocytomas and oligodendrogliomas are the most common tumors with focal cortical signal abnormality.
- Contusions occur in characteristic locations with focal edema, swelling, and hemorrhage.

Suggested Readings

Koeller KK, Rushing EJ. From the archives of the AFIP: Oligodendroglioma and its variants: radiologic-pathologic correlation. Radiographics. 2005; 25(6):1669–1688

O'Brien WT. Imaging of CNS infections in immunocompetent host. J Am Osteopath Coll Radiol. 2012; 1(1):3–9

Case 154

Paul M. Sherman

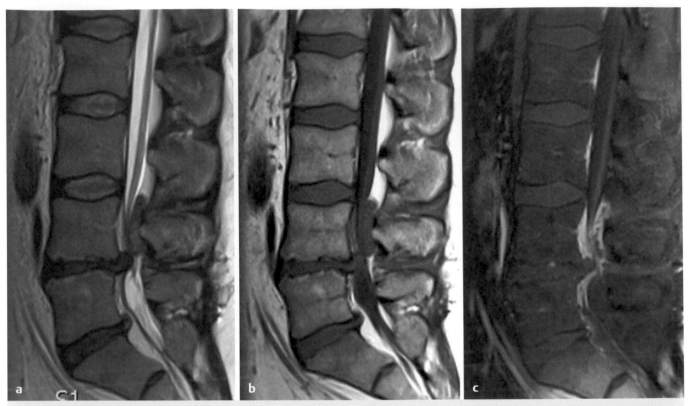

Fig. 154.1 (a) Sagittal T2 image demonstrates disc extrusions at the L4–L5 greater than L5–S1 levels, as well as a large ovoid lesion within the posterior epidural space at the L4 level. The posterior epidural lesion has intermediate to increased T2 signal intensity. **(b)** Sagittal T1 image confirms the epidural location based on its relationship to the surrounding epidural fat. **(c)** Sagittal postcontrast T1 image with fat suppression reveals enhancement along the periphery of the disc extrusions, within the ventral epidural venous plexus, and along the margins of the posterior epidural lesion. Relative increased signal intensity within the visualized sacrum corresponds to loss of fat suppression.

■ Clinical Presentation

Back pain and radiculopathy (►Fig. 154.1).

■ Key Imaging Finding

Epidural spinal mass

■ Top 3 Differential Diagnoses

- **Disc extrusion**. Disc extrusion refers to herniations with migration of the disc fragment within the anterior epidural space. There is often disc desiccation and height loss with intact endplates. The extruded fragment is usually similar in signal intensity and in continuity with the parent disc, unless it becomes sequestered. Although sequestered discs often remain in the anterior epidural space, they may occasionally migrate laterally or even posteriorly. There may be peripheral enhancement. Epidural hematomas may be seen in association with acute disc extrusions.
- **Epidural hematoma**. Epidural hematomas may occur spontaneously or result from trauma, transient venous hypertension (cough), iatrogenia, or coagulopathy. They are most often due to rupture of the epidural venous plexus. Most occur within the dorsal thoracolumbar spine in adults and cervicothoracic spine in children. They are generally biconvex and surrounded by epidural fat. Acute hemorrhage is T1 isointense, while subacute or chronic is most often T1 hyperin-

tense. Hemorrhage is variable in T2 signal intensity depending on the composition of blood products. On gradient echo imaging, hemorrhagic blood products are often hypointense. Peripheral enhancement is common; focal enhancement may represent extravasation.
- **Epidural abscess**. Epidural abscesses are commonly associated with disc osteomyelitis. They most often occur anteriorly and are associated with paraspinal phlegmon or abscess formation. They may result from hematogenous dissemination of a distant infection or direct inoculation from surgical procedures or epidural anesthesia. The latter are less common and occur dorsally. *Staphylococcus aureus* (70–75%) is the most common organism; *Mycobacterium tuberculosis* most often occurs in immunocompromised patients. *S. aureus* infections are centered at the disc space, while *TB* spondylitis results in relative sparing of the disc. Epidural abscesses follow fluid signal with peripheral rim and adjacent dural enhancement.

■ Additional Differential Diagnoses

- **Metastatic disease**. Epidural foci from metastatic disease are often contiguous with a pedicle or posterior vertebral body lesion. A pathologic compression fracture may be present. The masses are typically T1 hypointense and variable in T2 signal intensity with diffuse or heterogeneous enhancement depending on the presence of necrosis or hemorrhage. Common primary tumors include breast, lung, and prostate carcinoma. Non-Hodgkin lymphoma may also present as an extradural mass. Lymphoma is typically iso- to hyperdense on computed tomography (CT), isointense on T1, and variable on T2 sequences with intense homogeneous enhancement.
- **Epidural lipomatosis**. Lipomatosis refers to abnormal proliferation of epidural fat. It is most commonly seen in the tho-

racolumbar spine. Causative etiologies include excessive steroids (exogenous or endogenous) and obesity, although it may also be idiopathic. The lesions follow fat signal on all sequences and do not enhance. There may be compression of the spinal canal and neural structures.
- **Synovial cyst**. Synovial cysts result from degenerative facet disease and most commonly occur in the lumbar spine. They may extend into the posterolateral epidural space or through the neural foramen. The cyst follows fluid signal and has a T2 hypointense margin. Peripheral enhancement may be seen, as can hemorrhage or calcification. Patients commonly present with pain or radiculopathy.

■ Diagnosis

Disc extrusions anteriorly with a sequestered disc posteriorly

✓ Pearls

- Disc extrusions occur anterior to the thecal sac and commonly follow the signal intensity of the parent disc.
- Epidural hematomas are most often dorsal and may occur spontaneously or due to an inciting event.

- Epidural abscesses have rim enhancement and most commonly are associated with disc osteomyelitis.
- Synovial cysts result from degenerative facet disease and may compress the posterolateral thecal sac.

Suggested Readings

Chhabra A, Batra K, Satti S, Patel S, et al. Spinal epidural space: anatomy, normal variations and pathological lesions on MR imaging. Neurographics. 2005; 1(26):1–13

Case 155

Paul M. Sherman

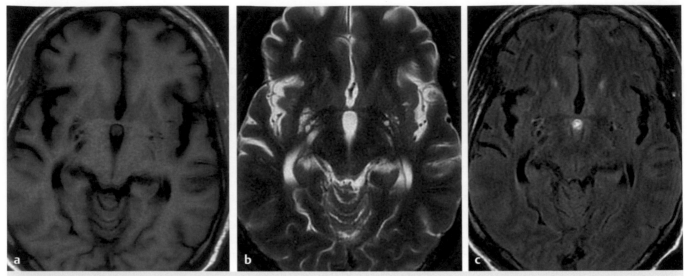

Fig. 155.1 **(a)** Axial T1, **(b)** T2, and **(c)** FLAIR images through the brain demonstrate multiple foci of CSF signal intensity in the basal ganglia and anterior perforated substance bilaterally. The FLAIR sequence **(c)** reveals increased signal intensity along the periphery of many of the lesions. There is diffuse atrophy, more than expected for patient's age.

■ Clinical Presentation

A 42-year-old man with progressive fatigue, somnolence, and decreased responsiveness (▶Fig. 155.1).

■ Key Imaging Finding

Prominent periventricular/basal ganglia cystic lesions

■ Top 3 Differential Diagnoses

• **Virchow–Robin (VR) spaces**. VR spaces are pial-lined perivascular spaces that surround perforating arteries extending from the subarachnoid space into the parenchyma. They occur in the deep gray/white matter (inferior one-third of the basal ganglia/anterior perforated substance); along medullary veins, most often in the periatrial regions; and within the midbrain. VR spaces are 2 to 5 mm in size; giant VR spaces are ≥1.5 cm. They follow cerebrospinal fluid (CSF) signal intensity, although occasionally atypical perivascular spaces may have minimal surrounding fluid-attenuated inversion recovery (FLAIR) signal.

• **Ischemia**. Lacunar infarcts are small areas of encephalomalacia from occlusion of perforating vessels. Common locations include the basal ganglia (upper two-thirds), thalami, internal/external capsules, pons, and periventricular white matter. Acutely, lacunar infarcts demonstrate restricted diffusion. In the subacute phase, enhancement may be seen. Chronic lacunes follow CSF signal intensity with variable surrounding gliosis. Lacunar infarcts occur most often in elderly patients with microvascular ischemic disease. In neonates, prenatal or perinatal insults result in periventricular leukomalacia (PVL), characterized by signal abnormality and volume loss in the periatrial white matter. Regions of necrosis result in cystic PVL with surrounding gliosis.

• **Infection**. *Cryptococcus* is an opportunistic fungal infection which affects immunosuppressed patients, especially those with AIDS. The infection affects the meninges and spreads through the subarachnoid and perivascular spaces, which become distended. The most common finding is multiple T2 hyperintense lesions in the basal ganglia with surrounding gliosis. Restricted diffusion and enhancement may be seen. Larger lesions are referred to as "gelatinous pseudocysts" and most often occur in the basal ganglia. Cryptococcomas are solid or ring-enhancing masses which most often involve the deep gray matter. Neurocysticercosis is a parasitic infection caused by the pork tapeworm (*Taenia solium*). It is the most common cause of epilepsy in endemic regions. In the initial vesicular stage, the cystic lesions are isointense to CSF, mimicking VR spaces. A hyperintense eccentric scolex may be seen (hyperdense by computed tomography [CT]). In the colloidal and granular stages, there is ring and nodular enhancement with surrounding edema. Calcification occurs in the nodular stage. Lesions may involve the gray/white junction (most common), subarachnoid space, and ventricles.

■ Additional Differential Diagnoses

• **Mucopolysaccharidoses (MPS)**. MPS are inherited disorders characterized by enzyme deficiencies which result in accumulation of glycosaminoglycan (GAG). Clinically, patients suffer from mental and motor retardation. Imaging reveals macrocephaly and dilated perivascular spaces because of accumulation of GAG. The dilated PV spaces are similar to CSF signal intensity; however, the surrounding white matter demonstrates confluent regions of increased T2/FLAIR signal abnormality, likely representing gliosis or de/dysmyelination.

• **Neuroepithelial cyst**. Neuroepithelial cysts are nonenhancing parenchymal cysts with minimal or no surrounding signal abnormality, similar to VR spaces. They most often occur within the cerebral hemispheres, thalami, brainstem, and choroidal fissures. They are smooth, round, unilocular, and follow CSF signal intensity on all sequences. There is no communication with the ventricles.

• **Cystic neoplasm**. Cystic tumors may occur within the deep gray and white matter. Unlike VR spaces, neoplasms have solid components and often demonstrate enhancement and surrounding vasogenic edema.

■ Diagnosis

Infection (*Cryptococcus* in an AIDS patient)

✓ Pearls

• VR spaces are perivascular spaces which occur in characteristic locations and follow CSF signal intensity.

• Lacunar infarcts and infection (*Cryptococcus*) mimic VR spaces but often have surrounding signal abnormality.

• MPS result in mental and motor retardation; dilated PV spaces have adjacent, confluent signal abnormality.

Suggested Readings

Kwee RM, Kwee TC. Virchow-Robin spaces at MR imaging. Radiographics. 2007; 27(4):1071–1086

Part 7

Pediatric Imaging

7

Case 156

Thomas Ray Sanchez

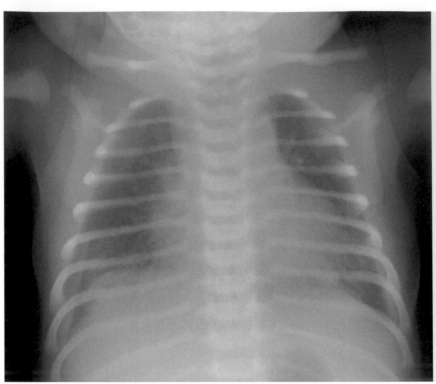

Fig. 156.1 Frontal chest radiograph shows bilateral diffuse granular opacities with small bilateral pleural effusions.

■ Clinical Presentation

A 4-day-old neonate with tachypnea and grunting (▶ Fig. 156.1).

■ Key Imaging Finding

Neonatal lung disease with diffuse granular opacities

■ Top 3 Differential Diagnoses

- **Surfactant deficiency**. Surfactant deficiency is the most common cause of respiratory distress in preterm infants, especially in those born before 34 weeks of gestation and who weigh less than 1,500 g. It occurs because immature lungs are often unable to produce enough surfactant to keep alveoli open for effective air exchange. Clinical manifestations of grunting, nasal flaring, subcostal retractions, tachypnea, and cyanosis are seen shortly after delivery and almost always within the first 8 hours of life. Radiographs typically show diffusely hazy and low lung volumes with air bronchograms. The granularity results from diffuse alveolar collapse, while the air bronchograms represent normal air-filled prealveolar airways. In severe cases (extreme prematurity and very low birth weight), assisted ventilation along with surfactant application may be needed to achieve acceptable gas exchange. When intubated, the lungs often appear well aerated. Potential complications of positive pressure include pulmonary interstitial emphysema, pneumomediastinum, and pneumothorax. Chronic intubation and oxygen administration may eventually result in bronchopulmonary dysplasia.

- **Transient tachypnea of the newborn (TTN; retained fetal fluid)**. TTN is the most common cause of respiratory distress in neonates. Transient and benign, TTN occurs when immature lymphatic vessels cannot absorb residual lung fluid quickly. It is exacerbated with caesarian section because of absence of the thoracic squeeze associated with vaginal deliveries, which normally helps clear fetal lung fluid. Patients demonstrate clinical improvement within 48 hours of birth, and radiographs normalize within 72 hours. Radiographs typically demonstrate central streaky opacities and small pleural effusions (with fluid in the minor fissure). More severe cases demonstrate pulmonary vascular congestion and air-space opacities. Lung volumes are typically normal to increased. Treatment is limited to supportive care and observation.

- **Neonatal pneumonia**. Bacterial pneumonias, especially those caused by group B *Streptococcus*, predominate in the neonatal period. The more common route of infection is through the birth canal, especially after early rupture of membranes in mothers who are febrile and positive for group B *Streptococcus*. Radiographic findings of diffuse haziness and granularity may mimic surfactant deficiency. Pleural effusions are rare in surfactant deficiency but are seen in as many as two-thirds of patients with neonatal pneumonia. With adequate antibiotic therapy, complications such as empyema, pulmonary abscess, and pneumatocele are unusual but may occur, especially with delayed treatment.

■ Diagnosis

Neonatal pneumonia

✓ Pearls

- Surfactant deficiency is the most common cause of respiratory distress in preterm infants.
- Surfactant deficiency presents with low lung volumes and diffuse granular opacities.

- TTN is transient with rapid clinical improvement; radiographs are normal at 72 hours.
- Neonatal pneumonia may mimic surfactant deficiency but often has pleural effusions.

Suggested Readings

Agrons GA, Courtney SE, Stocker JT, Markowitz RI. From the archives of the AFIP: Lung disease in premature neonates: radiologic-pathologic correlation. Radiographics. 2005; 25(4):1047–1073

Hermansen CL, Lorah KN. Respiratory distress in the newborn. Am Fam Physician. 2007; 76(7):987–994

Pramanik AK, Rangaswamy N, Gates T. Neonatal respiratory distress: a practical approach to its diagnosis and management. Pediatr Clin North Am. 2015; 62(2):453–469

Case 157

James B. Odone

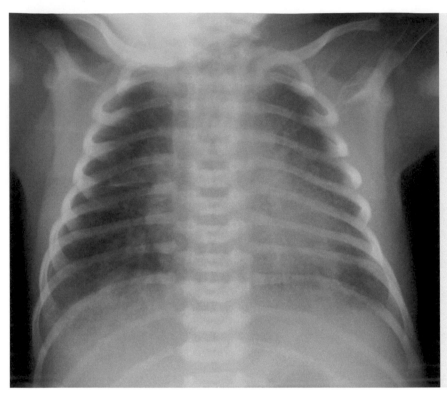

Fig. 157.1 Frontal chest radiograph demonstrates hyperinflation, increased interstitial markings and vasculature, and small pleural effusions.

■ Clinical Presentation

Term neonate born by cesarean section with respiratory distress (▶Fig. 157.1).

■ Key Imaging Finding

Neonatal lung disease with increased lung volumes

■ Top 3 Differential Diagnoses

- **Transient tachypnea of the newborn (TTN).** TTN usually manifests as tachypnea in term neonates who have undergone a cesarean section or precipitous birth. The lack of vaginal squeeze results in retained fetal lung fluid, which is slow to be cleared by the immature lymphatic system. Radiographic features include normal to increased lung volumes with bilateral diffuse patchy air-space disease and normal heart size. Perihilar linear densities and pleural effusions (often manifested by fluid in the minor fissure) are common. Air-space disease, when present, is similar in appearance to pulmonary edema and clears within 3 days of delivery. The typical clinical course is mild. If radiographic findings persist, alternative diagnoses such as cardiac disease or neonatal pneumonia should be considered. Follow-up radiographs are generally unnecessary in an otherwise healthy infant.
- **Meconium aspiration.** Meconium aspiration typically occurs in term or postterm neonates with in utero or peripartum fetal distress. The aspirated meconium causes a chemical pneumonitis and regions of airway obstruction that result in moderate to severe respiratory distress. The diagnosis is suspected clinically when amniotic fluid is stained with meconium. Radiographic appearance includes hyperinflation with patchy, asymmetric air-space disease and ropy perihilar opacities. Pleural effusions may be present, as well as areas of postobstructive atelectasis. Pneumothoraces are common (may occur in up to 40% of cases).
- **Neonatal pneumonia.** Neonatal pneumonia may result in respiratory distress in neonates. Radiographs typically demonstrate hyperinflation, as well as patchy, perihilar, or diffuse air-space disease. Pleural effusions may be seen. Occasionally, however, chest radiographs may be normal in the setting of neonatal pneumonia. Exposure to the infectious agent may occur in utero or in the perinatal period. Causative organisms include *Listeria*, *Escherichia coli*, and *Klebsiella*. Beta-hemolytic Streptococcal pneumonia is a separate entity that typically presents with low lung volumes and is thus not included in this differential. The infection typically resolves over a short period of time with the correct antibiotic therapy.

■ Additional Differential Diagnoses

- **Congenital heart disease.** Congenital heart disease commonly presents with respiratory distress, parenchymal opacities, and hyperexpanded lungs. Radiographic features may include cardiomegaly and pulmonary vascular congestion, depending on the underlying etiology. Diagnostic considerations in an acyanotic infant include shunt lesions and congestive heart failure. Considerations in a cyanotic infant include transposition of the great arteries, truncus arteriosus, total anomalous pulmonary venous return, tricuspid atresia, and single ventricle.

■ Diagnosis

Transient tachypnea of the newborn

✓ Pearls

- TTN is a self-limiting process that should resolve within 3 days.
- Meconium aspiration typically presents with patchy asymmetric air-space disease in hyperinflated lungs.
- Air-block complications (e.g., pneumothorax) must be carefully searched for with meconium aspiration.
- Neonatal pneumonia can mimic most other disease processes on chest X-ray; it may also appear normal.

Suggested Readings

Agrons GA, Courtney SE, Stocker JT, Markowitz RI. From the archives of the AFIP: Lung disease in premature neonates: radiologic-pathologic correlation. Radiographics. 2005; 25(4):1047–1073

Haney PJ, Bohlman M, Sun CC. Radiographic findings in neonatal pneumonia. AJR Am J Roentgenol. 1984; 143(1):23–26

Lobo L. The neonatal chest. Eur J Radiol. 2006; 60(2):152–158

Case 158

Karen M. Ayotte

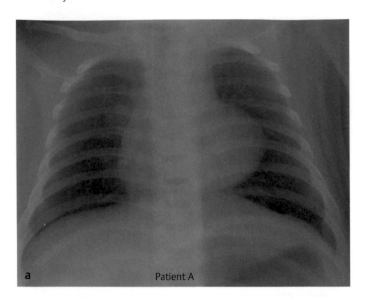

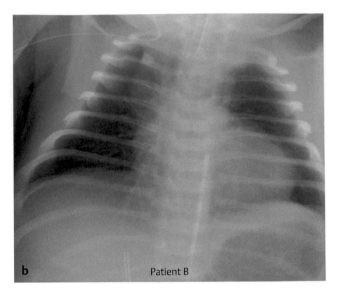

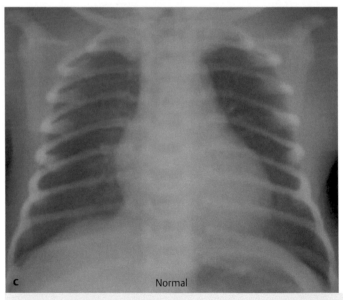

Fig. 158.1 **(a, b)** Frontal chest radiographs from different patients with the same disease process demonstrate a concave pulmonary artery shadow on the left with elevation of the cardiac apex, resulting in a "boot-shaped" heart. Relative oligemia is present. **(c)** A normal infant chest radiograph is provided for comparison.

■ Clinical Presentation

Cyanotic infants (▶Fig. 158.1**a,b**). Image **c** is normal for comparison.

Key Imaging Finding

Cyanotic infant with decreased pulmonary flow

Top 3 Differential Diagnoses

- **Tetralogy of Fallot (TOF).** TOF is the most common cyanotic heart condition in children. The four components which define this anomaly include right ventricular outflow tract obstruction (pulmonic stenosis), ventriculoseptal defect, overriding aorta, and right ventricular hypertrophy. Deficiency of the main pulmonary artery segment and elevation of the cardiac apex as the result of right ventricular hypertrophy lead to the classic radiographic appearance of a "boot-shaped" heart. Pulmonary vascularity is usually decreased, but the severity varies. The aortic arch is on the right in 25% of patients.
- **Pulmonary atresia.** The primary anatomic defect in pulmonary atresia is underdevelopment of the right ventricular outflow tract and pulmonary valve. When present with a ventricular septal defect (VSD), this anomaly is considered a severe variant of TOF, with similar radiographic findings. When the ventricular septum is intact, there is an obligatory right to left

shunt at the atrial level. Although the radiographic appearance varies, severe cardiomegaly is commonly seen. Pulmonary vascularity is normal to decreased and dependent on a patent ductus arteriosus (PDA).
- **Tricuspid atresia.** In tricuspid atresia, there is no direct path for blood flow between the right atrium and right ventricle. As a result, there is a right to left shunt at the atrial level, usually through a patent foramen ovale. Pulmonic blood flow is dependent on the presence of a VSD and/or PDA. Associated anomalies occur in up to 30% of affected patients (most commonly transposition of the great arteries). In isolated tricuspid atresia with a small VSD, chest radiographs demonstrate a normal or small heart with decreased pulmonary blood flow. However, when a large VSD is present, there is usually cardiomegaly and increased pulmonary blood flow. A right-sided aortic arch is present in about 10% of patients.

Additional Differential Diagnoses

- **Double-outlet right ventricle.** Double-outlet right ventricle occurs when both the aorta and pulmonary outflow tracts arise from the right ventricle. With 16 described variants, the radiographic appearance varies. Some forms mimic TOF with pulmonary oligemia and diminished left hilar shadow.
- **Ebstein anomaly.** Ebstein anomaly consists of apical displacement of the tricuspid valve, resulting in atrialization of the right ventricle. Tricuspid regurgitation with stasis of blood flow within the right atrium leads to massive right-sided cardiomegaly with a "box-shaped" heart and pulmonary oligemia. A right to left shunt at the atrial level is common.

Diagnosis

Tetralogy of Fallot

✓ Pearls

- TOF is the most common cyanotic congenital heart disease.
- TOF is characterized by pulmonic stenosis, VSD, right ventricular hypertrophy, and an overriding aorta.
- Pulmonary atresia with a VSD is considered a severe variant of TOF.
- Ebstein anomaly leads to massive right-sided cardiomegaly with a "box-shaped" heart.

Suggested Readings

Ferguson EC, Krishnamurthy R, Oldham SA. Classic imaging signs of congenital cardiovascular abnormalities. Radiographics. 2007; 27(5):1323–1334

Kellenberger CJ, Yoo SJ, Büchel ER. Cardiovascular MR imaging in neonates and infants with congenital heart disease. Radiographics. 2007; 27(1):5–18

Lapierre C, Déry J, Guérin R, Viremouneix L, Dubois J, Garel L. Segmental approach to imaging of congenital heart disease. Radiographics. 2010; 30(2):397–411

Schweigmann G, Gassner I, Maurer K. Imaging the neonatal heart--essentials for the radiologist. Eur J Radiol. 2006; 60(2):159–170

Case 159

Karen M. Ayotte

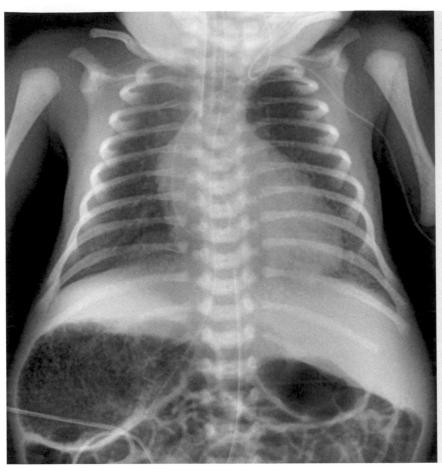

Fig. 159.1 Frontal chest radiograph shows mild cardiomegaly and markedly increased pulmonary vascularity. There is a left-sided aortic arch. The lungs are hyperinflated. Abdominal situs inversus is present, with the hepatic shadow on the left and the gastric bubble on the right. Multiple support tubes and lines are noted.

■ Clinical Presentation

A 2-day-old infant with cyanosis (▶ Fig. 159.1).

■ Key Imaging Finding

Cyanotic infant with increased pulmonary vascularity

■ Top 3 Differential Diagnoses

- **Transposition of the great arteries (TGA)**. In d-TGA (dextro-TGA), the aorta arises from the right ventricle and the pulmonary trunk arises from the left ventricle. Without a source for admixture (patent foramen ovale [PFO], ventricular septal defect [VSD], or patent ductus arteriosus [PDA]), this anatomy is incompatible with life. The classic radiographic appearance is characterized by cardiomegaly, a narrowed mediastinum ("egg on string"), and increased pulmonary vascularity. However, this appearance is rarely encountered because of prompt treatment. Occasionally, a relative normal radiographic appearance may be seen in the setting of TGA.
- **Truncus arteriosus**. Truncus arteriosus results from failure of division of the primitive single truncal vessel into the aorta and main pulmonary artery. This uncommon lesion accounts for only 1% of cases of congenital heart disease. There is always a large, high VSD. The degree of pulmonary blood flow is initially variable, depending on pulmonary resistance. When pulmonary resistance drops, usually by day 2 to 3 of life, pulmonary blood flow often dramatically increases. The combination of cardiomegaly, a right-sided arch (30% of cases), and increased pulmonary vascularity suggests the diagnosis.
- **Total anomalous pulmonary venous return (TAPVR)**. In TAPVR, none of the pulmonary veins connect normally with the left atrium; instead, they drain into the right heart via various venous connections. There are three types, classified by the location of pulmonary venous drainage: supracardiac, cardiac, and infracardiac. Supracardiac is the most common and may result in the "snowman" configuration of the heart because of an enlarged superior vena cava (SVC) and left vertical vein. In the cardiac type, pulmonary veins drain via the coronary sinus. With infracardiac TAPVR, pulmonary veins drain below the diaphragm into the portal veins or inferior vena cava. This subtype is associated with heterotaxy and presents radiographically with severe pulmonary edema and a normal heart size. In all three types, intracardiac shunting occurs via a PFO. Radiographic and clinical features vary.

■ Additional Differential Diagnoses

- **Tricuspid atresia**. In tricuspid atresia, there is no direct path for blood flow between the right atrium and right ventricle. However, there is a right to left shunt at the atrial level, usually through a PFO. Pulmonic blood flow depends on the presence of a VSD and/or PDA. With a large VSD, there is cardiomegaly and increased pulmonary flow.
- **Single ventricle**. Single ventricle is a rare anomaly in which the interventricular septum is absent. The nomenclature describing this diagnosis can be confusing, indicating specific associated anatomy. Patients without pulmonic stenosis demonstrate cardiomegaly, an enlarged main pulmonary artery, and increased pulmonary blood flow.

■ Diagnosis

Transposition of the great vessels

✓ Pearls

- TGA shows parallel configuration of outflow tracts with an "egg on a string" appearance on chest X-ray.
- Severe pulmonary edema with a normal heart size is the classic appearance of infradiaphragmatic TAPVR.
- An enlarged SVC and left vertical vein result in the "snowman" configuration in supracardiac TAPVR.

Suggested Readings

Ferguson EC, Krishnamurthy R, Oldham SA. Classic imaging signs of congenital cardiovascular abnormalities. Radiographics. 2007; 27(5):1323–1334

Lapierre C, Déry J, Guérin R, Viremouneix L, Dubois J, Garel L. Segmental approach to imaging of congenital heart disease. Radiographics. 2010; 30(2):397–411

Schweigmann G, Gassner I, Maurer K. Imaging the neonatal heart--essentials for the radiologist. Eur J Radiol. 2006; 60(2):159–170

Case 160

Karen M. Ayotte

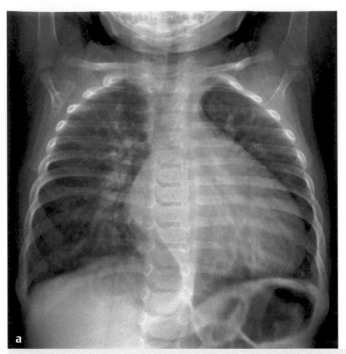
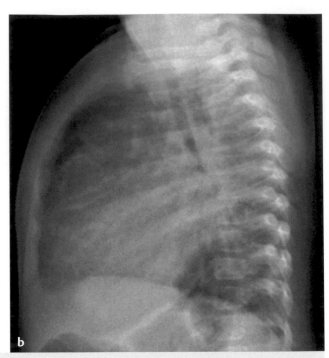

Fig. 160.1 **(a)** Frontal and **(b)** lateral chest radiographs show global cardiomegaly, as well as increased and sharply defined pulmonary vasculature. The lungs are hyperinflated, a common finding in patients with congenital heart disease.

■ **Clinical Presentation**

A 6-month-old acyanotic boy with a heart murmur (▶ Fig. 160.1).

■ Key Imaging Finding

Shunt vascularity

■ Top 3 Differential Diagnoses

- **Ventricular septal defect (VSD)**. VSD is the most common of the four causes of acyanotic shunt vascularity, and is the second most common congenital cardiac malformation after bicuspid aortic valve. Radiographs may be normal when the defect is small. Larger defects are associated with gross cardiomegaly, increased number and size of visualized, well-defined, "sharp" pulmonary vessels (i.e., shunt vascularity), an enlarged main pulmonary artery, and an enlarged left atrium. Pulmonary hyperinflation is common. Patients typically present after 6 weeks of age with failure to thrive and a murmur on physical exam (pulmonary vascular resistance drops at this time, allowing the left-to-right shunt of VSD to manifest). As with any left-to-right shunt, if untreated, VSD may lead to severe pulmonary hypertension with eventual reversal of flow across the shunt, referred to as Eisenmenger physiology.
- **Atrial septal defect (ASD)**. As with small VSDs, radiographic findings may be absent with ASDs. Larger ASDs, however, are associated with mild cardiomegaly, normal-to-enlarged main pulmonary artery, and shunt vascularity. In contrast to an isolated VSD, the left atrium is not enlarged with an ASD. Patients with ASD usually present at an older age than those with VSD, since there is relatively decreased blood flow across the shunt. ASDs are more likely to be clinically occult, and therefore, patients are more likely to have severe pulmonary hypertension at presentation.
- **Patent ductus arteriosus (PDA)**. The ductus arteriosus normally closes in the immediate perinatal period. Failure to close results in continued shunting of blood across the ductus. As an isolated lesion, PDA is commonly seen in premature infants. Radiographic findings include variable degrees of cardiomegaly and shunt vascularity. Over time, left atrial and left ventricular enlargement may develop. When associated with more complex congenital heart disease, PDA may be necessary for survival.

■ Additional Differential Diagnoses

- **Atrioventricular canal defect**. This defect is also commonly referred to as an endocardial cushion defect. It is characterized by failure of the atrial and ventricular septum to develop fully; the mitral and/or tricuspid valves are abnormal as well. Nearly 50% of patients have trisomy 21. As with other left-to-right shunts, radiographic findings include cardiomegaly, pulmonary artery enlargement, and shunt vascularity.

■ Diagnosis

Ventricular septal defect

✓ Pearls

- VSD is the most common septal defect; larger lesions result in cardiomegaly and shunt vascularity.
- Patients with ASD typically present at a later age than VSD because of decreased flow across the shunt.
- PDA commonly occurs in premature infants, as well as patients with complex congenital heart disease.
- Nearly half of patients with an atrioventricular canal (endocardial cushion) defect have trisomy 21.

Suggested Readings

Ferguson EC, Krishnamurthy R, Oldham SA. Classic imaging signs of congenital cardiovascular abnormalities. Radiographics. 2007; 27(5):1323–1334

Kellenberger CJ, Yoo SJ, Büchel ER. Cardiovascular MR imaging in neonates and infants with congenital heart disease. Radiographics. 2007; 27(1):5–18

Lapierre C, Déry J, Guérin R, Viremouneix L, Dubois J, Garel L. Segmental approach to imaging of congenital heart disease. Radiographics. 2010; 30(2):397–411

Schweigmann G, Gassner I, Maurer K. Imaging the neonatal heart--essentials for the radiologist. Eur J Radiol. 2006; 60(2):159–170

Case 161

Rebecca Stein-Wexler

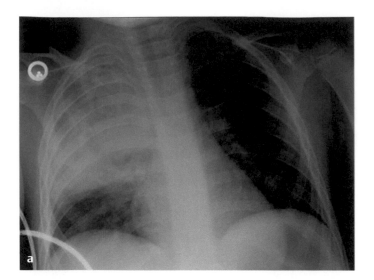
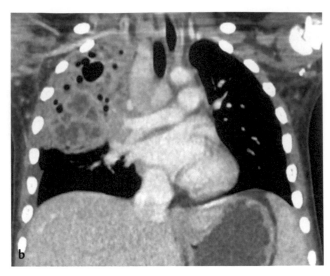
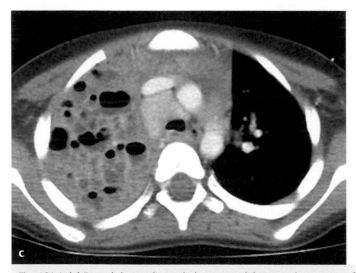

Fig. 161.1 (a) Frontal chest radiograph shows consolidation and expansion of the right upper lobe. **(b)** Coronal reformatted and **(c)** axial contrast-enhanced CT images show a mass that consists of multiple fluid- and gas-filled variably sized cysts. Most are less than 2 cm in diameter.

■ Clinical Presentation

A 4-year-old boy with cough and fever (▶Fig. 161.1).

■ Key Imaging Finding

Pulmonary mass

■ Top 3 Differential Diagnoses

- **Round pneumonia**. Round pneumonia presents as a well-defined pulmonary opacity in children up to 8 years of age, most often in the superior segment of a lower lobe. Usually caused by *Streptococcus pneumoniae*, the inflammatory process is confined because collateral pathways of air flow are less developed in this age group. In the appropriate clinical setting, a follow-up chest radiograph is suggested to ensure resolution with antibiotic therapy.
- **Congenital pulmonary airway malformation (CPAM)**. Part of the spectrum of bronchopulmonary foregut malformations, CPAM is often diagnosed in utero. Older patients may present with respiratory distress or recurrent pneumonia. CPAM consists of abnormal proliferation of respiratory elements that communicate with the tracheobronchial tree. It is differentiated into three types (I: cysts ≥ 2 cm, most common; II: many smaller cysts, associated with congenital anomalies; III: grossly solid but truly microcystic). In infants, the mass may appear solid on radiographs, although often it is occult; a solid or cystic mass is seen in older children. Computed tomography (CT) demonstrates air- or fluid-filled cysts or a solid lesion, depending upon the type. Resection is generally recommended because of increased risk of infection and malignancy.
- **Sequestration**. Pulmonary sequestration is a congenital lesion consisting of dysplastic and nonfunctioning lung tissue with systemic arterial supply. It connects with the tracheobronchial tree only when superinfected. It most often occurs in the left lower lobe. Frequently diagnosed in utero, this too can present with respiratory distress or pneumonia. Extralobar sequestration presents early in life, drains into the systemic venous system, and has its own pleural covering, whereas intralobar sequestration presents later in life with recurring infections, drains into the pulmonary venous system, and lacks a pleural covering. Both appear as a solid mass unless they contain areas of CPAM or have become superinfected, when tissue breakdown permits communication with the bronchial tree.

■ Additional Differential Diagnoses

- **Bronchogenic cyst**. The bronchogenic foregut duplication cyst typically presents as a solitary, discrete mediastinal mass, but it occasionally occurs in the medial lung parenchyma. It may contain simple or complex fluid, and its wall is typically thin unless superinfected. Mass effect on mediastinal structures may cause dysphagia or respiratory distress; older children may complain of chest pain.
- **Pleuropulmonary blastoma**. This rare, aggressive, primitive pleural-based or parenchymal neoplasm presents as a large (>5 cm) cystic, solid, or mixed soft-tissue mass. Pleural effusion is common, and the disease is often initially diagnosed as pneumonia. Childhood cancers are common in close relatives.

■ Diagnosis

Congenital pulmonary airway malformation (mixed, types I and II)

✓ Pearls

- Round pneumonia presents in children up to 8 years of age because of less developed collateral air flow.
- CPAMs communicate with the airway and are classified based on their cystic and/or solid makeup.
- Sequestrations have systemic arterial supply and are further classified according to venous drainage.
- Sequestrations are much more common in the lower lobes, especially on the left.

Suggested Readings

Newman B. Congenital bronchopulmonary foregut malformations: concepts and controversies. Pediatr Radiol. 2006; 36(8):773–791

Restrepo R, Palani R, Matapathi UM, Wu YY. Imaging of round pneumonia and mimics in children. Pediatr Radiol. 2010; 40(12):1931–1940

Yikilmaz A, Lee EY. CT imaging of mass-like nonvascular pulmonary lesions in children. Pediatr Radiol. 2007; 37(12):1253–1263

Case 162

William T. O'Brien, Sr.

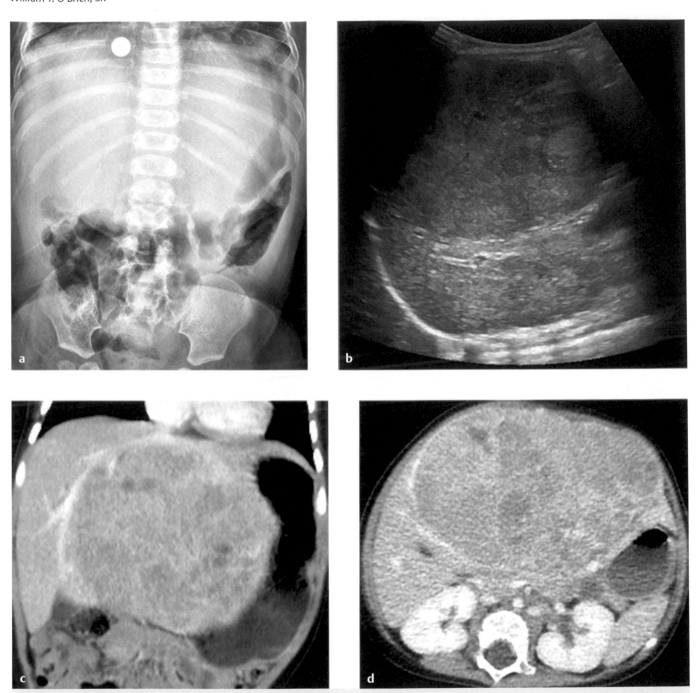

Fig. 162.1 (a) Abdominal radiograph shows mass effect displacing bowel. (b) US of the liver shows a large, ill-defined, heterogeneous mass. Contrast-enhanced (c) coronal and (d) axial CT images reveal a heterogeneous mass with foci of intense enhancement and cystic areas. The mass stretches and displaces the hepatic vasculature.

■ Clinical Presentation

A 12-month-old male infant with hepatomegaly on physical exam (▶Fig. 162.1).

■ Key Imaging Finding

Liver mass in an infant

■ Top 3 Differential Diagnoses

- **Hepatoblastoma.** Hepatoblastoma is the most common primary hepatic neoplasm in infancy, with the vast majority of cases occurring within the first 3 years of life. Patients usually present with a painless abdominal mass. Greater than 90% of patients have elevated levels of alpha-fetoprotein (AFP), a useful discriminator. The lesions are typically large, solitary, heterogeneous, and well-circumscribed, although they may also appear ill-defined. They are hypodense on computed tomography (CT), with calcifications in about 50% of cases. The calcifications are "chunky," compared to fine or coarse calcifications of hemangioendothelioma. Solid elements enhance slightly. On ultrasound (US), hepatoblastomas are heterogeneous with regions of calcification.
- **Hemangioendothelioma.** Hemangioendothelioma is a vascular hepatic lesion that occurs in neonates, with approximately 90% of cases presenting within the first 6 months of life. When large, they can be associated with high-output cardiac failure from vascular shunting. The lesions are often large, heterogeneous, and hypodense to surrounding normal liver parenchyma on CT. Calcifications are common and are typically described as fine or coarse. Enhancement is the rule, although the pattern varies depending on lesion size and number. Vascular shunting may result in enlargement of the suprahepatic aorta and decreased caliber of the infrahepatic aorta.
- **Mesenchymal hamartoma.** Mesenchymal hamartomas are uncommon benign hepatic masses that typically present in infancy. The masses are typically large, well-circumscribed, cystic, and multi-loculated. If there are solid components, the imaging appearance resembles hepatoblastoma or hemangioendothelioma.

■ Additional Differential Diagnoses

- **Metastases.** Neuroblastoma metastases typically arise from primary adrenal lesions, although the primary site may occur anywhere along the sympathetic chain. Metastatic foci are commonly heterogeneous secondary to hemorrhage and calcification. Metastatic foci from Wilms tumor (less common than from neuroblastoma) are hypodense on CT.
- **Abscess.** Large hepatic abscesses may rarely mimic primary hepatic lesions. Like abscesses elsewhere, they are hypodense on CT with peripheral enhancement. Abscesses result from hematogenous or direct spread from the primary site of infection.
- **Hematoma.** Hepatic hematomas vary in size and appearance based on the mechanism of injury and extent of trauma. They are usually hypodense to surrounding normal liver parenchyma on CT. Care should be taken to exclude areas of active extravasation of contrast. Follow-up imaging will show regression.

■ Diagnosis

Hepatoblastoma

✓ Pearls

- Hepatoblastoma is the most common primary hepatic malignancy of infancy and has elevated AFP levels.
- Hemangioendothelioma may be associated with vascular shunting and high-output cardiac failure.
- Mesenchymal hamartoma is usually large, multiloculated, and cystic.
- Neuroblastoma and Wilms tumor are the most common malignancies to metastasize to the liver.

Suggested Readings

Helmberger TK, Ros PR, Mergo PJ, Tomczak R, Reiser MF. Pediatric liver neoplasms: a radiologic-pathologic correlation. Eur Radiol. 1999; 9(7):1339–1347

Woodward PJ, Sohaey R, Kennedy A, Koeller KK. From the archives of the AFIP: a comprehensive review of fetal tumors with pathologic correlation. Radiographics. 2005; 25(1):215–242

Case 163

Karen M. Ayotte

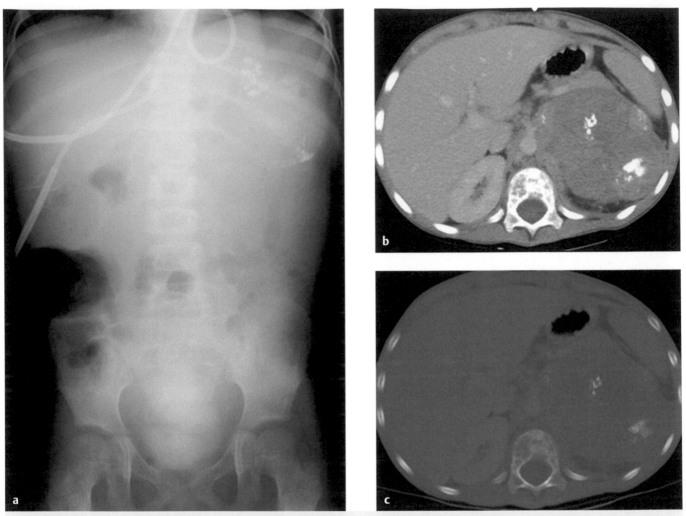

Fig. 163.1 (a) Abdominal radiograph shows coarse calcifications in the left upper quadrant with inferior displacement of the left renal silhouette. (b) Axial contrast-enhanced CT shows a predominantly hypodense mass with chunky calcifications and limited enhancement in the left upper quadrant. (c) Bone windows confirm the presence of calcification.

■ Clinical Presentation

A 5-year-old girl with profuse watery diarrhea (▶ Fig. 163.1).

■ Key Imaging Finding

Suprarenal mass in a child

■ Top 3 Differential Diagnoses

- **Neuroblastoma**. Neuroblastoma is a malignant tumor of primitive neural crest cells. This tumor accounts for approximately 10% of all pediatric neoplasms. Average age at diagnosis is approximately 2 years, and nearly all cases are diagnosed by age 10. Affected children are typically quite ill. They may present with paraneoplastic syndromes, including profuse, watery diarrhea because of vasoactive intestinal peptide secretion. The tumor may arise anywhere along the sympathetic chain, but it usually arises from the adrenal gland. Imaging features include an infiltrative soft-tissue mass that commonly calcifies, encases rather than invades vessels, and metastasizes to liver and bone.
- **Pheochromocytoma**. Approximately 70% of pheochromocytomas arise from the adrenal gland. These tumors are rare in children, usually presenting with hypertension. Most occur spontaneously, but incidence is increased in patients with multiple endocrine neoplasia and von Hippel–Lindau syndromes. These tumors are usually MIBG avid and are classically very bright on T2-weighted magnetic resonance (MR) images. On computed tomography (CT), the tumors are typically large and heterogeneous, with avid solid enhancement and regions of necrosis or cystic change. Fewer than 10% have calcifications.
- **Subdiaphragmatic sequestration**. Although far more common in the lower lobes, pulmonary sequestrations may occur in a subdiaphragmatic, usually left, suprarenal location. Always extralobar, they drain into the systemic venous system. As with all sequestrations, arterial supply is directly from the aorta.

■ Additional Differential Diagnoses

- **Adrenal hemorrhage**. In the perinatal period, adrenal hemorrhage is a significantly more common cause of a suprarenal mass than is neuroblastoma. In the absence of trauma, however, it is uncommon in older children. Classic ultrasound imaging findings are a hypo- or anechoic, avascular suprarenal mass, although in the acute phase hemorrhage may appear complex. On computed tomography (CT), adrenal hemorrhage is hyperdense acutely and becomes iso- to hypodense over time. Serial imaging shows progressive decrease in size, often eventually leading to radiographically evident focal calcification.
- **Adrenocortical carcinoma**. Although a rare tumor of childhood, adrenocortical carcinomas are more common than simple adenomas. They are usually hormonally active. The tumors are typically greater than 5 cm in diameter at presentation. Internal necrosis and calcification are common, yielding an irregular, heterogeneous mass.
- **Congenital adrenal hyperplasia (CAH)**. CAH represents a heterogeneous group of autosomal recessive disorders that typically include an underlying enzyme deficiency. It is a clinical diagnosis with confirmatory laboratory testing. Imaging demonstrates bilateral diffuse or nodular adrenal enlargement.

■ Diagnosis

Neuroblastoma

✓ Pearls

- Neuroblastoma is malignant, commonly calcifies, encases vessels, and metastasizes to liver and bone.
- Adrenal hemorrhage is common in the perinatal period and decreases in size over time.
- Pediatric pheochromocytomas are most common in children with underlying syndromes.

Suggested Readings

Balassy C, Navarro OM, Daneman A. Adrenal masses in children. Radiol Clin North Am. 2011; 49(4):711–727, vi

Nour-Eldin NE, Abdelmonem O, Tawfik AM, et al. Pediatric primary and metastatic neuroblastoma: MRI findings: pictorial review. Magn Reson Imaging. 2012; 30(7):893–906

Paterson A. Adrenal pathology in childhood: a spectrum of disease. Eur Radiol. 2002; 12(10):2491–2508

Case 164

John P. Lichtenberger III

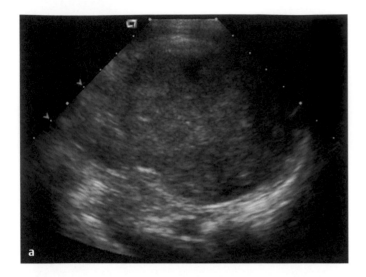
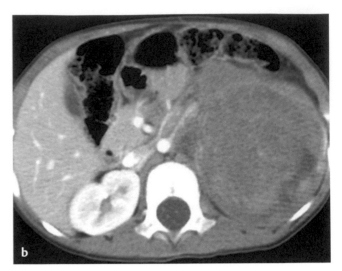
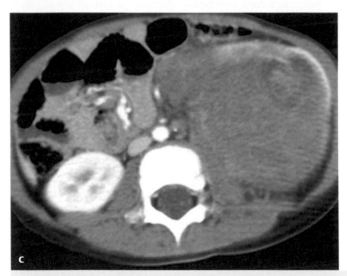

Fig. 164.1 (a) Transverse ultrasound of the kidney shows a large heterogeneous mass. **(b,c)** Axial contrast-enhanced computed tomography (CT) images show a partially circumscribed and heterogeneously enhancing left renal mass. The mass/thrombus extends into the left renal vein and inferior vena cava **(b)**. **(c)** Renal tissue stretches around the mass, resulting in the "claw sign," which confirms renal origin.

■ Clinical Presentation

A 3-year-old with asymptomatic abdominal mass on exam (▶Fig. 164.1).

■ Key Imaging Finding

Solid renal mass in a child

■ Top 3 Differential Diagnoses

- **Wilms tumor**. Wilms tumor is the most common renal malignancy of childhood, with peak incidence at 3 years of age. Patients often present with an abdominal mass. Wilms tumor is characteristically a well-defined, round mass arising from the renal cortex with local mass effect. The tumor generally enhances to a lesser degree than the surrounding renal parenchyma. Renal origin is confirmed by noting compressed renal parenchyma along the margin of the tumor, referred to as the "claw sign." When large, these tumors may appear heterogeneous and partially cystic with internal necrosis and hemorrhage. Calcification is relatively uncommon. Intratumoral fat is extremely rare. Wilms tumor spreads locally through the ipsilateral renal vein, via lymphatics to local lymph nodes, and hematogenously to the liver, lungs, and bones. Associated syndromes include WAGR (Wilms tumor, aniridia, genital anomalies, and mental retardation) and Beckwith–Wiedemann syndrome. Staging is surgical.

- **Nephroblastomatosis**. Persistence of nephrogenic rests is termed nephroblastomatosis. These lesions typically present as bilateral, confluent, plaquelike or rounded, peripheral solid renal masses in infants. Annual surveillance is required to exclude malignant degeneration to Wilms tumor.

- **Lymphoma**. Although primary renal lymphoma is rare, secondary involvement is common. Patients may present with multiple bilateral homogeneous hypodense parenchymal masses (most common), a solitary renal mass, or diffuse infiltration of the renal parenchyma. Bulky adjacent extrarenal lymphadenopathy is a diagnostic clue.

■ Additional Differential Diagnoses

- **Mesoblastic nephroma**. Mesoblastic nephroma is a hamartomatous solid tumor of the kidney and represents the most common solid renal mass in neonates. Mean age at presentation is 2 months. Patients are typically asymptomatic except for a palpable mass, although hypercalcemia may occasionally be detected clinically. Since mesoblastic nephroma is indistinguishable from Wilms tumor based on imaging findings, treatment is surgical.

- **Renal cell carcinoma (RCC)**. RCC is relatively rare in childhood, except in the setting of von Hippel–Lindau disease. Patients are typically older and present with flank pain or hematuria. Imaging findings most commonly reveal a hypervascular renal mass. Calcification is seen in 25% of cases. RCC spreads locally through the ipsilateral renal vein, via lymphatics to local lymph nodes, and hematogenously to the liver, lungs, and bones.

■ Diagnosis

Wilms tumor

✓ Pearls

- Wilms tumor is the most common renal malignancy of childhood with a peak incidence at 3 years of age.
- Wilms tumor may spread by direct extension (renal vein), lymphatic spread, and hematogenous spread.

- Mesoblastic nephroma is a benign, hamartomatous lesion with a peak incidence at 2 to 3 months of age.
- Nephroblastomatosis is usually bilateral and may degenerate into Wilms tumor.

Suggested Readings

Geller E, Kochan PS. Renal neoplasms of childhood. Radiol Clin North Am. 2011; 49(4):689–709, vi

Lowe LH, Isuani BH, Heller RM, et al. Pediatric renal masses: Wilms tumor and beyond. Radiographics. 2000; 20(6):1585–1603

McHugh K. Renal and adrenal tumours in children. Cancer Imaging. 2007; 7:41–51

Siegel MJ, Chung EM. Wilms tumor and other pediatric renal masses. Magn Reson Imaging Clin N Am. 2008; 16(3):479–497, vi

Case 165

William T. O'Brien, Sr.

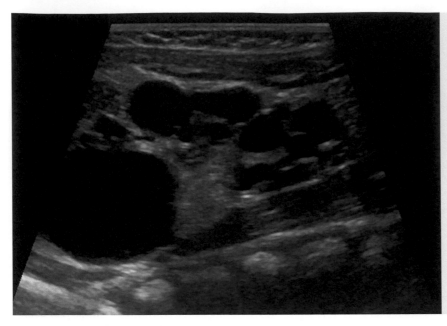

Fig. 165.1 Longitudinal US of the left kidney shows renal enlargement with multiple circumscribed anechoic lesions. The right kidney appeared normal (not shown).

■ Clinical Presentation

Newborn male with left-sided palpable abdominal mass on routine physical examination (▶Fig. 165.1).

■ Key Imaging Finding

Unilateral cystic kidney

■ Top 3 Differential Diagnoses

- **Hydronephrosis.** Hydronephrosis is the most common cause of a renal mass in a child. Unilateral disease is most often due to ureteropelvic junction (UPJ) obstruction or extrinsic compression on the ureter; bilateral hydronephrosis is usually due to bladder outlet obstruction (posterior urethral valves in boys). On ultrasound (US), the cystic lesions communicate centrally at the renal pelvis, a key distinguishing factor.
- **Multicystic dysplastic kidney (MCDK).** MCDK is thought to result from intrauterine obstruction of the fetal renal collecting system or altered induction of renal tissue because of an abnormal UPJ. Sonographic findings include multiple cysts

of varying sizes that do not communicate with one another. The affected renal segment is nonfunctioning. The other kidney should be closely evaluated, since contralateral anomalies (such as UPJ obstruction) are common.
- **Multilocular cystic nephroma (MLCN).** MLCN is a rare entity with a bimodal age distribution that affects young males and older adult females. Patients present with a multiloculated cystic renal mass that characteristically herniates into the renal pelvis/collecting system. Septations within the lesion may enhance on computed tomography (CT). The lesions are surgically resected.

■ Additional Differential Diagnoses

- **Cystic Wilms tumor.** Wilms tumor represents the most common childhood renal malignancy, with a peak incidence at 3 years of age. Patients typically present with a large, heterogeneous, solid abdominal mass, but Wilms tumor may occasionally be cystic. Local spread includes the renal vein, inferior vena cava, and lymph nodes; distant metastases include the lungs, liver, and bones. Rarely, both kidneys may be involved. Unlike neuroblastoma, Wilms tumor invades vessels rather than encasing them. Wilms tumor is typically sporadic but may be associated with cryptorchidism, hemihypertrophy, aniridia, Drash (Wilms tumor, congenital nephropathy, and gonadal dysgenesis with ambiguous genitalia), and other syndromes.

- **Autosomal dominant polycystic kidney disease (ADPKD).** ADPKD usually presents in late adolescence or early adulthood with hypertension or hematuria, but it may occasionally be seen in infants. The kidneys are enlarged with multiple bilateral cortical and medullary cysts of varying sizes. Cysts also occur in the liver and pancreas. Approximately 10% of patients have intracranial berry aneurysms.
- **Renal abscess.** Renal abscesses are rare but serious complications of urinary tract infections. They usually occur in children with chronic infections from persistent vesicoureteral reflux. US shows an ill-defined hypoechoic region, usually at the corticomedullary junction; focal abscesses are hypodense on CT.

■ Diagnosis

Multicystic dysplastic kidney

✓ Pearls

- Hydronephrosis is the most common cause of a renal mass in childhood.
- MCDK consists of multiple noncommunicating cysts with increased incidence of contralateral anomalies.

- MLCN has a bimodal age distribution and characteristically herniates into the renal pelvis.
- Wilms tumor, the commonest renal malignancy of childhood, may occasionally be cystic.

Suggested Readings

Avni FE, Hall M. Renal cystic diseases in children: new concepts. Pediatr Radiol. 2010; 40(6):939–946

Chung EM, Conran RM, Schroeder JW, Rohena-Quinquilla IR, Rooks VJ. From the radiologic pathology archives: pediatric polycystic kidney disease and

other ciliopathies: radiologic-pathologic correlation. Radiographics. 2014; 34(1):155–178

Lowe LH, Isuani BH, Heller RM, et al. Pediatric renal masses: Wilms tumor and beyond. Radiographics. 2000; 20(6):1585–1603

Case 166

Karen M. Ayotte

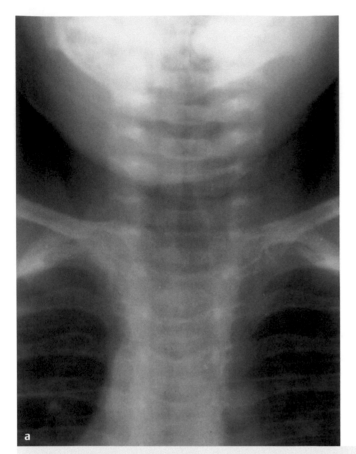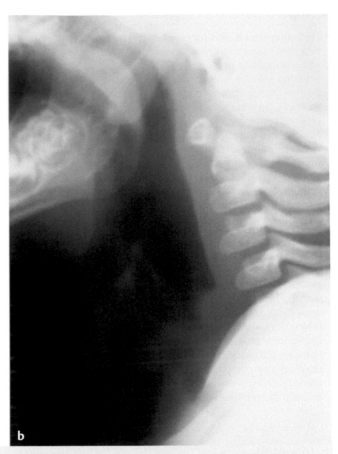

Fig. 166.1 **(a)** Frontal and **(b)** lateral radiographs of the neck reveal subglottic tracheal narrowing with loss of the normal shouldering of the airway on the frontal view, referred to as the "steeple sign." The lateral view also demonstrates overdistention of the hypopharynx **(b)**. The aryepiglottic folds and prevertebral soft-tissue contours are normal.

■ Clinical Presentation

Toddler with stridor (▶ Fig. 166.1).

■ Key Imaging Finding

Toddler with stridor and airway narrowing

■ Top 3 Differential Diagnoses

- **Croup (laryngotracheobronchitis)**. Croup is the most common cause of upper airway obstruction in children between 6 months and 3 years of age, with a peak incidence at around 1 year. The radiographic hallmark is subglottic airway narrowing manifested by loss of the normal shouldering of the upper airway on the frontal projection, referred to as the "steeple" sign. The lateral view commonly demonstrates overdistention of the hypopharynx, as well as narrowing of the subglottic airway.
- **Epiglottitis**. This potentially life-threatening disease affects patients older than those with croup. When the diagnosis is suspected, a provider capable of managing the child's airway should be immediately available during imaging. The radio-graphic hallmark is epiglottic enlargement (thumb sign) on the lateral view, as well as thick aryepiglottic folds. Epiglottitis may mimic croup on a frontal view.
- **Retropharyngeal abscess**. Space-occupying processes in the prevertebral and retropharyngeal soft tissues may exert mass effect on the airway, causing dyspnea and stridor. The differential diagnosis of widened prevertebral soft tissues includes abscess, hemorrhage, lymphadenopathy, and pseudothickening. If physiologic pseudothickening is suspected, a repeat inspiratory exam with the neck fully extended may resolve the dilemma. Airway fluoroscopy may also be employed to clarify difficult cases.

■ Additional Differential Diagnoses

- **Bacterial tracheitis**. Bacterial tracheitis is characterized by exudative plaques that adhere to the tracheal walls. Because of their flat, longitudinal configuration, they may be seen only on one view. Asymmetric subglottic airway narrowing may resemble the radiographic appearance of croup. However, patients with bacterial tracheitis are typically older (6–10 years old) and more toxic. Adherent mucus in the airway commonly mimics the plaques of bacterial tracheitis but should clear on repeat exam after coughing.
- **Aspirated foreign body**. Both aspirated and ingested foreign bodies may cause abnormal airway contours on radiographs, as well as present with dyspnea and stridor. Radioopaque foreign bodies are readily identified, whereas radiographic diagnosis of the more common nonopaque foreign bodies is problematic. Direct visualization may be necessary. Air trapping may be seen distal to the affected airway segment.
- **Hemangioma**. Hemangiomas tend to cause variably asymmetric airway narrowing and are commonly detected before age 1 year. When subglottic, the patient's symptoms may mimic other more common etiologies of stridor. Radiographs show asymmetric mass effect narrowing the airway.

■ Diagnosis

Croup

✓ Pearls

- Croup is most common in children younger than 3 years; the "steeple" sign is seen on frontal radiographs.
- Epiglottitis is potentially life-threatening; lateral radiographs show epiglottic thickening (thumb sign).
- Retropharyngeal abscesses present with prevertebral soft-tissue swelling.
- Foreign body aspiration must always be considered in a child with stridor.

Suggested Readings

John SD, Swischuk LE. Stridor and upper airway obstruction in infants and children. Radiographics. 1992; 12(4):625–643, discussion 644

Yedururi S, Guillerman RP, Chung T, et al. Multimodality imaging of tracheobronchial disorders in children. Radiographics. 2008; 28(3):e29

Case 167

Sandra L. Wootton-Gorges

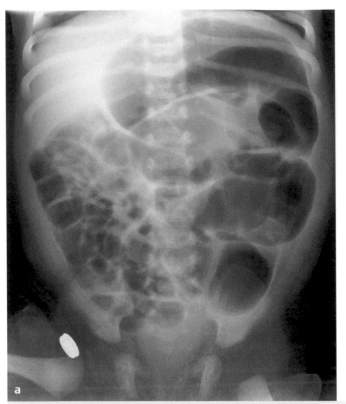
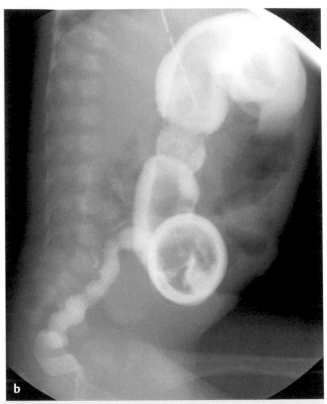

Fig. 167.1 (a) Supine abdominal radiograph shows multiple dilated bowel loops throughout the abdomen, but no rectal gas. (b) There is no evidence of extraluminal gas. Water-soluble contrast enema shows a narrow rectal caliber, with a transition zone at the distal sigmoid. The colon proximal to this point is distended and filled with meconium.

■ Clinical Presentation

A 35-week gestational age newborn boy with abdominal distension and bilious residuals after feeding. He has not passed meconium at 30 hours of age (▶Fig. 167.1).

■ Key Imaging Finding

Distal bowel obstruction in a neonate

■ Top 3 Differential Diagnoses

- **Functional immaturity of the colon**. Functional immaturity includes small left colon and meconium plug syndrome. This common cause of low bowel obstruction is associated with prematurity, infants whose mothers received magnesium sulfate or opiates during labor, and infants of diabetic mothers. Infants present with failure to pass meconium, abdominal distension, and/or vomiting. Abdominal radiographs show diffuse bowel distension. Contrast enema defines a normal rectum and a meconium plug in the rectosigmoid colon. The left colon may be small in caliber to the splenic flexure. No organic obstruction is seen. The stooling pattern becomes normal after the contrast enema stimulates passage of meconium.
- **Hirschsprung disease (HD)**. HD results from failure of complete craniocaudal migration of intramural ganglion cells. The aganglionic segment cannot relax, resulting in distal bowel obstruction. Symptoms may include constipation, abdominal distension, and/or bilious vomiting. About 2% of patients with Down syndrome have HD. Radiographs show distal bowel obstruction. A transition zone between the spastic, narrow distal colon and the dilated more proximal colon is defined at contrast enema, usually in the rectosigmoid region. Rarely HD affects the entire colon (resembling a "lead pipe"). Suction biopsy confirms absence of ganglion cells below the transition zone.
- **Ileal atresia/stenosis**. Ileal atresia/stenosis probably results from focal intrauterine ischemic injury. Neonates present with low bowel obstruction. Contrast enema is very helpful in defining the normally positioned microcolon, which results from colonic nonuse.

■ Additional Differential Diagnoses

- **Meconium ileus**. Meconium ileus may be the first sign of cystic fibrosis. Tenacious meconium blocks the terminal ileum and right colon, resulting in low bowel obstruction. Radiographs may show a lack of fluid–fluid levels, as well as a soap-bubble appearance in the right lower quadrant. A contrast enema defines meconium pellets in the distal ileum and right colon, as well as the smallest of microcolons. Diagnostic water-soluble enema may also be therapeutic, allowing meconium pellets to pass.
- **Anal atresia-anorectal malformations**: Anal atresia is an important cause of low bowel obstruction in infants. It is usually clinically evident. It is important to evaluate for associated renal and spinal cord anomalies in these babies, and to differentiate between high and low atresias.

■ Diagnosis

Hirschsprung disease

✓ Pearls

- Functional immaturity of the colon is associated with prematurity and infants of diabetic mothers.
- HD is due to aganglionosis; the transition point is usually in the rectosigmoid region.
- Ileal atresia is thought to result from intrauterine ischemia; there is microcolon because of nonuse.
- Meconium ileus occurs in cystic fibrosis and shows extreme microcolon with meconium pellets in the ileum.

Suggested Readings

Berrocal T, Lamas M, Gutieérrez J, Torres I, Prieto C, del Hoyo ML. Congenital anomalies of the small intestine, colon, and rectum. Radiographics. 1999; 19(5):1219–1236

Rao P. Neonatal gastrointestinal imaging. Eur J Radiol. 2006; 60(2):171–186
Vinocur DN, Lee EY, Eisenberg RL. Neonatal intestinal obstruction. AJR Am J Roentgenol. 2012; 198(1):W1–10

Case 168

Rebecca Stein-Wexler

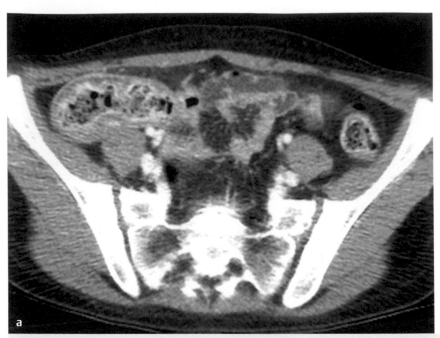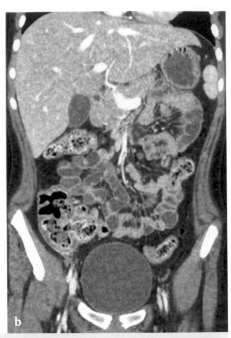

Fig. 168.1 (a) Contrast-enhanced axial CT of the pelvis demonstrates circumferential, symmetric, marked thickening of the wall of the cecum. There is mild heterogeneous enhancement and slight surrounding inflammation. (b) The coronal reformatted CT shows involvement of the proximal ascending colon as well, but bowel elsewhere is normal.

■ Clinical Presentation

An 11-year-old girl with history of acute myelocytic leukemia, status post bone marrow transplant, now presenting with fever and severe diarrhea (▶Fig. 168.1).

■ Key Imaging Finding

Bowel wall thickening in an immunocompromised child

■ Top 3 Differential Diagnoses

- **Pseudomembranous colitis.** Pseudomembranous colitis results from overgrowth of *Clostridium difficile* and usually occurs in patients receiving antibiotics. The colonic wall is markedly thickened secondary to mucosal and submucosal edema that creates central hypodensity. The disease usually affects the entire colon, but occasionally only the right colon is involved. The "accordion sign" results from intraluminal fluid extending between pseudomembranes and edematous haustra. Pericolonic fat is relatively spared.
- **Neutropenic colitis/typhlitis.** This inflammatory and necrotizing colitis occurs in neutropenic children and typically involves the entire right colon. However, it may be limited to the cecum or include the terminal ileum. Most common in those with acute leukemia, it presents with fever, diarrhea, and tenderness. The classic appearance is circumferential, symmetric mural thickening that is hypodense on unenhanced computed tomography (CT) and enhances heterogeneously. Pericolonic inflammatory stranding is common, and intramural pneumatosis may occur. Contrast enema is contraindicated because of perforation risk. Perforation and sepsis result in the high mortality rate of 40 to 50% in patients treated medically.
- **Graft-versus-host disease (GVHD).** GVHD occurs when marrow T-lymphocytes damage recipient epithelial cells. Older children are at increased risk. Patients typically present with diarrhea, hepatomegaly, ascites, and resultant abdominal distension. Mucosal ulceration and destruction occur, followed by replacement of mucosa with vascular granulation tissue. This results in the typical CT appearance of intense mucosal enhancement along with dilatation affecting the entire small and large bowel. On small bowel follow-through (SBFT), the contrast-filled bowel has a "ribbonlike" appearance. Treatment consists of increased immunosuppression, and outcomes are usually good.

■ Additional Differential Diagnoses

- **Posttransplant lymphoproliferative disorder.** This disorder ranges from lymphoid hyperplasia to malignant proliferation and is associated with reactivation of Epstein–Barr virus in the setting of chronic immunosuppression. It typically occurs in recipients of organ transplants. There is circumferential bowel wall thickening, sometimes accompanied with aneurysmal dilatation. Lymphadenopathy, solid masses, and hepatosplenomegaly also occur. Early diagnosis and treatment are essential.
- **Shock bowel.** Shock bowel, or hypoperfusion complex, causes diffuse bowel wall enhancement and thickening, along with abnormally intense enhancement of solid organs. The bowel enhancement pattern is similar to GVHD, but shock bowel occurs with major trauma and usually spares the colon.

■ Diagnosis

Neutropenic colitis

✓ Pearls

- In the setting of severe colitis, contrast enema is contraindicated because of risk of perforation.
- Pseudomembranous colitis is due to *C. difficile* overgrowth; the accordion sign may be seen on imaging.

- Neutropenic colitis occurs in immunosuppressed patients and most often involves the cecum/right colon.
- GVHD presents with intense mucosal enhancement on CT and a "ribbonlike" appearance on SBFT.

Suggested Readings

Khoury NJ, Kanj V, Abboud M, Muwakkit S, Birjawi GA, Haddad MC. Abdominal complications of chemotherapy in pediatric malignancies: imaging findings. Clin Imaging. 2009; 33(4):253–260

Lee V, Cheng PS, Chik KW, Wong GW, Shing MM, Li CK. Autoimmune hypothyroidism after unrelated haematopoietic stem cell transplantation in children. J Pediatr Hematol Oncol. 2006; 28(5):293–295

Levine DS, Navarro OM, Chaudry G, Doyle JJ, Blaser SI. Imaging the complications of bone marrow transplantation in children. Radiographics. 2007; 27(2):307–324

Case 169

John P. Lichtenberger III

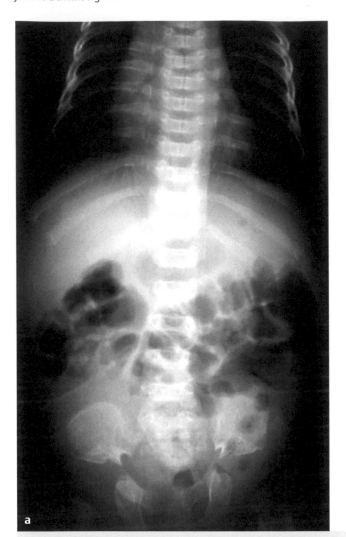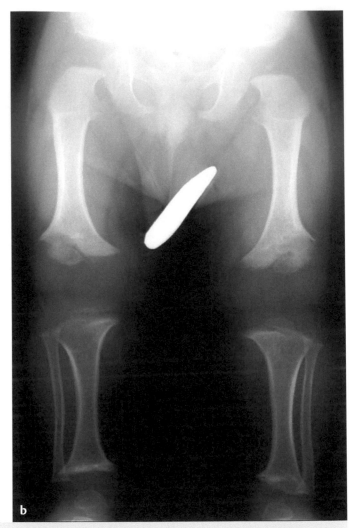

Fig. 169.1 **(a)** Frontal radiograph of the chest and abdomen demonstrates decreased interpediculate distances at the lower lumbar spine. Ribs are short and thick, and the pelvis has "tombstone" iliac bones secondary to decreased acetabular angles and a "champagne-glass" pelvic inlet. **(b)** Frontal radiograph of the lower extremities shows rhizomelic limb shortening, broad and relatively lucent femoral necks, and inverted "V" configuration of the distal femurs.

■ Clinical Presentation

Growth and skeletal abnormalities (▶Fig. 169.1).

■ Key Imaging Finding

Skeletal dysplasia

■ Top 3 Differential Diagnoses

- **Achondroplasia**. The most common nonlethal dysplasia, achondroplasia is an autosomal dominant disease characterized by skeletal abnormalities attributable to decreased cartilage matrix production and endochondral ossification. Rhizomelic (proximal) limb shortening, metaphyseal flaring, and decreased interpediculate distance within the lower lumbar spine are common findings. Short iliac bones with decreased acetabular angles have been described as having a "tombstone" appearance, and the inner pelvic contour has a "champagne-glass" configuration. The small skull base and foramen magnum may result in brainstem compression. Spine anomalies result in varying degrees of spinal stenosis. **Hypochondroplasia** is a less severe form of achondroplasia in which findings are mild and may be limited to the spine.

- **Thanatophoric dysplasia**. Thanatophoric dysplasia is the most common lethal skeletal dysplasia. Also characterized by rhizomelic (proximal) limb shortening, additional radiographic features include strikingly short ribs resulting in a narrow thorax and poor ventilation, platyspondyly, and small iliac bones. Abnormal bowing and shortening of the femurs result in a characteristic "telephone receiver" appearance. This entity is uniformly fatal in the neonatal period.
- **Jeune syndrome**. In Jeune syndrome, also known as asphyxiating thoracic dysplasia, the thorax is long and bell-shaped, with short, horizontal ribs and flared anterior ends. This configuration results in early respiratory compromise. Dysplastic acetabuli resembling an upside-down trident are often seen. There is associated acromelic (distal) limb shortening.

■ Additional Differential Diagnoses

- **Ellis–van Creveld syndrome**. Hair, nail, and teeth abnormalities are clinical hallmarks of this syndrome (also known as chondroectodermal dysplasia). Radiographic features include acromelic (distal) limb shortening, short ribs, cone-shaped epiphyses, and postaxial polydactyly. Congenital heart disease is the major cause of morbidity.
- **Chondrodysplasia punctata**. This skeletal dysplasia is characterized by rhizomelic limb shortening and multifocal stippling in epiphyses, apophyses, and the spine.

■ Diagnosis

Achondroplasia

✓ Pearls

- Achondroplasia is the most common nonlethal skeletal dysplasia; it is autosomal dominant and rhizomelic.
- Achondroplasia shows decreased interpediculate distance, "champagne-glass" pelvis, and "tombstone" iliacs.

- Thanatophoric dysplasia is uniformly fatal and reveals platyspondyly and "telephone receiver" femurs.
- Jeune syndrome (asphyxiating thoracic dysplasia) presents with a bell-shaped thorax and trident acetabuli.

Suggested Readings

Glass RB, Norton KI, Mitre SA, Kang E. Pediatric ribs: a spectrum of abnormalities. Radiographics. 2002; 22(1):87–104

Lemyre E, Azouz EM, Teebi AS, Glanc P, Chen MF. Bone dysplasia series. Achondroplasia, hypochondroplasia and thanatophoric dysplasia: review and update. Can Assoc Radiol J. 1999; 50(3):185–197

Parnell SE, Phillips GS. Neonatal skeletal dysplasias. Pediatr Radiol. 2012; 42(Suppl 1):S150–S157

Case 170

Karen M. Ayotte

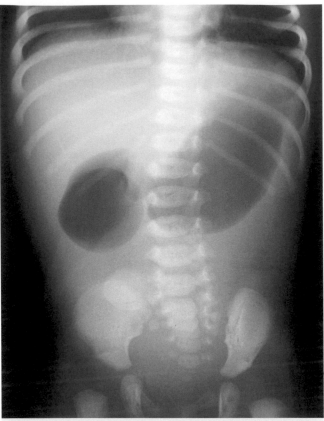

Fig. 170.1 Frontal radiograph of the abdomen demonstrates high-grade obstruction of the duodenum with a "double bubble" configuration of the proximal duodenum and stomach. There is no definite bowel gas distal to the level of obstruction.

■ Clinical Presentation

Newborn with bilious emesis (▶ Fig. 170.1).

■ Key Imaging Finding

"Double bubble" sign

■ Top 3 Differential Diagnoses

- **Malrotation/midgut volvulus.** Midgut volvulus is a surgical emergency that occurs when bowel twists around a narrow mesenteric pedicle in the setting of malrotation. When the diagnosis is suggested, expedited work-up is mandatory to minimize morbidity and mortality. The classic presentation is bilious emesis in an infant in the first month of life with partial duodenal obstruction. However, both clinical presentation and radiographic findings vary, and the radiographic appearance of volvulus ranges from normal to complete duodenal obstruction, mimicking duodenal atresia. An upper gastrointestinal (UGI) examination is needed to establish the course of the duodenum and proximal small bowel. In the setting of malrotation, the duodenal–jejunal junction (ligament of Treitz) fails to cross to the left of midline and/or is located inferior to the pylorus. With volvulus, the proximal bowel demonstrates a "corkscrew" appearance.
- **Duodenal atresia/stenosis.** Both duodenal atresia and duodenal stenosis result from a failure of recanalization of the

duodenum, either partial (stenosis) or complete (atresia). The classic radiographic presentation is the "double bubble" sign. In patients with complete atresia, there is usually no gas distal to the dilated duodenum. Patients present with vomiting in the first few hours of life. In 80%, emesis is bilious, but if the obstruction is proximal to the ampulla of Vater it will be nonbilious. The degree of duodenal dilation is usually marked, implying longstanding obstruction. There is an increased incidence of associated abnormalities, including a 30% incidence of Down syndrome. Duodenal stenosis may present in older patients.

- **Annular pancreas.** Annular pancreas often coexists with duodenal atresia or stenosis. Annular pancreas may present in infancy with duodenal obstruction or in adulthood with chronic nausea and vomiting. Cross-sectional imaging shows a soft-tissue mass contiguous with the pancreas, encircling the duodenum. UGI typically shows circumferential narrowing of the second portion of the duodenum.

■ Additional Differential Diagnoses

- **Duodenal web.** Intraluminal duodenal webs cause a variable degree of obstruction, and thus patients may present as older children or even adults. With severe obstruction in an infant, however, the radiographic appearance resembles other causes of duodenal obstruction. UGI may show circumferential narrowing of the duodenum or a variable-sized aperture, allowing

a restricted amount of contrast material to pass distally. Over time, the web may stretch, leading to a "windsock" appearance.

- **Preduodenal portal vein.** A preduodenal portal vein may obstruct the duodenum. It is usually accompanied by malrotation or other anomalies.

■ Diagnosis

Duodenal atresia

✓ Pearls

- Malrotation with midgut volvulus is a surgical emergency requiring immediate diagnosis and intervention.
- An UGI establishes the course of the duodenum and position of the ligament of Treitz.

- Duodenal atresia classically presents with the "double bubble" sign; 30% of patients have Down syndrome.
- Annular pancreas results in circumferential narrowing of the second portion of the duodenum.

Suggested Readings

Berrocal T, Lamas M, Gutieérrez J, Torres I, Prieto C, del Hoyo ML. Congenital anomalies of the small intestine, colon, and rectum. Radiographics. 1999; 19(5):1219–1236

Mortelé KJ, Rocha TC, Streeter JL, Taylor AJ. Multimodality imaging of pancreatic and biliary congenital anomalies. Radiographics. 2006; 26(3):715–731

Rao P. Neonatal gastrointestinal imaging. Eur J Radiol. 2006; 60(2):171–186

Strouse PJ. Disorders of intestinal rotation and fixation ("malrotation"). Pediatr Radiol. 2004; 34(11):837–851

Case 171

Karen M. Ayotte

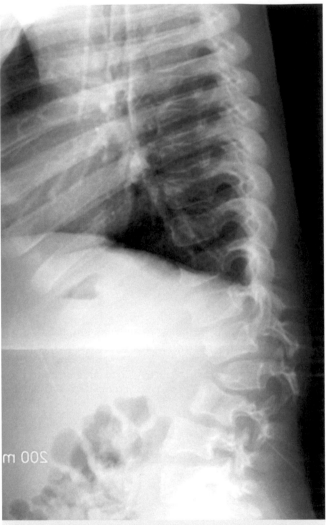

Fig. 171.1 Lateral spine radiograph shows concavity of the posterior vertebral bodies (vertebral scalloping), most pronounced from L2–L5. There is also beaking of the midportion of L2 with focal kyphosis centered at this level.

■ Clinical Presentation

Child with hepatosplenomegaly and coarse facial features (▶Fig. 171.1).

■ Key Imaging Finding

Posterior vertebral body scalloping

■ Top 3 Differential Diagnoses

- **Dural ectasia**. Dural ectasia refers to enlargement or widening of the dural sac. Common causes include connective tissue disorders, such as Marfan and Ehlers–Danlos syndromes, and neurofibromatosis type 1 (NF-1). The weakened dura transmits pressure along the posterior aspect of the vertebral bodies with resultant posterior vertebral body scalloping. In patients with NF-1, masses such as neurofibromas and thoracic meningoceles may also cause posterior vertebral body scalloping. Patients with Marfan and Ehlers–Danlos syndromes are prone to connective tissue abnormalities elsewhere, such as aneurysm formation. NF-1 patients may have cutaneous and neurological manifestations of the disease.
- **Mucopolysaccharidosis (MPS)**. MPSs are inherited disorders caused by deficiencies in lysosomal enzymes necessary to break down certain complex carbohydrates. This leads to excessive accumulation and deposition of lysosomal glycosaminoglycans. Patients often present with short stature, craniofacial abnormalities, and in some cases mental retardation. There are multiple variants of MPSs, with Hurler and Morquio being most common. Both Hurler and Morquio syndromes are associated with diffuse posterior vertebral scalloping, but the mechanism is not well established. Those with Hurler syndrome also demonstrate anterior beaking of the inferior aspect of the vertebral body, while patients with Morquio syndrome have anterior beaking in the midportion of the vertebral body. An enlarged, J-shaped sella is classically seen with Hurler syndrome.
- **Skeletal dysplasia/achondroplasia**. Achondroplasia is a common skeletal dysplasia, with autosomal dominant inheritance. Radiographic findings include a large skull with narrow foramen magnum, spinal stenosis, squared iliac wings, progressively decreasing interpediculate distance in the lumbar spine, flat acetabuli, short metacarpals, and short ribs. Posterior vertebral body scalloping is common and believed to be an adaptive response to congenital spinal stenosis. Posterior scalloping is also associated with metatropic dwarfism and osteogenesis imperfecta.

■ Additional Differential Diagnoses

- **Spinal tumor**. Intrathecal tumors may cause increased pressure within the spinal canal, leading to compensatory posterior vertebral body scalloping. The level of the vertebral scalloping typically corresponds to the location of the tumor. Common primary spinal cord tumors include ependymoma (most common primary cord tumor in adults) and astrocytoma (most common spinal cord tumor in children). Intradural extramedullary tumors include nerve sheath tumors, meningiomas, and metastases. Lipomas, dermoids/epidermoids, and perineural cysts may also lead to mass effect and vertebral body scalloping.
- **Normal variant**. When mild and not associated with other skeletal abnormalities, posterior vertebral body scalloping may be a normal variant. Patients are typically followed after other causes are excluded.

■ Diagnosis

Mucopolysaccharidosis (Morquio syndrome)

✓ Pearls

- Dural ectasia with posterior vertebral body scalloping may be seen with connective tissue disorders and NF-1.
- MPS (Hurler and Morquio) presents with posterior scalloping and anterior beaking of the vertebral body.
- Intrathecal tumors may show posterior vertebral body scalloping as a result of bony remodeling.
- Mild posterior vertebral body scalloping may be a normal developmental variant.

Suggested Readings

Lachman R, Martin KW, Castro S, Basto MA, Adams A, Teles EL. Radiologic and neuroradiologic findings in the mucopolysaccharidoses. J Pediatr Rehabil Med. 2010; 3(2):109–118

Wakely SL. The posterior vertebral scalloping sign. Radiology. 2006; 239(2):607–609

Case 172

Sandra L. Wootton-Gorges

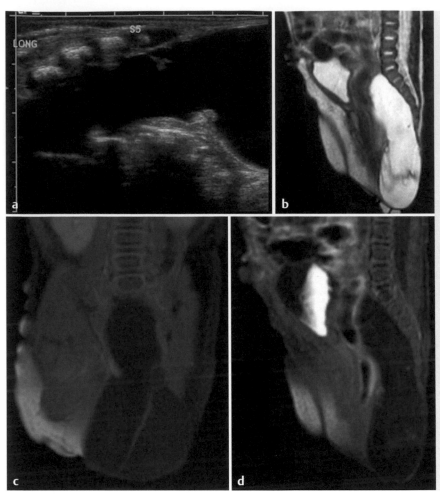

Fig. 172.1 **(a)** Longitudinal US of the spine demonstrates a cystic presacral mass that extends dorsally to a subcutaneous position. **(b)** Sagittal T2 MRI demonstrates a hyperintense mass with multiple septations. The mass is **(c)** hypointense on coronal T1 imaging and **(d,** sagittal T1 fat suppressed) does not enhance. The spine appears normal.

▪ Clinical Presentation

Term infant girl with buttocks and perineal mass (▶Fig. 172.1).

■ Key Imaging Finding

Cystic presacral mass

■ Top 3 Differential Diagnoses

• **Sacrococcygeal teratoma (SCT)**. SCTs are rare tumors that arise from multipotential cells and contain all three germ layers. They are the most common tumor of the caudal region in infants and may be extrapelvic, intrapelvic, or mixed. Most that present in the first few months of life are benign, but the risk of malignancy increases with advancing age. Cystic lesions and those that occur in girls are more often benign. Calcifications are seen in 60% of cases, varying in appearance. The tumors typically appear heterogeneous and variably cystic and solid, fatty, and calcific depending on their composition. Magnetic resonance imaging (MRI) best demonstrates the tumor extent and defines the degree of spinal involvement. The coccyx must be resected to help prevent recurrence.

• **Rectal duplication cyst**. Rectal duplication cysts account for 5% of enteric duplication cysts. They are spherical, thin-walled, uni- or multilocular cystic lesions that may communicate with the rectal lumen. Their walls contain smooth muscle, and they are lined with rectal mucosa, resulting in alternating hypo- and hyperechoic layers of the "gastrointestinal signature."

• **Anterior sacral meningocele (ASM)**. ASMs are rare herniations of cerebrospinal fluid (CSF)-distended meninges through a sacral foramen or defect. MRI is the best modality to define the lesion, but computed tomography (CT) may be useful to demonstrate the bony defect. ASMs may be associated with genitourinary and/or anorectal malformations, as well as neurofibromatosis type 1. They may also occur as part of the Currarino triad (anorectal malformation, sacral osseous defect [scimitar sacrum], and presacral mass).

■ Additional Differential Diagnoses

• **Lymphatic malformation**. Macrocystic lymphatic malformations are fluid-filled lymphatic spaces resulting from malconnection of lymphatic vessels with the central lymphatic system. They appear as thin-walled, uni- or multilocular cystic masses with enhancing walls and septa.

• **Dermoid cyst**. Dermoid cysts are developmental lesions that rarely occur in the presacral region. These cystic masses contain dermal elements, sebaceous and sweat glands with mucoid fluid, and a "fatty" appearance on imaging. Associated malformations include anorectal and osseous defects as part of the Currarino triad.

• **Ovarian cyst**. Ovarian cysts are common in neonatal girls and may be very large. They result from maternal hormonal stimulation of the ovarian follicles. Ultrasound confirms the cyst's ovarian origin. Cysts > 5 cm are at increased risk of torsion. Often midline, they are prerectal rather than presacral.

■ Diagnosis

Sacrococcygeal teratoma

✓ Pearls

• SCTs are the most common caudal region tumor in infants; appearance varies based on composition.
• SCTs may be intrapelvic, extrapelvic, or both; they may also demonstrate intraspinal extension.

• ASMs are CSF herniations through neural foramina or bony defects; they may have associated anomalies.
• Ovarian cysts are relatively common in neonatal girls; larger lesions are at risk of torsion.

Suggested Readings

Kocaoglu M, Frush DP. Pediatric presacral masses. Radiographics. 2006; 26(3):833–857

Pai DR, Ladino-Torres MF. Magnetic resonance imaging of pediatric pelvic masses. Magn Reson Imaging Clin N Am. 2013; 21(4):751–772

Shah RU, Lawrence C, Fickenscher KA, Shao L, Lowe LH. Imaging of pediatric pelvic neoplasms. Radiol Clin North Am. 2011; 49(4):729–748, vi

Case 173

Karen M. Ayotte

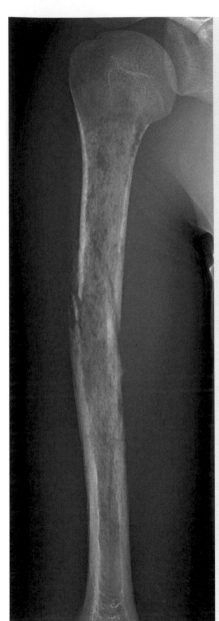

Fig. 173.1 Radiograph of the humerus shows a mixed permeative and moth-eaten appearance of the diaphysis, with a wide zone of transition. There is a pathological fracture and ill-defined, aggressive periostitis.

■ Clinical Presentation

College athlete with increasing arm pain (▶Fig. 173.1).

■ Key Imaging Finding

Aggressive lesion in a long bone

■ Top 3 Differential Diagnoses

- **Osteomyelitis.** Osteomyelitis has such a wide spectrum of radiographic appearances (including a normal appearance in early stages) that it is difficult—if not impossible—to conclusively exclude osteomyelitis on radiographs alone. A clinical history of fever or recent infection is helpful, but not specific. Common radiologic findings include lytic lesions with varying degrees of aggressive features, bone resorption, periostitis, sclerotic nidus, draining cloaca, and subcutaneous gas. The degree of sclerosis within and around the lesion varies depending on the organism, duration of infection, and age and overall health of the patient. Computed tomography (CT) and magnetic resonance imaging (MRI) are most useful if the clinical diagnosis is in doubt or if medical treatment fails.
- **Osteosarcoma.** Osteosarcoma is the most common primary bone malignancy of childhood, with a peak incidence at 10 to 20 years of age. The classic appearance is an aggressive lesion in the metaphysis of a long bone, with abnormal new bone proliferation. Highly aggressive lesions, however, may appear predominantly lytic. The more unusual telangiectatic osteosarcoma may have fluid–fluid levels, resembling an aneurysmal bone cyst. MRI is useful for detecting nearby "skip" lesions. Nuclear medicine bone scan (or positron emission tomography [PET] CT) is especially helpful during initial work-up to detect metastatic foci.
- **Ewing sarcoma.** Ewing sarcoma is the second most common primary bone malignancy of childhood, with a peak incidence of 10 to 15 years of age. The classic appearance is a lytic, medullary-based metadiaphyseal lesion in a long bone with aggressive periosteal reaction. However, the appearance ranges from purely lytic to predominantly sclerotic. Large soft-tissue masses are common. Long bone lesions are more common in younger patients; flat bone origin is more common in adolescents and young adults. Patients often present with pain. Constitutional findings, such as fever and elevated inflammatory markers, are common. MRI is critical for local staging.

■ Additional Differential Diagnoses

- **Langerhans cell histiocytosis (LCH).** LCH may present as solitary or multifocal lytic bone lesions. The radiographic appearance is notoriously variable. Therefore, LCH is a reasonable diagnostic consideration for many bone lesions, benign or aggressive, in patients younger than 30 years.
- **Metastases.** Secondary malignancies commonly affect bones via hematogenous dissemination. Leukemia is the most common entity to affect long bones in pediatric patients. Other common neoplasms that metastasize to bone include neuroblastoma and lymphoma. Metastatic foci typically present as lytic foci with a permeative or moth-eaten appearance. Lymphoma may arise in bone as a primary lesion.

■ Diagnosis

Lymphoma

✓ Pearls

- Osteosarcoma usually presents as an aggressive metaphyseal long bone lesion with bone proliferation.
- Ewing sarcoma typically presents as a lytic medullary lesion with aggressive periosteal reaction.
- Osteomyelitis has a wide variety of imaging appearance; history of fever is helpful but not specific.
- Bone scan is useful to evaluate for metastases, multifocal lesions, or skip lesions; MRI is useful for staging.

Suggested Readings

Kaste SC. Imaging pediatric bone sarcomas. Radiol Clin North Am. 2011; 49(4):749–765, vi–vii

Khanna G, Bennett DL. Pediatric bone lesions: beyond the plain radiographic evaluation. Semin Roentgenol. 2012; 47(1):90–99

Nichols RE, Dixon LB. Radiographic analysis of solitary bone lesions. Radiol Clin North Am. 2011; 49(6):1095–1114, v

Wyers MR. Evaluation of pediatric bone lesions. Pediatr Radiol. 2010; 40(4):468–473

Case 174

Rebecca Stein-Wexler

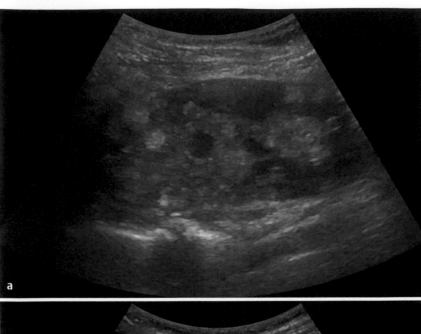

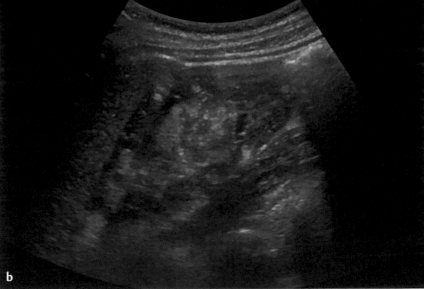

Fig. 174.1 Longitudinal US images of the (a) right and (b) left kidneys show multiple echogenic masses replacing much of the parenchyma. The kidneys are enlarged. On the right, there is a dominant mass measuring about 4 cm in the lower pole, whereas on the left a similar mass is in a more central location.

▪ Clinical Presentation

A 12-year-old girl with abdominal pain and anemia (▶ Fig. 174.1).

■ Key Imaging Finding

Multiple noncystic renal masses in a child

■ Top 3 Differential Diagnoses

- **Multifocal pyelonephritis**. Multifocal pyelonephritis usually results from an ascending infection. Lesions are often ill-defined and, if due to reflux, more common in upper and lower poles. Ultrasound (US) appearance varies and is often normal. Computed tomography (CT) and magnetic resonance imaging (MRI) may show hypoenhancing masses or patchy striations extending to the periphery.
- **Lymphoma/leukemia**. Renal lymphoma typically occurs in the setting of multiorgan involvement with non-Hodgkin lymphoma, especially Burkitt. The most common appearance is multiple parenchymal masses leading to renal enlargement. Diffuse renal infiltration, a single intrarenal mass, or an invasive extrarenal mass occur less frequently. Lesions are hypoechoic at US and show little enhancement on CT or MRI. Renal leukemia appears as relatively homogeneous renal enlargement.

- **Tuberous sclerosis (TS)**. TS is a systemic autosomal dominant disorder characterized by multiple hamartomas and benign tumors affecting the brain, skin, lungs, kidneys, eyes, heart, and elsewhere. The most common renal lesion is an angiomyolipoma (AML), which contains varying amounts of fat, abnormal vessels, and smooth muscle; renal cysts and (rarely) renal cell carcinoma also occur. The vast majority of sporadic cases of AML are solitary. Approximately 20% of cases occur in association with phakomatoses, particularly TS. In TS, AMLs occur at an earlier age and are often larger, multiple, and bilateral, increasing in size around puberty. Catastrophic hemorrhage, usually in tumors > 4 cm, may be fatal and potentially prevented by prophylactic embolization. AMLs are echogenic on US without shadowing. Fat-containing lesions are easier to characterize on CT and MRI, where they show fat attenuation/signal intensity.

■ Additional Differential Diagnoses

- **Nephroblastomatosis**. Multifocal or diffuse islands of primitive blastemal tissue after 36 weeks' gestational age result in nephroblastomatosis. The lesions may be single or multiple. Strongly associated with Wilms tumor, nephroblastomatosis is seen in 40% of patients with unilateral Wilms tumor and almost all of those with synchronous or metachronous disease. They also accompany a variety of syndromes, including Beckwith–Wiedemann, trisomy 18, sporadic aniridia, Drash (Wilms tumor, congenital nephropathy, and gonadal dysgenesis with ambiguous genitalia), and WAGR (Wilms tumor, aniridia, gen-

ital anomalies, and mental retardation). Up to 5% of patients with nephroblastomatosis will develop Wilms tumor. The kidneys may be enlarged, and US typically shows indistinct corticomedullary differentiation and sometimes focal hypoechoic areas. The lesions are homogeneous on CT and do not enhance. Although the lesions may be heterogeneous on MRI prior to administration of contrast, with gadolinium they appear more uniform than Wilms tumor.
- **Wilms tumor**. Although usually isolated, Wilms tumor may present with multiple masses ("synchronous").

■ Diagnosis

Tuberous sclerosis with multiple angiomyolipomas

✓ Pearls

- AMLs are common in children with TS and more likely to be multiple, bilateral, and large.
- AMLs larger than 4 cm are at increased risk of catastrophic hemorrhage.

- Renal lymphoma most often appears as multiple bilateral masses (vs. diffuse infiltration or a focal mass).
- Nephroblastomatosis is strongly associated with Wilms tumor, especially if Wilms tumor is multifocal.

Suggested Readings

Gee MS, Bittman M, Epelman M, Vargas SO, Lee EY. Magnetic resonance imaging of the pediatric kidney: benign and malignant masses. Magn Reson Imaging Clin N Am. 2013; 21(4):697–715

Geller E, Kochan PS. Renal neoplasms of childhood. Radiol Clin North Am. 2011; 49(4):689–709, vi

Lowe LH, Isuani BH, Heller RM, et al. Pediatric renal masses: Wilms tumor and beyond. Radiographics. 2000; 20(6):1585–1603

Siegel MJ, Chung EM. Wilms tumor and other pediatric renal masses. Magn Reson Imaging Clin N Am. 2008; 16(3):479–497, vi

Case 175

Arvind Sonik

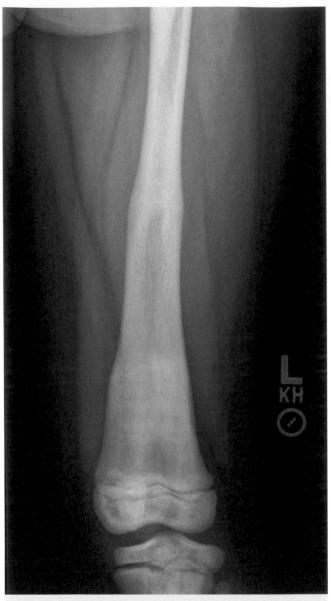

Fig. 175.1 Frontal radiograph of the left femur shows expansion of the distal metadiaphysis with loss of normal contour, resulting in Erlenmeyer flask deformity. The bone is sclerotic with alternating metaphyseal bands.

■ **Clinical Presentation**

A 7-year-old girl with leg pain (▶ Fig. 175.1).

■ Key Imaging Finding

Erlenmeyer flask deformity

■ Top 3 Differential Diagnoses

- **Osteopetrosis**. Osteopetrosis is an inherited disorder caused by failure of osteoclast function; this results in accumulation of primary spongiosa in the medullary spaces. In addition to Erlenmeyer flask deformity, findings include increased bone density, encroachment on the medullary space, bone-in-bone appearance, and alternating dense and lucent metaphyseal bands. Complications include fractures, anemia, and thrombocytopenia.
- **Fibrous dysplasia**. Fibrous dysplasia may be monostotic or polyostotic. Lesions typically arise in the central part of the bone and are expansile; they rarely involve the epiphysis. Density varies depending on the amount of osseous and fibrous tissue, but the classic lesion has a ground-glass matrix. Pathologic fracture is the most common complication. The polyos-

totic form of the disorder is more aggressive and often affects one side of the body. Associated disorders include McCune–Albright (precocious puberty and café-au-lait spots) and Mazabraud (intramuscular myxomas) syndromes.
- **Gaucher disease**. Gaucher disease is a rare, heritable metabolic disorder caused by deficiency of a lysosomal enzyme. The deficiency leads to accumulation of glucosylceramide in reticuloendothelial cells, which infiltrate marrow spaces. Radiographs demonstrate osteopenia, medullary expansion, and remodeling. Complications include bone infarcts, avascular necrosis (AVN), and pathologic fractures. Magnetic resonance imaging (MRI) may be useful to determine the extent of marrow infiltration. Infiltrating cells have signal similar to hematopoietic marrow.

■ Additional Differential Diagnoses

- **Hemoglobinopathy**. The most common hemoglobinopathies include sickle cell disease and the thalassemias. Bony changes in these conditions are due to marrow hyperplasia and vascular occlusion. Marrow hyperplasia results in osteopenia, hair-on-end appearance of the skull, and remodeling. Vascular occlusion may cause AVN, bone infarcts, and dactylitis. Physeal involvement may lead to growth disturbance.
- **Multiple hereditary exostoses**. Osteochondromatosis is an autosomal dominant dysplasia. As with solitary lesions, the cortex of the lesions is continuous with the underlying bone. Lesions that cause Erlenmeyer flask deformity tend to be sessile rather that pedunculated. Complications include growth disturbance, pain due to compression of neurovascular bundles, and—rarely—malignant transformation.

■ Diagnosis

Osteopetrosis

✓ Pearls

- Osteopetrosis results from osteoclast failure, leading to dense but fragile bones.
- Fibrous dysplasia may be monostotic or polyostotic; the classic lesion has a ground-glass matrix.
- Hemoglobinopathies (sickle cell and thalassemias) result in marrow hyperplasia, expansion, and infarcts.
- Sessile lesions associated with multiple hereditary exostoses may cause Erlenmeyer flask deformity.

Suggested Readings

Ihde LL, Forrester DM, Gottsegen CJ, et al. Sclerosing bone dysplasias: review and differentiation from other causes of osteosclerosis. Radiographics. 2011; 31(7):1865–1882

Katz R, Booth T, Hargunani R, Wylie P, Holloway B. Radiological aspects of Gaucher disease. Skeletal Radiol. 2011; 40(12):1505–1513

Khanna G, Bennett DL. Pediatric bone lesions: beyond the plain radiographic evaluation. Semin Roentgenol. 2012; 47(1):90–99

States LJ. Imaging of metabolic bone disease and marrow disorders in children. Radiol Clin North Am. 2001; 39(4):749–772

Case 176

Karen M. Ayotte

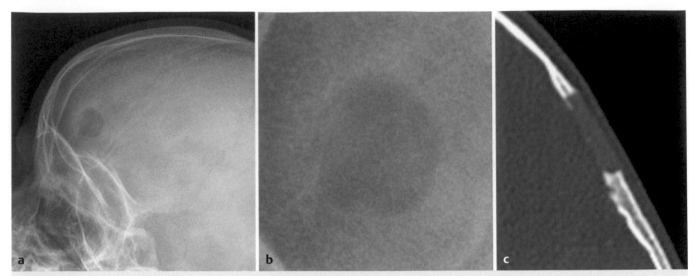

Fig. 176.1 **(a)** Lateral skull radiograph and **(b)** coned-down image over the frontal bone show a solitary lytic lesion with well-defined, nonsclerotic borders. **(c)** Computed tomography (CT) better shows well-defined margins.

■ Clinical Presentation

A 20-month-old boy with headache (▶Fig. 176.1).

■ Key Imaging Finding

Lytic skull lesion in a child

■ Top 3 Differential Diagnoses

- **Langerhans cell histiocytosis (LCH).** The skull is the most common site of osseous involvement in LCH. The classic lesion is well-defined and lytic, without sclerotic borders. A "beveled" edge appearance, or "hole within hole," results from greater involvement of the inner than outer table of the skull. LCH may also present as a round, radiolucent skull defect with a central dense nidus or sequestrum of intact bone, referred to as a "button sequestrum." The most common clinical symptoms include pain, palpable mass, and/or systemic symptoms.
- **Epidermoid cyst.** Epidermoid cysts result from abnormal deposition of epithelial rests within the diploic space during development. They are the second most common etiology for solitary skull lesions that lead to biopsy in the pediatric population. When an epidermoid cyst involves the diploic space,

the radiographic appearance overlaps with that of LCH. Epidermoid cysts are typically well-defined, expansile lesions without a central matrix. The rim may or may not be sclerotic. The magnetic resonance imaging (MRI) appearance is characteristic, demonstrating increased signal intensity of diffusion-weighted imaging.
- **Neoplasm.** Leukemia, Ewing sarcoma, and metastatic neuroblastoma can each produce poorly defined osteolytic lucencies in all bones, including the skull. Metastatic deposits in the skull cause lytic destruction and bony expansion. Localized areas of bone destruction in leukemia are frequently surrounded by normal bone and likely represent tumor metastases. These lesions tend to have an aggressive imaging appearance.

■ Additional Differential Diagnoses

- **Infection.** Osteomyelitis has a wide range of imaging manifestations, ranging from normal to mimicking an aggressive neoplasm. In the skull, bony destruction may lead to a lytic lesion, typically with poorly defined margins. There may be overlying soft-tissue edema. Subacute and chronic infection may present radiographically as a round, radiolucent, more well-defined skull defect with a central dense nidus or sequestrum of necrotic bone. This "button sequestrum" serves as a nidus for infection.
- **Leptomeningeal cyst.** The term leptomeningeal cyst (growing skull fracture) signifies a well-defined bone defect that arises when traumatic laceration of the dura exposes the bone to the pulsations of cerebrospinal fluid (CSF) within the subarachnoid space. Pulsatile pressure gradually widens the fracture line. Leptomeningeal cysts are an uncommon complication of skull fractures (<1%) and are most common in children under 3 years of age.

■ Diagnosis

Langerhans cell histiocytosis

✓ Pearls

- Langerhans cell histiocytosis classically presents as a lytic skull lesion with nonsclerotic, beveled margins.
- Langerhans cell histiocytosis and osteomyelitis may have "button sequestra."

- Common metastatic skull lesions in children include neuroblastoma and leukemia.
- A leptomeningeal cyst (growing skull fracture) is caused by CSF pulsations after disruption of the dura.

Suggested Readings

D'Ambrosio N, Soohoo S, Warshall C, Johnson A, Karimi S. Craniofacial and intracranial manifestations of langerhans cell histiocytosis: report of findings in 100 patients. AJR Am J Roentgenol. 2008; 191(2):589–597

Gibson SE, Prayson RA. Primary skull lesions in the pediatric population: a 25-year experience. Arch Pathol Lab Med. 2007; 131(5):761–766

Glass RBJ, Fernbach SK, Norton KI, Choi PS, Naidich TP. The infant skull: a vault of information. Radiographics. 2004; 24(2):507–522

Krasnokutsky MV. The button sequestrum sign. Radiology. 2005; 236(3):1026–1027

Case 177

Rebecca Stein-Wexler

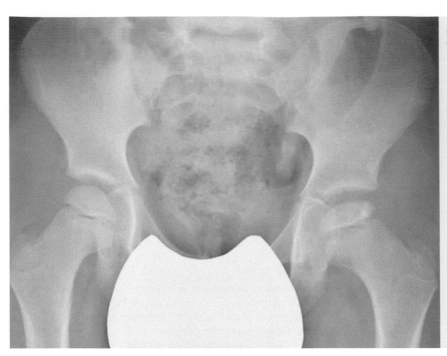

Fig. 177.1 Frontal radiograph of the pelvis shows flattening and sclerosis of the left femoral head.

■ Clinical Presentation

A 5-year-old boy with a limp (▶Fig. 177.1).

■ Key Imaging Finding

Avascular necrosis (AVN) of the femoral head

■ Top 3 Differential Diagnoses

- **Legg-Calvé-Perthes (LCP)**. LCP disease is most common between ages 5 and 8 years and is more common in boys. About 10% of cases are bilateral. Patients typically have no history of trauma and present with a limp and decreased range of motion. Necrosis of the femoral head results from impaired epiphyseal blood supply across the physis. Magnetic resonance imaging (MRI) allows earliest detection, demonstrating linear hypointensity on coronal T1-weighted sequences. In more advanced cases, T2-weighted sequences allow assessment of articular cartilage. Initial radiographs may show an effusion, thinning of the subchondral plate, and a relatively lucent epiphysis. The epiphysis then becomes denser, inhomogeneous, and fragmented. The paraphyseal metaphysis may become cystic. In the reparative stage, normal bone replaces sclerotic bone, and the femoral head appears smoother and less heterogeneous. Femoral head contour as well as congruence between the femoral head and the acetabulum determine long-term prognosis.

- **Traumatic injury**. Traumatic injury to the fragile blood vessels that traverse the physis may result in femoral head ischemia and subsequent AVN. This may result directly from a specific traumatic episode or from reduction of a dislocated hip. In the latter setting, risk for AVN may be proportional to the degree of flexion and abduction.

- **Sickle cell disease (SSD)**: Sickled erythrocytes occlude vessels, and subsequent hypoxemia further increases vascular distortion, exacerbating the resultant ischemia. The femoral and humeral heads are commonly involved, along with the vertebral endplates and the diametaphyseal region of the long bones.

■ Additional Differential Diagnoses

- **Corticosteroid use**. Corticosteroid use predisposes to AVN because of a variety of mechanisms, including demineralization and occlusion of small vessels by fat emboli. Risk is greatest with high doses and relatively short duration treatment. Corticosteroid-induced AVN is more likely to be bilateral.

- **Gaucher disease**. Gaucher disease manifests as inability to clear glucosylceramide from the reticuloendothelial system. Resultant increased pressure occludes interosseous sinusoids, leading to infarction. In addition to the complication of AVN, radiographic findings include osteopenia, medullary expansion, and bony remodeling.

- **Meyer dysplasia.** Meyer dysplasia affects the proximal femoral epiphyses, which appear irregular and small. It occurs in 2- to 4-year-olds, especially boys. It is painless and often bilateral. The radiographic appearance mimics AVN.

■ Diagnosis

Legg–Calvé–Perthes disease

✓ Pearls

- MRI is more sensitive than radiography for detecting early AVN.
- LCP disease results in AVN in the absence of trauma; it is more common in boys and is usually unilateral.

- Trauma may cause AVN by disrupting blood supply to the femoral head.
- SSD causes vascular occlusion and resultant AVN; corticosteroid use predisposes to bilateral AVN.

Suggested Readings

Dillman JR, Hernandez RJ. MRI of Legg-Calve-Perthes disease. AJR Am J Roentgenol. 2009; 193(5):1394–1407

Dwek JR. The hip: MR imaging of uniquely pediatric disorders. Magn Reson Imaging Clin N Am. 2009; 17(3):509–520, vi

Mankin HJ. Nontraumatic necrosis of bone (osteonecrosis). N Engl J Med. 1992; 326(22):1473–1479

Case 178

Sandra L. Wootton-Gorges

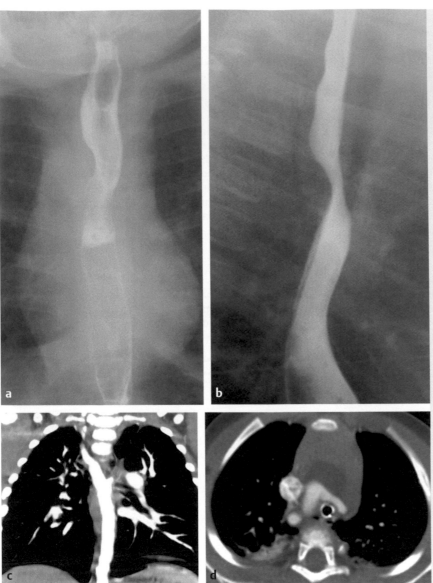

Fig. 178.1 (a) Frontal and (b) lateral views from an esophagram show a large, high, right-sided impression and smaller, lower, left-sided impression on the esophagus on the frontal view. There is a posterior impression on the esophagus on the lateral view (b). (c) Coronal contrast-enhanced reformatted CT shows a dominant right-sided arch and the distal extent of a smaller left-sided arch, also demonstrated on the (d) axial CT.

■ **Clinical Presentation**

A 15-month-old boy with long history of stridor (▶Fig. 178.1).

■ Key Imaging Finding

Vascular anomaly with esophageal and tracheal compression

■ Top 3 Differential Diagnoses

- **Aberrant right subclavian artery (RSCA).** Aberrant RSCA is a common isolated arch anomaly (1% of the population) that is rarely symptomatic. In this anomaly, the RSCA is the last branch of the left aortic arch. It courses behind the esophagus toward the right upper chest, causing posterior indentation on the esophagus during an esophagram. It is not considered a complete vascular ring.
- **Double aortic arch.** Double aortic arch is the most common symptomatic arch anomaly. It is an isolated anomaly in which two aortic arches are present. The right arch is higher and larger in 75% of cases. The two arches join posteriorly to form the (usually left-sided) descending aorta. The arches thus encircle and may compress the esophagus and trachea, resulting in stridor or problems with feeding. Because the trachea

is fixed between the two smaller aortic arches, it is midline in position on chest X-ray. The esophagram will show posterior and bilateral lateral indentation on the esophagus, as well as narrowing of the trachea. Magnetic resonance imaging (MRI) and contrast-enhanced computed tomography (CT) are excellent modalities to define this vascular anomaly and its effects on surrounding structures.

- **Right aortic arch with aberrant left subclavian artery (LSCA).** In this right aortic arch anomaly, the LSCA arises from the diverticulum of Kommerell and passes posterior to the esophagus to the left upper extremity. The ductal ligament extends from the LSCA to the left pulmonary artery, completing this often-symptomatic vascular ring.

■ Additional Differential Diagnoses

- **Pulmonary sling.** In this anomaly, the left pulmonary artery arises from the right pulmonary artery and passes between the trachea and esophagus on its way to the left lung. On upper GI examination, there is an anterior indentation on the esophagus and posterior indentation on the trachea. Associated tracheobronchial anomalies, such as complete tracheal rings, are common and may significantly contribute to respiratory symptoms.

- **Innominate artery compression syndrome.** Compression of the trachea by the crossing innominate artery is a rare cause of respiratory compromise in infants. The innominate artery origin or course may be anomalous in these cases. The patients have a normal left aortic arch. It is uncertain whether this constitutes a real entity, or whether symptoms result from underlying tracheal maldevelopment. Surgical reimplantation or suspension may help relieve tracheal narrowing and respiratory symptoms.

■ Diagnosis

Double aortic arch

✓ Pearls

- Aberrant RCSA is a common anomaly that is rarely symptomatic and is not considered a complete ring.
- Double aortic arch and right arch with aberrant LSCA are the most common symptomatic vascular rings.

- An aberrant LSCA (from a right aortic arch) arises from the diverticulum of Kommerell.
- Pulmonary sling (aberrant origin of the left pulmonary artery) is associated with complete tracheal rings.

Suggested Readings

Castañer E, Gallardo X, Rimola J, et al. Congenital and acquired pulmonary artery anomalies in the adult: radiologic overview. Radiographics. 2006; 26(2):349–371

Hernanz-Schulman M. Vascular rings: a practical approach to imaging diagnosis. Pediatr Radiol. 2005; 35(10):961–979

Kellenberger CJ. Aortic arch malformations. Pediatr Radiol. 2010; 40(6):876–884

Oddone M, Granata C, Vercellino N, Bava E, Tomà P. Multi-modality evaluation of the abnormalities of the aortic arches in children: techniques and imaging spectrum with emphasis on MRI. Pediatr Radiol. 2005; 35(10):947–960

Case 179

Karen M. Ayotte

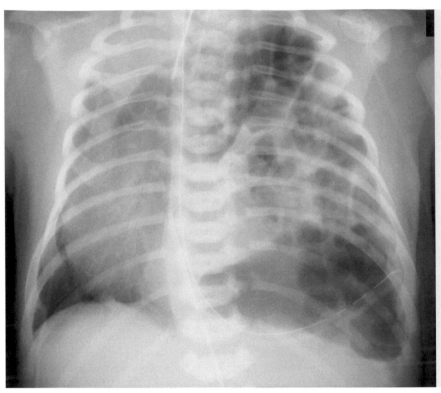

Fig. 179.1 Frontal chest radiograph shows the trachea and mediastinum shifted to the right because of a large, multiloculated cystic mass occupying the entire left thorax. The left lung is compressed, but visualized portions of the right are well aerated. The esophageal catheter ends in the gastric bubble in the left lower chest.

■ Clinical Presentation

A 3-week-old infant with persistent cough (▶Fig. 179.1).

■ Key Imaging Finding

Cystic pulmonary mass

■ Top 3 Differential Diagnoses

- **Congenital lobar emphysema (CLE)**. CLE constitutes progressive overexpansion of a pulmonary lobe secondary to obstruction of normal airflow, usually because of varying degrees of bronchial underdevelopment or obstruction. In prenatal life, the lung is filled with fluid. Perinatally, the radiographic appearance varies as the fluid within the affected lobe is gradually replaced with air. The most common location is the left upper lobe, followed by the right middle and right upper lobes. Parenchyma, vessels, and bronchi are present but attenuated. Patients often present in the neonatal period with respiratory distress. Definitive treatment consists of surgical resection of the affected lobe.
- **Congenital pulmonary airway malformation (CPAM)**. CPAM is a hamartomatous proliferation of terminal bronchioles at the expense of alveolar development. Most of these masses have both cystic and solid components, resulting in varied imaging appearances. The lesions communicate with the tracheobronchial tree and tend to aerate early in life. Internal flu-

id–fluid levels may be seen in the absence of superimposed infection. CPAMs are classified into three types: type 1 consists of one or more cysts >2 cm in size; type 2 has cysts <2 cm in size; and type 3 is essentially solid. Definitive management is surgical, although the approach to asymptomatic or incidentally discovered lesions is controversial.
- **Congenital diaphragmatic hernia**. Congenital defects in the diaphragm may lead to intrathoracic herniation of solid and hollow organs of the upper abdomen. Left-sided defects are much more common than those on the right. Herniations may appear cystic or solid at birth. If most of the herniated contents are bowel, fluid attenuation will fade as the bowel aerates. Most children present as neonates secondary to respiratory distress. Prognosis depends on the degree of pulmonary hypoplasia, as well as the presence of associated anomalies. Surgical consultation is required, regardless of the apparent defect size.

■ Additional Differential Diagnoses

- **Necrotizing pneumonia**. When necrosis or pulmonary abscess complicates parenchymal consolidation, the appearance may mimic other cystic lesions. Necrotizing pneumonia is more common in the lower lobes. The cysts may be solitary or multiple, as large as 10 cm, and filled with air, fluid, or both. Conservative management is often successful in otherwise healthy children.
- **Tension pneumothorax**. Especially sharp definition of the mediastinum, an asymmetrically deep costophrenic sulcus, and featureless unilateral hyperlucency suggest an anterior pneumothorax. Mediastinal shift indicates the presence of tension, which is considered a surgical emergency.

■ Diagnosis

Congenital diaphragmatic hernia

✓ Pearls

- Prognosis for most chest masses is based primarily on the degree of resultant pulmonary hypoplasia.
- CLE most commonly occurs within the left upper lobe, followed by the right middle and right upper lobes.
- CPAMs are categorized by the size of cystic components.
- CDH may mimic cystic or solid primary thoracic masses and is more common on the left.

Suggested Readings

Biyyam DR, Chapman T, Ferguson MR, Deutsch G, Dighe MK. Congenital lung abnormalities: embryologic features, prenatal diagnosis, and postnatal radiologic-pathologic correlation. Radiographics. 2010; 30(6):1721–1738

Newman B. Congenital bronchopulmonary foregut malformations: concepts and controversies. Pediatr Radiol. 2006; 36(8):773–791

Taylor GA, Atalabi OM, Estroff JA. Imaging of congenital diaphragmatic hernias. Pediatr Radiol. 2009; 39(1):1–16

Case 180

Arvind Sonik

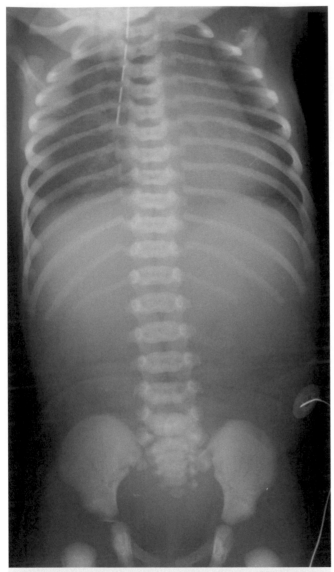

Fig. 180.1 Supine radiograph of the chest and abdomen shows an esophageal catheter ending in a lucent pouch just below and to the right of the carina. The abdomen is gasless.

■ Clinical Presentation

A 1-day-old infant not tolerating oral feedings (▶ Fig. 180.1).

■ Key Imaging Finding

Difficulty feeding and passing an enteric tube

■ Top 3 Differential Diagnoses

- **Tracheoesophageal (TE) fistula/esophageal atresia (EA).** EA is classified based on the presence and location, or absence, of a TE fistula. Proximal EA with a fistula between the airway and the distal esophageal segment is the most common type. EA is often associated with additional anomalies of the gastrointestinal (GI) tract. Cardiac, renal, and vertebral anomalies (including the VACTERL complex) are associated less frequently. Evaluation includes chest radiography after advancement of a feeding catheter to the level of the atresia, along with abdomen radiography to evaluate for intestinal air. Without a fistula, the abdomen will be gasless. If an H-type fistula is suspected (typically in older children with cough while feeding), an upper GI study is indicated, preferably with isosmolar water-soluble contrast. Esophageal webs are considered a variant of EA and may be associated with a TE fistula. On esophagograms, webs appear as thin, transverse, or oblique filling defects.

- **Foreign body.** Foreign bodies may become lodged in relatively narrow regions of the esophagus, including the level of the thoracic inlet, aortic arch, and less commonly the gastroesophageal (GE) junction. Esophagrams may be useful when a nonopaque foreign body is suspected. Disk batteries should be considered in the differential diagnosis of a round radioopaque foreign body and constitute a medical emergency because of their corrosive properties.
- **Esophageal duplication cyst.** Esophageal duplications generally manifest as cysts, usually right sided and in the posterior mediastinum. They are rarely complete, and they rarely communicate with the esophagus. Duplication cysts are near water attenuation on computed tomography (CT) and show no central enhancement. On magnetic resonance imaging (MRI), they are bright on T2 and variable on T1 sequences, depending on the amount of proteinaceous material.

■ Additional Differential Diagnoses

- **Vascular ring.** The most common vascular anomalies to cause dysphagia are complete vascular rings: (1) double aortic arch; and (2) right aortic arch with aberrant left subclavian artery and left ligament arising from the descending aorta. Esophagrams demonstrate a posterior indentation of the esophagus on lateral and oblique views and bilateral compression on the frontal. The double aortic arch is more common than the right arch with aberrant left subclavian artery. A left aortic arch with an aberrant right subclavian artery is the most common anomaly of the aortic arch, but this is an incomplete vascular ring and thus rarely symptomatic.

■ Diagnosis

Esophageal atresia without fistula

✓ Pearls

- EA is classified based on the presence and location, or absence, of a TE fistula.
- Proximal EA with a fistula between the airway and the distal esophagus is most common.

- Foreign bodies typically become lodged at the thoracic inlet, aortic arch, and (less often) GE junction.
- Complete vascular rings may cause esophageal compression and dysphagia.

Suggested Readings

Berrocal T, Torres I, Gutiérrez J, Prieto C, del Hoyo ML, Lamas M. Congenital anomalies of the upper gastrointestinal tract. Radiographics. 1999; 19(4):855–872

Lee NK, Kim S, Jeon TY, et al. Complications of congenital and developmental abnormalities of the gastrointestinal tract in adolescents and adults: evaluation with multimodality imaging. Radiographics. 2010; 30(6):1489–1507

Rao P. Neonatal gastrointestinal imaging. Eur J Radiol. 2006; 60(2):171–186

Part 8

Ultrasound Imaging

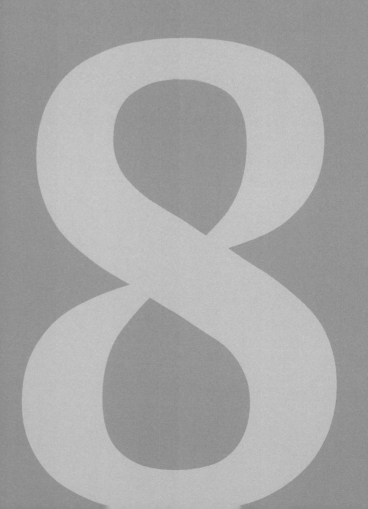

Case 181

Sima Naderi

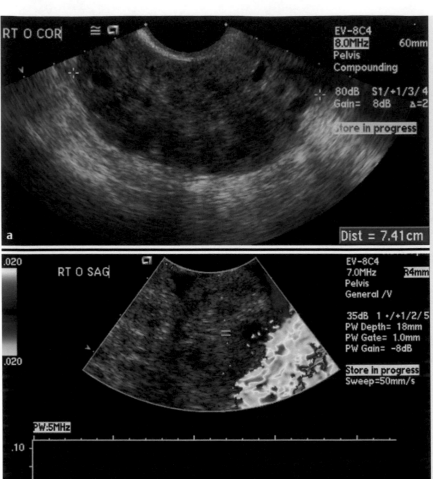

Fig. 181.1 (a) Grayscale endovaginal ultrasound image demonstrates an enlarged right ovary with heterogeneous parenchyma and multiple small follicles, many of which are located along the periphery. (b) There is no significant flow demonstrated on color or pulsed Doppler interrogation.

■ Clinical Presentation

A 17-year-old girl with acute-onset severe right-sided pelvic pain (▶Fig. 181.1).

■ Key Imaging Finding

Enlarged ovary

■ Top 3 Differential Diagnoses

- **Ovarian torsion**. Torsion of the ovary represents a gynecological surgical emergency. It is caused by partial or complete rotation of the ovarian pedicle on its ligamentous axis. Torsion can occur at any time in life but is most common during the fertile years. Predisposing factors include an ipsilateral adnexal mass and pregnancy, which accounts for up to 20% of cases. Prepubertal females can torse a normal ovary because of adnexal mobility. Sonographic findings are variable. The torsed ovary is commonly enlarged, up to 28 times the normal size, with multiple peripheral follicles, the "string of pearls" sign. The parenchyma can be heterogeneous because of edema, hemorrhage, or necrosis. A lead mass may be appreciated. Free fluid in the pelvic cul de sac is also a common finding. Color and spectral Doppler examination may show absent flow in the affected ovary. However, the presence of blood flow does not exclude torsion, as it may be incomplete or intermittent, resulting in increased diastolic flow in the edematous ovary. If there are venous and arterial waveforms in the setting of severe pain, the size of the ovary could indicate torsion. Commonly, venous flow is lost first, followed by arterial flow. Diag-

nosis requires the appropriate clinical setting of severe acute onset of pelvic pain.
- **Ovarian neoplasm**. Ovarian tumors, both benign and malignant, can result in enlargement of the ovary. Differentiating features compared to ovarian torsion include patient's age and clinical presentation. There is an increased risk of malignancy with increasing patient age and increasing size of the mass greater than 10 cm. As with other masses, ovarian tumors predispose patients to torsion. Findings suggesting neoplasm include thickened septations (>2–3 mm), solid components, vegetations, and increased vascular flow. Free fluid is not as helpful as it can be seen in all three of the top differentials.
- **Pelvic inflammatory disease (PID)/tubo-ovarian abscess**. The diagnosis of PID is made in the appropriate clinical setting of fever, cervical motion tenderness, and vaginal discharge. The dilated fallopian tube can best be differentiated from a cystic adnexal mass by transvaginal ultrasound (US). Tubo-ovarian abscess appears as a complex multiloculated mass with through transmission, scattered internal echogenicity, and increased vascularity. Ovarian enlargement may be seen in advanced presentations.

■ Additional Differential Diagnoses

- **Hemorrhagic cyst**. The sonographic appearance of a hemorrhagic cyst depends on the time of hemorrhage. Classically, the complex cyst forms lacelike internal echoes. As the clot retracts, a fluid–fluid level can be seen, or the echogenic clot

can settle at the dependent portion of the cyst. The key differentiating feature from malignancy is the lack of flow within the retractile clot on color Doppler.

■ Diagnosis

Ovarian torsion

✓ Pearls

- Ovarian torsion commonly presents as acute and severe adnexal tenderness with an enlarged ovary.
- Ovarian neoplasms are unlikely to cause acute pain and more likely to be malignant with advanced age.

- PID occurs in the appropriate clinical setting; the dilated fallopian tube may best be detected on transvaginal US.
- Hemorrhagic cysts classically present with lacelike pattern of internal echoes in a cystic mass.

Suggested Readings

Chang HC, Bhatt S, Dogra VS. Pearls and pitfalls in diagnosis of ovarian torsion. Radiographics. 2008; 28(5):1355–1368

Case 182

William T. O'Brien, Sr.

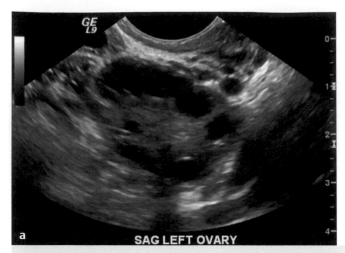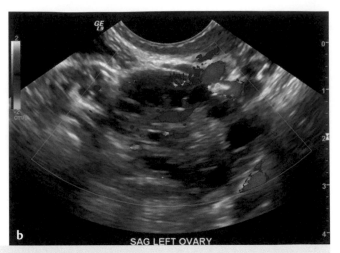

Fig. 182.1 (a) Sagittal grayscale and (b) color sonographic images through the left ovary demonstrate an enlarged ovary with multiple peripheral follicles. Flow is demonstrated within the ovary. Arterial and venous waveforms (not shown) were normal.

■ Clinical Presentation

A 24-year-old woman with irregular menses and pain (▶ Fig. 182.1).

■ **Key Imaging Finding**

Enlarged ovary with multiple peripheral follicles

■ **Top 3 Differential Diagnoses**

• **Ovarian torsion**. Ovarian torsion is the result of the ovary twisting about its vascular axis. Torsion is most common in premenopausal women but may occur at any age when a pathologic lead point (such as an ovarian mass) is present. Patients typically present with severe pelvic pain. As the torsion occurs, venous outflow is first decreased, resulting in an enlarged ovary (>12 mL) with heterogeneous echotexture. As the edema progresses, arterial inflow is decreased. Hemorrhage, necrosis, and infarction may occur if left untreated. The presence of flow within the ovary is of limited diagnostic value as the mere presence of flow does not exclude torsion. In cases of intermittent torsion, the ovary may actually be hyperemic. The absence of flow, however, is highly suggestive of torsion. Torsion may present sonographically as an enlarged edematous ovary with peripheral follicles.

• **Polycystic ovarian syndrome (PCOS)**. PCOS, also referred to as Stein–Leventhal syndrome, is a clinical syndrome which is only suggested by sonography consisting of obesity, hirsutism, amenorrhea or irregular menses, and infertility. The syndrome is associated with a variety of endocrine disturbances, including increased androgen production. Classic sonographic findings consist of enlarged ovaries with multiple peripheral follicles (10 or more) of similar size (usually <5 mm) in a "string of pearls" configuration. The ovaries may have a thick echogenic capsule. Treatment is directed at restoring fertility through fertility medications.

• **Ovarian hyperstimulation syndrome (OHS)**. Ovarian stimulation from fertility medications results in the maturation of multiple follicles during the menstrual cycle. Rarely, the ovaries may be overstimulated, resulting in enlarged ovaries with numerous enlarged peripheral follicles, ascites, and pleural effusions, referred to as OHS. When severe, the condition may be life threatening because of fluid and electrolyte imbalances. The syndrome typically occurs when the dosage of medications is increased and the ovaries may be massively enlarged (up to 15–20 cm). Treatment consists of correcting electrolyte imbalances and discontinuance of fertility medications.

■ **Diagnosis**

Polycystic ovarian syndrome

✓ **Pearls**

• Ovarian torsion must be considered with enlarged ovaries and pain; flow does not exclude the diagnosis.
• PCOS presents clinically with obesity, hirsutism, irregular menses, and infertility.

• Findings in PCOS include enlarged ovaries with greater than 10 peripheral follicles.
• OHS presents with enlarged ovaries with peripheral follicles, ascites, and pleural effusions.

Suggested Readings

Chang HC, Bhatt S, Dogra VS. Pearls and pitfalls in diagnosis of ovarian torsion. Radiographics. 2008; 28(5):1355–1368

Laing FC, Allison SJ. US of the ovary and adnexa: to worry or not to worry? Radiographics. 2012; 32(6):1621–1639, discussion 1640–1642

Case 183

William T. O'Brien, Sr.

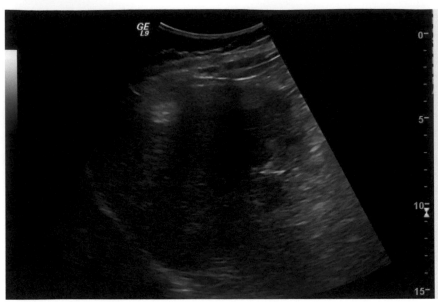

Fig. 183.1 Sonographic image through the right hepatic lobe demonstrates a well-circumscribed homogeneously echogenic lesion.

■ Clinical Presentation

Adult woman with an incidental finding on a study for right upper quadrant pain (▶Fig. 183.1).

■ Key Imaging Finding

Echogenic liver mass

■ Top 3 Differential Diagnoses

- **Hemangioma**. Hemangiomas are the most common hepatic neoplasm & second most common benign lesions following simple cysts. They are more common in women and typically asymptomatic. Classic imaging findings on ultrasound (US) are of a well-defined homogeneously echogenic mass. Larger lesions may be more heterogeneous. A common appearance is the "reverse target" sign with a centrally hypoechoic mass with a peripheral echogenic rim. Computed tomography (CT) or magnetic resonance imaging (MRI) may be helpful in confirming the diagnosis.
- **Focal fatty infiltration**. Fatty infiltration of the liver is common and most often due to obesity. Other etiologies include alcoholism and glycogen storage disease. It usually results in diffuse increased echogenicity but may also occur focally. Focal fatty infiltration presents as geographic echogenic regions, most commonly located along the falciform ligament/gallbladder fossa and portal confluence. This typical distribution of focal fatty infiltration is thought to be due to the venous drainage of this region. MRI is usually diagnostic in cases where the US findings are not characteristic.
- **Hepatocellular carcinoma (HCC)**. HCC is the most common primary hepatic malignancy with an increased incidence in patients with chronic liver disease, typically cirrhotics. Patients may present with a single lesion, multiple lesions, or diffuse hepatic involvement. HCC has a variety of appearances on US; the most common manifestation is a dominant hypervascular lesion with smaller satellite foci. Portal or hepatic vein invasion is common. MRI can be helpful in difficult cases, since HCC typically displays increased T2 signal intensity. Clinically, HCC is associated with elevated alpha-fetoprotein.

■ Additional Differential Diagnoses

- **Metastases**. Common primary neoplasms with liver metastases include lung, breast, and gastrointestinal malignancies. Lesions are often multiple; they may also be diffusely infiltrative. The most common US appearance is a target lesion that is centrally echogenic and peripherally hypoechoic.
- **Focal nodular hyperplasia (FNH)**. FNH is an uncommon lesion that typically presents in young females. It is composed of hepatocytes and classically contains a central scar. US findings include an isoechoic mass with central scar and a spoke wheel pattern of flow. Rarely, the lesions may be echogenic.

Since FNH is composed of hepatocytes, it may show uptake on sulfur colloid imaging.
- **Hepatic adenoma (HA)**. HA is a benign lesion predominantly seen in women (90%). Most often they are solitary but may occasionally be multiple, especially in patients with glycogen storage disease. HA have an increased frequency and risk of rupture with the use of oral contraceptives. They have variable appearances on US but are most commonly isoechoic. Fat content may result in increased echoes.

■ Diagnosis

Hemangioma

✓ Pearls

- Hemangiomas are the most common benign hepatic neoplasms; they are circumscribed and echogenic.
- Focal fatty infiltration appears as geographic regions of increased echoes in characteristic locations.
- HCC and metastases have a variety of imaging appearances on US and occur in at-risk patients.

Suggested Readings

Caturelli E, Pompili M, Bartolucci F, et al. Hemangioma-like lesions in chronic liver disease: diagnostic evaluation in patients. Radiology. 2001; 220(2):337–342

Prasad SR, Wang H, Rosas H, et al. Fat-containing lesions of the liver: radiologic-pathologic correlation. Radiographics. 2005; 25(2):321–331

Case 184

Charles A. Tujo

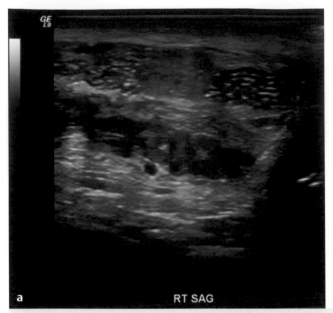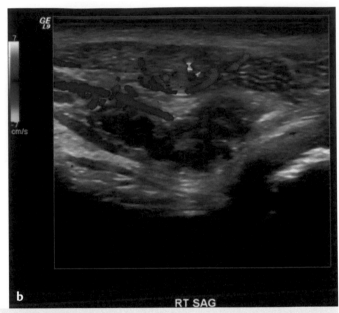

Fig. 184.1 Longitudunal gray scale **(a)** and color **(b)** images through the right epididymis (superficial structure) reveal an echogenic solid appearing mass with suggestion of increased through transmission and intrinsic color flow.

■ Clinical Presentation

Young adult man with chronic scrotal pain (▶ Fig. 184.1).

■ Key Imaging Finding

Epididymal mass

■ Top 3 Differential Diagnoses

- **Epididymal cyst or spermatocele**. Epididymal cysts are benign lesions that occur anywhere along the epididymis. They are anechoic with increased through transmission and no associated color flow. They may have septations when larger in size. Spermatoceles look similar; however, they more commonly contain internal echoes, and they tend to be found in the region of the epididymal head. Both entities are benign, though they can present as a palpable mass
- **Adenomatoid tumor**. Adenomatoid tumors are benign, and represent the most common extratesticular scrotal neoplasm and the most common primary tumor of the epididymis. They can occur anywhere along the epididymis, but are more commonly seen in the region of the epididymal tail; they can also occur in the tunica albuginea or along the spermatic cord. Rarely, they can extend into an intratesticular location, mimicking a true intratesticular neoplasm. These masses tend to be echogenic; however, the appearance on ultrasound (US) is variable.
- **Papillary cystadenoma**. Papillary cystadenomas are uncommon benign lesions that tend to occur in the setting of von Hippel–Lindau (VHL) disease, which is a phakomatosis. VHL is associated with cystic lesions in a variety of locations, including the pancreas and epididymis. On US, papillary cystadenomas are cystic with fine septations. They can be bilateral, which is virtually pathognomonic of VHL.

■ Additional Differential Diagnoses

- **Leiomyoma**. Leiomyomas represent the second most common primary tumor of the epididymis, following adenomatoid tumor. As there is smooth muscle within both the scrotum and the extratesticular portions of the scrotal contents, leiomyomas can occur in multiple locations, including the epididymis. Leiomyomas are solid lesions that tend to be well defined and heterogeneously hypoechoic with or without cystic components or calcification. On pathologic examination, there is a characteristic whorled appearance. There is a low risk for malignant transformation.

■ Diagnosis

Adenomatoid tumor

✓ Pearls

- Adenomatoid tumors are the most common solid extratesticular, scrotal neoplasm.
- Epididymal cysts and spermatoceles are commonly found along the epididymis and are typically palpable.
- Papillary cystadenomas are uncommon scrotal masses that have an increased incidence with VHL.
- Leiomyomas involve smooth muscle and are typically solid with or without cysts and calcifications.

Suggested Readings

Dogra VS, Gottlieb RH, Oka M, Rubens DJ. Sonography of the scrotum. Radiology. 2003; 227(1):18–36

Kim W, Rosen MA, Langer JE, Banner MP, Siegelman ES, Ramchandani P. US MR imaging correlation in pathologic conditions of the scrotum. Radiographics. 2007; 27(5):1239–1253

Woodward PJ, Schwab CM, Sesterhenn IA. From the archives of the AFIP: extratesticular scrotal masses: radiologic-pathologic correlation. Radiographics. 2003; 23(1):215–240

Case 185

David J. Weitz

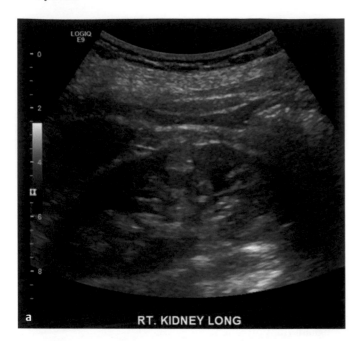

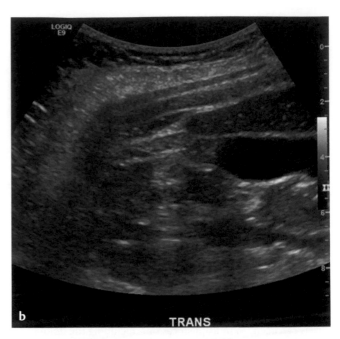

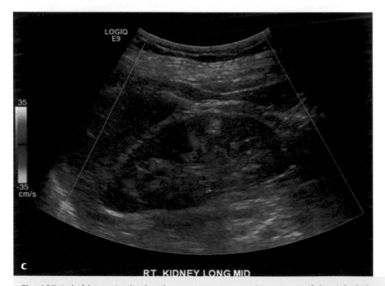

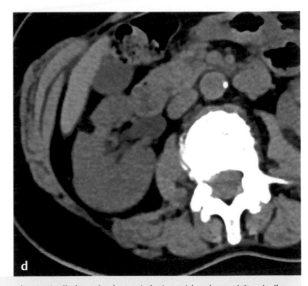

Fig. 185.1 **(a,b)** Longitudinal and transverse sonographic images of the right kidney reveal a cortically based echogenic lesion with echogenicity similar to peripelvic fat. **(c)** Color flow image demonstrates no significant intralesional flow with vessels surrounding lesion. **(d)** Noncontrast axial CT image through the upper abdomen demonstrates a sharply marginated hypodense fatty mass located within the interpolar right kidney.

■ Clinical Presentation

A 73-year-old woman with hepatitis C for hepatoma screening (►Fig. 185.1).

■ Key Imaging Finding

Echogenic renal mass

■ Top 3 Differential Diagnoses

- **Angiomyolipoma (AML).** AMLs are benign renal hamartomas—masses of normal tissue appearing in an abnormal location. Small AMLs are usually incidental discoveries in the work-up of other conditions, as they rarely produce symptoms. They are soft, pliable, and may grow large before symptoms prompt evaluation. Pain is usually from vessel rupture, as larger lesions (>4 cm) are prone to aneurysm formation. On ultrasound (US), these masses are usually found at the renal cortex and have a homogeneously echogenic appearance with posterior acoustic shadowing. Because of their overlapping US appearance with renal cell carcinoma (RCC), conclusive imaging with computed tomography (CT) or magnetic resonance imaging (MRI) is generally needed to demonstrate fat, which is considered pathognomonic for AML. Solitary AMLs are sporadic and found most frequently in adult women, while multiple AMLs are known to occur in the setting of tuberous sclerosis (TS). In the above case, the patient did not have a formal diagnosis of TS.
- **Renal cell carcinoma.** All solid renal masses are suspect for RCC, because it is the most common solid renal mass and its US appearance may mimic just about any other lesion. Patients present with hematuria, weight loss, anemia, and occasionally paraneoplastic syndromes. Risk factors include tobacco, long-term dialysis, and von Hippel–Lindau disease. Larger RCCs are most commonly echogenic; however, RCC can present as an echogenic, hypoechoic, or isoechoic mass. RCCs may appear as complex masses containing calcifications, cystic components, hemorrhage, or necrosis. Because these tumors are highly vascular, flow within a renal lesion lends support for RCC and can be particularly helpful in the detection of hard-to-identify isoechoic lesions. RCC spreads via lymphatics to local lymph nodes, direct spread to the ipsilateral renal vein and inferior vena cava, and hematogenously to distant sites.
- **Complex cyst.** US is considered the modality of choice for confirming a simple renal cyst which requires no further imaging. Complex cysts, on the other hand, may mimic a solid mass on US, prompting follow-up sonography, further imaging with CT or MRI, or intervention. These lesions are often the result of internal hemorrhage or protein and may demonstrate low-level echogenicity, fluid-debris levels, internal clot, calcification, or septations. The differential would include an infected cyst or abscess, a multiseptated cyst, and RCC, all of which may be sonographically indistinguishable. Thick septations (>2 mm), internal flow, vegetation, calcification, and demonstration of interval growth are highly suspicious findings for malignancy. The Bosniak classification using CT is a widely accepted standard for placing US indeterminate lesions into a medical or surgical category; however, MRI is gaining popularity and may be especially helpful for small lesions.

■ Diagnosis

Angiomyolipoma

✓ Pearls

- On US, AMLs have a homogeneously echogenic echotexture with posterior acoustic shadowing.
- Given the highly variable appearance of RCCs at US, all solid renal masses are suspect for RCC.

- US is the preferred modality to confirm a simple cyst; complex cystic renal lesions are nonspecific.

Suggested Readings

Hartman DS, Choyke PL, Hartman MS. From the RSNA refresher courses: a practical approach to the cystic renal mass. Radiographics. 2004; 24(Suppl 1):S101–S115

Siegel CL, Middleton WD, Teefey SA, McClennan BL. Angiomyolipoma and renal cell carcinoma: US differentiation. Radiology. 1996; 198(3):789–793

Case 186

William T. O'Brien, Sr.

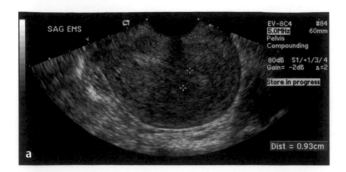
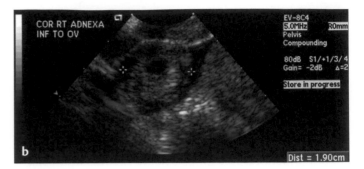
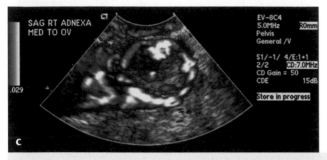

Fig. 186.1 (a) Longitudinal/sagittal sonographic image through the uterus demonstrates a normal endometrial echo complex without evidence of an intrauterine gestational sac. (b) Imaging through the right adnexa reveals a round adnexal mass with a thick hyperechoic rim and a small central hypoechoic region. (c) The mass demonstrates increased peripheral flow in a "ring of fire" pattern.

■ Clinical Presentation

A 24-year-old woman with severe right adnexal pain, vaginal spotting, and a positive human chorionic gonadotropin (HCG) (▶Fig. 186.1).

■ Key Imaging Finding

Complex cystic adnexal mass with positive HCG

■ Top 3 Differential Diagnoses

• **Ectopic pregnancy**. Ectopic pregnancy is the result of implantation of the conceptus outside the endometrial canal, usually within the fallopian tube. It is currently the most common cause of pregnancy-related mortality in the first trimester. Risk factors include prior ectopic pregnancy, pelvic inflammatory disease, tubal ligation, and fertility medications or interventions. Patients present in the first trimester with pain and/or vaginal bleeding. Ultrasound is the diagnostic modality of choice. Intrauterine sonographic findings include the lack of an intrauterine pregnancy (except in the exceedingly rare case of heterotopic pregnancy) or the presence of a pseudogestational sac. Cornual pregnancies must be considered when the gestational sac is present in the lateral upper portion of the uterus with less than 5 mm between the gestational sac and external uterine wall. Cervical ectopics also occur and must be carefully excluded, especially in the setting of the cervical phase of an abortion in progress. Extrauterine sonographic findings include a complex cystic adnexal mass with increased vascularity and/or complex free fluid (hemorrhage). An ectopic pregnancy classically has a thick echogenic rim representing the edematous tube with a central hypoechoic region—the gestational sac. The echogenic rim is more echoic than ovarian or uterine tissue. Peripheral flow in a "ring of fire" pattern is characteristic with a low-resistance waveform. Sonographic findings must be correlated with HCG levels, especially when the levels are below the expected threshold for visualization of a gestational sac (1,000–2,000 IU).

• **Corpus luteal cyst**. The key differential diagnosis in the setting of a suspected ectopic pregnancy is a corpus luteal cyst. Although it may not always be possible to differentiate between the two, the corpus luteal cyst arises from (rather than adjacent to) the ovary and has a thinner outer echogenic layer that is similar in echotexture to normal ovarian parenchyma. Additionally, the peripheral flow is not as avid; however, this observation is not always reliable. The presence of an anechoic, rather than hypoechoic, central fluid collection favors a corpus luteal cyst over ectopic pregnancy.

• **Hemorrhagic cyst**. Although hemorrhagic cysts typically present as cystic masses with lacelike internal echoes, they may occasionally mimic ectopic pregnancy both clinically and sonographically. Imaging findings that mimic ectopic pregnancy include a thick echogenic rim, as well as the presence of hemoperitoneum. In the setting of a positive HCG, these characteristics would be highly suggestive of ectopic pregnancy.

■ Diagnosis

Ectopic pregnancy

✓ Pearls

• Ectopic pregnancy must be considered if no intrauterine gestation is seen in an HCG-positive patient.

• A corpus luteal cyst may be indistinguishable from an ectopic pregnancy.

• Shared features of a hemorrhagic cyst and ectopic gestation are a thick echogenic rim and hemoperitoneum.

Suggested Readings

Frates MC, Visweswaran A, Laing FC. Comparison of tubal ring and corpus luteum echogenicities: a useful differentiating characteristic. J Ultrasound Med. 2001; 20(1):27–31, quiz 33

Dighe M, Cuevas C, Moshiri M, Dubinsky T, Dogra VS. Sonography in first trimester bleeding. J Clin Ultrasound. 2008; 36(6):352–366

Stein MW, Ricci ZJ, Novak L, Roberts JH, Koenigsberg M. Sonographic comparison of the tubal ring of ectopic pregnancy with the corpus luteum. J Ultrasound Med. 2004; 23(1):57–62

Case 187

Charles A. Tujo

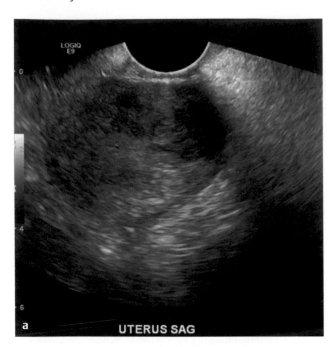
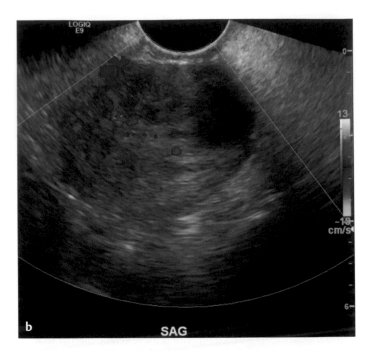
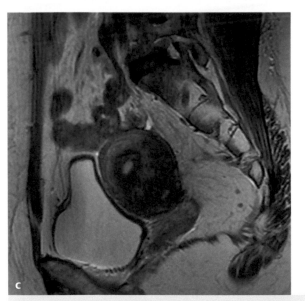
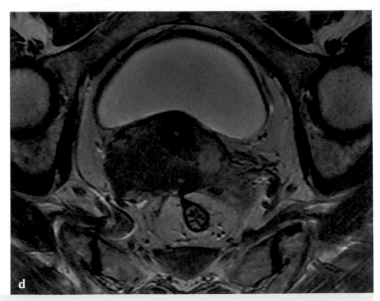

Fig. 187.1 (a) Longitudinal grayscale and (b) color flow sonographic images demonstrate a heterogeneously hypoechoic mass in the posterior uterus. (c) Sagittal T2 and (d) axial MR images reveal the junctional zone to measure >10 mm. Corresponding to the sonograms, there is a poorly defined hypointense region in the posterior uterine myometrium with glandular elements of increased T2 cystic foci.

■ Clinical Presentation

A 49-year-old premenopausal woman with pelvic pain, enlargement of the uterus, and heavy bleeding (►Fig. 187.1).

■ **Key Imaging Finding**

Hypoechoic uterine mass

■ **Top 3 Differential Diagnoses**

- **Leiomyoma (LM).** LMs are the most common uterine masses, considered the great mimicker in the pelvis because of their variable appearance. They are benign tumors composed of estrogen-dependent smooth muscle and connective tissue. They most often present as discrete uterine masses but may also be infiltrative, resulting in an enlarged, heterogeneous uterus. When focal, ultrasound (US) depicts a well-defined hypoechoic uterine mass with posterior acoustic shadowing. However, when these tumors outgrow their blood supply and degenerate, US findings may include echogenic shadowing foci from calcific degeneration or cystic regions of central necrosis. They are often described as subserosal, submucosal, or intramural based on their location. LMs are usually asymptomatic, but patients may present with abnormal or dysfunctional uterine bleeding, pain, or less commonly infertility. Magnetic resonance imaging (MRI) may be helpful for treatment planning of symptomatic fibroids, as well as to differentiate a diffuse fibroid uterus from adenomyosis. On MRI, LMs characteristically demonstrate low T2 signal intensity.
- **Adenomyoma.** Adenomyosis is defined by endometrial tissue displaced within the myometrium of the uterus, or endometriosis of the uterus. Clinical manifestations are frequent and include dysmenorrhea, menorrhagia, and in some cases infertility. Adenomyosis is frequently missed on sonography because its appearance is nonspecific; thus, MRI is required for confirmation. The imaging appearance generally reflects its focal or diffuse pattern within the myometrium. An ill-defined focal echogenic mass suggests focal adenomyosis. Diffuse adenomyosis and myometrial fibroids are difficult to distinguish sonographically, as both cause increased uterine heterogeneity. One clue to identify diffuse adenomyosis on US is asymmetric uterine enlargement of the anterior and posterior walls. Myometrial cysts, when present, are fairly specific for adenomyosis. On MRI, adenomyosis results in focal or diffuse thickening of the junctional zone (often >12 mm). Myometrial cysts, on the other hand, display characteristic increased T2 signal intensity.
- **Endometrial carcinoma (EC).** The most common gynecologic malignancy in North America, EC is caused by factors that predispose women to unopposed estrogen stimulation. Postmenopausal uterine bleeding in an otherwise asymptomatic woman is considered a sentinel sign of malignancy until proven otherwise. On US, a thickened endometrium in a postmenopausal woman (>5 mm) is an early sign of EC, and a biopsy is indicated. US findings of more advanced disease include an enlarged heterogeneous uterus, irregular lobulated endometrial margins or loss of endometrial–myometrial borders, and/or a large endometrial fluid collection. When EC invades the myometrium, the appearance can mimic other myometrial processes.

■ **Diagnosis**

Adenomyoma

✓ **Pearls**

- LMs are described on US as focal or diffuse in a subserosal, intramural, or submucosal location.
- Adenomyoma may be sonographically challenging, but is suggested with a hypoechoic mass.
- Biopsy is warranted in a woman with postmenopausal bleeding and a thickened endometrial stripe.

Suggested Readings

Byun JY, Kim SE, Choi BG, Ko GY, Jung SE, Choi KH. Diffuse and focal adenomyosis: MR imaging findings. Radiographics. 1999; 19(Spec No):S161–S170

Fleischer AC. Transvaginal sonography of endometrial disorders: an overview. Radiographics. 1998; 18(4):923–930

Mogavero G, Sheth S, Hamper UM. Endovaginal sonography of the nongravid uterus. Radiographics. 1993; 13(5):969–981

Case 188

David J. Weitz

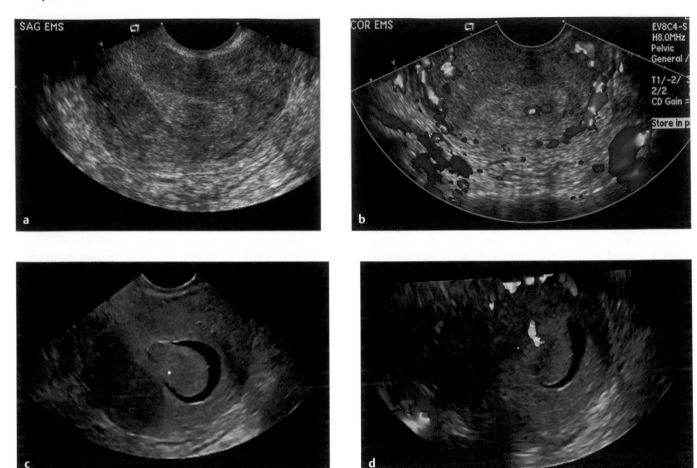

Fig. 188.1 **(a)** Grayscale and **(b)** color images from a transvaginal ultrasound of the uterus reveal an abnormally thickened endometrial stripe. Further work-up with saline infusion sonohysterogram shows **(c)** an echogenic predominately homogeneous endometrial polypoid mass with **(d)** a vascular stalk captured on Doppler flow imaging.

■ Clinical Presentation

A 42-year-old woman with "intermittent spotting between menstrual cycles" (▶Fig. 188.1).

■ Key Imaging Finding

Thickened endometrial stripe

■ Top 3 Differential Diagnoses

- **Endometrial hyperplasia**. Endometrial hyperplasia is a common cause of abnormal uterine bleeding. Hyperplasia is linked to unopposed estrogen stimulation (e.g., tamoxifen) and may progress to endometrial carcinoma (EC). The most common appearance is a uniformly thickened echogenic endometrium with or without cysts; however, ultrasound (US) is nonspecific and biopsy may be required.
- **Endometrial polyps**. Endometrial polyps can occur in young adults, but they are a frequent source of bleeding in postmenopausal women. US may show echogenic endometrial thickening. The presence of a vascular stalk is helpful, but not pathog-

nomonic. Hysterosonography, the preferred imaging exam for endometrial masses, will confirm a polyp as a pedunculated echogenic mass outlined by fluid.
- **Endometrial carcinoma**. An endometrial stripe greater than 5 mm is abnormal in postmenopausal women and should prompt an investigation to exclude malignancy. Although the appearance is variable, suspicion for EC should be raised when the endometrium is thickened, irregular, poorly marginated, or if there is disruption of the endometrial–myometrial border. Advanced EC may obstruct the endometrial canal, resulting in hydrometra or invade the myometrium.

■ Additional Differential Diagnoses

- **Submucosal fibroids**. Submucosal fibroids are the least common but most symptomatic type of fibroid. They generally appear as hypoechoic shadowing subendometrial masses. Given their submucosal location, they may be outlined by a more echogenic endometrium. They can protrude deep into the endometrial canal, mimicking a polyp, which makes hysterosonography a useful tool to differentiate between these entities.
- **Retained products of conception (RPOC)**. RPOC is an uncommon complication (1–2%) of pregnancy that should be suspected in recent postpartum women or recently terminated pregnancies with persistent vaginal bleeding and pelvic pain. US commonly reveals an endometrial mass with or without

Doppler flow. If flow is present, a high-velocity low-resistance Doppler signature is suggestive of RPOC. Other findings include a round fluid collection or an embryo-containing gestational sac.
- **Gestational trophoblastic disease (GTD)**. GTD ranges from a benign mole to choriocarcinoma. It is suspected in women with high beta HCG levels, abnormal bleeding, uterine size greater than dates, and preeclampsia. US features include an enlarged uterus, a thick echogenic endometrial canal, and through transmission; however, an additional finding of ovarian "theca lutein" cysts is highly suggestive.

■ Diagnosis

Endometrial polyp

✓ Pearls

- Endometrial hyperplasia commonly causes abnormal uterine bleeding and may progress to malignancy.
- Endometrial polyps can be confirmed by hysterosonography, a preferred exam for endometrial lesions.

- Findings for EC include a thick irregular endometrium or disruption of the endo/myometrial border.
- GTD is suspected with elevated β-HCG, abnormal bleeding, size greater than dates, and preeclampsia.

Suggested Readings

Botsis D, Papagianni V, Makrakis E, Aravantinos L, Creatsas G. Sonohysterography is superior to transvaginal sonography for the diagnostic approach of irregular uterine bleeding in women of reproductive age. J Clin Ultrasound. 2006; 34(9):434–439

Middleton WD, Kurtz AB, Hertzberg BS. Ultrasound: The Requisites. St. Louis, MO: Mosby; 2004

Case 189

David J. Weitz

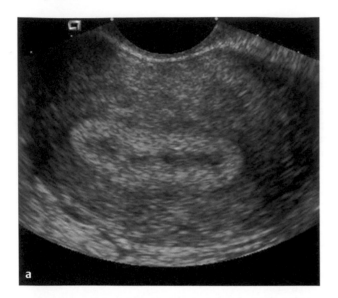 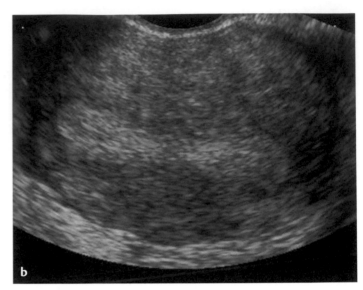

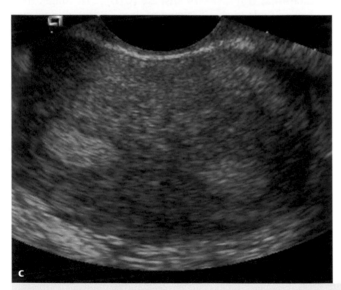

Fig. 189.1 (a–c) Transverse sonographic images demonstrate a thickened endometrial echo complex that begins to divide in the uterine body **(b)**. Two distinct and separated endometrial stripes are present in the uterine fundus **(c)**.

■ Clinical Presentation

Premenopausal woman with dysfunctional uterine bleeding (▶Fig. 189.1).

■ **Key Imaging Finding**

Uterine anomaly

■ **Top 3 Differential Diagnoses**

- **Bicornuate uterus.** Uterine anomalies are found in approximately 0.5% of the general population. Incomplete fusion of the Müllerian ducts results in a bicornuate uterus and may manifest either as two uterine horns, two cervices, and one vagina (bicornuate bicollis); or as two uterine horns, one cervix, and one vagina (bicornuate unicollis). The uterine cornua in a bicornuate uterus can be hypoplastic, which may infrequently lead to fertility problems. If a rudimentary "functional" horn does not communicate with the other horn, symptomatic hydrometrocolpos may occur. On ultrasound (US), the endometrium is usually widely divided and evaluation of the fundus reveals a midline uterine dimple at least 1 cm deep. Accuracy with 3D coronal US approaches that of magnetic resonance imaging (MRI), the imaging gold standard. Treatment, if needed, is metroplasty. Any uterine anomaly should prompt a search for renal anomalies (agenesis and ectopia), as uterine and renal anomalies frequently coexist because of their close relationship during development.
- **Didelphys uterus.** Uterine didelphys results from the failure of paired embryonic Müllerian (paramesonephric) ducts to fuse during fetal female development, resulting in two separate uteri, two cervices, and two vaginas. US should be performed in the secretory phase, because the endometrial stripe is thick and easily identified. US will reveal two separate and distinct uteri most often with widely separated uterine cornua. Fertility problems are unusual with this anomaly which is usually discovered incidentally.
- **Septated uterus.** Failure of the median uterine septum to regress during development results in a septated uterus. Unlike uterine didelphys which contains separate uterine cavities, a septated uterus is characterized by a thin septum which divides a single uterine cavity. Fertility problems occur frequently, since the fibrous septum generally will not support an embryo if implantation occurs on the relatively avascular septum. While sometimes difficult, it is important to make the imaging distinction between septated and bicornuate anomalies, since treatment options differ. While an involved metroplasty is required for a bicornuate uterus, a septated uterus is treated by a transvaginal hysteroscopic resection of the septum. On US, a narrowly divided endometrial echo complex is seen, but unlike a bicornuate anomaly, the fundal contour is normal, flat, or dimpled less than 1 cm.

■ **Additional Differential Diagnoses**

- **Arcuate uterus.** An arcuate uterus is generally considered a normal variant. This is an asymptomatic uterine variation with no observed complications. Sonographically, there may be a small indentation of the uterine fundus, but the uterine cavity is normal, leading to no fertility problems. As above, MRI is the imaging gold standard, but US may be the end point if findings are straightforward.

■ **Diagnosis**

Bicornuate uterus

✓ **Pearls**

- US reveals a bicornuate uterus as a widely divided endometrial echo complex and midline dimple > 1 cm.
- A didelphys uterus has two separate uteri, two cervices, and two vaginas; it is usually discovered incidentally.

- A septated uterus is the most common uterine anomaly associated with infertility.
- An arcuate uterus causes no complications and is characterized by a small uterine fundal indentation.

Suggested Readings

Middleton WD, Kurtz AB, Hertzberg BS. Ultrasound: The Requisites. St. Louis, MO: Mosby; 2004

Troiano RN, McCarthy SM. Mullerian duct anomalies: imaging and clinical issues. Radiology. 2004; 233(1):19–34

Case 190

Anokh Pahwa

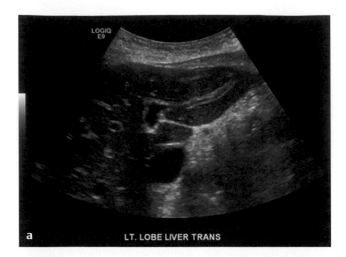

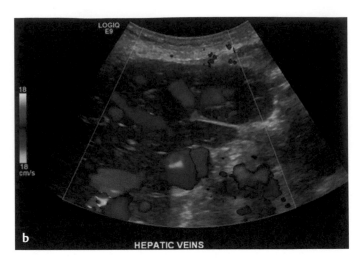

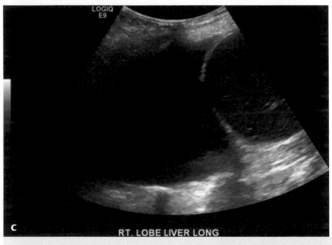

Fig. 190.1 **(a)** Transverse sonographic image through the liver demonstrates increased echogenicity in the region of the portal triads, referred to as a "starry sky" appearance. **(b)** Color flow image demonstrates robust flow in a prominently sized IVC. **(c)** Grayscale longitudinal image of the right hepatic lobe and lower thorax demonstrates a right-sided pleural effusion.

■ Clinical Presentation

An 86-year-old woman with new onset heart failure and transaminitis (▶Fig. 190.1).

■ Key Imaging Finding

"Starry sky" liver

■ Top 3 Differential Diagnoses

- **Acute hepatitis**. Although usually sonographically undetectable, acute hepatitis is a common cause of the "starry sky" appearance of the liver on ultrasound. Fibrosis of the portal venous walls leads to increased echogenicity of the portal triads. The "starry sky" appearance is secondary to this increased echogenicity of the portal triads in conjunction with decreased parenchymal echogenicity as a result of intralobular inflammatory edema. Chronic hepatitis is more likely to present with contrary findings, including coarsened parenchymal echotexture and decreased visualization of the portal triads.
- **Hepatic congestion**. Hepatic congestion is typically secondary to right-sided heart failure or less commonly inferior vena cava (IVC) or hepatic vein occlusion (Budd–Chiari syndrome). Ultrasound findings of passive hepatic congestion include hepatomegaly with IVC and hepatic vein enlargement. In right-sided heart failure, Doppler waveforms demonstrate

increased pulsatility within the hepatic and portal veins as a result of transmittance of right heart pressures. Rarely, the liver demonstrates a "starry sky" appearance.
- **Infiltrating neoplasm**. Both metastatic disease to the liver and primary hepatocellular carcinoma (HCC) can present as diffuse/infiltrative masses. Occasionally, diffuse tumor infiltration results in decreased echogenicity of the hepatic parenchyma, mimicking the "starry sky" appearance on ultrasound. Secondary involvement of the liver may occur with breast or lung carcinoma, as well as leukemia/lymphoma, to name a few entities. Diffuse HCC and diffuse metastatic disease can both lead to a nonspecific, heterogeneous, and multinodular-appearing liver. The presence of advanced cirrhosis decreases the sensitivity of ultrasound in detecting hepatic masses by 50%, particularly when diffuse.

■ Additional Differential Diagnoses

- **Toxic shock syndrome (TSS)**. TSS is a multisystem toxin-mediated disease most commonly caused by *Staphylococcus aureus*. TSS presentation can be varied, but the hallmarks include rapid-onset fever, hypotension, rash, vomiting, and diarrhea. In the liver, TSS can cause inflammation of the portal venous tracts, leading to a "starry sky" liver on ultrasound.
- **Biliary or portal venous gas**. Gas within the biliary ducts or portal veins results in increased echogenicity of the portal triads, which may mimic the "starry sky" appearance on ultrasound. Key differentiating features include the mobility of echoes (gas) during real-time examination, as well as the usually normal echotexture of the underlying hepatic parenchyma.

■ Diagnosis

Hepatic congestion due to congestive heart failure

✓ Pearls

- Acute hepatitis is the most common cause of the "starry sky" appearance on ultrasound.
- Hepatic congestion presents with hepatomegaly, dilated IVC/hepatic veins, and rarely a "starry sky" liver.
- Infiltrating neoplasms may decrease the hepatic echogenicity, mimicking a "starry sky" liver.
- Biliary or portal venous gas can be distinguished from a "starry sky" liver by mobility of the echoes.

Suggested Readings

Abu-Judeh HH. The "starry sky" liver with right-sided heart failure. AJR Am J Roentgenol. 2002; 178(1):78

Kurtz AB, Rubin CS, Cooper HS, et al. Ultrasound findings in hepatitis. Radiology. 1980; 136(3):717–723

Lieberman J, Bryan P, Cohen A. Toxic shock syndrome: sonographic appearance of the liver. AJR Am J Roentgenol. 1981; 137:606–607

Middleton WD, Kurtz AB, Hertzberg BS. Ultrasound: The Requisites. St. Louis, MO: Mosby; 2004

Case 191

Charles A. Tujo

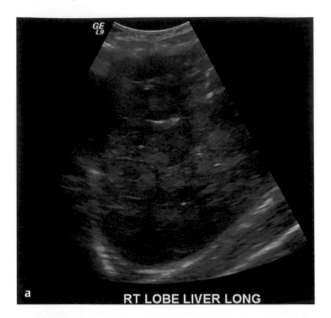

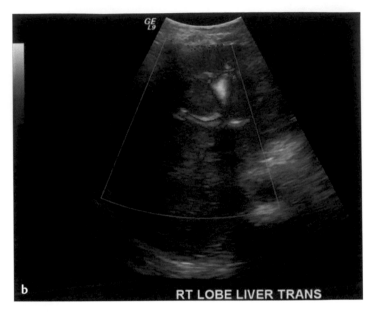

RT LOBE LIVER LONG

RT LOBE LIVER TRANS

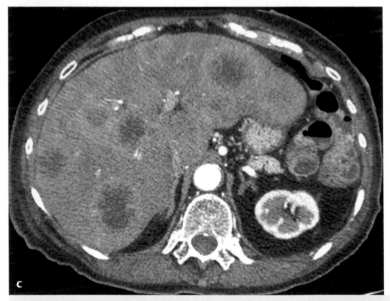

Fig. 191.1 **(a)** Grayscale ultrasound image of the right hepatic lobe reveals multiple heterogeneously echogenic lesions. **(b)** Power Doppler image shows displacement of vessels by one of the lesions. **(c)** Axial contrast-enhanced CT image through the midportion of the liver demonstrates multiple hypodense, peripherally enhancing masses.

■ Clinical Presentation

An 84-year-old woman with abdominal pain and elevated lipase and LDH (▶ Fig. 191.1).

■ Key Imaging Finding

Multiple echogenic liver masses

■ Top 3 Differential Diagnoses

- **Metastatic disease.** Multiple echogenic masses in the liver should prompt assessment for a gastrointestinal (GI) primary, such as colon cancer, which is the most common neoplasm to spread to the liver. GI malignancies contain a high amount of mucin, which accounts for the increased echoes. Other possibilities include breast, lung, pancreatic islet cell, carcinoid, and renal, which result in increased echoes because of their increased vascularity. Metastatic foci may have a peripheral hypoechoic halo. Computed tomography (CT) and magnetic resonance imaging (MRI) should be utilized to further characterize lesions and evaluate for complications, such as tumoral thrombus in the portal vein. Ultrasound (US) or CT can be used for image-guided biopsy.
- **Hepatocellular carcinoma (HCC).** HCC may present as an echogenic liver mass or present with multifocal liver disease. Surrounding cirrhotic nodules may be present. Risk factors for HCC include alcoholism, liver cirrhosis, and hepatitis B and C. Sonography is commonly utilized to screen for HCC in patients with risk factors. Sonography should be accompanied by cross-sectional imaging in the setting of a patient with hepatitis and increased tumoral markers, such as alpha-fetoprotein. The imaging appearance of HCC may be focal, nodular, or infiltrative. Smaller lesions are typically hypoechoic, whereas larger lesions are more heterogeneous or echogenic when fatty changes or hemorrhage are present. Lesions often have a peripheral low echogenicity halo (target lesion), especially in the setting of cirrhosis or fatty sparring.
- **Lymphoma.** In the unusual case that lymphoma involves the liver, it is more likely to be the non-Hodgkin variant. Patterns on US include multiple nodules, large masses, or diffusely infiltrating disease. Most commonly, US reveals small hypoechoic nodules or target lesions. A simple or complex "cystic" liver lesion in the setting of lymphoma should be considered suspicious. Other secondary findings include splenomegaly, hepatomegaly with or without discreet masses, and abdominal lymphadenopathy.

■ Additional Differential Diagnoses

- **Hepatic abscesses.** Liver abscesses have a variety of US appearances, including presentation as target or echogenic lesions. Given that multiple hepatic lesions are most often associated with malignancy, abscesses should be suspected in the appropriate clinical setting. Diagnosis is confirmed by percutaneous drainage.

■ Diagnosis

Metastatic disease (breast cancer)

✓ Pearls

- HCC is the most common primary hepatic malignancy and occurs in at-risk patient populations.
- Metastases commonly cause multiple liver lesions; GI and hypervascular primaries are often echogenic.
- US patterns of lymphoma include multiple nodules/masses or diffusely infiltrating tumor.
- Hepatic abscesses may be identified as target lesions and should be favored with signs of infection.

Suggested Readings

Castroagudín JF, Molina E, Abdulkader I, Forteza J, Delgado MB, Domínguez-Muñoz JE. Sonographic features of liver involvement by lymphoma. J Ultrasound Med. 2007; 26(6):791–796

Rubaltelli L, Savastano S, Khadivi Y, Stramare R, Tregnaghi A, Da Pian P. Targetlike appearance of pseudotumors in segment IV of the liver on sonography. AJR Am J Roentgenol. 2002; 178(1):75–77

Kim Y, Jung C, Jeong WK, et al. Hyperechoic hepatic nodules: correlation of findings from sonography, CT, and pathologic analysis. J Clin Ultrasound. 2004; 32(8):399–410

Case 192

David J. Weitz

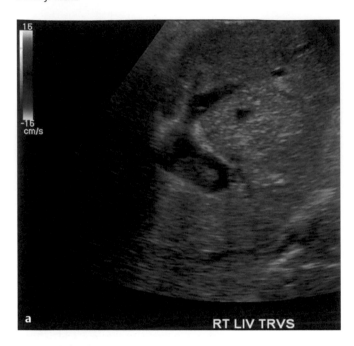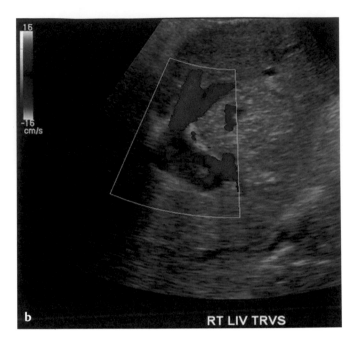

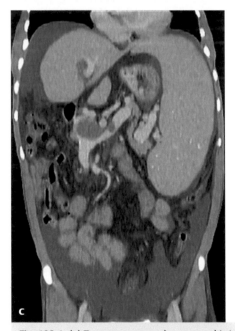

Fig. 192.1 **(a)** Transverse grayscale sonographic image through the liver demonstrates an isoechoic intraluminal filling defect (thrombus) within the main portal vein. **(b)** Color Doppler image delineates hepatopetal flow coursing around thrombus, as well as vascularity within the thrombus itself. **(c)** Reformatted contrast-enhanced computed tomography (CT) image in the coronal plane reveals the extent of thrombus which fills and expands the main portal vein and extends into the splenic vein. Additional CT findings include a nodular liver contour, massive splenomegaly, ascites, and varices, consistent with cirrhosis and portal hypertension. Additional imaging (not shown) revealed an infiltrating hepatic mass consistent with hepatocellular carcinoma in the setting of chronic liver disease.

■ Clinical Presentation

Increasing abdominal girth in an adult man with chronic liver disease (▶Fig. 192.1).

■ **Key Imaging Finding**

Portal vein thrombosis

■ **Top 3 Differential Diagnoses**

• **Tumor thrombus**. Tumor invasion of the portal vein is most commonly caused by hepatocellular carcinoma. Malignancies such as cholangiocarcinoma, gallbladder carcinoma, pancreatic carcinoma, gastric carcinoma, and metastases are less common offenders. Ultrasound (US) can diagnose tumor invasion accurately by demonstrating flow within the thrombus. It is important to note, however, that in some cases tumor thrombus may be hypovascular without detectable flow. Additional supportive findings include portal venous enlargement or expansion, which favors a neoplastic process over bland thrombus.

• **Hepatic cirrhosis with portal hypertension (HTN)**. In the United States, alcoholism is the most common cause of cirrhosis; however, longstanding fibrosis of any etiology will lead to portal HTN with sluggish portal flow or frank bland thrombus.

US usually demonstrates echogenic intraluminal clot in the portal vein; however, acute thrombus may also be hypo- or anechoic. In chronic portal HTN, collateral circulation may be seen as tortuous gastric, esophageal, and splenic varices. The development of collaterals within the porta hepatis is called cavernous transformation. Portal vein enlargement (>13 mm), ascites, and splenomegaly support the diagnosis of portal HTN. Reversal of portal flow (hepatofugal) or a recanalized umbilical vein is virtually diagnostic of portal HTN.

• **Periportal infection/inflammation**. Abundant literature supports the development of portal vein thrombosis in a variety of infectious and inflammatory conditions. The inflammatory process causes stasis of flow and subsequent clot formation. Common causes include sepsis, cholangitis, hepatitis, pancreatitis, and occasionally appendicitis.

■ **Additional Differential Diagnoses**

• **Hypercoagulable conditions**. Acquired hypercoagulable states include pregnancy, prolonged immobilization, medications (oral contraceptive pills), tobacco use, and underlying malignancy. Inherited conditions may summate with other risk factors, unmasking an underlying hypercoagulable state resulting in portal venous thrombosis. For example, factor V

Leiden, protein C, or protein S deficiencies may become clinically evident when combined with external risk factors.

• **Trauma/iatrogenic**. Portal vein thrombosis may occur in the setting of trauma or as a complication of medical procedures. Common iatrogenic causes of portal vein thrombosis include umbilical catheter placement in neonates and patients undergoing orthotopic liver transplant.

■ **Diagnosis**

Tumor thrombus (hepatocellular carcinoma) in the portal vein

✓ **Pearls**

• US can accurately demonstrate tumor invasion of the portal vein by revealing thrombus vascularity.

• Portal flow reversal and umbilical vein recanalization are diagnostic of portal HTN.

• Sepsis, cholangitis, hepatitis, pancreatitis, and other inflammatory etiologies can cause venous thrombosis.

• Iatrogenic causes of portal vein thrombosis include umbilical catheter placement and liver transplant.

Suggested Readings

Middleton WD, Kurtz AB, Hertzberg BS. Ultrasound: The Requisites. St. Louis, MO: Mosby; 2004

Rumack CM, Wilson SR, Charboneau JW. Diagnostic Ultrasound. 3rd ed. St. Louis, MO: Mosby; 2005

Tessler FN, Gehring BJ, Gomes AS, et al. Diagnosis of portal vein thrombosis: value of color Doppler imaging. AJR Am J Roentgenol. 1991; 157(2):293–296

Case 193

Sima Naderi

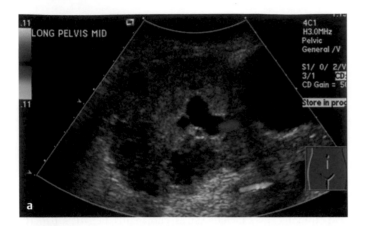

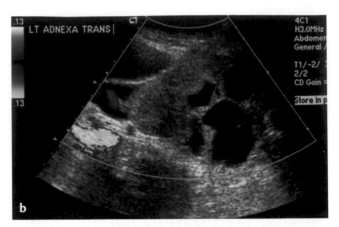

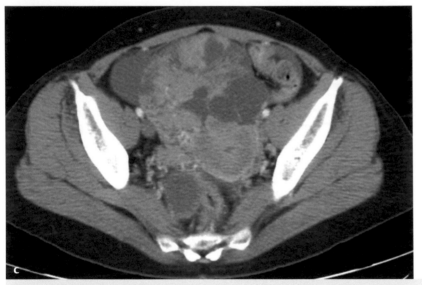

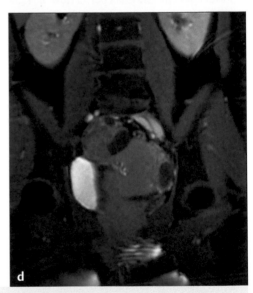

Fig. 193.1 Color transabdominal ultrasound image of **(a)** the pelvis and **(b)** left adnexa demonstrates a left solid and cystic adnexal mass with regions of flow. **(c)** Axial contrast-enhanced CT image demonstrates a corresponding heterogeneously enhancing solid and cystic midline pelvic mass. **(d)** Contrast-enhanced T1 fat-saturated coronal MR image of the pelvis demonstrates an enhancing multilobulated cystic and solid mass.

■ Clinical Presentation

A 49-year-old woman with tightening in the pelvis and a palpable mass on exam suspected as a fibroid. Human chorionic gonadotropin (HCG) is negative (▶Fig. 193.1).

■ Key Imaging Finding

Cystic adnexal mass with negative HCG

■ Top 3 Differential Diagnoses

- **Ovarian neoplasm.** Ninety percent of ovarian malignancies are epithelial neoplasms. The remaining are germ cell tumors, sex cord–stromal tumors, and metastatic tumors. Malignant masses are associated with advanced age, nulliparity, and a positive family history. Ultrasound (US) is the initial study of choice for evaluating the adnexa. However, US is not able to definitively differentiate benign ovarian neoplasms, such as serous cystadenoma or mucinous cystadenoma, from malignant. An ovarian mass has a higher incidence of being malignant when larger than 10 cm or contains more complex US features, such as irregular walls, thickened septations > 2 mm, vegetations, or solid echogenic components. Peritoneal carcinomatosis and malignant ascites can also be present. Doppler findings may be helpful, but should be interpreted in association with mass morphology. Malignant tumors are regularly staged with computed tomography (CT).
- **Hemorrhagic cyst.** Functional cysts such as follicular or corpus luteal cysts can have internal hemorrhage. Clinically, patients may complain of acute onset of unilateral adnexal pain. Appearance is quite variable depending on the stage of the clot, but acute hemorrhage appears as a complex echogenic mass with through transmission. As the hemorrhage ages, the mass characteristically shows lacelike internal echoes. As the clot retracts, fluid–fluid levels can be seen, or the echogenic clot can settle in the dependent portion of the cyst, which can mimic a papillary projection of malignancy. This is readily differentiated, however, by the lack of flow within the clot on color Doppler. Hemorrhagic cysts typically are not greater 3 cm, and if so, may warrant follow-up to confirm decrease in size or resolution.
- **Tubo-ovarian abscess (TOA).** TOA is usually suspected based on the clinical presentation of pelvic pain and localized adnexal tenderness in an ill-appearing patient. If significantly dilated and redundant, the fallopian tube can mimic a cystic adnexal mass. As the infection spreads, the ovaries enlarge and the margins of pelvic structures become indistinct, such that inflammation may prevent the vaginal transducer from separating the ovary and tube. Distorted anatomy can make US challenging to interpret.

■ Additional Differential Diagnoses

- **Endometrioma.** Unlike the rapid onset of pain seen with hemorrhagic cysts, chronic pelvic pain is a frequent complaint with endometriosis. Endometriomas most commonly implant on the ovary. They are characteristically thick-walled cystic lesions with homogeneous low-level echoes characterized as a "chocolate cyst." US may show a complex mass similar to a hemorrhagic cyst. Some endometriomas can appear solid or have thick septa mimicking an ovarian neoplasm. Magnetic resonance imaging (MRI) can be helpful by demonstrating chronic blood products seen as T2 hypointensity (shading).

■ Diagnosis

Ovarian neoplasm (mucinous cystadenoma)

✓ Pearls

- US findings for malignancy include solid portions, papillary projections, thick septations, and large size.
- Hemorrhagic cysts change over time and are associated with acute adnexal tenderness.
- TOA is painful and should be suspected in ill-appearing patients with a history of pelvic inflammatory disease.
- Endometriomas classically have thick walls and low level echoes on US with T2 shading on MRI.

Suggested Readings

Fried AM, Kenney CM, III, Stigers KB, Kacki MH, Buckley SL. Benign pelvic masses: sonographic spectrum. Radiographics. 1996; 16(2):321–334

Middleton WD, Kurtz AB, Hertzberg BS. Ultrasound: The Requisites. St. Louis, MO: Mosby; 2004

Laing FC, Allison SJ. US of the ovary and adnexa: to worry or not to worry? Radiographics. 2012; 32(6):1621–1639, discussion 1640–1642

Case 194

Eleanor L. Ormsby

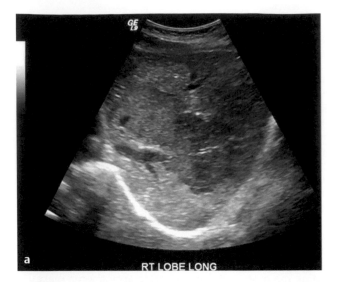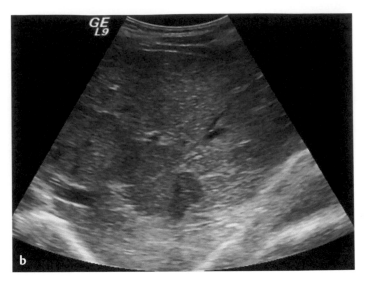

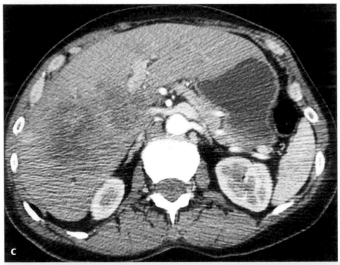

Fig. 194.1 **(a, b)** Longitudinal grayscale ultrasound images through the right hepatic lobe demonstrate multiple hypoechoic masses. **(c)** Contrast-enhanced axial CT image through the liver in soft-tissue window shows multiple corresponding low-density masses.

■ Clinical Presentation

A 71-year-old woman status post mastectomy with elevated liver enzymes (▶Fig. 194.1).

■ **Key Imaging Finding**

Multiple hypoechoic liver masses

■ **Top 3 Differential Diagnoses**

- **Neoplasm**. **Metastatic disease** is the most common malignancy to involve the liver and usually presents with multiple masses involving both hepatic lobes. They can have a variety of ultrasound (US) appearances, including the classic target appearance with an echogenic center and hypoechoic halo, as well as multiple uniformly hypoechoic masses. **Hepatocellular carcinoma** (HCC) is the most common primary hepatic malignancy and may present as solitary, multifocal, or diffuse and infiltrating masses with variable echogenicity. HCC usually occurs in the setting of chronic liver disease or cirrhosis. **Lymphoma** is a homogeneous tumor which produces hypoechoic lesions in the liver. US appearance may mimic a cyst. Given the overlapping nature of these neoplasms, tissue diagnosis is often required.
- **Multifocal abscesses**. Multifocal abscesses in the liver commonly appear as complex fluid collections with mixed echo-

genicity and thick-walled cysts. Abscesses typically do not demonstrate intralesional flow, although commonly they have increased flow along the peripheral margins in adjacent liver parenchyma. They can also mimic solid hepatic masses with variable echogenicity, especially early in the disease process. Patients with multifocal abscesses are clinically symptomatic with fever, leukocytosis, and pain.
- **Candidiasis**. Fungal infections of the liver usually occur in the immunocompromised and are most commonly *Candida*. Although it usually causes small lesions (microabscesses), larger lesions may occur. These typically have a target appearance with a central echogenicity and a peripheral hypoechoic halo, but may also occasionally appear as hypoechoic masses. Healed lesions may calcify appearing echogenic.

■ **Additional Differential Diagnoses**

- **Hematoma**. Hepatic hematomas can be traumatic or iatrogenic. They can appear as complex cystic lesions or hypoechoic masses. Acute hematomas are often isoechoic to liver parenchyma and produce only subtle alterations in hepatic echogenicity. However, as they become progressively more liquefied, they appear more hypoechoic and cystic. There should be no blood flow on color Doppler imaging.
- **Diffuse fatty infiltration with focal fatty sparing**. With diffuse fatty infiltration of the liver, there is uniformly increased echogenicity. Under normal circumstances, liver parenchyma

is only slightly more echogenic than the renal cortex. Fatty infiltration is recognized by seeing marked discrepancy between the echogenic liver and less echogenic kidney. In many cases, there will be focal areas of spared normal liver parenchyma that appear hypoechoic with respect to the fatty infiltrated parenchyma. These can be mistaken for focal hypoechoic lesions. Knowledge of the usual location of focal sparing, such as adjacent to the gallbladder fossa, falciform ligament, and porta hepatis, helps differentiate this entity.

■ **Diagnosis**

Neoplasm (breast carcinoma metastases)

✓ **Pearls**

- Multiple hypoechoic masses are nonspecific and may be seen in primary or secondary hepatic neoplasms.
- In the clinical setting of infection, multiple masses within the liver are suggestive of pyogenic abscesses.

- Although microabscesses are more common, *Candida* may produce multiple hypoechoic liver lesions.

Suggested Readings

Middleton WD, Kurtz AB, Hertzberg BS. Ultrasound: The Requisites. St. Louis, MO: Mosby; 2004

Prasad SR, Wang H, Rosas H, et al. Fat-containing lesions of the liver: radiologic-pathologic correlation. Radiographics. 2005; 25(2):321–331

Case 195

David J. Weitz

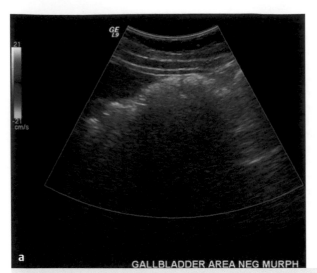
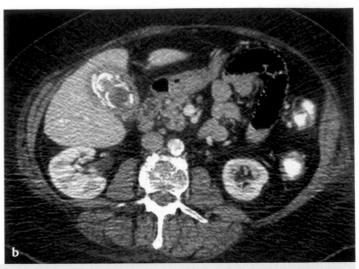

Fig. 195.1 **(a)** Right upper quadrant ultrasound image shows an echogenic curved focus in the gallbladder fossa with extensive posterior shadowing. **(b)** Corresponding axial CT image reveals a thin layer of calcification in the gallbladder with additional calcified stones.

■ Clinical Presentation

An 85-year-old woman with right upper quadrant pain (▶Fig. 195.1).

■ **Key Imaging Finding**

Echogenic foci in gallbladder wall

■ **Top 3 Differential Diagnoses**

- **Porcelain gallbladder.** Porcelain gallbladder derives its name from the gross appearance at surgery, described as a brittle-appearing gallbladder with bluish tint. A calcium-encrusted gallbladder wall occurs as a result of chronic inflammation which, in large part, explains the very high association of gallstones and porcelain gallbladder. Porcelain gallbladder is considered to be asymptomatic, most often discovered incidentally. Once diagnosed, however, surgical removal is warranted because of an increased risk of gallbladder carcinoma. On ultrasound (US), the gallbladder wall appears as a highly reflective curvilinear interface with associated posterior shadowing and nonvisualization of the gallbladder lumen. If the sound beam is able to penetrate the calcification within the near wall, the posterior gallbladder wall will be visualized, distinguishing this entity from a stone-filled gallbladder where a back wall is absent. The diagnosis of porcelain gallbladder should prompt a search for a gallbladder mass, liver lesions, or lymphadenopathy. Wall calcification may be confirmed with plain film or computed tomography (CT).
- **Emphysematous cholecystitis (EC).** EC is a rare complication of acute cholecystitis and is considered a surgical emergency. There is a high association of EC with older diabetic men. The etiology is thought to be from vascular compromise, which leads to the production of gas in the gallbladder wall by bacteria such as *Escherichia coli*. Progression to gallbladder gangrene and perforation is much higher in EC than in uncompli-

cated acute cholecystitis. Early on, patients may complain of right upper quadrant pain. If gallbladder perforation occurs, temporary symptom relief is followed by generalized abdominal pain, usually from life-threatening peritonitis. On US, the normal appearance of the gallbladder is replaced by a curvilinear echogenic line and dirty shadowing in the gallbladder fossa. Ring down artifact, seen with gas and not calcification, is helpful to differentiate EC from a stone-filled gallbladder or porcelain gallbladder. Gas extending into the gallbladder lumen can appear as mobile bright foci. Other findings include gallbladder calculi, wall thickening, and pericholecystic fluid. If US findings are nonspecific, CT is exquisite for distinguishing between the entities above.
- **Adenomyomatosis.** Adenomyomatosis, a type of hyperplastic cholecystosis, is a relatively common benign finding affecting the gallbladder. Pathologically, there is muscular thickening of the gallbladder wall and deposition of cholesterol crystals into intramural diverticula, termed Rokitansky–Aschoff sinuses. US typically shows a thickened gallbladder wall in asymptomatic patients. Punctate echogenic reflectors with comet tail artifact in the gallbladder wall are considered a specific finding. Because gas will also produce a similar appearing artifact, that is, ring down, care must be taken not to mistake this entity for EC. Therefore, it is important to note that adenomyomatosis is most often an incidental finding in contradistinction to the ill presentation noted in patients afflicted with EC.

■ **Diagnosis**

Porcelain gallbladder with underlying gallstones

✓ **Pearls**

- The diagnosis of porcelain gallbladder should prompt a cholecystectomy because of its association with malignancy.
- EC, seen in significantly ill older diabetics, is suggested by mobile comet tail artifact in the gallbladder wall.

- Adenomyomatosis also produces comet tail reflectors but is found in fairly asymptomatic patients.

Suggested Readings

Hanbidge AE, Buckler PM, O'Malley ME, Wilson SR. From the RSNA refresher courses: imaging evaluation for acute pain in the right upper quadrant. Radiographics. 2004; 24(4):1117–1135

Middleton WD, Kurtz AB, Hertzberg BS. Ultrasound: The Requisites. St. Louis, MO: Mosby; 2004

Rosenthal SJ, Cox GG, Wetzel LH, Batnitzky S. Pitfalls and differential diagnosis in biliary sonography. Radiographics. 1990; 10(2):285–311

Case 196

Sima Naderi

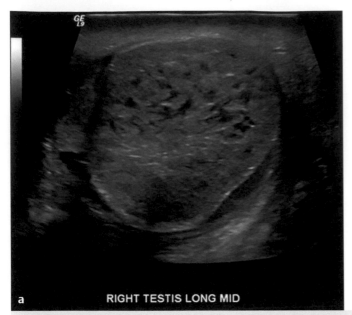
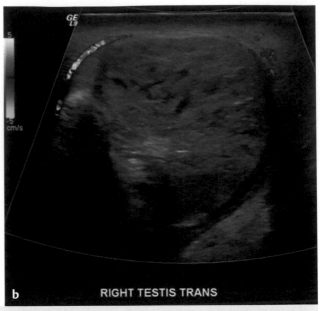

Fig. 196.1 **(a)** Grayscale and **(b)** color Doppler imaging of the right testicle demonstrates an enlarged, heterogeneous left testicle with abnormal orientation and absent internal blood flow.

■ Clinical Presentation

A 17-year-old boy with acute-onset right testicular pain (►Fig. 196.1).

■ Key Imaging Finding

Enlarged painful testicle

■ Top 3 Differential Diagnoses

- **Testicular torsion**. Torsion of the testicle occurs most commonly in the setting of the bell-clapper deformity. In this anomaly, the tunica vaginalis completely surrounds the testis, epididymis, and part of the spermatic cord, and there is no attachment of the testis to the posterior scrotal wall. Prompt diagnosis is needed. If surgery is performed within 6 hours of the onset of torsion/pain, there is improved chance of salvaging the testicle. Within the first 6 hours of torsion, grayscale imaging can show an enlarged testicle with normal echogenicity. As ischemia continues, the testicle becomes heterogeneous and hypoechoic. Color Doppler is a useful ultrasound (US) function to diagnose torsion and demonstrates absent or significantly decreased blood flow in the affected testicle compared with the contralateral testicle. The number of twists of the spermatic cord determines testicular viability. Complete torsion, or greater than 540-degree twisting, results in arterial occlusion. With partial torsion, or less than 360-degree twisting, the venous outflow is obstructed, resulting in arterial flow still visualized on Doppler examination, but with decreased diastolic flow. If spontaneous detorsion occurs, the resultant hyperemic testes may mimic orchitis.

- **Epididymo-orchitis**. Epididymo-orchitis is the key differential diagnosis in the adult patient with acute scrotal pain and swelling. The inflammatory disease usually involves the epididymis initially and spreads to the testis. The epididymis is enlarged, with decreased echogenicity and increased vascularity. Typical findings of orchitis include testicular enlargement and decreased echogenicity. In contrast to testicular torsion, the testicle has increased vascularity. If there is progression to testicular abscess, the complex fluid collections will have peripheral hyperemia. A potential pitfall is severe orchitis, which can cause global ischemia, mimicking testicular torsion.

- **Testicular hematoma/fracture**. While testicular injury is in the differential of the enlarged painful testicle, there is typically a history of trauma. Sonographic findings include focal areas of increased and decreased testicular echogenicity because of areas of hemorrhage or infarction, as well as testicular contour irregularity. The testis may also appear distorted. If the surrounding tunica albuginea remains intact, surgery is not needed. However, if there is evidence of testicular rupture, emergent surgery is required to salvage the testicle.

■ Diagnosis

Testicular torsion

✓ Pearls

- The testis is enlarged and hypoechoic in acute torsion; decreased or absent testicular flow is diagnostic.
- In contradistinction to torsion, epididymo-orchitis results in a hyperemic epididymis and testicle.

- Testicular injury may appear similar to torsion or orchitis on US but is seen in the setting of trauma.
- Missed or delayed torsion can present with an edematous testicle, decreased echoes, and peripheral flow.

Suggested Readings

Woodward PJ, Sohaey R, O'Donoghue MJ, Green DE. From the archives of the AFIP: tumors and tumorlike lesions of the testis: radiologic-pathologic correlation. Radiographics. 2002; 22(1):189–216

Zagoria RJ, Dyer R, Brady C. Genitourinary Imaging: The Requisites. 3rd ed. Philadelphia, PA: Elsevier Inc.; 2016

Case 197

David J. Weitz

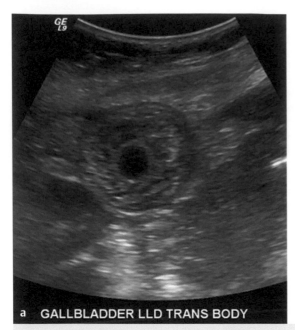
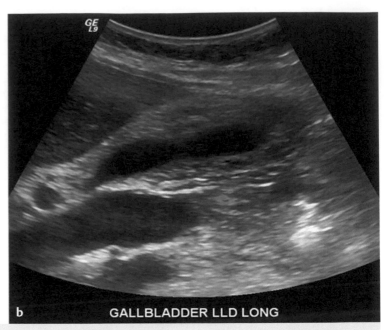

Fig. 197.1 Diffuse and marked thickening of the gallbladder wall is demonstrated in **(a)** transverse and **(b)** longitudinal ultrasound images of the gallbladder. Notice the absence of gallbladder calculi, the concentric striated appearance of an edematous gallbladder wall, and the increased caliber of the inferior vena cava **(b)**.

■ Clinical Presentation

Vague abdominal pain in an elderly woman (▶Fig. 197.1).

■ Key Imaging Finding

Gallbladder (GB) wall thickening

■ Top 3 Differential Diagnoses

- **Acute cholecystitis**. Acute cholecystitis is usually a consequence of cystic duct obstruction from an impacted calculus leading to GB enlargement and pain. A hydropic GB with intraluminal calculi and a sonographic Murphy sign allows a confident diagnosis of cholecystitis. Wall thickening (>3 mm) is often present, but is not specific. Other supportive findings include pericholecystic fluid and GB wall hyperemia. Acalculus cholecystitis typically occurs in critically ill patients who produce "hyperviscous" obstructive sludge. Hepatobiliary scanning, computed tomography (CT), and now magnetic resonance imaging/magnetic resonance cholangiopancreatography (MRI/MRCP) are often used for complicated cases.
- **Gallbladder wall edema**. A striated sonographic appearance of the GB wall containing pockets of fluid in the absence of a sonographic Murphy sign is more characteristic of GB wall edema rather than acute cholecystitis. GB wall thickening in generalized edematous states includes congestive heart failure (CHF), hypoproteinemia, renal failure, advanced liver disease, and lymphatic obstruction secondary to portal lymphadenopathy or mass.
- **Secondary inflammation**. Apart from primary GB disease, there are focal and systemic inflammatory conditions which may evoke GB wall inflammation. Pancreatitis, hepatitis, and pyelonephritis are common diseases which may secondarily inflame the GB wall. In AIDS patients, diffuse wall thickening may be a consequence of the primary HIV virus or opportunistic infections (e.g., *Cytomegalovirus* [CMV], *Cryptosporidium*).

■ Additional Differential Diagnoses

- **Gallbladder carcinoma**. Asymmetric GB wall thickening or a large mass in the GB lumen or fossa is suspicious for malignancy. Doppler is useful in differentiating neoplasm from nonvascular tumefactive sludge, as well as assessing for vascular invasion or adenopathy in the setting of GB carcinoma. GB carcinoma is closely associated with gallstones, and there is an increased risk in patients with porcelain GB.
- **Gallbladder polyp**. Polyps are asymptomatic nonshadowing nonmobile masses growing from the GB wall, which may simulate focal wall thickening. Color or power Doppler is a useful tool to demonstrate a vascular pedicle. While not considered true tumors, polyp resection is warranted with a diameter >1 cm.
- **Adenomyomatosis**. This idiopathic condition results in diffuse or focal thickening of the muscular wall and overgrowth of GB mucosa. Ring-down artifact arising from echogenic foci in the GB wall on ultrasound is considered pathognomonic and reflects the deposition of cholesterol crystals into mucosal diverticuli (Rokitansky–Aschoff sinuses). This is a benign finding and usually incidentally discovered.

■ Diagnosis

Gallbladder wall edema (CHF)

✓ Pearls

- The diagnosis of cholecystitis is made by demonstrating GB calculi and a sonographic Murphy sign.
- A thickened striated appearance to the GB wall without a sonographic Murphy sign suggests edema.
- Inflammatory conditions such as hepatitis and pancreatitis may secondarily thicken the GB wall.
- Asymmetric GB wall thickening is unusual in benign conditions and should raise the suspicion for cancer.

Suggested Readings

Rumack CM, Wilson SR, Charboneau JW. Diagnostic Ultrasound. 3rd ed. St. Louis, MO: Mosby; 2005

van Breda Vriesman AC, Engelbrecht MR, Smithuis RH, Puylaert JB. Diffuse gallbladder wall thickening: differential diagnosis. AJR Am J Roentgenol. 2007; 188(2):495–501

Case 198

Eleanor L. Ormsby

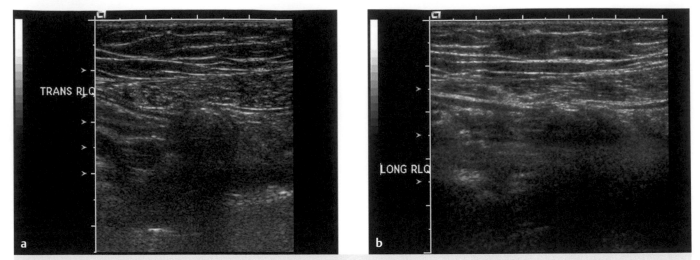

Fig. 198.1 **(a)** Transverse and **(b)** longitudinal sonographic images through the RLQ demonstrate a thickened blind-ending tubular structure measuring 12 mm in diameter with adjacent echogenic fat. On the transverse view **(a)**, there is a luminal filling defect with posterior acoustic shadowing.

■ Clinical Presentation

A 10-year-old boy with right lower quadrant (RLQ) pain (►Fig. 198.1).

■ Key Imaging Finding

RLQ mass in a child

■ Top 3 Differential Diagnoses

- **Appendicitis**. The primary criterion for the diagnosis of appendicitis is an appendiceal diameter greater than 6 mm on ultrasound (US) with compression. The measurement is made from outer wall to outer wall. In some patients, an intraluminal appendicolith, typically with posterior shadowing, may be detected. Other associated findings are inflamed echogenic periappendiceal fat, loculated periappendiceal fluid collections, and hyperemia on color Doppler imaging.
- **Intussusception**. Intussusception can be idiopathic or secondary to a pathologic lead point. Possible lead points include a Meckel diverticulum, lymphoma, inspissated feces in cystic fibrosis, or bowel wall hemorrhage in Henoch–Schönlein purpura. On a transverse US image, it appears as a donut with multiple altering echogenic and hypoechoic layers because of the presence of overlapping mucosal and muscular layers of the intussuscipiens and the intussusceptum with interposed fat. On longitudinal or sagittal imaging, it can resemble a pseudokidney. Lack of blood flow in the intussusception increases the likelihood of necrosis, which would suggest the need for surgical intervention.
- **Enteric duplication cyst**. Duplication cysts typically present as a rounded fluid-filled mass displacing the adjacent bowel. They may contain ectopic gastric mucosa which can cause hemorrhage, focal bowel wall thickening, and/or inflammation. The ileum is the most common site of involvement.

■ Additional Differential Diagnoses

- **Mesenteric adenitis**. Mesenteric adenitis is a diagnosis of exclusion where multiple enlarged and clustered lymph nodes are seen just anterior to the right psoas muscle without evidence of appendicitis. This entity can coexist with inflammation of the terminal ileum and cecum and generally has a self-limited clinical course.
- **Adnexal mass in a female**. In young females, RLQ pain may be secondary to ovarian or adnexal pathology. Common etiologies include ovarian torsion with or without an associated mass, ruptured ovarian cyst, hemorrhagic cyst, endometrioma, infectious process (tubo-ovarian abscess), and ectopic pregnancy.
- **Meckel diverticulum**. Meckel diverticulum is an omphalomesenteric duct anomaly which can cause pain because of bleeding from ectopic gastric mucosa, focal inflammation, perforation, or intussusception. Meckel scan using Tc-99m pertechnetate is useful for detecting diverticula that contain ectopic gastric mucosa.

■ Diagnosis

Acute appendicitis

✓ Pearls

- Appendicitis is diagnosed by observing a noncompressible tubular mass in the RLQ > 6 mm in diameter.
- Lead points for intussusception include Meckel diverticulum, lymphoma, or hemorrhage.
- Enteric duplication cysts present as round fluid-filled masses occurring most commonly in the ileum.
- Adnexal masses in women may mimic appendicitis, emphasizing the relevance of age and clinical history.

Suggested Readings

Middleton WD, Kurtz AB, Hertzberg BS. Ultrasound: The Requisites. St. Louis, MO: Mosby; 2004

Ripollés T, Martinez-Perez MJ, Morote V, Solaz J. Diseases that simulate acute appendicitis on ultrasound. Br J Radiol. 1998; 71(841):94–98

Case 199

David J. Weitz

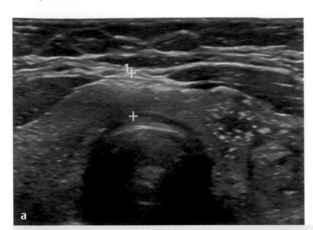 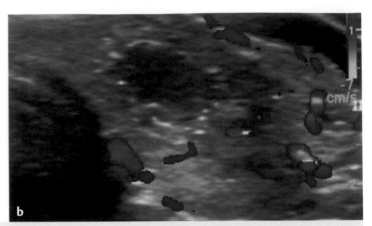

Fig. 199.1 **(a)** Transverse grayscale US image of thyroid gland demonstrates diffuse thickening and nodularity in a multinodular gland. Scattered echogenic foci are seen within a hypoechoic nodule in the medial anterior left lobe. **(b)** Coned-down color Doppler image of the same nodule reveals a predominately hypoechoic echotexture with punctate nonshadowing echogenic foci, representing microcalcifications. Although flow is observed at the periphery of an ill-defined nodule border, no flow is demonstrated centrally.

■ Clinical Presentation

Palpable thyroid nodule in a middle-aged woman (▶ Fig. 199.1).

■ Key Imaging Finding

Thyroid mass

■ Top 3 Differential Diagnoses

- **Benign thyroid nodule.** Thyroid nodules are very common in the adult population and their prevalence increases with age. The vast majority of nodules are benign and are categorized as hyperplastic (most common), colloid cysts, or adenomas. Common features shared by benign nodules include rim or egg-shell calcification, cystic components, and a thin hypoechoic halo. Glandular hyperplasia can result in nonneoplastic nodules, whereas adenomas are true neoplasms. Both are indistinguishable from malignant nodules via ultrasound (US). Hyperplastic nodules and adenomas may be entirely solid or partially cystic. Echogenicity is variable and ranges from hyper- to hypoechoic. Coarse peripheral calcification may obscure the nodule secondary to extensive shadowing. Colloid nodules contain inspissated colloid (echogenic foci with comet-tail artifact) which reliably differentiates them from microcalcifications (echogenic foci without comet tail artifact) which are suspect for thyroid malignancy.
- **Thyroid malignancy.** Risk factors include male, age < 20 or >60, history of head/neck radiation, and positive family history. Patients may present with pain or hoarseness. Common thyroid cancer types include papillary, follicular, medullary, anaplastic, Hürthle cell, lymphoma, and mixed. Differentia-

tion of a benign nodule from thyroid cancer cannot reliably be made with US. However, microcalcifications in a hypoechoic solid nodule are very suspicious for thyroid malignancy, most commonly papillary cancer. Malignant nodules often have irregular borders. Enlarged cystic or calcified lymph nodes in the neck with a suspect thyroid nodule are suggestive of local extension of thyroid cancer. Flow patterns are nonspecific, but an avascular nodule is more likely to be benign. Size, number of nodules, and growth are less helpful in classification. Indeterminate and suspicious nodules may require fine needle aspiration (FNA).
- **Parathyroid adenoma.** Normal parathyroid glands are rarely visualized on routine thyroid exams because of their small size, but US is useful for suspected parathyroid adenomas. On US, they appear as solid hypoechoic ovoid masses posterior to the thyroid gland. US is helpful to identify ectopic adenomas. Since these tumors are highly vascular, Doppler technique is a useful search tool. US may be combined with parathyroid scintigraphy and sometimes computed tomography (CT) or magnetic resonance imaging (MRI) to improve localization accuracy.

■ Additional Differential Diagnoses

- **Thyroglossal duct cyst (TDCs).** The most common congenital neck mass, TDCs occur from failure of the epithelial tract of the developing thyroid to involute. Cysts may arise anywhere along the tract which runs midline from the tongue base (foramen cecum) to the thyroid gland; the majority are found be-

low the hyoid bone where they are characteristically embedded in strap musculature. Commonly, these lesions will have a homogeneously hypoechoic (or anechoic) appearance in the midline with a smooth circumscribed border. Below the hyoid bone, they are often paramidline.

■ Diagnosis

Thyroid malignancy (papillary thyroid carcinoma)

✓ Pearls

- The presence of colloid crystals in a thyroid nodule is a reliable sign of benignity.
- A hypoechoic nodule containing microcalcifications raises suspicion for thyroid malignancy.

- US may be used to localize parathyroid adenomas, and is commonly combined with other modalities.
- TDCs are usually midline, homogeneously hypoechoic, and defined by a smooth circumscribed border.

Suggested Readings

Hoang JK, Lee WK, Lee M, Johnson D, Farrell S. US Features of thyroid malignancy: pearls and pitfalls. Radiographics. 2007; 27(3):847–860, discussion 861–865

Middleton WD, Kurtz AB, Hertzberg BS. Ultrasound: The Requisites. St. Louis, MO: Mosby; 2004

Case 200

Anokh Pahwa

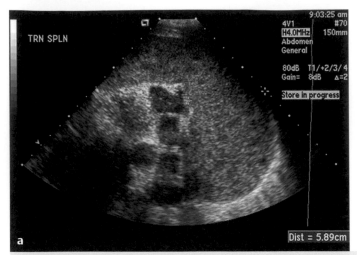
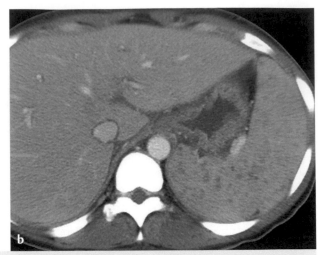

Fig. 200.1 **(a)** Transverse sonographic image through the left upper quadrant demonstrates innumerable small hypoechoic foci involving the spleen diffusely. **(b)** Contrast-enhanced axial CT image in the same patient confirms the findings, showing multiple hypodense splenic lesions.

■ Clinical Presentation

A 26-year-old HIV-positive woman with cough and fever (►Fig. 200.1).

■ Key Imaging Finding

Multiple splenic hypoechoic foci

■ Top 3 Differential Diagnoses

• **Fungal abscess (candidiasis).** Most commonly occurring in immunocompromised patients, fungal abscesses are multifocal and can be caused by *Candida*, *Aspergillus*, or *Cryptococcus*. They are typically characterized by multiple "target" lesions on ultrasound, consisting of a hypoechoic central nidus of necrosis surrounded by an echogenic ring of viable fungal elements. When this lesion is surrounded by a peripheral hypoechoic zone of inflammatory change, it is referred to as a "wheel-within-a-wheel" pattern.

• **Diffuse lymphoma.** Lymphoma is the most common malignant neoplasm of the spleen. It may manifest as unifocal, multifocal, or diffuse disease involvement. Splenomegaly is commonly, but not invariably, present. While ultrasound is insensitive for diffuse splenic lymphoma, the finding of multiple hypoechoic foci with indistinct borders in a patient with known lymphoma is highly specific for splenic involvement.

• **Granulomatous disease.** Similar to fungal abscesses, active granulomatous disease can present as multiple hypoechoic splenic lesions that can calcify over time. The most frequent granulomatous disease to involve the spleen in the United States is histoplasmosis, but in immunocompromised patients, *Mycobacterium tuberculosis* or *Pneumocystis jirovecii* can have similar imaging characteristics. Discrete small hypoechoic splenic nodules can also be seen with sarcoidosis.

■ Additional Differential Diagnoses

• **Metastatic disease.** Metastatic disease to the spleen is relatively rare and generally only seen in advanced disease with widespread metastatic involvement. While 50% of splenic metastases are secondary to malignant melanoma, other primaries malignancies include carcinomas from lung, breast, and colon. US appearance can be quite variable, but the lesions are most typically hypoechoic with low-level internal echoes. These findings correlate to cystic masses with internal necrosis. A surrounding hypoechoic halo is thought to be a sign of aggressiveness.

■ Diagnosis

Granulomatous disease (miliary tuberculosis)

✓ Pearls

• Fungal abscesses are fairly uncommon and nearly always occur in immunocompromised patients.

• Splenic lymphoma has a variable sonographic appearance and is suggested with appropriate history.

• Granulomatous disease of the spleen presents as hypoechoic nodules which often calcify over time.

• Splenic metastases most often result from melanoma, lung, breast, and colon primary malignancies.

Suggested Readings

Chen MJ, Huang MJ, Chang WH, et al. Ultrasonography of splenic abnormalities. World J Gastroenterol. 2005; 11(26):4061–4066

Urrutia M, Mergo PJ, Ros LH, Torres GM, Ros PR. Cystic masses of the spleen: radiologic-pathologic correlation. Radiographics. 1996; 16(1):107–129

Case 201

Anokh Pahwa

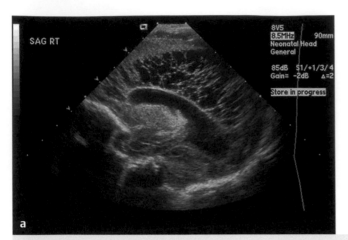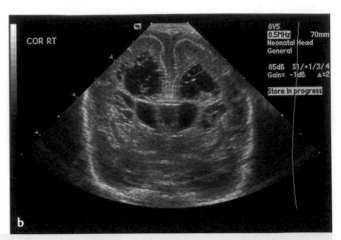

Fig. 201.1 **(a)** Longitudinal/sagittal and **(b)** coronal ultrasound images of the head demonstrate marked cystic changes in the posterior and lateral periventricular white matter with sparing of the cortex.

■ Clinical Presentation

One-month-old premature girl born at 29 weeks of gestation
(►Fig. 201.1).

■ Key Imaging Finding

Periventricular cysts

■ Top 3 Differential Diagnoses

- **Periventricular leukomalacia.** Periventricular leukomalacia (PVL) is defined as ischemic injury to the periventricular white matter in the preterm infant. White matter in the preterm infant is poorly vascularized and sensitive to ischemic and infectious injury. In addition, the lack of autoregulation in preterm brains leaves these watershed areas at risk. The typical distribution includes the deep white matter dorsal and lateral to the lateral ventricles, particularly involving the optic and acoustic radiations with sparing of the cortex. Infants born at less than 32 weeks of gestation are at the highest risk. Immediate neonatal head ultrasound (US) may be normal. Earliest findings are vague echogenic changes which may progress to multicystic involvement (cystic PVL) in severe cases. Prognosis is poor with cystic PVL, and large bilateral cysts (>10 mm) are highly predictive of development of cerebral palsy.

- **Subependymal cysts.** Subependymal cysts may be congenital or acquired. Acquired subependymal cysts are secondary to germinal matrix hemorrhage in preterm infants. The germinal matrix is a highly vascular structure near the head of the caudate nucleus which regresses near term. Infants born at less than 32 weeks of gestation should be screened with a head US for germinal matrix hemorrhage at 4 and 7 days.
- **Infection.** With the exception of herpes simplex, which an infant acquires during passage through the birth canal, TORCH infections affect a fetus by transplacental transmission. Head US can reveal a variety of findings, from microcephaly or hydranencephaly secondary to early gestational infection to porencephalic cysts and periventricular calcifications (CMV and toxoplasmosis) with infections later in gestation. Cysticercosis leads to multiple cysts which usually calcify.

■ Additional Differential Diagnoses

- **Choroid plexus cysts.** Choroid plexus cysts can vary in size and be solitary or multiple. They arise from the body of the choroid but may protrude into the ventricle. While choroid plexus cysts can be seen in a small percentage (<5%) of normal pregnancies, there is a greater-than-expected association with aneuploidy, particularly trisomy 18, particularly when multiple, bilateral, and/or large (>1 cm). Their presence on prenatal US should trigger a search for associated anatomic defects. In

an otherwise normal infant, however, there is no clinical significance to a choroid plexus cyst.
- **Porencephaly.** Porencephaly describes a CSF-filled cavity adjacent to and possibly communicating with the ventricles. It is secondary to encephalomalacia from any destructive process (e.g., ischemia, hemorrhage, infection) occurring in the third trimester or postnatally. There may be wall calcifications.

■ Diagnosis

Periventricular leukomalacia

✓ Pearls

- Early signs of PVL include echogenic foci in the deep white matter that may lead to cystic changes.
- US is used to screen preterm infants (<32 weeks) for germinal matrix hemorrhage in the first 7 days of life.

- TORCH infections in the neonate are associated with a variety of sequelae, including cyst formation.
- Choroid plexus cysts are usually incidental findings, but there is an association with aneuploidy.

Suggested Readings

Blickman H. Pediatric Radiology: The Requisites. St. Louis, MO: Mosby; 1998

Epelman M, Daneman A, Blaser SI, et al. Differential diagnosis of intracranial cystic lesions at head US: correlation with CT and MR imaging. Radiographics. 2006; 26(1):173–196

Middleton WD, Kurtz AB, Hertzberg BS. Ultrasound: The Requisites. St. Louis, MO: Mosby; 2004

Case 202

David J. Weitz

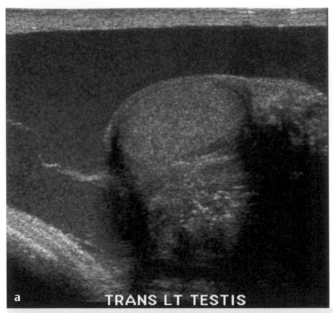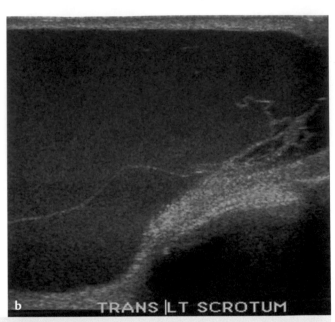

Fig. 202.1 (a, b) Transverse ultrasound images through the left scrotum reveal a large predominately hypoechoic fluid collection with fine free-floating septations superimposed on a background of uniform low level echoes.

■ Clinical Presentation

Enlarged painful scrotal mass in a young adult man after vasectomy 1 month earlier (▶Fig. 202.1).

■ Key Imaging Finding

Complex extratesticular fluid collection

■ Top 3 Differential Diagnoses

- **Varicocele.** Abnormal dilatation of the spermatic cord veins (pampiniform plexus) is defined as a varicocele. Classically, patients will present with a palpable mass in the scrotum that has the consistency of a "bag of worms." Larger varicoceles may be painful, but most are asymptomatic and generally discovered during a fertility evaluation where varicoceles are a well-established cause of male infertility. Seen in approximately 15% of men, varicoceles result from valvular incompetence. Most varicoceles (85%) are left sided because of increased venous pressure from an asymmetrically longer left testicular vein that drains into a higher pressure system (i.e., the left renal vein), whereas on the right the testicular vein drains directly into the inferior vena cava. An isolated right varicocele should prompt a search for a retroperitoneal mass or adenopathy. On ultrasound (US), testicular veins (usually in the superior lateral scrotum) dilated more than 2 mm are suspect, but demonstration of flow reversal during color Doppler interrogation is diagnostic. Other supporting findings on US include serpiginous tubular structures in the scrotum and a greater than 1 mm change in caliber post-Valsalva (or supine to standing).
- **Hematocele:** A scrotal hematocele can be characterized as a type of complex hydrocele in which blood products collect within and separate the visceral and parietal layers of the tunica vaginalis. Hematoceles are most commonly posttraumatic (including iatrogenic), but may occur in the setting of scrotal tumors or torsion. In early stages, hematoceles are more uniformly echogenic or mildly heterogeneous, often with reactive hyperemia of the scrotum and epididymis. Skin thickening from edema is common. Over time, septations, fluid-fluid levels, or low-level echoes often develop on a background of hypoechoic fluid. US is the initial study of choice in the evaluation of acute scrotal injury.
- **Pyocele.** Like a hematocele, a pyocele falls into the category of a complex hydrocele. A pyocele represents an infectious extratesticular fluid collection, most commonly a complication of epididymo-orchitis or retrograde spread of cystitis. US appearance may vary, but most pyoceles are complex fluid collections indistinguishable from hematoceles. Color Doppler may reveal reactive hyperemia of the scrotal wall, and vascular engorgement of the epididymis. US should always be correlated with clinical findings. Patients with a pyocele typically present with fever, leukocytosis, and acute scrotal pain. On clinical exam, the scrotum is painfully enlarged, often with overlying skin erythema. The presence of echogenic foci producing ring-down artifact is highly suggestive of gas, seen in the setting of life-threatening necrotizing fasciitis, or Fournier gangrene, most common in diabetics.

■ Diagnosis

Hematocele (iatrogenic)

✓ Pearls

- Varicoceles are diagnosed by noting an increase in vein caliber during Valsalva and reversal of flow.
- Hematoceles are usually the result of trauma; US is the preferred initial study.
- Pyoceles are complex extratesticular fluid collections distinguished from hematoceles by clinical history.

Suggested Readings

Deurdulian C, Mittelstaedt CA, Chong WK, Fielding JR. US of acute scrotal trauma: optimal technique, imaging findings, and management. Radiographics. 2007; 27(2):357–369

Dogra VS, Gottlieb RH, Oka M, Rubens DJ. Sonography of the scrotum. Radiology. 2003; 227(1):18–36

Kim W, Rosen MA, Langer JE, Banner MP, Siegelman ES, Ramchandani P. US MR imaging correlation in pathologic conditions of the scrotum. Radiographics. 2007; 27(5):1239–1253

Woodward PJ, Schwab CM, Sesterhenn IA. From the archives of the AFIP: extratesticular scrotal masses: radiologic-pathologic correlation. Radiographics. 2003; 23(1):215–240

Case 203

Charles A. Tujo

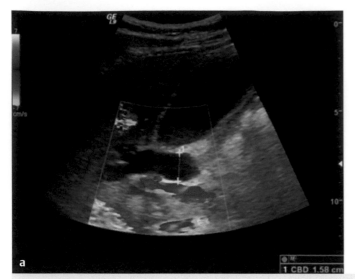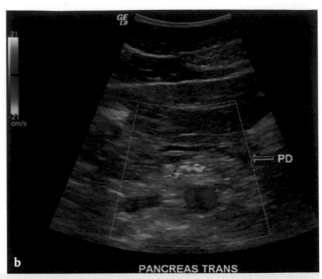

Fig. 203.1 **(a)** Right upper quadrant color flow ultrasound image at the level of the porta hepatis demonstrates a dilated common bile duct. **(b)** A color flow image through the body of the pancreas demonstrates a dilated pancreatic duct. This "double duct" appearance is used to describe concomitant dilatation of the common bile duct and pancreatic duct, and is suspicious for an obstructing mass at the convergence of the two ducts.

■ Clinical Presentation

A 66-year-old man with right upper quadrant pain; rule out biliary disease (▶ Fig. 203.1).

■ Key Imaging Finding

Double duct sign (dilatation of common bile and pancreatic ducts)

■ Top 3 Differential Diagnoses

- **Malignancy**. *Pancreatic adenocarcinoma* is the number one cause of malignant biliary obstruction. Sonographically, adenocarcinoma appears as a hypoechoic avascular mass. If located in the pancreatic head, common bile duct (CBD) dilatation is common. A "double duct sign" is seen when a pancreatic head mass obstructs and dilates both the pancreatic and CBDs. Unfortunately, ultrasound (US) cannot reliably distinguish neoplasm from pancreatitis. *Cholangiocarcinoma* is a rare biliary malignancy commonly seen in older men with painless jaundice and may be intrahepatic, hilar, or distal (common duct). A common appearance is proximal duct dilatation and abrupt tapering distally with or without ductal wall thickening. Less commonly seen is a hypoechoic polypoid mass expanding the CBD. Flow is usually absent. *Ampullary carcinoma* can result in dilation of the pancreatic and hepatic ductal system. However, this entity should be considered after careful exclusion of a pancreatic neoplasm. Malignancies are better evaluated with CT, MRI, and/or endoscopic US.
- **Choledocholithiasis**. Biliary calculi are the most common cause of CBD dilatation. A dilated CBD is often the primary or only finding on US, although occasionally the obstructing stone can be visualized. The CBD is considered dilated if >6 mm in patients younger than 70 years with 1 mm of dilatation allowed per decade thereafter. Primary choledocholithiasis is the formation of stones in the CBD from stasis, whereas secondary choledocholithiasis is the result of stone passage from the gallbladder and cystic duct. US may show an echogenic, rounded, intraluminal filling defect with posterior shadowing most often at the distal duct near the ampulla of Vater. If a calculus is present distally in the common duct near the sphincter of Oddi, the double duct configuration can be present.
- **Ampullary stenosis**. Ampullary stenosis is essentially a diagnosis of exclusion. It should be considered once other etiologies are excluded (e.g., obstructing mass or stone). Ampullary stenosis can result from instrumentation of the biliary system, to include endoscopic retrograde cholangiopancreatography (ERCP) or biopsy, as well as secondary to infectious or inflammatory processes, to include variants of cholangitis (e.g., primary sclerosing cholangitis).

■ Additional Differential Diagnoses

- **Cholangitis**. Acute cholangitis typically results from biliary obstruction, usually as a result of intraductal calculi causing bile stasis with subsequent infection. Postoperative biliary strictures, tumors, primary sclerosing cholangitis, and iatrogenic seeding are also potential etiologies of cholangitis. Classic symptoms include fever, right upper quadrant pain, and jaundice. On US, dilated intra- and extrahepatic bile ducts are commonly seen, as are intraductal calculi. Biliary sludge, ductal wall thickening, and hepatic abscesses are also supporting US features.

■ Diagnosis

Malignancy (pancreatic adenocarcinoma)

✓ Pearls

- Dilatation of the CBD and pancreatic duct (double-duct sign) should raise the suspicion for malignancy.
- On US, choledocholithiasis appears as ductal dilatation with an echogenic shadowing obstructive lesion.
- Classically described symptoms for acute cholangitis are fever, right upper quadrant pain, and jaundice.

Suggested Readings

Cronan JJ. US diagnosis of choledocholithiasis: a reappraisal. Radiology. 1986; 161(1):133–134

Rumack CM, Wilson SR, Charboneau JW. Diagnostic Ultrasound. 3rd ed. St. Louis, MO: Mosby; 2005

Shawker TH, Garra BS, Hill MC, Doppman JL, Sindelar WF. The spectrum of sonographic findings in pancreatic carcinoma. J Ultrasound Med. 1986; 5(3):169–177

Case 204

David J. Weitz

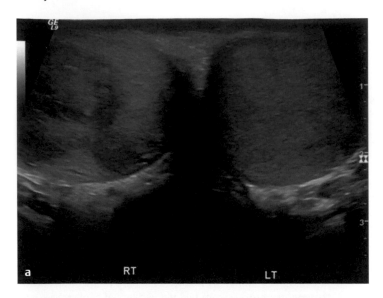
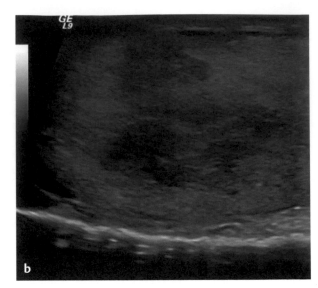
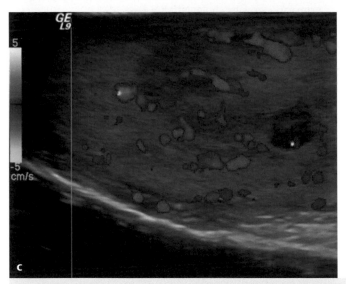

Fig. 204.1 **(a)** Transverse gray scale ultrasound image of both testicles demonstrates asymmetric enlargement of the right testicle which contains a lobulated heterogeneously mixed but predominantly hypoechoic mass. **(b)** Transverse view of the right testicle better depicts the hypoechoic region. **(c)** Doppler color image of the right testicle demonstrates vascular flow within the hypoechoic region.

■ Clinical Presentation

A 28-year-old man with an enlarged but painless testicle (▶Fig. 204.1).

■ Key Imaging Finding

Enlarged painless testis

■ Top 3 Differential Diagnoses

- **Testicular neoplasm**. Testicular neoplasms are the most common malignancy in young males. Thus, any testicular mass must be considered malignant in the absence of trauma or infection. The sentinel clinical symptom is painless enlargement or a palpable lump. A small number of patients do experience pain, however, from hemorrhage or infarct. Nearly all testicular neoplasms are germ cell tumors, most commonly being mixed germ cell tumors or seminomas. Other neoplasms include sex chord stromal tumors, metastases, lymphoma, and epidermoid cysts. Seminomas are classically homogeneously hypoechoic. Non-seminomatous tumors are heterogeneous and may contain coarse calcifications or cystic regions. Although controversial, microlithiasis may predispose to malignancy. Most tumors demonstrate vascularity, which may be normal or increased. It is important to scan the contralateral testis as bilateral tumors may be found with metastases, lymphoma, and rarely seminomas.
- **Lymphoma/leukemia**. Lymphoma of the testes is primarily a disease of older males, while leukemia is most often seen in children. Primary lymphoma/leukemia of the testes is rare, but because the blood–testes barrier hinders therapeutic concentrations of chemotherapeutic agents to the testes, it is a frequent site of recurrence. Ultrasound (US) findings include diffuse hypoechoic unilateral or bilateral testicular enlargement. Occasionally, US may demonstrate a focal hypoechoic mass. In the absence of other findings, diffuse or focal hypervascularity of the testes may help identify tumor in subtle cases. Involvement of the epididymis is common, which is generally enlarged and hypoechoic, but epididymal vascularity is usually normal. Patients are generally asymptomatic, distinguishing it from epididymo-orchitis.
- **Testicular cysts**. Testicular cysts are found in 8 to 10% of males. They may be located within the testicular parenchyma or arise from the tunica albuginea. Given that intratesticular masses are nearly always malignant, the importance of confirming a simple cyst cannot be overstated. Tunica albuginea cysts are small (generally <5 mm) and peripheral. Despite the small size, the majority of these cysts present as palpable abnormalities. Intratesticular cysts are not palpable and are usually located near the mediastinum testis, but may occur anywhere within the parenchyma. Because of their mediastinal location, they may originate from a dilated rete testis. An enlarged rete testis (tubular ectasia) is cystic transformation of the efferent ductules, located within the mediastinum. US shows a network of dilated tubular structures, often bilateral, replacing the mediastinum in the presence of epididymal head cysts.

■ Additional Differential Diagnoses

- **Epidermoid cyst.** Epidermoid cysts are well-defined, round, benign testicular lesions which may demonstrate characteristic alternating hyper and hypoechoic rings, appearing as "onion skinning." No abnormal color flow is associated with these lesions. Treatment of these lesions is wedge resection.

■ Pseudoaneurysm

Testicular neoplasm (Seminoma)

✓ Pearls

- Intratesticular mass in the absence of a known cause should be considered suspicious for malignancy.
- The testes are often a site of lymphoma/leukemia recurrence due to a drug-inhibiting blood–testis barrier.
- Testicular cysts are common benign testicular lesions that must be differentiated from cystic neoplasms.

■ Suggested Reading

Woodward PJ, Sohaey R, O'Donoghue MJ, Green DE. From the archives of the AFIP: tumors and tumorlike lesions of the testis: radiologic-pathologic correlation. Radiographics. 2002; 22(1):189–216

Case 205

Charles A. Tujo

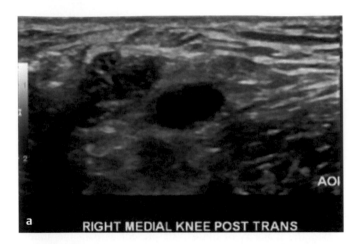
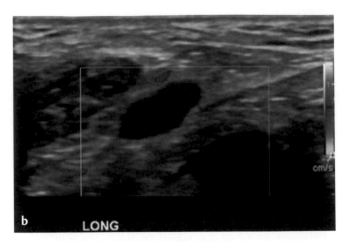

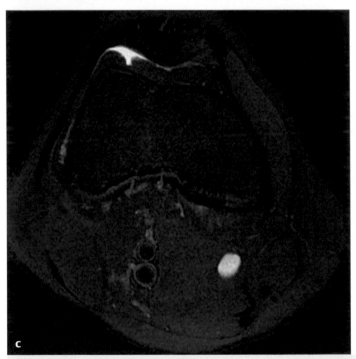
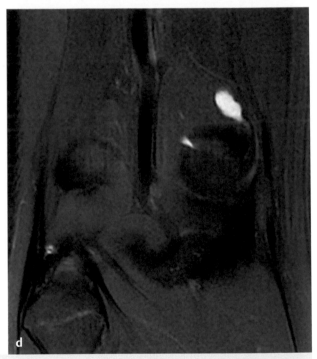

Fig. 205.1 **(a)** Transverse grayscale and **(b)** longitudinal color image of the right knee demonstrate an anechoic lesion between the medial head of the gastrocnemius and semimembranosus muscles without flow. **(c)** Axial and **(d)** coronal T2 fat-saturated images confirm a T2 hyperintense lesion between the medial head of the gastrocnemius and semimembranosus muscles.

■ **Clinical Presentation**

Young adult with right posterior knee pain (▶Fig. 205.1).

■ Key Imaging Finding

Popliteal cystic mass

■ Top 3 Differential Diagnoses

- **Popliteal cyst.** Popliteal or Baker cysts are common lesions. They are considered synonymous; however, some reserve the diagnosis of a Baker cyst only when there is a neck located between the medial head of the gastrocnemius and semimembranosus tendons. These lesions have a multitude of appearances ranging from simple to complex cysts with septations and/or echogenic components. Popliteal cysts are not solid lesions; therefore, they do not demonstrate any flow. They have been known to reach sizes of 3 to 5 cm in some patients and can compress adjacent structures, resulting in pain or a palpable mass. As most lesions are discovered incidentally, they do not require treatment or follow-up if asymptomatic.
- **Popliteal artery aneurysm.** Popliteal aneurysms are typically pulsatile lesions that are diagnosed when the popliteal artery reaches ≥7 mm. They are second in incidence and commonly seen in association with abdominal aortic aneurysms. When the aneurysm is patent, the diagnosis can be fairly easily made on color Doppler imaging, demonstrating internal flow and communication with the popliteal artery. However, should the popliteal artery be partially or fully thrombosed, this can reduce the diagnostic confidence by US and necessitate further cross-sectional imaging.
- **Synovial sarcoma.** The most common location for a synovial sarcoma is the knee. Synovial sarcomas appear as a heterogeneously hypoechoic masses on US that may contain solid mural nodular components and/or calcifications. They typically have a mixed-cystic and solid-type appearance. If a popliteal lesion has solid components or calcification, a Baker cyst is unlikely and additional cross-sectional imaging should be considered.

■ Additional Differential Diagnoses

- **Popliteal hemorrhage/hematoma.** Hematomas can present as palpable masses with appearances ranging from homogeneously hypoechoic to heterogeneous with echogenic foci and lace-like septations. There may even be a retractile clot simulating an underlying solid mass; however, there is no internal flow. Therefore, flow in a popliteal mass excludes hematoma, unless of course there is active hemorrhage with associated increase in size.

■ Diagnosis

Baker cyst

✓ Pearls

- Baker cyst are located between the medial head of the gastrocnemius and semimembranosus tendons.
- Popliteal aneurysms are pulsatile masses and are diagnosed when the artery reaches ≥7 mm.
- Synovial sarcoma is uncommon; however, it presents as a mixed cyst and solid mass with calcification.

Suggested Readings

Helbich TH, Breitenseher M, Trattnig S, Nehrer S, Erlacher L, Kainberger F. Sonomorphologic variants of popliteal cysts. J Clin Ultrasound. 1998; 26(3):171–176

Murphey MD, Gibson MS, Jennings BT, Crespo-Rodríguez AM, Fanburg-Smith J, Gajewski DA. From the archives of the AFIP: Imaging of synovial sarcoma with radiologic-pathologic correlation. Radiographics. 2006; 26(5):1543–1565

Wright LB, Matchett WJ, Cruz CP, et al. Popliteal artery disease: diagnosis and treatment. Radiographics. 2004; 24(2):467–479

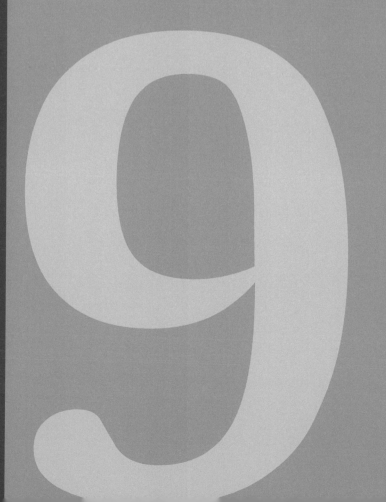

Part 9

Fetal Imaging

Case 206

Corinne D. Strickland

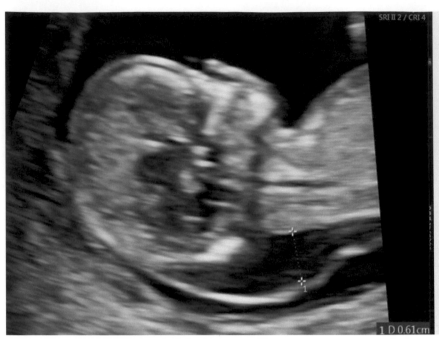

Fig. 206.1 Sagittal ultrasound image of a fetus at 12 weeks of gestational age reveals a nuchal translucency measuring over 3 mm.

■ Clinical Presentation

Screening ultrasound (US) of a 38-year-old G1P0 woman at 12 weeks of gestational age (►Fig. 206.1).

■ Key Imaging Finding

Nuchal translucency

■ Top 3 Differential Diagnoses

• **Trisomy 21**. Trisomy 21 (Down syndrome) is the most common disorder caused by chromosomal nondisjunction and is a frequent cause of mental retardation. Like other nondisjunction syndromes, the incidence of Down syndrome is increased with advanced maternal age. The most widely used screening method utilizes sonographic measurement of the fluid layer in the posterior fetal neck, known as the nuchal translucency (NT). Between 11 and 14 weeks of gestation, NT is normally less than 3 mm, and NT is frequently increased in fetuses with chromosomal abnormalities and/or congenital heart defects. NT measurement is combined with maternal age and two maternal serum markers to yield an estimated risk of trisomy 21. More reliable methods of screening for trisomy 21 combine these values with second trimester maternal serum markers, elevating the trisomy 21 detection rate of approximately 85% with a false-positive rate of 5%. Alternative noninvasive prenatal screening has been increasingly used, called *cell-free DNA* (cfDNA) and consists of the analysis of fetal DNA extracted from maternal blood with lower false-positive and false-negative rates than the sequential screen (NT combined with blood analysis). Definitive prenatal diagnosis, however, requires amniocentesis or chorionic villus sampling. Both of these methods carry a risk of fetal loss. Patients with Down syndrome may have associated abnormalities and findings on US, including cardiac defects, ventriculomegaly, duodenal atresia, pyelectasis, hyperechoic bowel, omphalocele, and short femora and humeri.

• **Turner syndrome**. Girls with Turner syndrome (monosomy XO) display short stature, ovarian dysgenesis, and variable learning difficulties. Congenital lymphedema is a common feature of the syndrome and may manifest as increased NT (often > 4.5 mm) on first trimester US. Cystic hygroma, a form of nuchal fluid collection caused by abnormal lymphatic development, may be identified in the first or second trimester.

• **Trisomy 18**. Trisomy 18 (Edward syndrome) is the second most common chromosomal nondisjunction syndrome. Affected infants rarely survive beyond the first year of age. Sonographic findings include increased NT in the first trimester, cystic hygroma, growth restriction, abnormal extremities (clenched hands, overlapping digits), and choroid plexus cysts.

■ Additional Differential Diagnoses

• **Trisomy 13**. Trisomy 13 (Patau syndrome) is characterized by holoprosencephaly, cleft lip and palate, polydactyly, and renal and cardiac anomalies. Occasionally, nuchal translucency may be seen on first trimester US. Survival beyond a few months of life is rare.

■ Diagnosis

Trisomy 21

✓ Pearls

• Down syndrome is the most common cause of increased nuchal translucency during first trimester US.
• Down syndrome is characterized by mental retardation, as well as cardiac, central nervous system, gastrointestinal, and skeletal defects.

• Turner syndrome is characterized by short stature, ovarian dysgenesis, and cystic hygromas.
• Trisomy 18 presents with cystic hygromas, clenched fists with overlapping digits, and choroid plexus cysts.

Suggested Readings

Cuckle HS, Malone FD, Wright D, et al. Contingent screening for Down syndrome--results from the FaSTER trial. Prenat Diagn. 2008; 28(2):89–94

Fong KW, Toi A, Salem S, et al. Detection of fetal structural abnormalities with US during early pregnancy. Radiographics. 2004; 24(1):157–174

Tanriverdi HA, Hendrik HJ, Ertan AK, Axt R, Schmidt W. Hygroma colli cysticum: prenatal diagnosis and prognosis. Am J Perinatol. 2001; 18(8):415–420

Case 207

Corinne D. Strickland

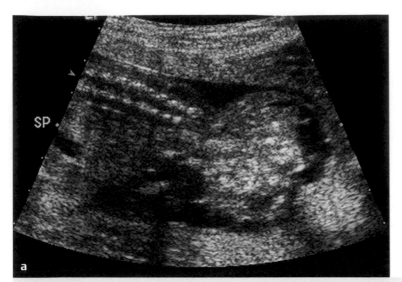
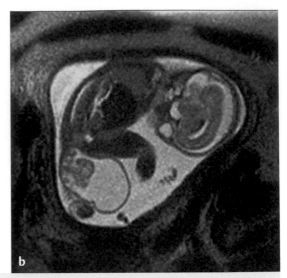

Fig. 207.1 (a) Longitudinal ultrasound image of the lower fetal spine in gray scale demonstrates a heterogeneous cystic and solid mass arising from the distal fetal spine. (b) Fetal MR image better demonstrates the mass arising from the sacrum.

■ Clinical Presentation

Abnormal ultrasound findings in G1P0 woman at 20 weeks of pregnancy (▶Fig. 207.1).

■ Key Imaging Finding

Sacral mass

■ Top 3 Differential Diagnoses

- **Sacrococcygeal teratoma.** Sacrococcygeal teratoma is the most common fetal neoplasm, with an incidence of 1 in 40,000. The neoplasm represents an extragonadal germ cell tumor resulting from aberrant migration of primordial germ cells. Ultrasound reveals a solid, cystic, or mixed sacrococcygeal mass. Type I lesions are entirely external, type IV lesions are entirely intrapelvic, and types II and III lesions have both internal and external components. Histologically, sacrococcygeal teratomas contain all three germ cell layers. Most tumors are benign; however, primarily internal tumors are more likely to contain malignant elements. Large, solid sacrococcygeal teratomas are associated with a worse prognosis than predominantly cystic masses, due to increased vascularity and arteriovenous shunting within the tumors that may lead to hydrops fetalis and maternal mirror syndrome (edema similar to hydrops but affecting the mother).

- **Myelomeningocele and variants.** MR imaging is the preferred imaging modality for neural tube defects due to its superior demonstration of neural elements. On prenatal ultrasonography, both open and closed neural tube defects may appear as sacrococcygeal masses. Myelomeningocele and myelocele are open neural tube defects that occur most commonly at the lumbosacral level, and they are usually associated with a Chiari II malformation. Anterior meningocele is a presacral, closed neural tube defect involving herniation of a cerebrospinal fluid–filled dural sac through a bony sacral defect. Anterior meningoceles may be difficult to differentiate from a cystic sacrococcygeal teratoma.
- **Rhabdomyosarcoma.** Rhabdomyosarcoma is an aggressive, malignant soft-tissue tumor that accounts for 4 to 8% of all pediatric neoplasms. Occurrence within the presacral space usually represents extension of a mass originating from the genitourinary tract.

■ Additional Differential Diagnoses

- **Duplication Cyst.** Duplication cysts are congenital enteric cysts that may arise anywhere along the alimentary tract but are most common within the ileum. Duplication cysts of the rectum are rare but should be considered in the differential diagnosis of a cystic presacral mass.

■ Diagnosis

Sacrococcygeal teratoma

✓ Pearls

- Sacrococcygeal teratoma is the most common fetal neoplasm; it may be cystic, solid, or mixed.
- Myelomeningocele is usually associated with intracerebral findings of Chiari II malformation.

- Rhabdomyosarcoma within the presacral space is often due to extension from the genitourinary tract.

Suggested Readings

Kocaoglu M, Frush DP. Pediatric presacral masses. Radiographics. 2006; 26(3):833–857

Rossi A, Biancheri R, Cama A, Piatelli G, Ravegnani M, Tortori-Donati P. Imaging in spine and spinal cord malformations. Eur J Radiol. 2004; 50(2):177–200

Woodward PJ, Sohaey R, Kennedy A, Koeller KK. From the archives of the AFIP: a comprehensive review of fetal tumors with pathologic correlation. Radiographics. 2005; 25(1):215–242

Case 208

Corinne D. Strickland

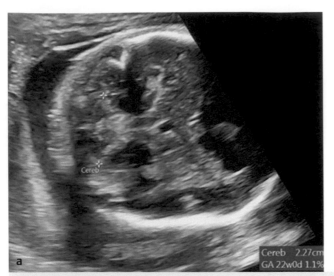
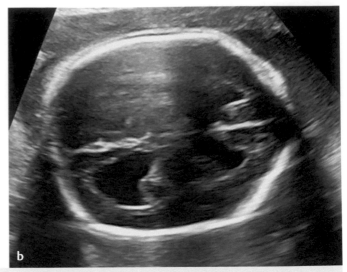

Fig. 208.1 (a) Axial ultrasound image of the fetal posterior fossa demonstrates a posterior fossa malformation with an abnormal "banana-shaped" configuration of the cerebellum. No fluid is seen in the cisterna magna and the cerebellum size is small for the gestational age. **(b)** An axial image more superiorly shows abnormal indentation of the frontal bones, referred to as a "lemon-shaped" head configuration, as well as ventriculomegaly.

■ Clinical Presentation

A 29-year-old woman at 26 weeks of gestation (►Fig. 208.1).

■ Key Imaging Finding

Posterior fossa malformation

■ Top 3 Differential Diagnoses

- **Chiari malformation.** The Chiari malformations are posterior fossa anomalies in which the cerebellar tonsils protrude through the foramen magnum. Chiari I, the mildest and most common malformation, may be asymptomatic or produce headache and cerebellar signs in adulthood. Chiari II, also known as Arnold-Chiari malformation, results from a primary defect of neural tube closure and is the most common cause of congenital hydrocephalus. The series of events resulting in Chiari II malformation include leakage of cerebrospinal fluid through a spinal defect that leads to collapse of the cerebral ventricles and underdevelopment of the posterior fossa. As the cerebellum develops within the small posterior fossa, the cerebellar tonsils herniate caudally, obstructing the outlets of the fourth ventricle and obliterating the cisterna magna. Associated signs on prenatal ultrasound (US) include ventriculomegaly, a "banana-shaped" cerebellum, and indentation of the frontal bones giving the skull a characteristic "lemon-shaped" appearance.

- **Dandy-Walker malformation.** A true Dandy-Walker malformation is defined by a triad of features: (1) partial or complete agenesis of the cerebellar vermis, (2) cystic dilatation of the fourth ventricle, and (3) enlargement of the posterior fossa with upward displacement of the tentorium cerebelli and torcula. The term "Dandy-Walker variant" is often used to describe a hypoplastic or absent inferior vermis. Such variants include a spectrum of cerebellar hypoplasia malformations. Fetal MR imaging can be useful for clarification of the underlying malformation.

- **Joubert syndrome.** Joubert syndrome is a rare autosomal recessive disorder characterized by hypoplasia or absence of the cerebellar vermis. Elongation of the superior cerebellar peduncles and increased depth of the interpeduncular fossa may be observed on MR imaging. These findings comprise the "molar tooth sign" that is characteristic for this condition.

■ Diagnosis

Chiari II malformation

✓ Pearls

- "Banana-shaped" cerebellum and "lemon-shaped" calvarium are US findings of Chiari II malformations.
- Dandy-Walker malformation is characterized by vermian agenesis with cystic fourth ventricular enlargement.

- Joubert syndrome presents with vermian aplasia/hypoplasia and a "molar tooth" brainstem configuration.

Suggested Readings

Fong KW, Toi A, Salem S, et al. Detection of fetal structural abnormalities with US during early pregnancy. Radiographics. 2004; 24(1):157–174

Niesen CE. Malformations of the posterior fossa: current perspectives. Semin Pediatr Neurol. 2002; 9(4):320–334

Oh KY, Rassner UA, Frias AE, Jr, Kennedy AM. The fetal posterior fossa: clinical correlation of findings on prenatal ultrasound and fetal magnetic resonance imaging. Ultrasound Q. 2007; 23(3):203–210

Case 209

Daniel Church

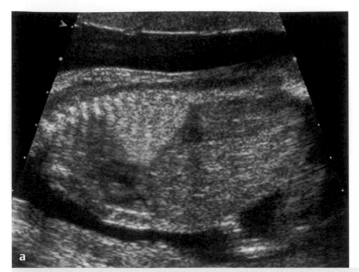 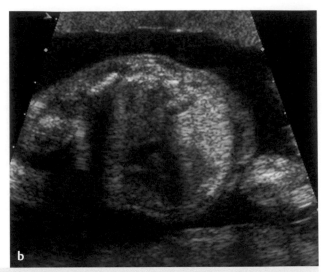

Fig. 209.1 **(a)** Longitudinal and **(b)** transverse ultrasound images of the fetus demonstrate the presence of an echogenic mass within the fetal chest.

■ Clinical Presentation

A 28-year-old G3P1 woman at 23 weeks of gestational age
(▶Fig. 209.1).

■ Key Imaging Finding

Hyperechoic thoracic mass

■ Top 3 Differential Diagnoses

• **Congenital pulmonary airway malformation (CPAM).** CPAM (previously known as cystic adenomatoid malformation or CCAM) constitutes most of the lung masses detected by prenatal imaging. CPAM is characterized by abnormal growth of the terminal respiratory bronchioles. Prenatal ultrasonography demonstrates a hyperechoic pulmonary mass with or without cystic elements of varying sizes. On pathology, masses with large cysts are classified as type 1; masses with medium-sized cysts are classified as type 2; and predominantly solid masses with nonvisible (microscopic) cysts are classified as type 3. CPAM is limited to one lobe or segment of the lung in 95% of cases. Prognosis depends on the size of the mass and the presence or absence of hydrops, which is likely to occur with large masses associated with mediastinal shift. CPAM may increase in size, but many will decrease in size during the third trimester.

• **Pulmonary sequestration.** Pulmonary sequestration represents aberrantly developed lung tissue that is perfused (receiving its blood supply primarily from the systemic circulation) but not ventilated (typically, there is no communication with the tracheobronchial tree). Prenatal ultrasonography demonstrates a relatively homogeneous hyperechoic pulmonary mass, and Doppler studies may demonstrate a systemic feeding vessel. Pulmonary sequestrations are most commonly located in the lung base. Sequestrations are classified as intra- or extralobar. Extralobar are more common than intralobar sequestrations in the fetus and newborn. Intralobar sequestrations are contained within the pleura of the normal lung, have a systemic arterial blood supply, and have venous drainage into the pulmonary veins. Extralobar sequestrations are found above or below the diaphragm and have their own pleural lining, systemic arterial supply, and systemic venous drainage.

• **Congenital lung overinflation (CLO).** CLO (also referred to as congenital lobar hyperinflation or CLH) represents a developmental anomaly of the bronchus resulting in a ball-valve phenomenon with subsequent lobar hyperinflation. Bronchial atresia is associated with CLO and CLO and usually occurs in the upper (left more common than right) or middle lobes. The masses may be opacified with fetal lung fluid at birth and gradually become more lucent as the fluid is cleared.

■ Additional Differential Diagnoses

• **Congenital diaphragmatic hernia (CDH).** CDH is the most common developmental abnormality of the diaphragm, with up to 90% of hernias occurring on the left side. The stomach, intestines, liver, and spleen may herniate into the chest. Prenatal ultrasonography demonstrates herniation of abdominal contents into the chest with contralateral mediastinal shift. Prognosis depends on hernia volume, herniated organs, hypoplasia of the lungs resulting from lung compression, and degree of pulmonary hypertension developed at birth.

■ Diagnosis

Congenital pulmonary airway malformation

✓ Pearls

• CPAM is the most common lung mass identified on prenatal US; it is classified by cystic/solid components.
• All sequestrations have systemic arterial supply; venous drainage pattern distinguishes the two types.

• CLO results from hyperinflation due to a ball-valve phenomenon; the LUL is most commonly involved.
• Up to 90% of CDHs occur on the left side; prognosis depends on the extent of pulmonary hypoplasia.

Suggested Reading

Bromley B, Parad R, Estroff JA, Benacerraf BR. Fetal lung masses: prenatal course and outcome. J Ultrasound Med. 1995; 14(12):927–936, quiz p1378

Case 210

Joyce F. Sung

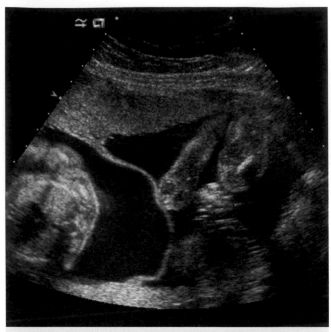

Fig. 210.1 Ultrasound image of the maternal uterus demonstrates a twin pregnancy with a thick membrane separating the two gestational sacs and a broad insertion into the maternal uterus, known as the twin "peak sign."

■ Clinical Presentation

A 31-year-old G1P0 woman with twin pregnancy (▶Fig. 210.1).

■ Key Imaging Finding

Twin development—chorionicity

■ Top 3 Differential Diagnoses

- **Dichorionic/Diamniotic twin pregnancy**. Dichorionic/diamniotic pregnancies may be dizygotic ("fraternal"), resulting from fertilization of two separate ova, or monozygotic ("identical"), resulting from division of a single zygote during the first 3 days following fertilization. Dizygotic pregnancies account for 80% of all twin pregnancies; thus, most dichorionic/diamniotic twins are dizygotic. Monozygotic dichorionic/diamniotic twins account for approximately 6 to 7% of all twin pregnancies. The dividing membrane separating the twin fetuses appears relatively thick on ultrasound (usually 2 mm or greater), because each twin is surrounded by its own amnion and chorion. A single fused placenta or two distinct placentas may be present. In the case of fused dichorionic placentas, a "twin peak" or "lambda" sign is visible on ultrasound, a result of placental tissue extending between the chorion layers of the dividing membrane. Risks associated with dichorionic/diamniotic twin pregnancy include growth restriction (25–30% risk), preterm (before 37 weeks) delivery (40%), and perinatal mortality (10–20%).
- **Monochorionic/Diamniotic twin pregnancy**. Monochorionic/diamniotic twins are always monozygotic, resulting from division of the zygote between 4 and 8 days following fertilization, and account for 13 to 14% of all twin pregnancies. Two embryos develop with separate amnionic sacs but are covered by a common chorion and share a single placenta. On ultrasonography, the dividing membrane appears thin (usually <2 mm). Monochorionic/diamniotic twins risk fetal growth restriction (50% risk), preterm delivery (60%), and perinatal mortality (30–40%). The diagnosis of monochorionicity is critical given that monochorionic twins are at risk for developing twin-to-twin transfusion syndrome (TTTS). TTTS results from unequal shunting across vascular anastomoses within the monochorionic twin placenta and is associated with a risk of fetal demise.
- **Monochorionic/Monoamnionic twin pregnancy**. Monochorionic/monoamnionic twin pregnancies are monozygotic twin pregnancies resulting from division of the zygote between 8 and 13 days following fertilization and account for <1% of all twin pregnancies. Two embryos share a single amnionic sac, as well as a single chorion and a single placenta. These twins are at particular risk for cord entanglement, which can result in fetal death. On ultrasound, no dividing membrane is seen. Additional risks associated with monoamnionic twins include fetal growth restriction (40%), preterm delivery (60–70%), and perinatal mortality (60%). Rarely, monochorionic/monoamnionic twin pregnancies may result in conjoined twins, resulting from division of the zygote after 13 days following fertilization.

■ Diagnosis

Dichorionic/Diamniotic twin pregnancy

✓ Pearls

- Characteristic US findings associated with a dichorionic twins include the "twin peak" or "lambda" sign.
- Monochorionic/diamniotic twins have a thin (<2 mm) separating membrane.
- Monoamnionic twins are at risk for cord entanglement, as well as increased perinatal morbidity/mortality.
- Division of the zygote after day 13 following fertilization results in conjoined twins.

Suggested Readings

Khalil A, Rodgers M, Baschat A, et al. ISUOG Practice Guidelines: role of ultrasound in twin pregnancy. Ultrasound Obstet Gynecol. 2016; 47(2):247–263

Case 211

Laura Varich

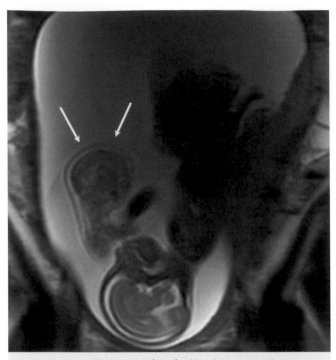

Fig. 211.1 Sagittal MR image of the fetal heads in a monochorionic diamniotic twin pregnancy demonstrates significant asymmetry in fetal size, and amount of amniotic fluid. The amniotic membrane of the underperfused fetus (*arrows*) surrounds closely the fetal head with decreased amniotic fluid around this fetus.

■ Clinical Presentation

A 30-year-old G2P1 woman with twin pregnancy at 22 weeks of gestational age (▶Fig. 211.1).

■ Key Imaging Finding

Twin pregnancy with asymmetric fetal sizes

■ Top 3 Differential Diagnoses

- **Twin–twin transfusion syndrome (TTTS).** In monochorionic twins (in which the two fetuses share the same placenta), there are known placental vascular anastomoses. In 35% of monochorionic twins, an imbalance in blood flow to the fetuses produces asymmetry in fetal size and amniotic fluid volume. The underperfused twin will demonstrate evidence of oligohydramnios and restricted growth. When the fluid is so severely restricted that the fetus is immobilized within its gestational sac, the fetus will appear in a static position, referred to as a "stuck twin." The twin with increased perfusion will demonstrate increased growth and polyhydramnios. Twin–twin transfusion syndrome is diagnosed when there is greater than a 20% discrepancy in estimated fetal weight (EFW) and a major difference in the volumes of amniotic fluid.
- **Fetal demise.** Twin pregnancies are associated with a four- to six-fold increase in mortality relative to singleton pregnancies.

In up to 20% of twin gestations identified in the first trimester, there will be demise of one twin prior to delivery. Asymmetry in size of the fetuses may be the first clue to demise of a twin. Absolute signs of demise are absence of fetal cardiac activity and fetal movement at the appropriate stage of fetal gestation (remember that it is important to always give the pregnancy the benefit of the doubt and obtain a repeat confirmatory scan). Other signs of fetal demise are overlapping cranial sutures, maceration and edema of the soft tissues, and decrease in size of the gestational sac.
- **Normal variation.** There can be some normal variation in the size of twin fetuses, especially in dizygotic twins (whose genetic makeup differs). However, discordance in EFW greater than 20% is considered abnormal and should be monitored closely.

■ Diagnosis

Twin–twin transfusion syndrome

✓ Pearls

- Twin–twin transfusion syndrome occurs in monochorionic twins and results from blood flow imbalances.
- The underperfused twin in twin–twin transfusion syndrome has oligohydramnios and restricted growth.

- The hyperperfused twin in twin–twin transfusion syndrome has polyhydramnios and increased growth.
- Fetal demise results in asymmetric sizes; absolute signs include lack of cardiac activity and movement.

Suggested Readings

Duncombe GJ, Dickinson JE, Evans SF. Perinatal characteristics and outcomes of pregnancies complicated by twin-twin transfusion syndrome. Obstet Gynecol. 2003; 101(6):1190–1196

Khalil A, Rodgers M, Baschat A, et al. ISUOG Practice Guidelines: role of ultrasound in twin pregnancy. Ultrasound Obstet Gynecol. 2016; 47(2):247–263

Case 212

Hedieh K. Eslamy

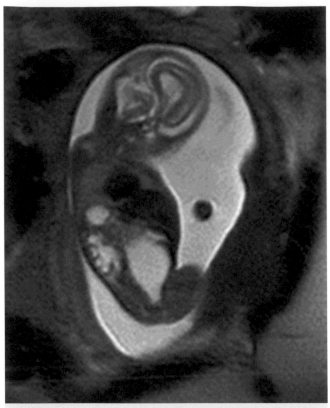

Fig. 212.1 T2-weighted sagittal MR image of a fetus demonstrates an enlarged urinary bladder with a dilated bladder neck and hydronephrosis involving the left kidney.

■ Clinical Presentation

A 19-year-old G1P0 woman with a 19-week gestational age male fetus (▶Fig. 212.1).

■ Key Imaging Finding

Enlarged bladder (megacystis)

■ Top 3 Differential Diagnoses

- **Posterior urethral valves (PUV).** The bladder is the first structure of the urinary tract visible in the pelvis, identifiable at approximately 9 to 10 weeks of embryonal life. Anomalies of the urinary tract may be suspected when the urinary bladder is enlarged or not visualized. Megacystis is defined as a urinary bladder >3 cm in length in the second trimester and >6 cm in length in the third trimester. The most common etiology of megacystis is bladder outlet obstruction. A male fetus with megacystis in the second or third trimester will almost invariably have posterior urethral valves (PUVs) as the cause of obstruction. Ultrasonographic findings of PUVs include megacystis, bladder wall thickening, hydroureter, variable degrees of hydronephrosis, renal dysplasia, urinary ascites, urinoma, oligohydramnios, and hypoplastic lungs secondary to mass effect.
- **Prune belly syndrome.** Megacystis within a fetus (usually male) in the first and early second trimesters may indicate prune belly syndrome. In this condition, the abdominal musculature is deficient or absent and genitourinary tract anomalies are present. Genitourinary findings include an enlarged thick-walled bladder, megaureter, hydronephrosis, and cryptorchidism. Complications include oligohydramnios and resultant pulmonary hypoplasia.
- **Megacystis microcolon intestinal hypoperistalsis (MMIH) syndrome.** Megacystis microcolon intestinal hypoperistalsis syndrome is a rare anomaly most often seen in female fetuses and characterized by a massively distended bladder and a small colon. Although the exact cause of this abnormality is not completely understood, it is thought to represent a form of neuropathy or myopathy. Ultrasound findings consist of nonobstructive megacystis and varying degrees of hydroureter and hydronephrosis. Unlike causes of bladder outlet obstruction, amniotic fluid is typically normal or increased. A microcolon may or may not be detected on sonography.

■ Additional Differential Diagnoses

- **Marked vesicoureteral reflux.** Marked vesicoureteral reflux may result in nonobstructive megacystis secondary to persistent and increased postvoid residuals due to reflux. It is seen more often in females. Patients typically have associated hydroureter and hydronephrosis when severe.

■ Diagnosis

Posterior urethral valves

✓ Pearls

- Megacystis in males is most commonly due to bladder outlet obstruction from posterior urethral valves.
- Prune belly syndrome consists of deficient abdominal musculature, urinary anomalies, and cryptorchidism.
- Nonobstructive causes of megacystis include MMIH syndrome and marked vesicoureteral reflux.

Suggested Readings

Callen PW. Ultrasonography in Obstetrics and Gynecology. 5th ed. Philadelphia, PA: Saunders; 2008

Montemarano H, Bulas DI, Rushton HG, Selby D. Bladder distention and pyelectasis in the male fetus: causes, comparisons, and contrasts. J Ultrasound Med. 1998; 17(12):743–749

Case 213

Joyce F. Sung

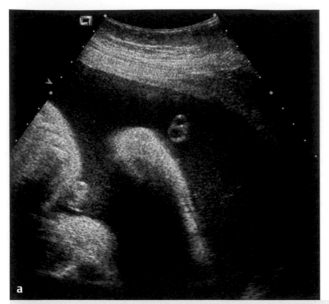 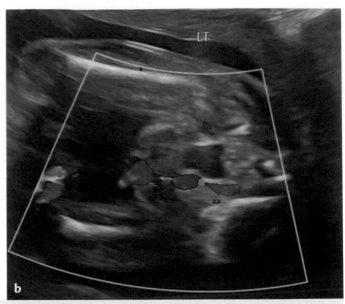

Fig. 213.1 (a) Fetal ultrasound image demonstrates two round hypoechoic foci within the umbilical cord, consistent with a two-vessel cord. Umbilical arteries are usually assessed with color Doppler in the transverse/axial plane through the fetal bladder. (b) Color Doppler ultrasound image demonstrates a single umbilical artery along the wall of the bladder.

■ Clinical Presentation

A 36-year-old G2P1 woman with a small fetus of 34 weeks of gestational age (▶Fig. 213.1).

■ **Key Imaging Finding**

Umbilical cord vascular abnormality

■ **Top 3 Differential Diagnoses**

- **Two-vessel cord**. The normal umbilical cord contains three vessels (two arteries and one vein), which can be verified on color Doppler by visualizing the two arteries on each side of the fetal bladder or by visualizing a cross-section of the umbilical cord demonstrating two arteries and one vein. A two-vessel cord (or single umbilical artery) occurs in 1% of pregnancies. It is important to evaluate the cord at the fetal end, as there may occasionally be only two vessels within the cord near the placental end, which is considered normal if three vessels are seen within the remainder of the cord. Although most often an incidental finding, an increase in fetal anomalies (especially cardiac and genitourinary) and chromosomal abnormalities has been reported in association with a two-vessel cord. Therefore, it is important to conduct a thorough anatomic survey when a two-vessel cord is found. Additionally, a two-vessel cord is associated with increased risk of growth restriction.

- **Cord hematoma**. Umbilical cord hematomas are usually iatrogenic in nature, resulting from invasive procedures such as amniocentesis or cordocentesis; they rarely occur spontaneously. As they are associated with a 50% risk of fetal demise, fetuses with a cord hematoma should be monitored closely with consideration for expectant delivery. On ultrasound, cord hematomas present as focal cord expansion with variable echogenicity ranging from hypo- to hyperechoic.

- **Cord hemangioma**. Cord hemangiomas are vascular tumors of endothelial cell origin, which most commonly occur near the placental cord insertion. They appear as hyperechoic and/or multicystic masses. Associated findings include polyhydramnios. The lesions may exert local mass effect within the cord, jeopardizing fetal blood flow and they may spontaneously hemorrhage.

■ **Additional Differential Diagnoses**

- **Wharton jelly cyst**. Wharton jelly is a substance, which insulates and supports umbilical cord vessels, protecting them from injury. A Wharton jelly cyst represents a focal thickening of Wharton jelly, which typically occurs close to the fetal cord insertion. These lesions are often associated with omphaloceles.

- **Umbilical cord varix**. An umbilical cord varix is a relatively uncommon anomaly characterized by focal dilatation of the umbilical vein, likely caused by weakness of the umbilical vein wall. It may occur anywhere within the cord or within the intrahepatic segment of the umbilical vein. The lesions cause local turbulent flow (and possible vascular steal phenomenon) and are prone to occlusion, which may result in fetal demise.

■ **Diagnosis**

Two-vessel cord

✓ **Pearls**

- Two-vessel cords are most often incidental but may be associated with anomalies and growth restriction.
- Umbilical cord hematomas are usually iatrogenic and are associated with a high risk of fetal demise.

- Umbilical cord hemangiomas are hyperechoic and/or multicystic; they may jeopardize fetal blood flow.
- An umbilical cord varix produces local turbulent flow and may thrombose, resulting in fetal demise.

Suggested Reading

Sherer DM, Anyaegbunam A. Prenatal ultrasonographic morphologic assessment of the umbilical cord: a review. Part I. Obstet Gynecol Surv. 1997; 52(8): 506–514, 515–523

Case 214

Hedieh K. Eslamy

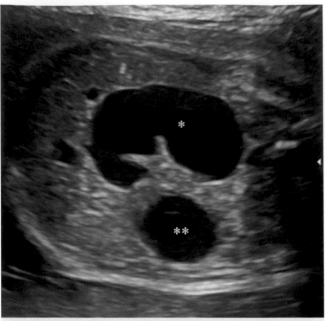

Fig. 214.1 Transverse ultrasound image of the fetal abdomen demonstrates a fluid-filled, distended stomach (*) and first portion of the duodenum (**).

■ Clinical Presentation

A 28-year-old G3P2 woman at 30 weeks of gestational age (▶Fig. 214.1).

■ Key Imaging Finding

"Double bubble" sign

■ Top 3 Differential Diagnoses

- **Congenital duodenal obstruction (duodenal atresia or stenosis).** Congenital duodenal obstruction is the most common cause of fetal small bowel obstruction, with an incidence of 1:5,000 to 1:10,000 live births. Duodenal atresia and stenosis occur secondary to failure of recanalization of the bowel, whereas atresia of the jejunum and ileum is related to vascular insult. Duodenal obstruction occurs in the second or third portion of the duodenum. The two fluid-filled bubbles demonstrated on obstetric ultrasound represent the dilated stomach and proximal duodenum. Approximately 70% of cases are associated with other structural anomalies, mainly of the gastrointestinal tract or heart, and 40% of cases have associated polyhydramnios. In fetuses found to have duodenal obstruction, approximately 30% will have Down syndrome

- **Annular pancreas.** Annular pancreas is the second most common condition to produce the characteristic "double bubble" sign. Annular pancreas is believed to result from failure of the embryonic pancreas to properly rotate around the duodenum, producing a ring of pancreatic tissue surrounding the second portion of the duodenum, causing varying degrees of duodenal obstruction. Polyhydramnios is present in obstructive cases; fetuses may also have restricted growth.

- **Intestinal malrotation with volvulus.** In the fetus, the gastrointestinal tract is initially located outside of the abdominal cavity. The bowel rotates as it is gradually withdrawn into the abdomen. In intestinal malrotation, the gastrointestinal tract fails to completely rotate. In general, the cecum and terminal ileum are displaced medially and superiorly, and the normal small bowel mesenteric attachment is lost. In these cases, the mesenteric attachment is a very short pedicle, allowing the bowel to twist around the superior mesenteric artery. Volvulus may be intermittent or persistent, causing vascular compromise with potential complications of bowel ischemia, necrosis, perforation, and gangrene.

■ Diagnosis

Congenital duodenal obstruction (duodenal atresia)

✓ Pearls

- "Double bubble" sign on ultrasound corresponds to dilated, fluid-filled stomach and proximal duodenum.
- Duodenal atresia is a failure of recanalization; it is associated with fetal anomalies and Down syndrome.

- Annular pancreas results in a ring of pancreatic tissue surrounding the second portion of the duodenum.
- Malrotation with volvulus can result in vascular compromise with resultant bowel ischemia and necrosis.

Suggested Reading

Traubici J. The double bubble sign. Radiology. 2001; 220(2):463–464

Case 215

Erika Rubesova

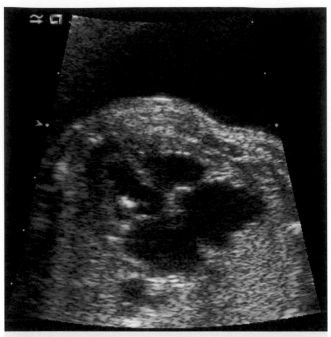

Fig. 215.1 Ultrasound image (four-chamber view) of the fetal heart demonstrates an echogenic focus in the left ventricle.

■ Clinical Presentation

A 34-year-old G3P2 woman at 21 weeks of gestational age (▶ Fig. 215.1).

■ Key Imaging Finding

Hyperechoic intracardiac focus

■ Top 3 Differential Diagnoses

- **Echogenic intracardiac focus (EIF)/Papillary muscle calcification**. An echogenic intracardiac focus is commonly seen in the left ventricle and is considered a normal variant in the patient population at low risk for chromosomal abnormalities. Its prevalence is three times higher in the Asian population. In the patient population at increased/high risk for chromosomal abnormalities (e.g., advanced maternal age), the presence of an EIF is a marker of increased risk of Down syndrome and Trisomy 13. In and of itself, however, it is not associated with cardiac anomalies.
- **Rhabdomyoma**. Rhabdomyomas are benign neoplasms, which are associated with tuberous sclerosis (TS) in 50 to 80% of cases. They are the most common benign cardiac tumors in infants and children. These tumors often appear as multiple hyperechoic round masses found during the second trimester.

The masses can grow until the third trimester but are then seen to regress during the later stages of pregnancy and first year of life; therefore, they have good prognosis. Very large tumors may cause outflow obstruction, alter valve function, and generate arrhythmias. Very small lesions may be difficult to detect with their only manifestation being an alteration in myocardial echogenicity.
- **Fibroma**. Cardiac fibromas are rare lesions, which usually appear on ultrasound as echogenic masses within the septal myocardium. They may undergo cystic transformation and do not usually regress. On MRI, the lesions are characteristically hypointense on T2-weighted sequences due to the presence of fibrous tissue. They have been described in association with other abnormalities, including Beckwith-Wiedeman syndrome and cleft palate.

■ Additional Differential Diagnoses

- **Teratoma**. Cardiac teratomas are rare and most often located within the pericardium; myocardial teratomas are extremely rare. The masses are often heterogeneous and large with marked mass effect and cardiac enlargement. They are composed of all three germ cell layers, often have cystic components, and may contain calcifications. They are associated with large pericardial effusions.

- **Hemangioma**. Cardiac hemangiomas are benign vascular lesions, which may involve the heart and/or pericardium. They are most frequently located within the right atrium and are associated with pericardial effusions. Ultrasound findings include a hyperechoic mass with cystic components. Hemangiomas are typically treated surgically.

■ Diagnosis

Echogenic intracardiac focus/papillary muscle calcification

✓ Pearls

- An EIF may be associated with increased risk of Down syndrome and Trisomy 13 in high-risk populations.
- Rhabdomyomas are the most common intracardiac tumors in the fetus and may be associated with TS.

- Cardiac fibromas typically occur along the septum and are characteristically hypointense on T2 MRI.
- Teratomas are large and heterogeneous; they often present with large pericardial effusions.

Suggested Readings

Coco C, Jeanty P, Jeanty C. An isolated echogenic heart focus is not an indication for amniocentesis in 12,672 unselected patients. J Ultrasound Med. 2004; 23(4):489–496

Case 216

Bo Yoon Ha

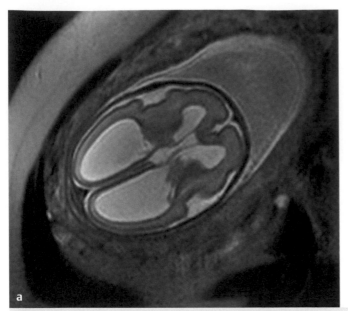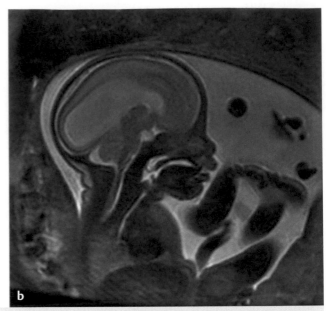

Fig. 216.1 **(a)** Axial and **(b)** sagittal T2-weighted MR images of the fetal brain demonstrate dilated third and lateral ventricles with a normal sized fourth ventricle.

■ Clinical Presentation

Follow-up of an abnormal ultrasound at 20 weeks of gestation in a 20-year-old G1P0 woman at 28 weeks of gestational age (▶Fig. 216.1).

■ Key Imaging Finding

Central nervous system (CNS) ventriculomegaly

■ Top 3 Differential Diagnoses

- **Ventriculomegaly**. Ventriculomegaly on prenatal imaging is defined as dilatation of the lateral ventricles over 10 mm in width as measured in the transverse plane at the atrial level. Slight asymmetry between the lateral ventricles can be normal. Follow-up imaging is typically performed in the third trimester to document stability. Mild ventriculomegaly without an underlying etiology may have a good outcome.
- **Congenital aqueductal stenosis**. Congenital aqueductal stenosis occurs at the aqueduct of Sylvius (between the third and fourth ventricles) and results in dilatation of the lateral and third ventricles with a normal sized fourth ventricle. It may be caused by webs/septations or secondary to prior intraventricular bleeding or infection. Adjacent masses can also rarely result in aqueductal stenosis or obstruction.

- **Chiari malformation**. The Chiari malformations are posterior fossa anomalies in which the cerebellar tonsils protrude through the foramen magnum. Chiari I malformations are associated with cervical spine abnormalities and cord syrinx (usually cervical); hydrocephalus may occur but is not nearly as common as with Chiari II malformations. Chiari II malformations consist of inferior cerebellar tonsillar displacement with crowding at the foramen magnum, a small posterior fossa, and hydrocephalus—all of which are secondary to a lumbosacral myelomeningocele. Prenatal ultrasound findings include ventriculomegaly, a "banana-shaped" cerebellum, "lemon-shaped" calvarium, and a lumbosacral myelomeningocele.

■ Additional Differential Diagnoses

- **Agenesis of the corpus callosum (ACC)**. ACC is an anomaly that may be partial or complete. It is often associated with other CNS or systemic malformations, including disorders of neuronal migration, hydrocephalus, midline lipoma, Chiari malformation, Dandy-Walker malformation, or interhemispheric cysts. Findings include parallel lateral ventricles, colpocephaly, and a high-riding third ventricle.
- **Dandy-Walker malformation**. Dandy-Walker malformation is a rare congenital malformation that involves the cerebellum and fourth ventricle. It is characterized by agenesis or hypoplasia of the cerebellar vermis, cystic dilatation of the fourth

ventricle, and enlargement of the posterior fossa. It is often associated with hydrocephalus, as well as other congenital CNS malformations, to include ACC.
- **Holoprosencephaly**. The result of incomplete or absent cleavage of the primitive forebrain into two cerebral hemispheres, holoprosencephaly is categorized into three types depending on severity: alobar, semilobar, and lobar. The alobar type is most severe with complete absence of division of the forebrain resulting in a monoventricle and fused cerebral hemispheres. The lobar type is the least severe with almost complete division of the hemispheres.

■ Diagnosis

Congenital aqueductal stenosis

✓ Pearls

- Mild ventriculomegaly without an underlying etiology may have a good outcome.
- Aqueductal stenosis may result from intrinsic webs or occur secondarily; the fourth ventricle is normal in size.

- Chiari II malformations (tonsillar displacement and myelomeningocele) commonly cause hydrocephalus.
- ACC results in a parallel configuration of the lateral ventricles, colpocephaly, and high-riding third ventricle.

Suggested Reading

D'Addario V, Pinto V, Di Cagno L, Pintucci A. Sonographic diagnosis of fetal cerebral ventriculomegaly: an update. J Matern Fetal Neonatal Med. 2007; 20(1):7–14

Case 217

Hedieh K. Eslamy

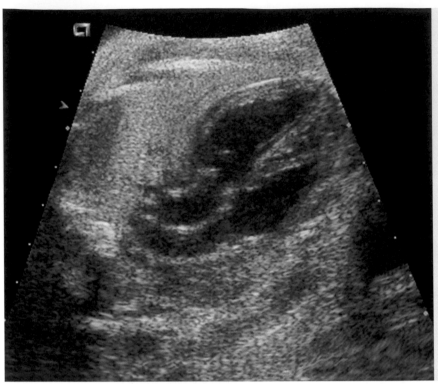

Fig. 217.1 Ultrasound image of the fetal heart demonstrates abnormal parallel configuration of the ventricular outflow tracts (they are not crossing as is normally expected).

■ Clinical Presentation

A 31-year-old G1P0 woman for fetal anatomy scan (▶Fig. 217.1).

■ **Key Imaging Finding**

Abnormal ventriculoarterial configuration

■ **Top 3 Differential Diagnoses**

- **Transposition of the great arteries (TGA).** TGA is divided into two subtypes: D-TGA and L-TGA. D-TGA is more common (5% of congenital heart disease) and consists of discordant ventriculoarterial connections (i.e., right ventricle connected to the aorta and left ventricle connected to the pulmonary trunk) with concordant atrioventricular connections (i.e., right atrium connected to the right ventricle and left atrium connected to the left ventricle). In most cases of TGA, the ventricular outflow tracts are parallel to each other. The aorta arises anterior and to the right of the left ventricular connection to the pulmonary artery. L-TGA is less common (1% of congenital heart disease) and has discordant ventriculoarterial and atrioventricular connections.
- **Tetralogy of Fallot (TOF).** The incidence of TOF is 3 to 5 per 10,000 live births; it is the most common cyanotic congenital heart anomaly. TOF occurs secondary to underdevelopment of the right ventricular outflow tract. The four components of this anomaly are right ventricular outflow tract stenosis, right ventricular hypertrophy, ventricular septal defect (VSD), and an over-riding aorta. Associated cardiac abnormalities include pulmonary artery branch stenosis or hypoplasia, absence of the pulmonary valve, right aortic arch, and anomalies of the origins of the coronary arteries.
- **Truncus arteriosus (TA).** In truncus arteriosis, a common arterial trunk arises from the base of the ventricles and gives rise to the aorta and pulmonary arteries, as well as the coronary arteries. TA constitutes approximately 2% of congenital cardiac anomalies and is associated with VSD (100%), right-sided aortic arch (30–40%), and DiGeorge syndrome (absent thymus and parathyroid glands).

■ **Additional Differential Diagnoses**

- **Double outlet right ventricle (DORV).** In DORV, both great arteries arise completely or predominantly from the morphologic right ventricle. DORV constitutes approximately 1 to 1.5% of congenital cardiac anomalies and is highly associated with a VSD. The relationship of the outflow tracts varies with a side-by-side configuration being most common.
- **Hypoplastic left heart syndrome.** Hypoplastic left heart syndrome refers to severe underdevelopment of the left heart due to mitral and aortic valve atresia. The heart is enlarged and the ascending aorta is hypoplastic with a threadlike configuration. Left-to-right shunting occurs at the atrial level. A patent ductus arteriosis is the only connection which allows for systemic circulation.

■ **Diagnosis**

Transposition of the great arteries

✓ **Pearls**

- Visualization of normal crossing ventricular outflow tracts is essential during a fetal survey.
- TOF consists of pulmonic stenosis, right ventricular hypertrophy, VSD, and over-riding aorta.
- TGA (D-TGA most common) results in a parallel configuration of the ventricular outflow tracts.
- TA consists of a common trunk giving rise to the aorta, pulmonary arteries, and coronary arteries.

Suggested Readings

Carvalho JS, Allan LD, Chaoui R, et al; International Society of Ultrasound in Obstetrics and Gynecology. ISUOG Practice Guidelines (updated): sonographic screening examination of the fetal heart. Ultrasound Obstet Gynecol. 2013; 41(3):348–359

Rajiah P, Mak C, Dubinksy TJ, Dighe M. Ultrasound of fetal cardiac anomalies. AJR Am J Roentgenol. 2011; 197(4):W747–60

Case 218

Bo Yoon Ha

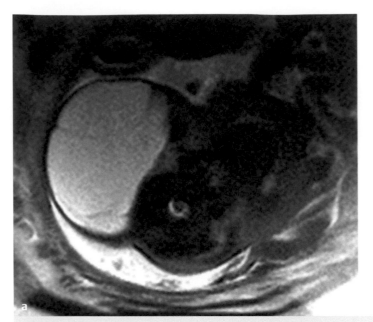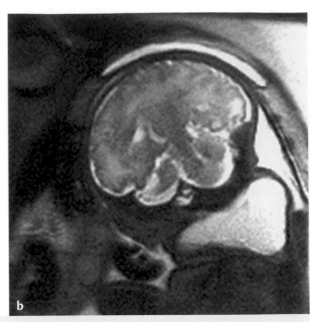

Fig. 218.1 (a) Axial and **(b)** sagittal T2-weighted MR images of the fetal head demonstrate a large, hyperintense cystic mass with internal septations in the posterolateral neck.

■ **Clinical Presentation**

A 21-year-old G2P1 woman with an abnormal ultrasound at 19 weeks of gestational age (▶Fig. 218.1).

■ Key Imaging Finding

Cystic posterior neck mass

■ Top 3 Differential Diagnoses

• **Cystic hygroma**. Cystic hygroma belongs to a group of diseases now recognized as lymphatic malformations. Almost 50% of cases of fetal cystic hygromas have an association with chromosomal disorders, such as Turner syndrome, although sporadic cases can occur. Ultrasound findings in fetal cystic hygroma can vary with gestational age. Increased nuchal translucency may be seen during the first trimester, with progression to a large, thin-walled, multiseptated cystic mass during the second trimester. Occasionally, cystic hygromas can become large and extend into the adjacent mediastinum, axillae, mouth, and chest. Cystic hygroma is most frequently diagnosed by fetal ultrasonography, with MR imaging used to further characterize the extent of involvement. Cystic hygromas may be associated with either oligohydramnios or hydrops.

• **Occipital encephalocele and cervical myelomeningocele**. Encephaloceles and myelomeningoceles are the most serious types of neural tube defects. Both conditions involve herniation of central nervous tissue and meninges through an osseous defect. In the case of encephalocele, brain tissue is herniated through a calvarial defect that is usually occipital in location. Myelomeningoceles can occur anywhere along the spinal canal, including the cervical region. Evaluation for an underlying calvarial or spinal defect is helpful in suggesting the diagnosis.

• **Cystic teratoma**. Teratomas are tumors derived from more than one germ cell layer (usually all three layers). The most common site of origin is sacrococcygeal, and tumor location is typically midline or paraxial. These tumors can also originate from sequestered midline embryonic cell rests in the mediastinum, retroperitoneum, and neck. Ultrasound findings are those of a cystic mass, which may contain septations, solid components, calcification, or fat.

■ Diagnosis

Lymphatic malformation (cystic hygroma)

✓ Pearls

• Cystic hygromas may be associated with chromosomal abnormalities, especially Turner syndrome.
• Encephaloceles and myelomeningoceles may present as neck masses with underlying osseous defects.

• Cystic teratoma is a cystic mass that may contain septations, solid components, calcification, and fat.

Suggested Readings

Mernagh JR, Mohide PT, Lappalainen RE, Fedoryshin JG. US assessment of the fetal head and neck: a state-of-the-art pictorial review. Radiographics. 1999; 19(Spec No):S229–S241

Tanriverdi HA, Hendrik HJ, Ertan AK, Axt R, Schmidt W. Hygroma colli cysticum: prenatal diagnosis and prognosis. Am J Perinatol. 2001; 18(8):415–420

Case 219

Daniel Church

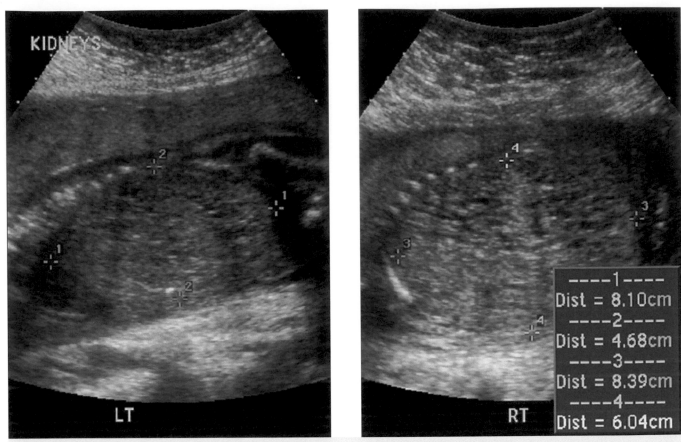

Fig. 219.1 Longitudinal sonographic images through the fetal abdomen demonstrate bilateral, enlarged, hyperechoic kidneys with loss of corticomedullary differentiation.

■ Clinical Presentation

A 24-year-old G1P0 woman at 24 weeks of gestational age (►Fig. 219.1).

■ **Key Imaging Finding**

Enlarged hyperechoic kidneys

■ **Top 3 Differential Diagnoses**

• **Autosomal recessive polycystic kidney disease (ARPKD).** ARPKD is a rare disorder, occurring in about 1 in 40,000 pregnancies. There is an association with congenital hepatic fibrosis and the severity of the renal abnormalities varies inversely with hepatic disease. Prenatal ultrasound demonstrates bilateral markedly enlarged echogenic kidneys. The medullary portion of the kidneys is affected and hyperechogenicity is confined to the pyramids with a preserved hypoechoic "halo" of cortical tissue. The majority of renal cysts are below the size resolution for sonography. In severe cases, oligohydramnios will not be apparent until after 16 weeks of gestation, when fetal urination becomes the major source of amniotic fluid. Associated pulmonary hypoplasia is often seen.

• **Trisomy 13.** Thirty percent of trisomy 13 fetuses have enlarged echogenic kidneys, similar to ARPKD. The list of anomalies occurring with this trisomy include cardiac defects, cystic hygroma, echogenic intracardiac focus, facial clefts, holoprosencephaly, intrauterine growth retardation (IUGR), microcephaly, neural tube defects, ocular anomalies, omphalocele, polydactyly, and ventriculomegaly.

• **Meckel-Gruber syndrome.** Meckel-Gruber is a rare and lethal syndrome consisting of an occipital encephalocele, postaxial polydactyly, and dysplastic cystic kidneys. The kidneys develop microscopic cysts that destroy the renal parenchyma and cause marked nephromegaly. Oligohydramnios is typical and associated pulmonary hypoplasia is often seen. In the presence of a normal karyotype, two out of three of the classic features are diagnostic of the syndrome.

■ **Additional Differential Diagnoses**

• **Autosomal dominant polycystic kidney disease (ADPKD).** Although usually diagnosed in adult life, ADPKD may also manifest in childhood or in the fetus. As this condition has an autosomal dominant inheritance pattern, one of the parents is likely to have the disease (although sporadic cases can occur). Therefore, the parental kidneys should be evaluated if the diagnosis is suspected in the fetus. Prenatal ultrasound will demonstrate enlarged echogenic kidneys. Cysts do not appear until late pregnancy and are not a dominant finding.

■ **Diagnosis**

Autosomal recessive polycystic kidney disease

✓ **Pearls**

• ARPKD results in markedly enlarged echogenic kidneys with a thin hypoechoic "halo" of preserved cortex.
• Trisomy 13 presents with echogenic kidneys similar to ARPKD, as well as other structural defects.

• Meckel-Gruber is characterized by an occipital encephalocele, polydactyly, and dysplastic cystic kidneys.

Suggested Readings

Callen PW. Ultrasonography in Obstetrics and Gynecology. 4th ed. Philadelphia, PA: W.B. Saunders Company; 2000

Fong KW, Toi A, Salem S, et al. Detection of fetal structural abnormalities with US during early pregnancy. Radiographics. 2004; 24(1):157–174

Case 220

Laura Varich

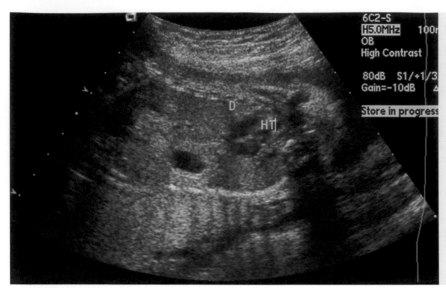

Fig. 220.1 Ultrasound image of the fetus in coronal plane with absence of amniotic fluid around the fetus.

■ Clinical Presentation

A 29-year-old G1P0 woman at 20 weeks of gestational age (▶Fig. 220.1).

■ Key Imaging Finding

Oligohydramnios. Oligohydramnios is the condition of decreased amniotic fluid volume relative to gestational age. This is defined subjectively by obvious lack of amniotic fluid, crowding of fetal parts, and poor fluid–fetal interface. Objectively, oligohydramnios is defined by an amniotic fluid index (AFI) of less than 5 cm and a maximum vertical pocket (MVP) of less than 1 to 2 cm. Amniotic fluid is necessary for normal lung development; therefore, fetuses with prolonged oligohydramnios will suffer from pulmonary hypoplasia at birth

■ Top 3 Differential Diagnoses

- **Bilateral renal failure or outlet obstruction**. In the second and third trimesters, fetal urination is an important contributor to amniotic fluid volume. Therefore, lack of urine production or inability to excrete urine produces fetal oligohydramnios. Specific causes of oligohydramnios include renal failure involving both kidneys (renal agenesis, renal dysplasia, muticystic dysplastic kidneys, and autosomal recessive polycystic kidney disease) and severe urinary outflow tract obstruction (especially posterior urethral valves). It is important to remember that renal causes of oligohydramnios may not become evident until after 16 weeks of gestation when fetal urination becomes a significant contributor to amniotic fluid volume.
- **Premature rupture of membranes (PROM)**. PROM is defined as rupture of the fetal membranes prior to the onset of labor. In the 10% of pregnancies affected by PROM at term, the obstetrician will choose to induce labor. In the 2% of preterm pregnancies affected by PROM, patients will be treated conservatively. In preterm cases, there may be a long latency period during which the fetus has decreased amniotic fluid (increasing the risk of pulmonary hypoplasia), as well as loss of the normal barrier to ascending infection (increasing the risk for chorioamnionitis).
- **Intrauterine growth restriction**. Decreased placental perfusion, which can result from various causes, will produce a hypoxic state within the fetus. When the fetus becomes hypoxic, there is redistribution of cardiac output, preserving blood flow to the brain. The remaining organs are consequently underperfused. The kidneys respond to this decreased vascular flow by decreasing urine output (prerenal renal failure), resulting in oligohydramnios.

■ Additional Differential Diagnoses

- **Fetal demise**. Intrauterine demise of the fetus will result in decreased size of the gestational sac, as amniotic fluid is no longer produced and begins to resorb. Other signs of fetal demise are routinely visible, including absence of fetal cardiac activity, absence of fetal movement, overlapping cranial sutures, and maceration and edema of the fetal soft tissues.

■ Diagnosis

Premature rupture of membranes

✓ Pearls

- Prolonged oligohydramnios, regardless of cause, will result in pulmonary hypoplasia.
- Renal causes of oligohydramnios may not be evident until the second trimester (typically after 16 weeks).
- Prolonged PROM (preterm) may result in pulmonary hypoplasia and increased risk of chorioamnionitis.
- IUGR secondary to hypoxia results in redistribution of cardiac output and decreased urine output.

Suggested Readings

Callen P. Ultrasound in Obstetrics and Gynecology. 5th ed. Saunders; Philadelphia, PA: 2008

Ott WJ. Reevaluation of the relationship between amniotic fluid volume and perinatal outcome. Am J Obstet Gynecol. 2005; 192(6):1803–1809, discussion 1809

Case 221

Hedieh K. Eslamy

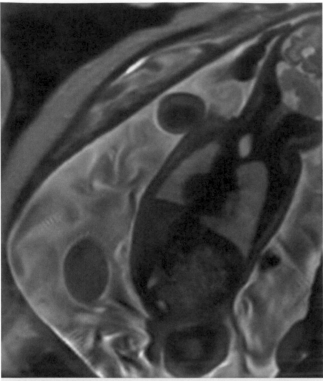

Fig. 221.1 Coronal T2-weighted MR image of the fetus demonstrates increased amniotic fluid and a high signal intensity pouch within the fetal neck.

■ Clinical Presentation

Increased uterine height for the 33 weeks of gestational age in a 33-year-old G2P1 woman (►Fig. 221.1).

■ Key Imaging Finding

Polyhydramnios. Polyhydramnios is an excessive accumulation of amniotic fluid (>1,500 mL). The balance of fluid flow into the amniotic sac (fetal urination and lung fluid production) and out of the amniotic sac (swallowing and intramembranous absorption) determines the volume of amniotic fluid. Polyhydramnios typically results from decreased fetal swallowing or increased fetal urination. On ultrasound, polyhydramnios can be diagnosed subjectively (the fetus in mid-to-late second or third trimester appears to float in the amniotic fluid, displaced away from the anterior uterine wall or placenta) or objectively (the deepest amniotic fluid volume pocket >8 cm or an amniotic fluid index >25 cm)

■ Top 3 Differential Diagnoses

• **Fetal gastrointestinal (GI) anomalies.** Fetal GI obstruction is the most common congenital anomaly to cause polyhydramnios. The abnormality usually occurs at or prior to the more proximal small bowel where water absorption occurs. Primary considerations include esophageal, duodenal, jejunal, or proximal ileal atresia.
• **Fetal central nervous system (CNS) anomalies.** Fetal CNS and associated chromosomal abnormalities were once a major cause of third trimester polyhydramnios; however, with the advent of second trimester anatomic screening and wide use of ultrasound, this is no longer the case. Major CNS structural defects associated with polyhydramnios include anencephaly, hydranencephaly, and encephalocele; however, any CNS anomaly that causes a lack of normal swallowing function can lead to polyhydramnios.
• **Maternal diabetes mellitus.** Fetal polyhydramnios is often seen in diabetic mothers with poorly controlled blood sugars. Polyhydramnios is likely related to fetal hyperglycemia causing osmotic diuresis and polyuria. There is typically associated fetal macrosomia; therefore, accurate assessments of fetal weight should be performed.

■ Additional Differential Diagnoses

• **Idiopathic polyhydramnios.** Idiopathic polyhydramnios refers to the presence of ultrasound findings of polyhydramnios in a nondiabetic mother and lack of discernible fetal cause of excess amniotic fluid. The condition is most often considered benign in the absence of other abnormalities, but the pregnancy should be closely monitored with follow-up imaging as necessary.
• **Fetal hydrops.** Fetal hydrops is characterized by abnormal fluid accumulation in at least two fetal cavities, to include placental enlargement, body wall edema, ascites, pericardial effusions, and/or pleural effusions. Polyhydramnios is often present. Hydrops is most often due to nonimmune causes (e.g., cardiovascular anomalies, intrauterine infection, or chromosomal abnormality) and less commonly due to circulating maternal antibodies against fetal red blood cells due to Rh incompatibility (immune hydrops).

■ Diagnosis

Fetal GI anomaly (esophageal atresia)

✓ Pearls

• Common fetal causes of polyhydramnios include GI and CNS anomalies, as well as fetal hydrops.
• Poorly controlled maternal diabetes may result in polyhydramnios and fetal macrosomia.
• Idiopathic polyhydramnios is typically considered a benign condition once other causes are excluded.

Suggested Readings

Alexander ES, Spitz HB, Clark RA. Sonography of polyhydramnios. AJR Am J Roentgenol. 1982; 138(2):343–346

Hill LM, Breckle R, Thomas ML, Fries JK. Polyhydramnios: ultrasonically detected prevalence and neonatal outcome. Obstet Gynecol. 1987; 69(1):21–25

Case 222

Joyce F. Sung

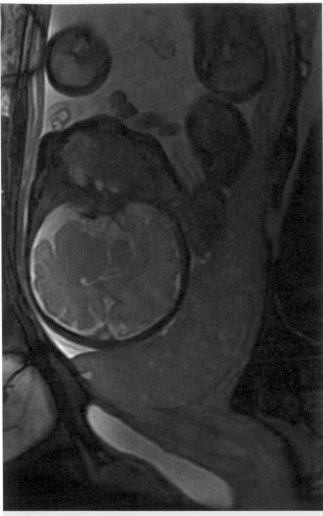

Fig. 222.1 Sagittal T2–weighted MR image of the maternal uterus demonstrates complete coverage of the cervix by the placenta.

■ Clinical Presentation

A 38-year-old G3P2 woman with vaginal bleeding at 34 weeks of gestational age (▶Fig. 222.1).

■ Key Imaging Finding

Placental location abnormality

■ Top 3 Differential Diagnoses

- **Placenta previa**. Placenta previa occurs when the placenta lies near or over the cervical internal os. There are four types of placenta previa: complete (the placenta completely covers the internal os), partial (the placenta partially covers the internal os), marginal (the placenta reaches the edge of but does not cover the internal os), and low-lying (the placenta lies close to but does not reach the edge of the internal os—usually defined as within 2 cm of the internal os on ultrasound). Risk factors include prior cesarean section, pregnancy termination, or uterine surgery, as well as multiparity, smoking, increased maternal age, cocaine use, and multiple pregnancies. Pregnancy complications associated with placenta previa include painless antepartum bleeding, intrapartum and postpartum hemorrhage, placental implantation abnormalities, and increased preterm delivery. Transvaginal ultrasound is more accurate in cases where the diagnosis is in question.
- **Placenta accreta/increta/percreta**. In placenta accreta, the placenta is abnormally adherent to the uterine myometrium. The depth of invasion into the uterine wall defines the two variants: *placenta increta* describes invasion into the myometrium, while *placenta percreta* describes invasion through the entire thickness of the myometrium and uterine serosa (invasion can even involve adjacent organs such as the bladder and rectum). Risk factors for placenta accreta include prior cesarean delivery or other uterine surgery. When placenta previa is present and is associated with a history of prior cesarean delivery or uterine surgery, ultrasound and MR imaging should be used to evaluate for placenta accreta. Suspicious ultrasonographic findings include irregularly shaped vascular spaces (lacunae) within the placenta, turbulent blood flow in the lacunae on Doppler imaging, thinning of the myometrium at the placental site, loss of retroplacental echolucency, protrusion of the placenta into the bladder, and increased vascularity between the uterine serosa and bladder. Clinically, it is important to make the diagnosis of accreta prior to delivery to plan for possible perinatal complications, including massive hemorrhage and disseminated intravascular coagulation (DIC).
- **Marginal insertion of the cord**. A marginal insertion is defined as insertion of the umbilical cord within 1 to 2 cm of the placental edge. Although some pathologic studies have suggested an association with growth restriction, a fairly recent study of sonographically identified marginal placental cord insertions in singleton pregnancies failed to demonstrate any association with fetal growth restriction.

■ Additional Differential Diagnoses

- **Velamentous insertion of the cord**. A cord insertion is considered velamentous when the cord inserts into the fetal membranes rather than into the placenta (1% of pregnancies). In this condition, the fetal vessels run through a portion of the membranes before reaching the placenta. If the fetal vessels cross the cervix, the condition is known as vasa previa. In vasa previa, rupture of the fetal membranes may cause vessel rupture and catastrophic fetal hemorrhage; therefore, cesarean section should be anticipated.

■ Diagnosis

Placenta previa

✓ Pearls

- Placenta previa refers to the placenta lying near or over the cervical os and is associated with hemorrhage.
- Placenta accreta refers to placental invasion into the uterine myometrium; it is associated with hemorrhage.

- Marginal insertion of the cord is described as cord insertion within 2 cm of the placental edge.
- Velamentous cord insertion occurs when the placenta inserts into the fetal membranes rather than placenta.

Suggested Reading

Wu S, Kocherginsky M, Hibbard JU. Abnormal placentation: twenty-year analysis. Am J Obstet Gynecol. 2005; 192(5):1458–1461

Case 223

Daniel Church

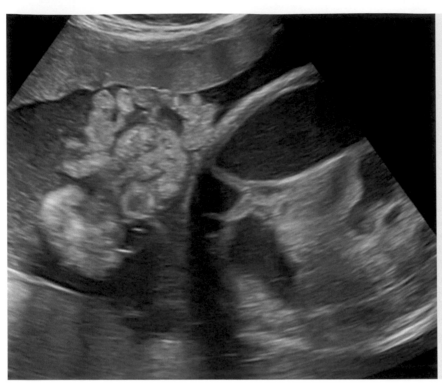

Fig. 223.1 Sagittal ultrasound image demonstrates a fetus with an anterior abdominal wall defect. The extra-abdominal loops of bowel are not contained within a membrane. The intra-abdominal loops of bowel are dilated.

■ Clinical Presentation

An 18-year-old G1P0 woman at 34 weeks of gestational age (▶Fig. 223.1).

■ Key Imaging Finding

Abdominal wall defect

■ Top 3 Differential Diagnoses

- **Omphalocele**. An omphalocele is an abdominal wall defect that results in herniation of abdominal contents into the base of the umbilical cord. Two layers of intact membranes (the peritoneum and the amnion) form a sac that separates the eviscerated organs from the amniotic fluid. Prenatal ultrasound demonstrates a midline defect with the umbilical cord at its apex. Associated anomalies are present in 67 to 88% of cases and include intestinal atresias, malrotation, cardiac anomalies, and chromosomal anomalies. Association with chromosomal anomalies is lower when the liver is herniated. The mortality rate of isolated omphalocele is 10%; it is much higher with associated anomalies.
- **Gastroschisis**. In gastroschisis, bowel loops herniate through a paraumbilical full-thickness abdominal wall defect into the amniotic cavity. Unlike omphaloceles, there is no surrounding membrane with gastroschisis. The defect is usually right-sided to the umbilical cord insertion, and the umbilical cord insertion is normal and separate from the defect. There is usually no association with chromosomal or other congenital anomalies. Incidence of gastroschisis is greater in young mothers. Gastroschisis mortality rates are lower than with omphalocele (<10%).
- **Limb–body wall complex**. Limb–body wall complex is a universally fatal condition, which has, as one component, a ventral wall anomaly (omphalocele) but can be differentiated from isolated omphalocele and gastroschisis by its other features. The associated findings include craniofacial defects, limb reductions, and spinal defects.

■ Additional Differential Diagnoses

- **Pentalogy of Cantrell**. The Pentalogy of Cantrell is a rare condition of unknown etiology. It consists of an omphalocele, ectopia cordis, diaphragmatic defect, pericardial defect, and cardiovascular malformation. It can be associated with other anomalies and chromosomal abnormalities. Prognosis depends on the severity of the multiple defects, especially cardiac.
- **Bladder and cloacal exstrophy**. Bladder exstrophy is a congenital malformation of unknown etiology which refers to exstrophy of the bladder through an abdominal wall (anteroinferior) defect, as well as musculoskeletal abnormalities. Findings include absence of a normal bladder, protruding soft-tissue mass, and pubic diastasis. Cloacal exstrophy is more severe and refers to defects involving the bladder and bowel.

■ Diagnosis

Gastroschisis

✓ Pearls

- Omphalocele has a membrane covering the herniated bowel; the cord inserts at the apex of the defect.
- Gastroschisis occurs to the right of midline and contains bowel loops without a membrane covering.
- Omphalocele has a high incidence of associated anomalies and a worse prognosis than gastroschisis.

Suggested Reading

Emanuel PG, Garcia GI, Angtuaco TL. Prenatal detection of anterior abdominal wall defects with US. Radiographics. 1995; 15(3):517–530

Case 224

Bo Yoon Ha

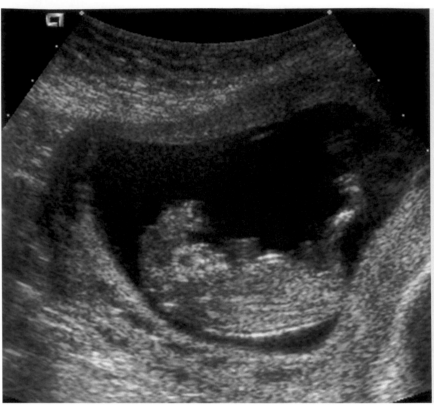

Fig. 224.1 Longitudinal ultrasound image of the fetus demonstrates absence of the fetal cranium and brain.

▪ Clinical Presentation

A 38-year-old G1P0 woman at 12 weeks of gestational age (▶Fig. 224.1).

■ Key Imaging Finding

Cranial/Calvarial defect

■ Top 3 Differential Diagnoses

- **Anencephaly**. Anencephaly is a lethal developmental anomaly of the central nervous system resulting from failure of closure of the rostral portion of the neural tube (neural tube defect, NTD). It may first be suspected due to elevated maternal serum alpha-fetoprotein (MSAFP). Ultrasound findings include reduction or absence of the cerebrum and cerebellum with preservation of a portion of the hindbrain. Tissue located above the orbits on ultrasound is referred to as angiomatous stroma. The diagnostic feature is the absence of the cranial bones (skull base is present) after 11 weeks of gestation when normal cranial ossification should be visible. Anencephaly, like other forms of NTD, is associated with chromosomal abnormalities, and risk of recurrence is increased in fetuses with previously affected sibling.
- **Acrania**. Acrania (also referred to as exencephaly) is characterized by partial or complete absence of the cranium. It results from failure of membranous bone formation (as seen with ectodermal migrational abnormalities) and is universally fatal. Although the underlying brain typically forms, to some degree, it is abnormal. The condition can be associated with anencephaly. Ultrasonography will demonstrate variable degrees of cranial absence, beginning in the first trimester.
- **Amniotic band syndrome**. Amniotic bands are thin fibrous bands that may be found within the amniotic sac which may be difficult to visualize on ultrasound or MRI. Amniotic band syndrome is a rare condition where the bands cause associated anomalies, including regions of constriction and amputation. The cranium may be involved with asymmetric amputation or disruption of normal bone formation. Amniotic band syndrome may be distinguished from other calvarial defects by noting asymmetric calvarial defects, the presence of underlying brain parenchyma, and evaluation for other sequela of amniotic band syndrome.

■ Additional Differential Diagnoses

- **Encephalocele or myelomeningocele**. Encephaloceles and myelomeningoceles are characterized by herniation of portions of the brain (encephalocele), spinal cord (myelomeningocele), nerves, cerebrospinal fluid (CSF), and meninges through a bony defect of the calvarium or spine, respectively. Encephaloceles are most common in the occipital region. They can be differentiated from anencephaly or acrania by the presence of a bony calvarium. Myelomeningoceles are the most serious form of spina bifida and can occur anywhere along the spinal cord. They most commonly occur within the lumbosacral spine, followed by the cervical spine. Associated findings may be identified within the fetal head, including ventriculomegaly, Chiari II malformation, and concavity of the frontal bones. MR imaging is useful to evaluate the level and extent of the myelomeningocele.

■ Diagnosis

Anencephaly

✓ Pearls

- Anencephaly is a defect with absence of normal brain and calvarial development above the orbits.
- Acrania is characterized by partial or complete absence of the calvarium due to failed bone formation.
- Amniotic band syndrome may result in constriction and amputations with asymmetric calvarial defects.
- Encephaloceles consist of herniated brain parenchyma through a calvarial defect; most are occipital.

Suggested Readings

Mangels KJ, Tulipan N, Tsao LY, Alarcon J, Bruner JP. Fetal MRI in the evaluation of intrauterine myelomeningocele. Pediatr Neurosurg. 2000; 32(3):124–131

McComb JG. Spinal and cranial neural tube defects. Semin Pediatr Neurol. 1997; 4(3):156–166

Case 225

Daniel Church

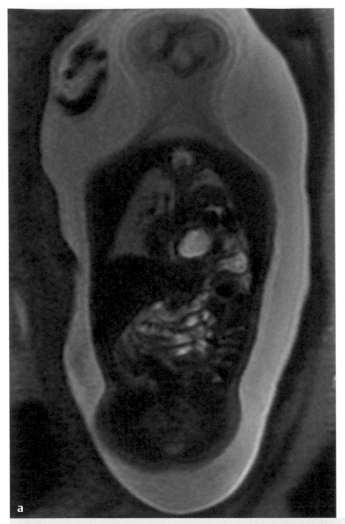
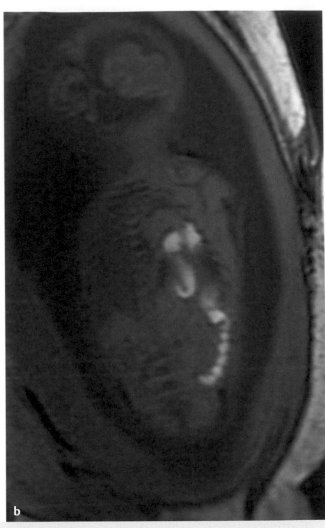

Fig. 225.1 (a) Coronal T2 and **(b)** T1 fetal MR images demonstrate herniation of the abdominal contents (stomach and bowel) into the left chest with mass effect on the mediastinum. The T1-weighted image shows the presence of meconium (bright on T1) within the herniated bowel.

■ Clinical Presentation

A 31-year-old G2P1 woman at 24 weeks of gestational age (▶ Fig. 225.1).

■ Key Imaging Finding

Diaphragm abnormality

■ Top 3 Differential Diagnoses

- **Congenital diaphragmatic hernia (CDH)**. CDH is the most common developmental abnormality of the diaphragm. Up to 90% occur on the left; Bochdalek (posterior) hernias far outnumber Morgagni (anterior) hernias. The stomach, intestines, liver, and spleen can all herniate into the chest. Prenatal ultrasound is the main modality for the prenatal diagnosis of CDH, demonstrating herniation of abdominal contents into the chest with contralateral mediastinal shift. CDH is associated with other congenital malformations in up to half of cases, with congenital heart disease being the most common. Prognosis depends on hernia volume, degree of mediastinal shift, pulmonary hypoplasia, solid organ herniation, as well as development of pulmonary hypertension postnatally. Intrathoracic liver in a left-sided CDH carries a worse prognosis. Lung-to-head ratio (LHR) is commonly used to predict prognosis and is the result of the product of two diameters of the contralateral lung measured on a four-chamber view of the heart, divided by the head circumference. Fetal MR imaging is a complementary method to ultrasound for evaluating the herniated organs and to measure the fetal lung volume.

- **Congenital pulmonary airway malformation (CPAM)**. CPAM (also known as cystic adenomatoid malformation or CCAM) constitutes more than 80% of lung masses detected by prenatal imaging. CPAM is characterized by excessive growth of the terminal respiratory bronchioles. Prenatal ultrasonography demonstrates a hyperechoic pulmonary mass with or without cystic elements of varying sizes. Occasionally, CPAMs may approximate the diaphragm, simulating a mass associated with a diaphragmatic hernia.

- **Pulmonary sequestration**. Pulmonary sequestration represents aberrantly developed lung tissue that is perfused (receiving its blood supply primarily from the systemic circulation) but not ventilated (typically, there is no communication with the tracheobronchial tree). Prenatal ultrasonography demonstrates a relatively homogeneous hyperechoic pulmonary mass, and Doppler studies may demonstrate a systemic feeding vessel. Pulmonary sequestrations are most commonly located in the medial lung base and are classified as intra- or extralobar. Given their common location with the medial lung bases, they may simulate a mass associated with a diaphragmatic hernia.

■ Additional Differential Diagnoses

- **Diaphragmatic eventration**. Congenital eventration of the diaphragm is caused by hypoplasia of the diaphragmatic muscle and is usually right sided. With an eventrated diaphragm, the abdominal components also shift superiorly. On axial imaging, the liver may be mistaken for a chest mass with an associated diaphragmatic defect. Sagittal imaging may help verify an intact but elevated diaphragm.

■ Diagnosis

Congenital diaphragmatic hernia

✓ Pearls

- CDH is the most common congenital diaphragmatic abnormality and is more common on the left.
- Prognosis of CDH depends on the severity of pulmonary compression and the presence of intrathoracic liver.

- CPAMs and sequestrations can simulate a mass associated with a diaphragmatic hernia.
- Diaphragmatic eventration is more common on the right; the liver may be mistaken for a thoracic mass.

Suggested Readings

Goldstein RB. Ultrasound evaluation of the fetal thorax. In: Callen PW, ed. Ultrasonography in Obstetrics and Gynecology. 4th ed. Philadelphia, PA: W.B. Saunders Company; 2000

Guibaud L, Filiatrault D, Garel L, et al. Fetal congenital diaphragmatic hernia: accuracy of sonography in the diagnosis and prediction of the outcome after birth. AJR Am J Roentgenol. 1996; 166(5):1195–1202

Case 226

William T. O'Brien Sr.

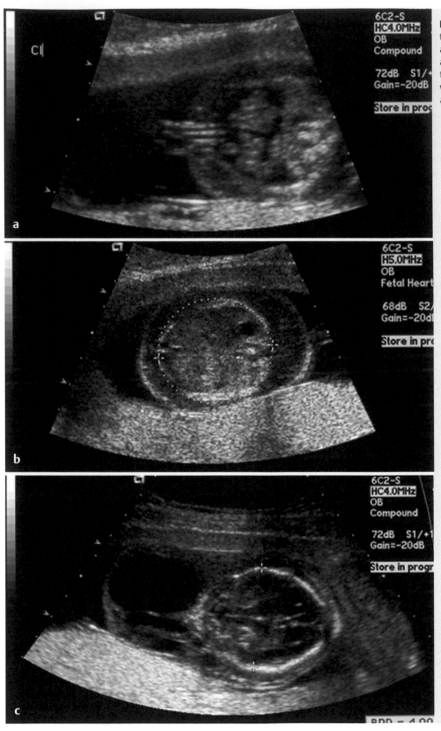

Fig. 226.1 (a, b) Transverse sonographic images through the fetal abdomen during a second trimester anatomy scan demonstrate diffuse body wall edema, as well as ascites. (c) Transverse sonographic image through the fetal head reveals diffuse scalp edema with a complex cystic hygroma along the posterior aspect of the neck and base of the skull.

■ Clinical Presentation

A 34-year-old G1P0 woman with abnormal triple screen (▶Fig. 226.1).

■ Key Imaging Finding

Fetal hydrops

■ Top 3 Differential Diagnoses

- **Cardiac anomalies**. Cardiovascular disease (including structural anomalies, cardiac arrhythmias, and high output failure) is the most common cause of fetal hydrops, accounting for approximately 25% of cases. Diagnostic findings on ultrasound include abnormal fluid accumulation in at least two fetal cavities to include the following: placental enlargement, body wall edema (anasarca), ascites, pericardial effusions, and/or pleural effusions. Abnormal fluid accumulation in a single cavity should not result in the diagnosis of hydrops fetalis. Once hydrops is found, a thorough anatomy scan should be performed to identify potentially treatable causes.
- **Chromosomal abnormalities**. Chromosomal abnormalities, to include Down syndrome, trisomy 18, trisomy 13, and Turner syndrome (XO), represent the most common genetic disorders that result in fetal hydrops. Often, secondary signs can be identified to suggest a genetic cause. In Down syndrome, secondary findings include a short or absent nasal bone, increased nuchal thickness, endocardial cushion defects, echogenic intracardiac focus, hyperechoic bowel, pyelectasis, and short limbs. The hallmark sonographic finding in trisomy 18 (Edward syndrome) is choroid plexus cysts. Other abnormalities include clenched fists with or without overlapping digits, clubfeet, rocker-bottom feet, nuchal translucency, two-vessel cord, and cardiac anomalies. Ultrasound findings in trisomy 13 (Patau syndrome) include holoprosencephaly, neural tube defects, cardiac anomalies, polydactyly, and enlarged hyperechoic kidneys. Turner syndrome is characterized by lymphatic malformations, to include a cervical cystic hygroma, aortic coarctation, cardiac defects, and renal abnormalities.
- **Infection**. Infections represent a relatively rare cause of fetal hydrops. Numerous viral, bacterial, and parasitic infections may result in fetal hydrops with the vast majority resulting from parvovirus B19, cytomegalovirus, toxoplasmosis, and syphilis.

■ Additional Differential Diagnoses

- **Immune hydrops**. Immune hydrops fetalis is the result of circulating maternal antibodies that destroy fetal red blood cells due to rhesus (Rh) incompatibility. Increased prenatal surveillance and application of the Rh immunoglobulin prophylaxis have drastically decreased the incidence of immune fetal hydrops. Today, immune hydrops is very uncommon.

■ Diagnosis

Chromosomal abnormality (Turner syndrome)

✓ Pearls

- Fetal hydrops is characterized by abnormal fluid accumulation in at least two fetal cavities.
- Nonimmune causes of hydrops are more common than immune hydrops due to Rh prophylaxis.
- Cardiac anomalies most commonly cause hydrops, followed by infection and chromosomal abnormalities.

Suggested Readings

Désilets V, Audibert F; Society of Obstetrician and Gynaecologists of Canada. Investigation and management of non-immune fetal hydrops. J Obstet Gynaecol Can. 2013; 35(10):923–938

Tercanli S, Gembruch U, Holzgreve W. Nonimmune hydrops fetalis: diagnosis and management. In: Callen PW, ed. Ultrasonography in Obstetrics and Gynecology. 5th ed. Philadelphia, PA: W.B. Saunders Company; 2008

Case 227

Erika Rubesova

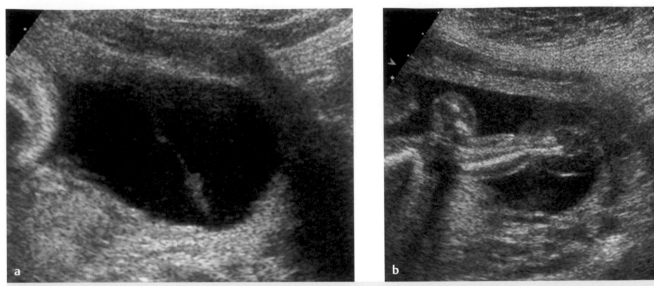

Fig. 227.1 (a) Fetal ultrasound image through the amniotic sac demonstrates an echogenic linear band within the amniotic fluid. (b) Ultrasound image of the fetal lower extremity reveals soft-tissue constriction and distal soft-tissue edema.

■ Clinical Presentation

Abnormal findings on fetal ultrasound at 20 weeks of gestation (▶Fig. 227.1).

■ Key Imaging Finding

Linear echoes within the amniotic fluid

■ Top 3 Differential Diagnoses

• **Amniotic band syndrome**. Amniotic bands typically criss-cross the uterus, may be attached to the fetus, and entangle and disrupt fetal parts. Bands may be difficult to visualize by ultrasound. The term "amniotic band syndrome" should be used only if there is an association with congenital anomalies such as limb constriction, amputation, lymphedema, and other multiple, bizarre congenital anomalies. This syndrome is relatively rare, and the etiology is not clear. The prognosis for fetuses with amniotic band syndrome is poor; however, in some circumstances, fetal surgery may be performed to free the fetus from some constrictive bands.

• **Synechiae (or amniotic shelves)**. Synechiae are thick bands that do not attach to the fetus and have no impact on the de-velopment. Most women with synechiae have a history of uterine instrumentation or uterine infection, resulting in intrauterine scars and adhesions. However, synechiae have also been reported in women with no prior history of uterine surgery or infection.

• **Chorioamniotic separation**. Chorioamniotic separation is considered normal before 16 weeks of gestation. Abnormal chorioamniotic separation may occur during the second and third trimesters. Prognosis depends on the degree of separation; small separations are usually clinically insignificant, having no effect on the pregnancy.

■ Additional Differential Diagnoses

• **Hemorrhage**. Bands of fibrin may be present following any bleeding within the amniotic cavity (such as following traumatic amniocentesis). Fibrin strands appear irregular, allow-ing for differentiation from chorioamniotic separation. They resolve with time and usually do not interfere with fetal development.

■ Diagnosis

Amniotic band syndrome

✓ Pearls

• Amniotic bands attach to the fetus and may be associated with fetal anomalies.
• Uterine synechiae appear thick and are attributed to adhesions; they have no effect on fetal development.

• Chorioamniotic separation is abnormal after 16 weeks; prognosis depends on the degree of separation.
• Fibrin strands from hemorrhage are irregular and resolve with time; they have no effect on development.

Suggested Readings

Callen P. Ultrasound in Obstetrics and Gynecology. 5th ed. Saunders; Philadelphia, PA: 2008

Middleton K. Hertzberg BS. Ultrasound: The Requisites. 2nd ed. St. Louis, MO: Mosby, Inc.; 2004

Case 228

Erika Rubesova

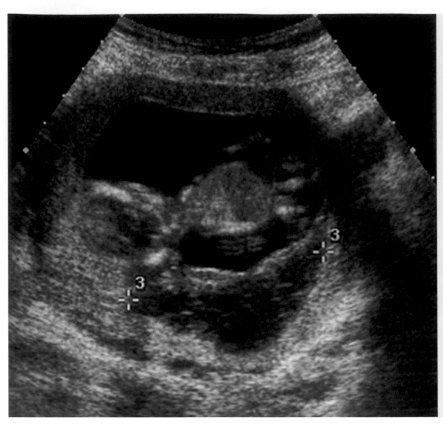

Fig. 228.1 Ultrasound images of the pelvis demonstrate a hypoechoic heterogeneous area between the maternal uterus and the chorion.

■ Clinical Presentation

A 30-year-old G3P2 woman at 13 weeks of gestational age (▶Fig. 228.1).

■ Key Imaging Finding

Placental abnormality/mass

■ Top 3 Differential Diagnoses

• **Subchorionic/Retroplacental hematoma**. The ultrasonographic features of retroplacental hematomas differ based on the age of the bleed. They appear hyperechoic in the acute phase and hypoechoic with no internal vascular flow at 1 to 2 weeks of age. The reported incidence is 5%, but many cases are not visualized on ultrasound. Retroplacental hematomas may cause placental abruption, a major cause of perinatal death. They are associated with maternal hypertension, preeclampsia, cigarette and cocaine use, blunt trauma, chorioamnionitis, obstruction of venous drainage, and cardiolipin antibodies.

• **Placental venous lakes**. Venous lakes result from perivillous fibrin deposition and appear as hypoechoic intraplacental lesions and are usually visualized under the fetal surface of the placenta. They occur in approximately 20% of pregnancies and are not associated with increased fetal morbidity or mortality.

• **Circumvallate placenta**. Circumvallate placenta is characterized by thickened chorioamniotic membranes at the periphery of the placenta. The placental edge has a rolled-up appearance on ultrasound. Complete circumvallation of the placenta is associated with increased risk for bleeding, intrauterine growth retardation (IUGR), perinatal mortality, placental abruption, and preterm labor.

■ Additional Differential Diagnoses

• **Succenturiate lobe**. A succenturiate lobe appears as a mass of placental tissue separate from the main placental mass. It occurs in 5% of pregnancies and is associated with placental infarction and velamentous insertion of the umbilical cord.

■ Diagnosis

Subchorionic hematoma

✓ Pearls

• Appearance of retroplacental hematomas varies based on age; they may not always be visualized on ultrasound.
• Large retroplacental hematomas may result in placental abruption, a leading cause of perinatal mortality.
• Venous lakes occur along the fetal surface of the placenta and do not increase morbidity or mortality.
• Circumvallate placenta and succenturiate lobes are placental variants with potential increased morbidity.

Suggested Reading

Trop I, Levine D. Hemorrhage during pregnancy: sonography and MR imaging. AJR Am J Roentgenol. 2001; 176(3):607–615

Case 229

Jeffrey P. Tan

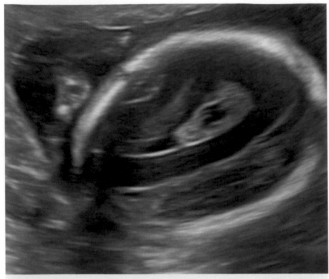

Fig. 229.1 Transverse/oblique sonographic image of the fetal head demonstrates unilateral choroid plexus cyst.

■ Clinical Presentation

A 34-year-old G1P0 woman at 20 weeks of gestational age (▶Fig. 229.1).

■ Key Imaging finding

Choroid plexus cyst

■ Top 3 Differential Diagnoses

- **Incidental finding**. Choroid plexus cysts are found incidentally in approximately 1 to 2% of the population. The sonographic appearance of choroid plexus cysts should be made on axial images of the lateral ventricles. Oblique coronal images may falsely interpose hypoechoic structures into the choroid simulating a cyst. Once identified, a detailed anatomy scan should be performed to evaluate for additional fetal abnormalities. An isolated choroid plexus cyst with otherwise normal fetal anatomy and a normal triple/quadruple screen is likely an incidental finding; the risk of amniocentesis in these cases may outweigh the potential benefit.
- **Trisomy 18 (Edward syndrome)**. Trisomy 18 or Edward syndrome is a relatively rare chromosomal abnormality with an incidence of 3 in 10,000 live births. The mortality rate is approximately 90% within the first year of life. Choroid plexus cysts can be found in approximately one-third of fetuses with trisomy 18. These fetuses usually present with intrauterine growth restriction. Additional abnormalities associated with trisomy 18 include cardiac defects, clubfeet, clenched fists with overlapping digits, facial defects, neural tube defects, radial ray abnormalities, and a two-vessel cord. As with other chromosomal abnormalities, a thickened nuchal translucency can be seen during first trimester imaging.
- **Trisomy 21 (Down syndrome)**. Trisomy 21 is the most common chromosomal anomaly and occurs more frequently with advanced maternal age. Although once thought to be associated with choroid plexus cysts, recent studies show that the incidence of choroid plexus cysts in Down syndrome is similar to that of the general population. Additional sonographic abnormalities associated with trisomy 21 include an increased first trimester nuchal translucency (>3 mm) or second trimester nuchal fold (>6 mm), ventriculomegaly, brachycephaly, flat facies, endocardial cushion defects, echogenic cardiac focus, hyperechoic bowel, duodenal atresia, pyelectasis, clinodactyly, hypoplasia of the fifth digit, short femur, and short humerus.

■ Diagnosis

Trisomy 18 (Edward syndrome)

✓ Pearls

- Choroid plexus cysts are typically incidental findings in the setting of otherwise normal fetal anatomy.
- Choroid plexus cysts do have an association with trisomy 18; associated anomalies are commonly seen.
- There is debate as to whether choroid plexus cysts are associated with trisomy 21.

Suggested Readings

Turner SR, Samei E, Hertzberg BS, et al. Sonography of fetal choroids plexus cysts: detection depends on cyst size and gestational age. J Ultrasound Med. 2003; 22:1219–1227

Dagklis T, Plasencia W, Maiz N, Duarte L, Nicolaides KH. Choroid plexus cyst, intracardiac echogenic focus, hyperechogenic bowel and hydronephrosis in screening for trisomy 21 at 11 + 0 to 13 + 6 weeks. Ultrasound Obstet Gynecol. 2008; 31(2):132–135

Case 230

Laura Varich

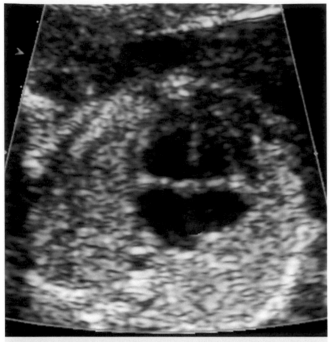

Fig. 230.1 Ultrasound four-chamber view of the fetal heart demonstrates a septal defect of the interventricular septum.

■ Clinical Presentation

A 30-year-old G3P2 woman at 18 weeks of gestational age (▶Fig. 230.1).

■ Key Imaging Finding

Ventricular septal defect

■ Top 3 Differential Diagnoses

- **Ventricular septal defect (VSD).** The fetal heart is optimally scanned between 18 and 22 weeks of gestation. An adequate fetal cardiac examination should include a four-chamber view and ventricular outflow views, at a minimum. The four-chamber view is used to evaluate chamber size, symmetry, situs, axis, valves, and integrity of the septum. Ventricular septal defects account for 20 to 40% of congenital cardiac defects. The abnormal communication between the ventricles results in a left-to-right shunt after birth. VSDs can typically be diagnosed on the four-chamber view; however, small, isolated VSDs are the most commonly missed congenital cardiac defects when using fetal ultrasonography. Color Doppler may be useful, increasing the sensitivity for detecting smaller abnormalities.
- **Endocardial cushion defect (ECD).** Endocardial cushion defects represent 2 to 7% of congenital heart defects. These defects involve both the lower atrial septum (ostium primum–type defect) and ventricular septum; they result from the failure of the endocardial cushion to fuse. Ultrasound has a high sensitivity for detection of this abnormality. Of patients with endocardial cushion defects, 30 to 40% will have Down syndrome.
- **Normal foramen ovale.** The foramen ovale is a normal fetal connection between the atria. The anatomic communication shunts a portion of oxygenated blood (from the placenta via the umbilical vein) to the systemic side of the heart, bypassing the fetal lungs. This directs more highly oxygen-saturated blood to vital organs, including the developing fetal brain. The foramen ovale is normally visualized as a flap valve at the upper atrial septum opening into the left atrium.

■ Diagnosis

Ventricular septal defect

✓ Pearls

- A fetal cardiac examination should at least consist of a four-chamber view and ventricular outflow views.
- Four-chamber view should assess chamber size, symmetry, situs, axis, valves, and integrity of the septum.
- VSD is a common congenital cardiac defect which results in a left-to-right shunt after birth.
- ECD affects the ventricular septum and lower atrial septum; it is associated with Down syndrome.

Suggested Readings

Barboza JM, Dajani NK, Glenn LG, Angtuaco TL. Prenatal diagnosis of congenital cardiac anomalies: a practical approach using two basic views. Radiographics. 2002; 22(5):1125–1137, discussion 1137–1138

, Lee W. Performance of the basic fetal cardiac ultrasound examination. J Ultrasound Med. 1998; 17(9):601–607

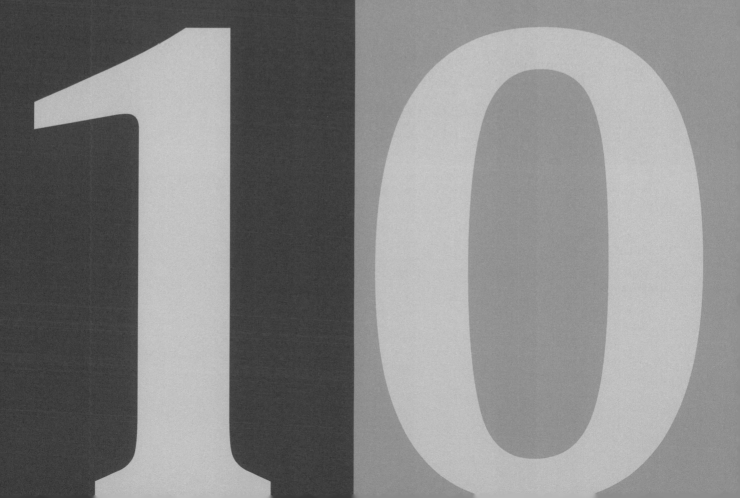

Part 10

Vascular and Interventional Radiology

Case 231

David D. Gover

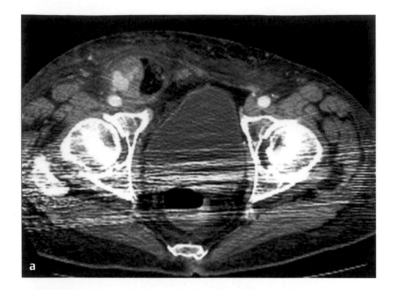
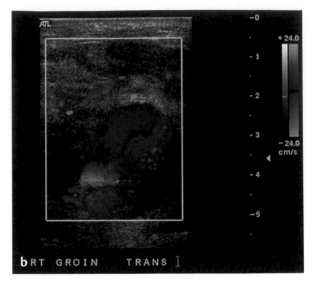
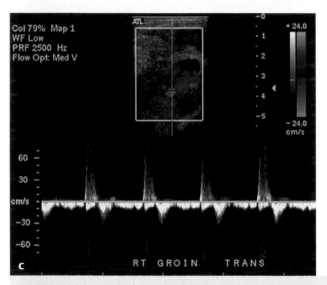

Fig. 231.1 **(a)** Contrast-enhanced axial CT image of the pelvis shows an inflammatory mass in the right groin with areas of contrast enhancement equal to the adjacent artery. Duplex ultrasound of the right groin reveals **(b)** a "yin-yang" color configuration within the right groin mass as well as **(c)** a "to-and-fro" waveform.

▪ Clinical Presentation

A 53-year-old man with right leg and groin pain after cardiac catheterization (▶Fig. 231.1).

■ Key Imaging Finding

Postprocedure arterial abnormality

■ Top 3 Differential Diagnoses

- **Hematoma**. The most frequent complication of diagnostic angiography, minor hematomas occur at rates up to 10% of cases and typically are self-limited. Major hematomas, defined as those requiring transfusion, surgical evacuation, or delay in discharge, occur in 0.5% of femoral punctures. Differentiating hematoma from pseudoaneurysm can be done by physical exam; however, confirmation with ultrasound is the norm.
- **Pseudoaneurysm**. Also known as false aneurysms, these areas of dilated vessel lack all three arterial layers. Therefore, blood flows out of the vessel, is contained by juxta-arterial tissues (connective tissue and hematoma), and is returned to the original vessel. This creates the classic "yin-yang" or "to-and-fro" appearance on ultrasonography. Causative etiologies include infection, trauma (both penetrating and blunt), and iatrogenia. Iatrogenic lesions form at a rate of 0.1 to 0.2% in diagnostic angiography and up to 2% in interventional cases. Risk factors include a "high" or "low" puncture of the femoral artery, the use of anticoagulants or antiplatelet agents, thrombocytopenia, use of thrombolytics, and large cannulas. On physical exam, the presence of a pulsatile mass is virtually diagnostic. The presence of a bruit is helpful, but is not specific, as other complications may present with a bruit (e.g., dissection, stenosis, arteriovenous fistula). Pseudoaneurysms are painful and may lead to rupture, embolization, or overlying skin ischemia. Treatment options include ultrasound-guided compression, percutaneous thrombin (or collagen) injection under ultrasound guidance, endoluminal coils or stent-graft placement, or surgery. Percutaneous options are usually the first-line treatments. Surgery is required with rapid expansion, distal ischemia, neurologic deficit, failure of percutaneous interventions, infection, or compromised soft-tissue viability.
- **Arteriovenous fistula (AVF)**. This abnormal communication between an artery and adjacent vein occurs secondary to access of ipsilateral vessels or unnoticed puncture of the vein when accessing the artery. Fistulae form rarely after diagnostic arteriography, at rates less than 0.2%. Clinically, patients complain of leg pain and swelling, and a bruit is audible on physical exam. Ultrasound interrogation will reveal arterialized flow in the adjacent vein extending centrally. The site of communication can usually be determined. Treatment options include stent-graft placement, coiling of the communication, or open surgery.

■ Diagnosis

Pseudoaneurysm

✓ Pearls

- Groin hematomas are the most common puncture site complication; the vast majority are self-limiting.
- Pseudoaneurysms present as pulsatile masses with a classic "yin-yang" or "to-and-fro" appearance on ultrasound.
- Arteriovenous fistulas most often result from inadvertent venous puncture during arterial access.
- AVFs reveal arterialized flow in the adjacent vein; they can be treated endovascularly or with surgery.

Suggested Readings

Lenartova M, Tak T. Iatrogenic pseudoaneurysm of femoral artery: case report and literature review. Clin Med Res. 2003; 1(3):243–247

Singh H, Cardella JF, Cole PE, et al; Society of Interventional Radiology Standards of Practice Committee. Quality improvement guidelines for diagnostic arteriography. J Vasc Interv Radiol. 2003; 14(9, Pt 2):S283–S288

Case 232

David D. Gover

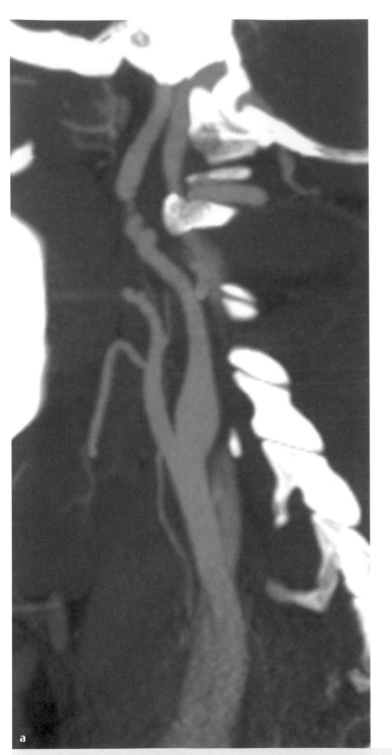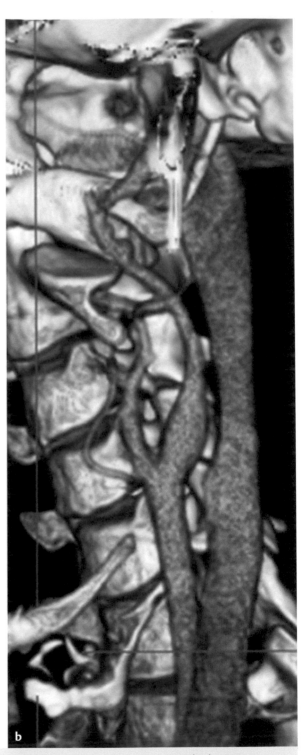

Fig. 232.1 **(a)** Oblique sagittal maximum intensity projection (MIP) and **(b)** 3D volume-rendered (VR) images from a CT angiography demonstrate alternating regions of stenosis and dilatation involving the right internal carotid artery with a "string of beads" appearance, as well as a focal region of high-grade stenosis. (Image courtesy of Richard Latchaw, MD.)

■ Clinical Presentation

A 42-year-old woman with incidental carotid bruits (▶ Fig. 232.1).

■ Key Imaging Finding

Carotid artery stenosis

■ Top 3 Differential Diagnoses

- **Atherosclerosis**. Atherosclerosis is the most common cause of carotid artery stenosis. It most often occurs in older individuals and is more advanced with smoking history, hypertension, hyperlipidemia, and diabetes. The carotid bifurcation and proximal internal carotid artery are the most common sites involved, although atherosclerosis may involve any segment, including intracranially. Doppler ultrasound is the initial screening study. Typical findings on ultrasound include visualization of plaque with vessel stenosis, elevated velocities, and turbulent flow with aliasing. MRA and CTA are used as confirmatory studies. Carotid endarterectomy (CEA) remains the treatment of choice in low-risk surgical candidates. Current guidelines recommend CEA for symptomatic lesions with greater than 50% stenosis (data from NASCET trial) or asymptomatic lesions with more than 60% stenosis (data from ACAS trial). Although many recent trials have shown a benefit of endovascular carotid stent placement with distal embolic protection devices in many patient populations, current guidelines recommend this treatment only for high-risk surgical patients with symptomatic lesions of ≥70% stenosis. High-risk surgical patients are defined as follows: clinically significant cardiac disease, severe pulmonary disease (if general anesthesia will be used),

recurrent stenosis after prior CEA, prior neck surgery or irradiation, contralateral recurrent laryngeal nerve paralysis, contralateral carotid artery occlusion, and surgically inaccessible lesions (high or low lesions).
- **Fibromuscular dysplasia (FMD)**. FMD is a dysplastic vascular disease, which primarily affects young women. The renal arteries are most commonly involved, followed by the carotid arteries. The disease results in vascular stenosis and resultant hypertension (renal artery) or stroke (internal carotid artery). Patients are at increased risk of aneurysms and dissections. The medial fibroplasia variant is the most common subtype and presents with the classic "string of beads" appearance due to alternating regions of stenosis and dilatation. Symptomatic lesions are treated with angioplasty.
- **Dissection**. Carotid artery dissection may be due to hypertension, trauma, iatrogenia, or even FMD. Most nontraumatic dissections can be managed medically with some form of anticoagulation and follow-up imaging (usually CTA) to ensure stability or resolution. Symptomatic lesions or lesions which progress despite medical management often require intervention, to include stent placement.

■ Additional Differential Diagnoses

- **Iatrogenic**. The most common iatrogenic causes of carotid stenosis include clamp injury during surgical procedures or vasculitis secondary to radiation therapy for head and neck

cancer. Treatment depends on symptoms and morphology of the lesions with endovascular therapy favored over surgical intervention.

■ Diagnosis

Fibromuscular dysplasia

✓ Pearls

- Atherosclerosis is the most common cause of carotid artery stenosis; it typically occurs in older individuals.
- Carotid stents are indicated for symptomatic lesions of ≥70% stenosis in high-risk surgical patients.

- FMD affects primarily young females; angioplasty is the primary treatment option for symptomatic lesions.
- Most dissections are due to hypertension or trauma; treatment depends on morphology and symptoms.

Suggested Readings

Gurm HS, Yadav JS, Fayad P, et al; SAPPHIRE Investigators. Long-term results of carotid stenting versus endarterectomy in high-risk patients. N Engl J Med. 2008; 358(15):1572–1579

Endarterectomy for asymptomatic carotid artery stenosis.Executive Committee for the Asymptomatic Carotid Atherosclerosis Study JAMA. 1995; 273:1421–1428

North American Symptomatic Carotid Endarterectomy Trial Collaborators. Beneficial effect of carotid endarterectomy in symptomatic patients with high-grade carotid stenosis. N Engl J Med. 1991; 325(7):445–453

Roffi M, Yadav JS. Carotid stenting. Circulation. 2006; 114(1):e1–e4

Case 233

Glade E. Roper

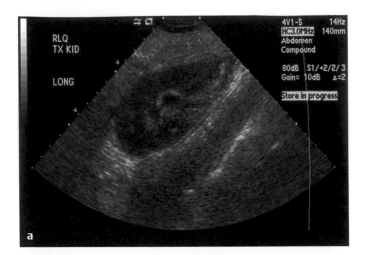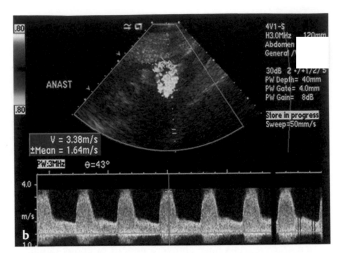

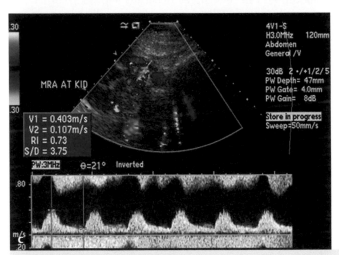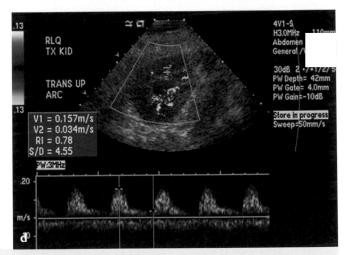

Fig. 233.1 (a) Grayscale US of a RLQ transplant kidney reveals subtle loss of corticomedullary differentiation and no peritransplant fluid. (b) Doppler US of the renal artery reveals turbulent flow with aliasing at the anastomosis of a transplant renal artery and the host iliac artery with maximum velocity >300 cm/s. (c) The more distal renal artery reveals parvus et tardus waveform. (d) Doppler US of intrarenal arcuate arteries reveals normal RI and moderate hydronephrosis. There was also hydroureter, though the distal ureter could not be interrogated due to patient body habitus.

■ Clinical Presentation

A 60-year-old woman post–renal transplant 6 weeks previously with rising creatinine (►Fig. 233.1).

■ Key Imaging Finding

Failing renal transplant with abnormal Doppler examination

■ Top 3 Differential Diagnoses

- **Acute tubular necrosis**. ATN is the most common cause of graft dysfunction within the first posttransplant week. Ultrasound (US) reveals an enlarged, swollen kidney with poor corticomedullary differentiation, elevated resistive indices (RI) within the kidney (0.8–0.9 equivocal, >0.9 requires further workup, often with biopsy), and a self-limited course with recovery of function in days to weeks. Imaging findings are nonspecific and overlap with transplant rejection.
- **Renal artery stenosis (RAS)**. RAS is a potentially treatable cause of transplant failure due to stricture at the anastomotic site. It is the most common vascular complication of renal transplant. US criteria include turbulent flow at the anasto-

motic site, peak systolic velocity >250 cm/s, and parvus/tardus waveform in the renal artery distal to the stenosis. Gold standard for diagnosis is angiography, though care must be taken to minimize contrast dose; CO2 may be used as a contrast agent.
- **Urinary obstruction**. Urinary obstruction is a relatively common transplant complication, as ureteral strictures form due to disruption of ureteral blood supply when performing the ureterovesical anastomosis. US reveals hydronephrosis. Cystoscopy and retrograde ureterography with ureteral stent placement may be diagnostic and therapeutic options.

■ Additional Differential Diagnoses

- **Transplant rejection**. Rejection occurs in 20 to 30% of cadaveric allograft recipients. Acute rejection is usually found in the first week; chronic rejection occurs in months to years. US findings overlap with ATN, though the RI may be normal in early acute rejection. Other possible findings include urothelial wall thickening, areas of hypoechogenicity due to infarction, and perinephric fluid if there is necrosis or hemorrhage. In chronic rejection, the graft becomes small and echogenic, classically with thinning of the cortices and sparing of the medullary pyramids. Biopsy is often required as imaging findings are nonspecific. Prognosis with early acute rejection is typically good, while the prognosis with chronic rejection is poor.
- **Renal vein thrombosis (RVT)**. RVT is a relatively uncommon complication of renal transplants, but is important to recog-

nize as it is a surgical emergency. It is most commonly due to mechanical obstruction. The transplanted kidney does not have venous collaterals; therefore, a delay in diagnosis may result in venous infarction. US demonstrates reversal of diastolic flow in a "to-and-fro" pattern.
- **Cyclosporine toxicity**. Cyclosporine has a constrictive effect on renal arterioles resulting in decreased perfusion. US findings are nonspecific and essentially unremarkable, with no change in RI or renal size. Effective renal plasma flow is reduced, which can be evaluated with nuclear medicine imaging. With chronic or more longstanding toxicity, the RI may be elevated.

■ Diagnosis

Renal artery stenosis

✓ Pearls

- ATN is the most common graft dysfunction in the first week posttransplant and is usually self-limited.
- RAS is most often due to stricture at the anastomotic site; it is the most common vascular complication.

- Acute transplant rejection occurs in the first week; chronic rejection occurs in months to years.

Suggested Readings

Federle MP, Jeffrey RB, Woodward PJ. Diagnostic Imaging: Abdomen. Salt Lake City, UT: Amirsys; 2004

Urban BA, Ratner LE, Fishman EK. Three-dimensional volume-rendered CT angiography of the renal arteries and veins: normal anatomy, variants, and clinical applications. Radiographics. 2001; 21(2):373–386, 549–555

Case 234

David D. Gover

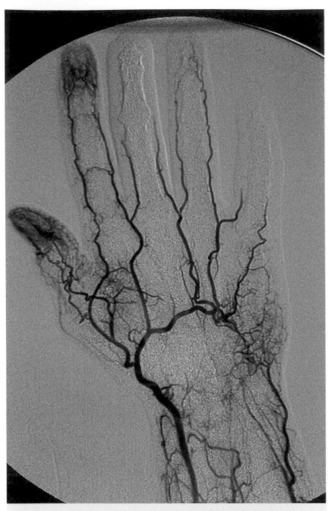

Fig. 234.1 Digital subtraction angiography of the right hand demonstrates multiple filling defects within the digital arteries, most pronounced within the third through fifth digits. There is underlying deformity of the third distal phalanx.

■ Clinical Presentation

A 38-year-old man with chronic unilateral hand pain and intermittent pallor (▶Fig. 234.1).

■ Key Imaging Finding

Digital artery occlusion/ischemia

■ Top 3 Differential Diagnoses

- **Raynaud syndrome**. Raynaud syndrome is a vasospastic disorder prompted by cold temperatures. Imaging findings include stenosis or occlusion of digital artery branches that are relieved by warming of the affected extremity or administration of a vasodilator. Although Raynaud syndrome is associated with scleroderma, other connective tissue disorders can produce similar clinical symptoms and radiographic findings.
- **Vasculitis**. Vasculitis may result in upper extremity ischemia and has a variety of etiologies, to include *systemic lupus erythematous*, *connective tissue disorders*, and *Buerger disease*. Imaging findings typically include stenosis or occlusion of arteries within the hand or wrist. Systemic steroids provide relief of acute episodes. Buerger disease (thromboangiitis obliterans) occurs predominantly in young male smokers and has a particular prevalence for the upper extremities. With chronic ischemia, "corkscrew collaterals" develop, which are classic for this entity. Symptoms are improved with smoking cessation.
- **Embolic disease**. Embolic disease may emanate from either the heart or within the vascular supply to the affected upper extremity. Cardiac emboli constitute the most common cause of acute upper extremity ischemia. Imaging findings include arterial occlusions most commonly within the small vessels of the hand(s). A cardiac source usually involves both upper extremities, while a source from a more proximal artery results in unilateral disease. The entire extremity should be evaluated to find lesions amenable to percutaneous interventions, and thrombolysis may be beneficial in certain circumstances.

■ Additional Differential Diagnoses

- **Thoracic outlet syndrome**. Thoracic outlet syndrome results from chronic compression of the upper extremity neurovascular structures secondary to abnormal insertion of scalene musculature or the presence of a cervical rib. Imaging findings include stenosis or occlusion of the subclavian artery, arterial injury (aneurysm or pseudoaneurysm), and distal emboli. If the angiography in the neutral position is normal, the angiography should be repeated with the affected extremity abducted and externally rotated. Percutaneous treatment may be beneficial, but the definitive treatment is surgical correction of the compressive lesion.
- **Trauma**: Frostbite or repetitive injury commonly involves the hands. *Frostbite* results in ischemia/occlusion of the digital arteries with sparing of the thumbs secondary to clenched fists with the digits protecting the thumbs. *Hypothenar hammer syndrome* is due to repetitive trauma and results in pseudoaneurysm formation along the hypothenar eminence with distal emboli to the digital arteries.
- **Atherosclerosis**: Atherosclerotic disease constitutes the most common cause of chronic upper extremity ischemia. Although any artery may be involved, the digital arteries are affected in patients with chronic hypertension, diabetes, and/or renal failure. Imaging findings include stenosis or occlusion of the arteries of the wrist, hand, or digits. The vascular supply of the entire extremity should be interrogated to find lesions amenable to percutaneous interventions.

■ Diagnosis

Thoracic outlet syndrome

✓ Pearls

- Raynaud syndrome is vasospasm due to cold temperatures; it is relieved with warming or vasodilators.
- Many vasculitides may cause digital artery occlusion; Buerger disease results in "corkscrew collaterals."
- Embolic disease from a proximal source (cardiac or thoracic outlet) may cause digital artery occlusion.

Suggested Readings

Raptis CA, Sridhar S, Thompson RW, Fowler KJ, Bhalla S. Imaging of the patient with thoracic outlet syndrome. Radiographics. 2016; 36(4):984–1000

Case 235

David D. Gover

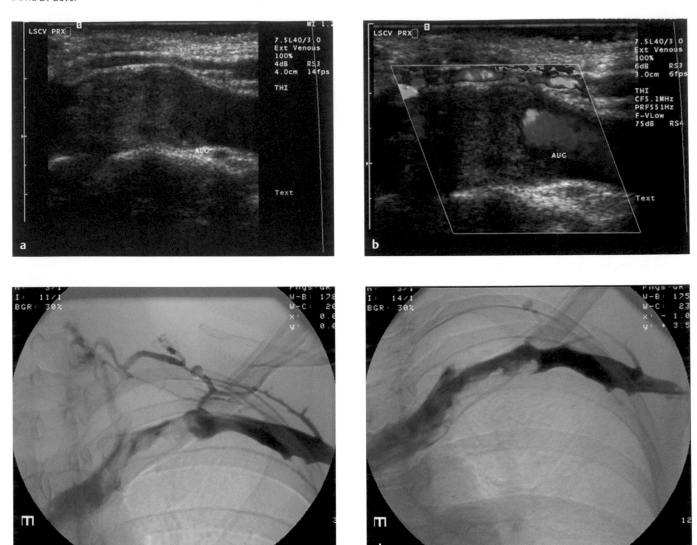

Fig. 235.1 **(a)** Grey scale and **(b)** color Doppler ultrasound images of the left subclavian vein reveal an echogenic focus within the vessel and expanding the lumen without flow. **(c)** Conventional venography reveals a corresponding filling defect with minimal contrast flow around the abnormality, as well as the presence of collateral vessels. **(d)** Venogram at the same level after overnight pharmacological thrombolysis and angioplasty demonstrates improved contrast opacification of the vessel with resolution of the collateral venous pathways.

■ Clinical Presentation

A 33-year-old woman with acute left arm swelling which began after wearing a new backpack (▶Fig. 235.1).

■ Key Imaging Finding

Subclavian vein occlusion

■ Top 3 Differential Diagnoses

- **Prior instrumentation/catheter placement**. Upper extremity deep venous thrombosis (DVT) accounts for nearly 10% of all DVT cases; most attribute this change to the use of chronic indwelling catheters and cardiac devices. Ultrasound is the initial exam of choice, followed by CT venography or conventional venography in equivocal cases. Contrast exam will reveal a filling defect or occlusion at areas of prior or current devices, along with collateral venous circulation. Management depends on symptoms, ability to receive anticoagulation, and clinical necessity of any medical devices weighted against the risk of thromboembolic disease. Treatment options include conservative measures, anticoagulation, thrombolysis, or all of the previously mentioned plus removal of the catheter or cardiac device.
- **Hypercoagulability**. Virchow's triad refers to a predisposition for venous thromboses secondary to trauma (intimal injury), stasis/immobility, and/or an underlying hypercoagulable state. Genetic conditions which result in a hypercoagulable state include factor V Leiden, antithrombin III, and protein S

or C deficiencies; acquired conditions include oral contraceptives, tobacco usage, and underlying malignancy. In cases of an inherited hypercoagulable state or underlying malignancy, lifelong anticoagulation is the usual treatment. Endovascular therapy with catheter-directed thrombolysis or angioplasty may be beneficial in many instances.
- **Paget-von Schroetter syndrome/Effort thrombosis**. Defined as primary thrombosis at the thoracic inlet, Paget-von Schroetter syndrome is usually found in young patients with cervical ribs, osseous deformity (e.g., tumor, trauma) of the clavicle or first rib, or myofascial narrowing. It may occasionally occur bilaterally. Definitive diagnosis is obtained through conventional venography with provocative maneuvers such as abduction with external rotation (caution as possible false-positive results may occur). Management consists of thrombolysis followed by anticoagulation of symptomatic lesions until definitive surgical decompression can be performed. Follow-up venography may yield persistent irregular stenosis that may require percutaneous transluminal angioplasty.

■ Diagnosis

Paget-von Schroetter syndrome

✓ Pearls

- Chronic indwelling catheters are the most common cause of upper extremity deep venous thrombosis.
- Virchow's triad refers to trauma (intimal injury), stasis/immobility, or underlying hypercoagulable state.

- Paget-von Schroetter syndrome results in venous thrombosis due to osseous or myofascial abnormalities.
- Definitive treatment of Paget-von Schroetter syndrome requires surgical intervention.

Suggested Readings

Demondion X, Herbinet P, Van Sint Jan S, Boutry N, Chantelot C, Cotten A. Imaging assessment of thoracic outlet syndrome. Radiographics. 2006; 26(6):1735–1750

Sheeran SR, Hallisey MJ, Murphy TP, Faberman RS, Sherman S. Local thrombolytic therapy as part of a multidisciplinary approach to acute axillosubclavian vein thrombosis (Paget-Schroetter syndrome). J Vasc Interv Radiol. 1997; 8(2):253–260

Case 236

David D. Gover

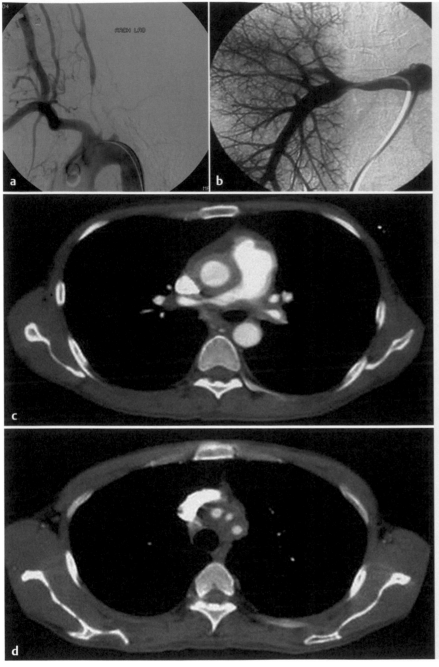

Fig. 236.1 **(a)** Digital subtraction angiogram (DSA) in the left anterior oblique (LAO) position shows long-segment, smooth stenosis of the proximal left common carotid and left subclavian arteries near their origins. **(b)** Selective DSA of the right pulmonary artery reveals a smooth, concentric, short-segment stenosis proximally. Contrast-enhanced CT images of the thorax at the level of **(c)** the pulmonary arteries and **(d)** great vessel origins confirm the angiographic findings, as well as demonstrate inflammatory thickening surrounding the involved vessels.

■ Clinical Presentation

A 27-year-old Asian woman with left arm pain (▶Fig. 236.1).

■ Key Imaging Finding

Great vessel stenosis

■ Top 3 Differential Diagnoses

- **Atherosclerosis**. Atherosclerosis is the most common cause of great vessel stenosis. Multiple vessels are usually involved. Patients are typically older and have risk factors such as hypertension, smoking, hyperlipidemia, and/or diabetes. Concomitant cardiovascular and peripheral vascular disease is common. Symptoms are related to the specific end organ being underperfused, and therapy is geared toward relief of said symptoms. Catheter-directed therapies are attempted due to the decreased morbidity compared with open surgery. Technical success rates exceed 95%. Long-term clinical success of angioplasty for stenosis and stent placement for occlusion ranges from 70 to 90%.
- **Vasculitis**. Great vessel and aortic vasculitis is usually secondary to primary conditions such as Takayasu or giant cell arteritis (GCA). Takayasu tends to affect younger, Asian female patients, and manifests clinically with malaise, arthralgias,

and gradual onset of extremity claudication. Clinical exam may reveal asymmetric pulses or blood pressure in the upper extremities. GCA typically is seen in older Caucasian females. Patients have fevers, polymyalgia rheumatica, facial or upper extremity claudication, visual disturbances, blindness, and generalized constitutional symptoms. The diagnosis of GCA is confirmed with temporal artery biopsy. Treatment of vasculitis consists of corticosteroid administration. Once acute flares have resolved, residual stenoses may be treated percutaneously should concordant symptoms persist.
- **Dissection**. Stanford A dissections may have false lumen extension into the origins of the great vessels. This can lead to end-organ hypoperfusion/stroke. Surgical management is the usual treatment. In nonsurgical patients, endoluminal options include stent or stent-graft placement at the leading intimal tear or fenestration of the intimal flap.

■ Additional Differential Diagnoses

- **Radiation**. Radiation therapy to the chest wall or neck may lead to multiple, smooth, long-segment strictures of affected vessels. History is the key to making this diagnosis. Treatments

are centered on endoluminal options for arch vessel involvement, given the high morbidity associated with surgical procedures, along with similar patency rates.

■ Diagnosis

Vasculitis (Takayasu arteritis)

✓ Pearls

- Atherosclerosis is the most common cause of great vessel stenosis and typically affects older individuals.
- GCA and Takayasu arteritis are common vasculitides affecting the great vessels; treatment is with steroids.

- Aortic dissections may involve the great vessels; Stanford A dissections are typically managed surgically.
- Radiation therapy to the neck results in long-segment strictures; endoluminal treatment is preferred.

Suggested Readings

Hadjipetrou P, Cox S, Piemonte T, Eisenhauer A. Percutaneous revascularization of atherosclerotic obstruction of aortic arch vessels. J Am Coll Cardiol. 1999; 33(5):1238–1245

Roane DW, Griger DR. An approach to diagnosis and initial management of systemic vasculitis. Am Fam Physician. 1999; 60(5):1421–1430

Zimpfer D, Czerny M, Kettenbach J, et al. Treatment of acute type a dissection by percutaneous endovascular stent-graft placement. Ann Thorac Surg. 2006; 82(2):747–749

Case 237

David D. Gover

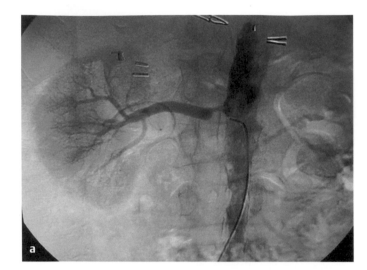

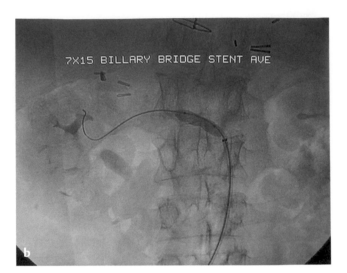

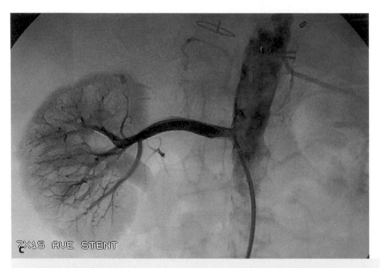

Fig. 237.1 **(a)** Selective right renal artery angiogram demonstrates an 80% ostial stenosis. Note the lack of filling to the left renal artery secondary to prior nephrectomy. **(b)** The proximal right renal artery lesion was crossed and a 7-mm balloon-expandable stent was placed. **(c)** Follow-up imaging post–stent placement demonstrates a properly placed stent without evidence of residual narrowing or complication.

■ Clinical Presentation

A 66-year-old man with prior left nephrectomy, worsening hypertension, and renal failure while on an ACE inhibitor. Images A and B are pretreatment; image C is posttreatment (▶ Fig. 237.1).

■ Key Imaging Finding

Renal artery stenosis

■ Top 3 Differential Diagnoses

- **Atherosclerosis.** The most common cause of renal artery stenosis, atherosclerotic plaques usually form at the ostia (first centimeter) of the renal artery due to disease of the aorta. Patients may be asymptomatic or suffer from renovascular hypertension, chronic renal failure, or episodes of flash pulmonary edema. In the setting of symptoms, intervention is usually offered. The mainstay intervention has become percutaneous stent placement. Despite a high technical success rate (>98%), clinical responses are variable and difficult to predict. For example, in the setting of renovascular hypertension, approximately one-third have improvement in blood pressure, one-third stabilize, and one-third continue to deteriorate. Reasons for failure include contrast-induced nephropathy, progressive nephrosclerosis, diffuse distal renal artery atherosclerotic disease, and atheroembolism. The theory of atheroembolism has led to the development of low-profile systems for interventions and distal embolic protection devices. Embolic protection appears safe to incorporate into the procedure but is still not widely accepted as a proven benefit. Finally, the decision to treat stenosis is somewhat controversial. Most current studies, although not definitive, show no benefit to stent placement over maximal medical management (especially with the use of statins for plaque stabilization or even regression). Although some espouse early treatment despite symptoms, most currently consider invasive intervention only in the setting of the symptoms mentioned previously.

- **Fibromuscular dysplasia (FMD).** Although relatively uncommon, FMD is the leading cause of curable hypertension and most often occurs in younger females. The most common form is that of medial fibroplasia (about 90% of all FMD), which has the typical angiographic appearance of a "string of beads" with alternating regions of stenosis and dilatation. The other subtypes may present with stenosis similar to atherosclerosis. Patients usually present with renovascular hypertension but are younger than is typical for atherosclerosis. Angioplasty is highly effective with 80% improvement in hypertension at 1 month and 93% at 2 years. Angioplasty can be repeated as needed with similar clinical results. Other medium-sized vessels may also be affected (e.g., internal carotid artery).

- **Dissection.** Dissections often begin in the aorta (ascending or descending) and affect the perfusion and origin caliber of the renal arteries. Additionally, iatrogenic dissection of the renal artery can occur with diagnostic angiography or endoluminal interventions. Treatment is based on the morphology of the dissection and clinical symptoms with operative therapy, fenestration, or stenting all utilized.

■ Diagnosis

Atherosclerosis

✓ Pearls

- Atherosclerosis is the most common cause of renal artery stenosis and typically involves the renal ostia.
- Despite technical success of renal artery stents for atherosclerotic lesions, clinical response is variable.

- FMD most often occurs in young females; lesions are treated with angioplasty, which is highly effective.
- Treatment of renal artery dissections is based on the morphology of the dissection and clinical symptoms.

Suggested Readings

Misra S, Gomes MT, Mathew V, et al. Embolic protection devices in patients with renal artery stenosis with chronic renal insufficiency: a clinical study. J Vasc Interv Radiol. 2008; 19(11):1639–1645

Kim HJ, Do YS, Shin SW, et al. Percutaneous transluminal angioplasty of renal artery fibromuscular dysplasia: mid-term results. Korean J Radiol. 2008; 9(1):38–44

van Bockel JH, Weibull H. Fibrodysplastic disease of the renal arteries. Eur J Vasc Surg. 1994; 8(6):655–657

Case 238

David D. Gover

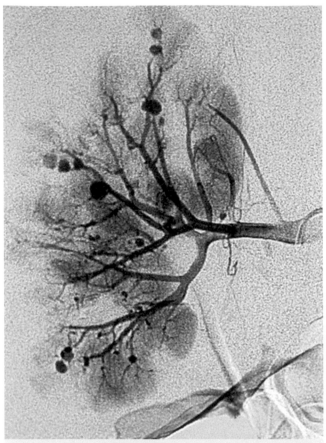

Fig. 238.1 Selective digital subtraction angiogram (DSA) of the right renal artery shows numerous small intraparenchymal aneurysms.

■ Clinical Presentation

A 44-year-old woman with hematuria (▶Fig. 238.1).

■ Key Imaging Finding

Intraparenchymal renal artery aneurysms

■ Top 3 Differential Diagnoses

- **Vasculitis**. Vascular inflammatory conditions are the major cause of intraparenchymal renal aneurysms. The most common condition to affect the small to medium sized renal arteries is *polyarteritis nodosa (PAN)*. This is usually idiopathic, but can be associated with cryoglobulinemia, leukemia, rheumatoid arthritis, Sjögren syndrome, and hepatitis B (mnemonic "CLASH"). Patients are usually middle aged suffering from peripheral neuropathy, intestinal ischemia, and livedo reticularis. Patients with *Wegener vasculitis* present with recurrent sinusitis or epistaxis, mucosal ulcerations, hemoptysis, tracheal stenosis, and eye involvement. Other vasculitides affecting the renal arteries include Takayasu and Churg-Strauss. Treatment involves corticosteroid administration, sometimes with the addition of less proven immunosuppressive therapy.
- **Mycotic/Septic emboli**. Sources of septic emboli include bacterial endocarditis (often associated with IV drug abuse), in-

fected valves, infected atrial thrombus, or noncardiac sources, and can lead to multiple renal pseudoaneurysms. Typical organisms are gram-positive bacteria (*Streptococcus* and *Staphylococcus* subspecies). Treatment is supportive, and antibiotic therapy is directed toward the offending organism accounting for susceptibility. If congestive heart failure occurs, valve replacement may be necessary.
- **Trauma**. Aneurysms are usually solitary with a history of recent blunt or penetrating trauma. Iatrogenic injury from endovascular procedures has led to an increase in this condition, with rupture being the most dreaded complication. Coils, stent-grafts, open surgical repair, or nephrectomy are effective treatment options depending on the anatomic location and clinical scenario.

■ Additional Differential Diagnoses

- **Ehlers-Danlos**. Ehlers-Danlos is a connective tissue disorder characterized by abnormal collagen synthesis, which results in skin hyperelasticity, joint hyperextensibility, and vascular fragility. Aneurysms can be seen in multiple vascular beds with mass effect or bleeding. Early diagnosis results in minimizing invasive vascular procedures, which can be catastrophic (especially in type IV Ehlers-Danlos).

- **Speed kidney**. Chronic oral amphetamine use (50 mg daily for 22 years to 200 mg daily for 2 years) may be an independent risk factor for multiple renal artery aneurysms. These patients have no other risk factors but present with multiple visceral artery aneurysms.

■ Diagnosis

Vasculitis (polyarteritis nodosa)

✓ Pearls

- PAN classically results in multiple aneurysms involving small and medium sized renal arteries.
- Mycotic/septic emboli may result from cardiac or noncardiac sources; multiple pseudoaneurysms are seen.

- Blunt or penetrating trauma, along with iatrogenia, may cause renal artery aneurysms.
- Chronic amphetamine usage predisposes patients to multiple renal artery aneurysms (speed kidney).

Suggested Readings

Bloch R, Hoffer E, Borsa J, Fontaine A. Ehlers-Danlos syndrome mimicking mesenteric vasculitis: therapy, then diagnosis. J Vasc Interv Radiol. 2001; 12(4):527–529

Nosher JL, Chung J, Brevetti LS, Graham AM, Siegel RL. Visceral and renal artery aneurysms: a pictorial essay on endovascular therapy. Radiographics. 2006; 26(6):1687–1704, quiz 1687

Roane DW, Griger DR. An approach to diagnosis and initial management of systemic vasculitis. Am Fam Physician. 1999; 60(5):1421–1430

Welling TH, Williams DM, Stanley JC. Excessive oral amphetamine use as a possible cause of renal and splanchnic arterial aneurysms: a report of two cases. J Vasc Surg. 1998; 28(4):727–731

Case 239

Glade E. Roper

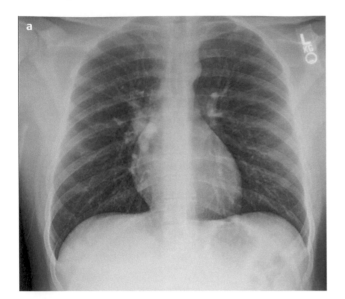

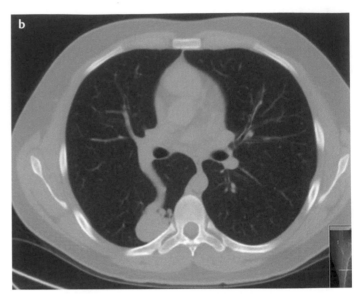

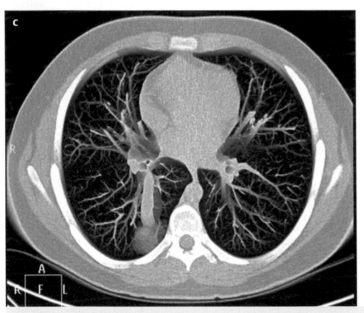

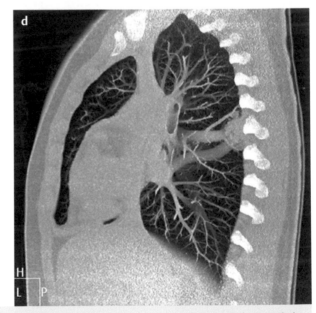

Fig. 239.1 **(a)** Frontal chest radiograph demonstrates rounded densities overlying the right hilum. **(b)** Axial CT image in lung window reveals a rounded peripheral mass within the superior segment of the right lower lobe with an enlarged feeding vessel. Contrast-enhanced maximum intensity projection images in the **(c)** axial and **(d)** sagittal planes postcontrast confirm the peripheral mass with an enlarged feeding artery and draining vein. (Images courtesy of Children's Hospital and Research Center Oakland.)

■ **Clinical Presentation**

Patient with cough (▶Fig. 239.1).

■ Key Imaging Finding

Hypervascular pulmonary mass

■ Top 3 Differential Diagnoses

- **Arteriovenous malformation (AVM)**. AVMs are anomalous connections between the pulmonary arteries and veins, which bypass the normal pulmonary capillary bed. Large AVMs can result in paradoxical emboli or high-output heart failure. AVMs may occur sporadically or be associated with Osler-Weber-Rendu syndrome, in which case they are multiple. CECT reveals a noncalcified, homogenously enhancing nodule with one or more feeding arteries and one or more draining veins. Angiography reveals opacification of the pulmonary veins on arterial injection of contrast. AVMs fed by an artery of greater than 3 mm and those contributing to paradoxical emboli or heart failure should be treated with coil embolization.
- **Bronchogenic carcinoma**. Lung cancer is the most common cause of cancer death in the United States. Adenocarcinoma is the most common subtype. Squamous and small cell subtypes are highly associated with tobacco usage. Nodules less

than 5 mm in diameter on CT have less than 1% chance of being malignant. Nodules larger than 7 mm can be interrogated for enhancement; nearly all of those with less than 15 HU of enhancement will be benign. Large, spiculated nodules and those with concurrent mediastinal lymphadenopathy are most concerning for cancer. PET imaging or biopsy can help establish a diagnosis and direct treatment in more difficult cases.
- **Hypervascular metastasis**. The lung is the most common site of metastatic disease; approximately 50% of cancer patients have lung metastases at autopsy. A solitary enhancing lung nodule may represent metastases from a hypervascular primary malignancy, such as malignant melanoma, sarcoma, carcinoid, or renal cell carcinoma. Thyroid carcinoma metastatic lesions are quite vascular and thus enhance avidly, but usually present as multiple lesions.

■ Additional Differential Diagnoses

- **Pulmonary carcinoid**. Carcinoid is an uncommon malignant tumor of bronchial neuroendocrine cells. Patients present between 30 and 60 years of age with a chronic cough and often with hemoptysis. Radiography reveals a smooth mass, usually centrally located, with or without postobstructive pneumonia. CT reveals a centrally located mass with avid contrast enhancement. Thirty percent of carcinoid tumors demonstrate calcification. Often times, there is a small endobronchial com-

ponent with a large extrabronchial component, referred to as the "tip of the iceberg" sign.
- **Pulmonary artery aneurysm**. Pulmonary artery aneurysms are relatively rare and are most commonly due to pulmonary hypertension, pulmonary infections (Rasmussen aneurysm with TB), or vasculitides. They may involve the main or more distal pulmonary artery branches, in which they may present as a hyperenhancing pulmonary nodule or mass.

■ Diagnosis

Arteriovenous malformation

✓ Pearls

- AVMs may occur sporadically or be multiple and associated with Osler-Weber-Rendu syndrome.
- Pulmonary neoplasms may appear as hypervascular masses, especially carcinoid.

- Rasmussen aneurysms occur secondary to pulmonary infection with TB; they are prone to hemorrhage.

Suggested Readings

Gossage JR, Kanj G. Pulmonary arteriovenous malformations. A state of the art review. Am J Respir Crit Care Med. 1998; 158(2):643–661

Swensen SJ, Viggiano RW, Midthun DE, et al. Lung nodule enhancement at CT: multicenter study. Radiology. 2000; 214(1):73–80

Case 240

David D. Gover

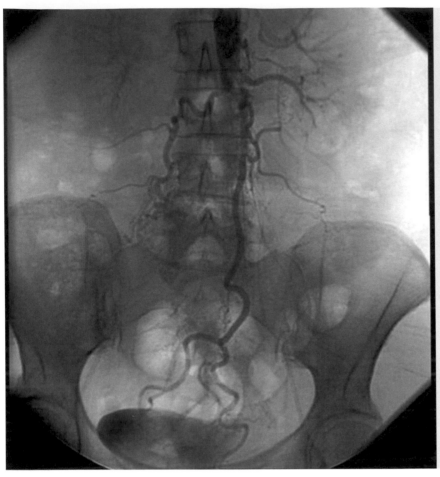

Fig. 240.1 Frontal angiogram of the abdominal aorta and pelvis from a left brachial artery access shows occlusion of the aorta below the level of the inferiormost left renal artery. Note the hypertrophied lumbar vessels that serve as collateral pathways reconstituting the external iliac vessels to supply the lower extremities.

■ Clinical Presentation

A 58-year-old woman with bilateral lower extremity claudication and diminished femoral pulses (▶Fig. 240.1).

■ Key Imaging Finding

Infrarenal aortic occlusion

■ Top 3 Differential Diagnoses

- **Atherosclerosis**. This distribution of occlusive disease is most often seen in smokers, presenting with claudication (80%), rest pain (25%), and tissue loss (15%). About 75% of men will be impotent. Add diminished or absent femoral pulses to complete the constellation of findings in Leriche syndrome. Preoperative CTA should be utilized to aid in management decisions. With long-segment disease (TASC C and D), surgical management usually entails aorto-bifemoral bypass. Operative mortality is around 5%, with 67% 5-year survival rates. Medical options are reserved for nonoperative candidates. Short-segment occlusive disease (TASC A and B), which is less common, can be managed with stent placement. Stent placement in the infrarenal aorta and iliac systems has a greater than 95% technical and clinical success, with a mean 30-day mortality of 0.5%. Primary patency rates are greater than 80% at 3 years. Patients are often placed on aspirin.
- **Thrombus/Embolus**. Clot may be formed in situ or come from a proximal source (e.g., cardiac). The underlying pathology is extremely important for management purposes. In the setting of a previously placed aorto-bifemoral bypass graft, the patient may present acutely with recurrence of symptoms. Endoluminal management is preferred and entails thrombolysis with probable perianastomotic angioplasty and/or stent placement. Embolus lodging in a region of aortic tapering may present with acute ischemia, requiring endoluminal thrombolysis or embolectomy (depending on clinical status). Thrombosis of an aneurysm can also occur (usually in hypercoagulable states) and may merit anything from emergent operative intervention to conservative management with surveillance. History and CTA are important steps in initial management and determination of appropriate therapy.
- **Vasculitis**. Takayasu arteritis can involve the aorta and its branches. Patients tend to be younger than those with atherosclerosis and typically have systemic clinical findings (e.g., fevers, fatigue, and malaise). Management of the vascular lesions should be delayed until the more fibrotic phase of the disease. When the ESR has normalized, the lesions can be handled similarly to atherosclerotic lesions with surgery or endovascular options. Appropriate treatment depends on the morphology of the lesions, as well as the clinical status of the patient (e.g., symptoms and comorbidities). Relapses can occur.

■ Additional Differential Diagnoses

- **Dissection**. Dissections may occur as a result of hypertension, trauma, or iatrogenia. Preoperative CTA helps make the diagnosis and also aids in management decisions. Medical management, endoluminal stent placement or fenestration, or open surgical repair have all been utilized, depending on the patient's symptoms and comorbidities.

■ Diagnosis

Atherosclerosis

✓ Pearls

- Atherosclerosis is a common cause of infrarenal aortic occlusion; treatment depends on lesion morphology.
- Clot may form in situ (thrombus) or result from proximal embolic sources, such as cardiac thrombi.
- Vasculitis involves younger patients with systemic findings; lesions are treated in the fibrotic phase.
- Dissections often occur from hypertension or trauma; treatment depends on symptoms and comorbidities.

Suggested Readings

Kim SH, Jeong JY, Kim YI, Choi YH, Chung JW, Hyung Park J. SCVIR 2002 Film Panel case 3: aortic occlusion secondary to intimal sarcoma. J Vasc Interv Radiol. 2002; 13(5):537–541

Ligush J, Jr, Criado E, Burnham SJ, Johnson G, Jr, Keagy BA. Management and outcome of chronic atherosclerotic infrarenal aortic occlusion. J Vasc Surg. 1996; 24(3):394–404, discussion 404–405

Uberoi R, Tsetis D. Standards for the Endovascular Management of Aortic Occlusive Disease. CIRSE; 2008

Case 241

David D. Gover

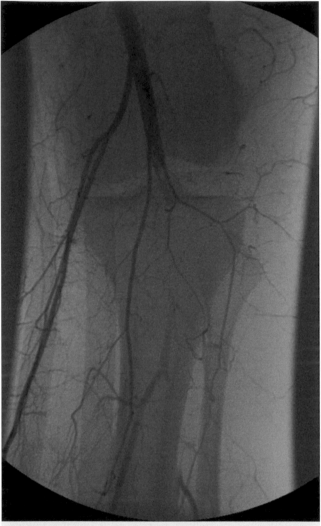

Fig. 241.1 Run-off angiogram of the left popliteal artery shows occlusion at the level of the knee with collateral vessels filling the tibial and peroneal vessels. Secondary findings include asymmetric widening of the medial joint compartment in comparison to the lateral compartment.

■ Clinical Presentation

A 38-year-old man with left leg pain (▶ Fig. 241.1).

■ Key Imaging Finding

Popliteal artery occlusion

■ Top 3 Differential Diagnoses

- **Atherosclerosis**. Atherosclerosis is the most common cause of popliteal artery stenosis and occlusion. Risk factors include hypertension, diabetes, smoking, and hyperlipidemia. Endothelial injury leads to a fibrotic plaque that can rupture or calcify, ultimately leading to narrowing and occlusion. Patients may present with claudication, rest pain, or tissue loss. Treatment is geared toward the morphology of the lesion and the symptoms. Medical management focuses on risk factors (e.g., hyperlipidemia) or symptoms (e.g., claudication). Interventions include angioplasty, stents/stent grafts, patch angioplasty, or bypass surgery. Overall, patient health plays an important role in the choice of intervention.

- **Embolism**. Emboli present acutely with pain or limb threat. Sources include the heart (e.g., arrhythmias) and proximal arterial lesions (AAA). Thrombolysis can be used if time allows versus thrombectomy.
- **Trauma**. Occlusion of the popliteal artery can be seen in blunt (e.g., motor vehicle accident) or penetrating trauma. A high index of suspicion is requisite given possible relocation of the knee joint prior to presentation, as well as preservation of the distal arterial pulse despite injury. Prompt and accurate diagnosis is required to limit morbidity, with angiography being the best exam. Surgical repair is almost always necessary.

■ Additional Differential Diagnoses

- **Thrombosed popliteal artery aneurysm**. Aneurysms are usually true (involving all layers) and degenerative (similar risk factors to atherosclerosis). Rarely, aneurysms form from connective tissue disorders, trauma, or vasculitis. Aneurysms are defined in the popliteal artery as focal areas of widening when compared to normal (8 mm in diameter or greater). Popliteal artery aneurysms are bilateral 50 to 70% of the time, and are associated with abdominal aortic aneurysms in 30 to 50% of cases. Patients may present with thrombosis, distal emboli (blue toe syndrome), or rupture (rare). Treatment is usually surgical, but stent-grafts have been used in patients at high operative risk.
- **Popliteal artery entrapment syndrome**. Narrowing of the vessel occurs due to an abnormal relationship of the artery to

the medial head of the gastrocnemius or popliteus, or sometimes due to muscle hypertrophy. Patients are usually young and athletic, presenting with claudication. In the proper setting, MR or angiography with the foot neutral and in flexion can be diagnostic. Treatment consists of myomectomy. Left untreated, permanent arterial narrowing will usually result.
- **Cystic adventitial disease**. This rare disease consists of mucoid cysts in the adventitia, leading to compression of the artery. Patients are usually middle-aged males with claudication. MRI best characterizes the lesion, showing the narrowing of the vessel and the mucinous cyst. Treatment options include cyst aspiration (with risk of recurrence), surgical resection with preservation of the artery, or patch angioplasty.

■ Diagnosis

Trauma (posterior knee dislocation)

✓ Pearls

- Atherosclerotic and embolic disease encompasses the majority of cases of popliteal artery occlusion.
- Traumatic occlusion of the popliteal artery is evaluated with angiography and treated surgically.

- Popliteal artery aneurysms are often bilateral and are associated with abdominal aortic aneurysms.
- Popliteal artery entrapment syndrome is due to abnormal relationship between the artery and musculature.

Suggested Readings

Wright LB, Matchett WJ, Cruz CP, et al. Popliteal artery disease: diagnosis and treatment. Radiographics. 2004; 24(2):467–479

Case 242

David D. Gover

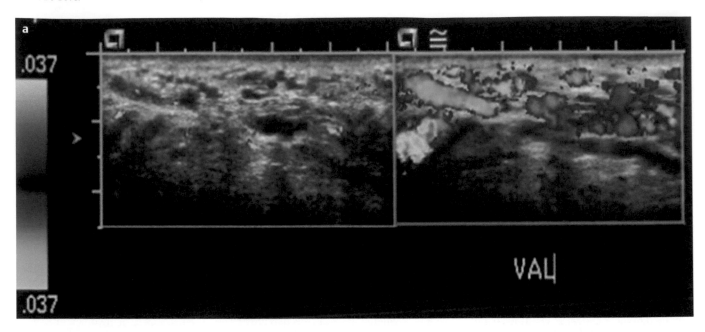

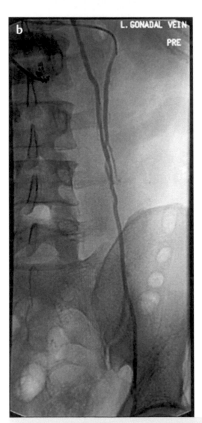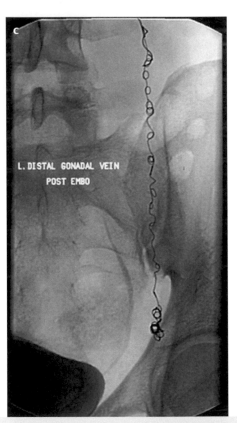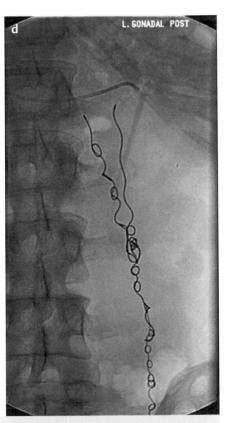

Fig. 242.1 **(a)** Color-Doppler ultrasound of the left scrotum reveals a vascular, extratesticular mass with increased flow during Valsalva maneuver, consistent with a varicocele. **(b)** On selective left gonadal venography, there is reflux of contrast to the level of the inguinal canal. Note the partial duplication of the vessel at the renal vein end. **(c)** Coil embolization is performed, **(d)** inclusive of the area of duplication.

■ Clinical Presentation

A 28-year-old man with painful left scrotal mass (▶Fig. 242.1).

■ Key Imaging Finding

Extratesticular mass

■ Top 3 Differential Diagnoses

• **Varicocele**. Varicoceles are usually caused by venous reflux of the ipsilateral gonadal vein and have been classically described as a "bag of worms" on scrotal physical examination. They enlarge or worsen with increased intraabdominal pressure (e.g., Valsalva maneuver). Unlike lower extremity varicosities that are caused by valvular incompetence (due to prior inflammatory or thrombotic events), varicoceles are usually the result of congenital absence of valves. Varicoceles lead to any combination of male infertility, testicular atrophy, and pain. The vast majority of varicoceles occur on the left side. An isolated right varicocele should prompt a search for a retroperitoneal mass. Treatment options include open, microsurgical, or laparoscopic varicocelectomy versus endoluminal ablation with a variety of materials (e.g., coils, Gelfoam, detergent sclerosants, balloons, or glue). Surgical failure rates range from 1 to 10% at 2 years with recurrence most likely due to anatomic variations and duplications that evade the surgeon (most in or near the inguinal canal). Endoluminal techniques may be employed as first-line or salvage procedures for symptomatic patients. Endoluminal measures carry the benefit of decreased complication rates, decreased morbidity, and quicker recovery times.

Pregnancy rates are similar (around 35%) for the partners of patients treated with surgical varicocele repair or embolization.

• **Pyocele/hematocele**. Pyoceles and hematoceles are abnormal collections of pus or blood in the scrotum, respectively. Both present on ultrasound as complex cystic lesions with internal septations and loculations without the blood flow and flow alterations seen with a varicocele. Hematoceles are usually secondary to trauma, surgery, or neoplasm. Pyoceles result from untreated epididymo-orchitis or rupture of an intratesticular abscess. Treatment is centered on the underlying cause.

• **Hydrocele**. A small amount of serous fluid collecting between the layers of the tunica vaginalis may be normal in an asymptomatic patient. Larger or symptomatic collections are abnormal. On ultrasound, these fluid collections are mostly anechoic with good through transmission. Abnormally large collections of fluid may be congenital (patent processus vaginalis), idiopathic, or the result of trauma, infection, torsion, or tumor; therefore, the presence of a hydrocele should prompt a search for underlying pathology.

■ Diagnosis

Varicocele

✓ Pearls

• Varicoceles result from reflux of the ipsilateral gonadal vein; they enlarge or worsen with Valsalva.
• An isolated right varicocele should prompt a search for a retroperitoneal mass.

• Pyoceles and hematoceles result in complex extratesticular fluid collections within the scrotum.
• Although often incidental, the presence of a hydrocele should prompt a search for underlying pathology.

Suggested Readings

Dogra VS, Gottlieb RH, Oka M, Rubens DJ. Sonography of the scrotum. Radiology. 2003; 227(1):18–36

Shlansky-Goldberg RD, VanArsdalen KN, Rutter CM, et al. Percutaneous varicocele embolization versus surgical ligation for the treatment of infertility: changes in seminal parameters and pregnancy outcomes. J Vasc Interv Radiol. 1997; 8(5):759–767

Sze DY, Kao JS, Frisoli JK, McCallum SW, Kennedy WA, II, Razavi MK. Persistent and recurrent postsurgical varicoceles: venographic anatomy and treatment with N-butyl cyanoacrylate embolization. J Vasc Interv Radiol. 2008; 19(4):539–545

Case 243

Wayne L. Monsky

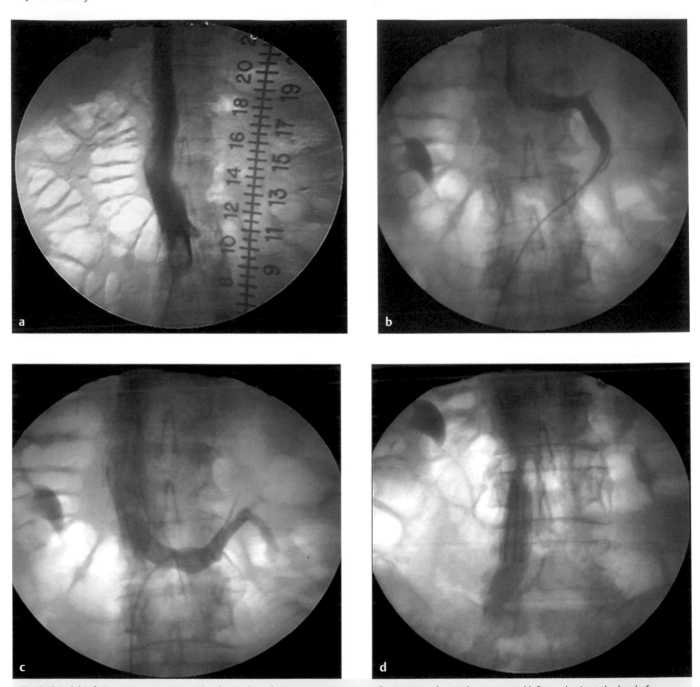

Fig. 243.1 **(a)** Inferior vena cava-gram with ruler in place demonstrates contrast refluxing into a lower than expected left renal vein at the level of the third lumbar vertebra (11-cm mark), as well as mixing/inflow at the level of the expected left and right renal veins (14–15-cm marks). Venogram with selected catheterization of **(b)** the left inferior and **(c)** superior renal veins confirms two separate regions of venous drainage on the left. **(d)** Postprocedure venogram demonstrates an IVC filter placed below the level where the most inferior portion of the left renal vein enters the IVC.

■ **Clinical Presentation**

Patient with lower extremity deep venous thrombosis and recent trauma (anticoagulation is contraindicated) (▶Fig. 243.1).

■ Key Imaging Finding

Inferior vena cava (IVC) vascular anomaly/abnormality

■ Top 3 Differential Diagnoses

- **Circumaortic/retroaortic left renal vein.** A circumaortic left renal vein occurs when both the left renal vein and the infrarenal segment of the left supracardinal vein persist, while a retroaortic renal vein occurs when only the left supracardinal vein persists. The circumaortic left renal vein is seen in 1.5 to 8.7% of the population, while retroaortic left renal veins are reported in 1.8 to 2.4%. In the circumaortic variant, vena cava-gram demonstrates the renal vein passing anterior to the aorta with a normal course, while the persistent left supracardinal vein courses posterior to the aorta and enters the IVC more inferiorly (typically L2 or L3 level). In the retroaortic variant, the left renal vein (persistent left supracardinal vein) also enters the IVC at a lower than expected level. Review of any prior cross-sectional imaging is useful. It is helpful to position the catheter tip within the left renal vein to best demonstrate these anatomic variants. These anomalies require filter placement inferior to the lower left renal vein IVC insertion. If placed above the insertion of these variant left renal veins, they serve as a collateral pathway for emboli to circumvent the filter, resulting in pulmonary embolism.

- **Megacava.** Megacava is defined when the IVC measures 28 mm or greater. The incidence may be as high as 3%. Placement of a Bird's nest filter within the infrarenal IVC or the placement of a filter within each common iliac vein would be required. A Bird's nest filter has been placed in a 42 mm IVC.

- **Duplicated inferior vena cava.** A duplicated IVC occurs when the embryonic right and left supracardinal veins persist. This is seen in 0.2 to 3% of the population. The right IVC is usually larger. The left common iliac vein drains into the left IVC, which in turn typically drains into the left renal vein. A catheter cannot be positioned within the left common iliac vein from a right femoral approach, since there is no direct communication between the IVCs. However, the catheter can be advanced into left common iliac vein from the left renal vein to demonstrate a duplicated IVC. When present, IVC filters must be placed in both IVCs. Alternatively, but less commonly, a single suprarenal filter can be placed. Placement of only a single infrarenal filter in the "normal" right IVC will not prevent contralateral pelvic and lower extremity emboli from reaching the lungs.

■ Additional Differential Diagnoses

- **Inferior vena cava thrombosis.** Free-floating iliofemoral or IVC thrombus has been associated with a significant rate of pulmonary embolism, and is considered an indication for IVC filter placement. In patients with nonocclusive IVC thrombus, the filter must be placed superior/cranial to the thrombus within the IVC. A suprarenal IVC filter may be placed if there is IVC thrombosis extending above the level of the renal veins, thrombus in the infrarenal IVC that does not leave enough room for the filter between the thrombus and renal veins, or in the setting of renal vein thrombosis.

■ Diagnosis

Circumaortic left renal vein

✓ Pearls

- Prior to filter placement, look for caval anomalies, thrombus, size of the IVC, and location of renal veins.
- With circumaortic or retroaortic left renal veins, a filter must be placed below the most inferior renal vein.

- Megacava is defined as 28 mm or greater; either a Bird's nest or bilateral iliac vein filters must be placed.
- With a duplicated IVC, a filter must either be placed in each IVC or a suprarenal filter must be placed.

Suggested Readings

Mejia EA, Saroyan RM, Balkin PW, Kerstein MD. Analysis of inferior venacavography before Greenfield filter placement. Ann Vasc Surg. 1989; 3(3):232–235

Case 244

Charlyne Wu

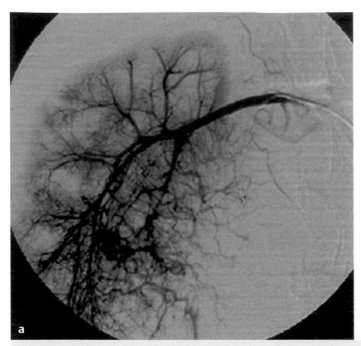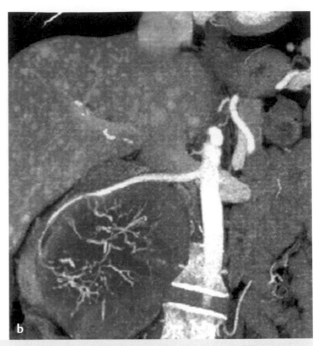

Fig. 244.1 **(a)** Digital subtraction angiography (DSA) of the right kidney demonstrates a hypervascular mass with tumor neovascularity particularly at the mid to lower pole. **(b)** Enhanced cortical phase, coronally reconstructed MIP CT image demonstrates a large right renal mass with central necrosis and neovascularity as reflected in image (a), along with multiple hypervascular hepatic metastatic lesions.

■ Clinical Presentation

A 50-year-old woman with hematuria (▶Fig. 244.1).

■ Key Imaging Finding

Hypervascular renal mass

■ Top 3 Differential Diagnoses

- **Renal cell carcinoma (RCC).** In adults, RCC comprises over 80% of all malignant renal masses. It is more common in older men and may be multiple when associated with von Hippel–Lindau disease. Angiographically, RCC most often has prominent neovascularity (94%) and shunting with or without venous invasion. On CT, RCC presents as a hypervascular mass. When large, they may become centrally necrotic. The central hypodensity in these instances should not be confused with fat, as is seen in benign angiomyolipomas (AMLs). The typical indication for angiographic intervention is usually 24-hour preoperative embolization of the tumor or kidney to decrease intraoperative hemorrhage. Devascularization with smaller particles for peripheral embolization is preferred, provided no arteriovenous shunts are present. Otherwise, alcohol ablation with balloon occlusion catheter or coils may be used. Smaller RCC can be treated with nephron-sparing surgery or RF (radiofrequency)/cryoablation. RCC commonly produces hypervascular hepatic metastases and lytic bone lesions.
- **Angiomyolipoma (AML).** AMLs are benign hamartomatous lesions that contain fat, smooth muscle, and blood vessels. The typical patient is female between 30 and 60 years old. Multiple bilateral lesions are found in up to 80% of patients with tuberous sclerosis. Large lesions (>4 cm) are prone to acute spontaneous hemorrhage. On CT, a fat-containing mass originating from the kidney is virtually pathognomonic. Angiography demonstrates neovascularity and bizarre aneurysms without vascular shunting. Embolization with permanent particles or alcohol is an excellent alternative to resection.
- **Oncocytoma.** Oncocytomas are solid benign renal neoplasms composed of oncocytes. They are usually asymptomatic, but may present with hematuria, flank pain, and/or an abdominal mass, mimicking RCC. The lesions are typically large (>5 cm) at presentation and have a pseudocapsule. On CT, the lesions are hypervascular, and up to one-third will have a central stellate scar. The classic angiographic finding is a "spoke wheel" arrangement of tumor vascularity. Although the diagnosis may be suggested by imaging findings, there is significant overlap with the findings of RCC.

■ Additional Differential Diagnoses

- **Arteriovenous malformation/fistula (AVM/AVF).** AVMs are congenital and rare in the absence of Osler–Weber–Rendu syndrome. AVFs are almost always acquired from trauma or iatrogenic causes. Angiography demonstrates enlarged feeding arteries and early draining veins. Symptoms include hematuria, hypertension, flank pain, or, less commonly, spontaneous retroperitoneal hemorrhage. Treatment options include percutaneous embolization with coils, glue, or alcohol.

■ Diagnosis

Renal cell carcinoma

✓ Pearls

- RCC is the most common renal tumor in adults; it is hypervascular with neovascularity and shunting.
- Large AMLs (>4 cm) are prone to hemorrhage secondary to neovascularity and bizarre aneurysms.
- Oncocytomas are solid benign renal neoplasms with a central scar and "spoke wheel" pattern of vascularity.
- AVMs are rare congenital lesions; AVFs occur secondary to trauma, including iatrogenic causes.

Suggested Readings

Davidson AJ, Hartman DS, Choyke PL, et al. Radiological assessment of renal masses: complications for patient care. Radiology. 2002; 297:1997

Federle MP, Jeffrey RB, Desser TS, et al. Diagnostic Imaging: Abdomen. Salt Lake City, UT: Amirsys; 2004

Israel GM, Bosniak MA. How I do it: evaluating renal masses. Radiology. 2005; 236(2):441–450

Kaufman JA, Lee MJ. Vascular & Interventional Radiology: The Requisites. Philadelphia, PA: Elsevier; 2004:6–11, 337–346

Case 245

Matthew J. Moore

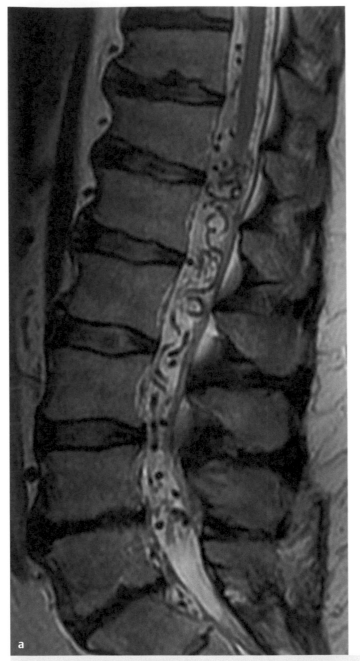 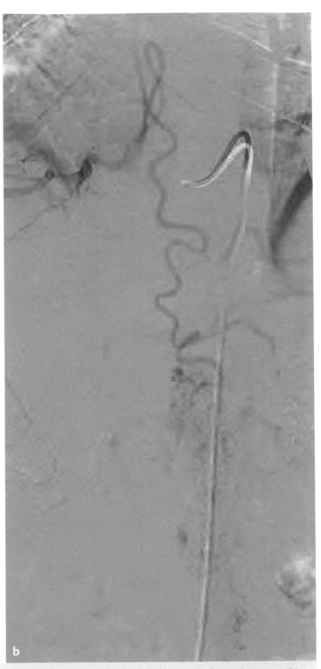

Fig. 245.1 **(a)** Sagittal T2-weighted MR image demonstrates multiple serpentine extramedullary, intradural vascular flow voids in the lumbar spine. **(b)** Subsequent spinal digital subtraction angiogram image during the arterial phase of a right T10 intercostal artery injection reveals an enlarged anterior spinal artery with early filling of a plexus of intradural veins from arteriovenous shunting.

■ Clinical Presentation

A 55-year-old man with progressive lower extremity weakness (▶ Fig. 245.1).

■ Key Imaging Finding

Prominent paraspinal flow voids

■ Top 3 Differential Diagnoses

- **Dural arteriovenous fistula (AVF).** There are four types of spinal arteriovenous shunt lesions. The most common (80%) is the Type I dural AVF, which is a direct arteriovenous connection (no intervening nidus) within the spinal dura mater itself. The lesion drains into distended and enlarged pial veins, which are seen as extramedullary, intradural serpentine flow voids on sagittal T2-weighted MRI or multiple enhancing serpentine vessels on sagittal T1 contrast-enhanced MRI. There may also be "flame-shaped" cord edema with sparing of the periphery, best seen on T2-weighted MRI. The lesions cause intramedullary venous hypertension leading to chronic ischemia, which results in clinical symptoms. These lesions typically present in the fifth or sixth decade, more commonly in men, with progressive lower extremity weakness, which is exacerbated by exercise. Spinal angiogram is the gold standard for accurate diagnosis and localization. Endovascular coiling is the treatment of choice. The Type IV AVF or "perimedullary

fistula" is the other true AVF, which may be indistinguishable from the Type I dural AVF on MRI.
- **Spinal cord arteriovenous malformation (AVM).** The other two types of spinal arteriovenous shunting include the true AVMs with an intervening nidus. These Type II and III AVMs will also present with vascular flow voids; however, you will see intramedullary in addition to extramedullary flow voids. The spinal Type II AVM is similar to a brain AVM. They commonly present with acute onset of symptoms due to subarachnoid hemorrhage. Type III, or juvenile AVMs, are rare lesions which occur in the first through third decades. The AVM has both intramedullary and extramedullary components.
- **Collateral venous flow from inferior vena cava (IVC) occlusion.** IVC occlusion may cause prominent collateral epidural or intradural veins. Look for a small or ill-defined IVC, or metal artifact in the IVC region due to filter. Common etiologies of IVC occlusion include trauma, extrinsic compression, tumor invasion, and hypercoagulable states.

■ Additional Differential Diagnoses

- **Spinal cord neoplasm with increased vascular flow.** Spinal flow voids can be seen with several spinal cord neoplasms. Hemangioblastoma is classically an expansile intramedullary mass with serpentine flow voids, often associated with a syrinx or cystic component and an enhancing mural nodule. Ependymomas, paragangliomas, and schwannomas can also be seen with flow voids related to increased vascular flow.
- **Cerebrospinal fluid (CSF) pulsations.** Normal CSF pulsations are seen dorsal to the cord on T2-weighted MR sequences. They have ill-defined margins, which easily differentiate them from the well-defined vascular flow voids seen with spinal arteriovenous shunt lesions. The lack of corresponding abnormality on non–T2-weighted sequences allow for identification of this common artifact.

■ Diagnosis

Dural arteriovenous fistula (Type I)

✓ Pearls

- Type I dural AVFs result in vascular shunting with chronic cord ischemia and progressive weakness.
- Spinal cord AVMs are similar to brain AVMs with a vascular nidus and arteriovenous shunting.
- Collateral epidural and intradural veins may be seen with IVC occlusion, simulating an AVF or AVM.
- Hemangioblastomas, ependymomas, and neurogenic tumors may have prominent paraspinal flow voids.

Suggested Readings

Rodesch G, Lasjaunias P. Spinal cord arteriovenous shunts: from imaging to management. Eur J Radiol. 2003; 46(3):221–232

Case 246

Matthew J. Moore

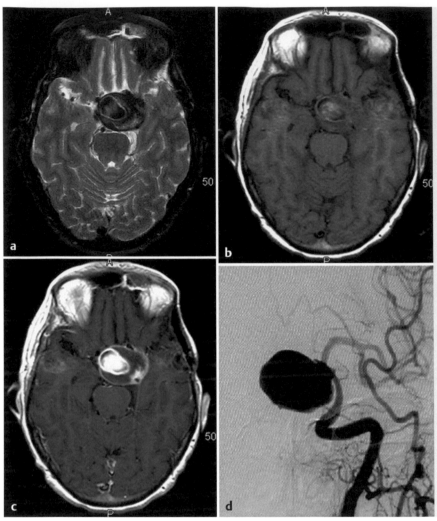

Fig. 246.1 (a) Axial T2-weighted image demonstrates a large predominantly hypointense suprasellar mass eccentric to the left with regions of increased signal internally. (b) Axial T1 precontrast image reveals a predominantly iso- to hypointense suprasellar mass with a circumscribed region of increased T1 signal medially. (c) Axial T1 postcontrast image demonstrates intense enhancement along the medial aspect of the suprasellar mass, as well as peripheral enhancement. Both T1 images (b, c) show pulsation artifact in association with the mass. (d) Frontal projection from a left carotid angiogram reveals a large (giant) aneurysm involving the cavernous segment of the left internal carotid artery. (The images are provided courtesy of Thomas Tomsick, MD, University of Cincinnati.)

■ Clinical Presentation

A 57-year-old woman presents with headache and blurred vision (▶Fig. 246.1).

■ Key Imaging Finding

Suprasellar mass in an adult

■ Top 3 Differential Diagnoses

- **Pituitary macroadenoma.** Upward extension of a pituitary macroadenoma (>10 mm) from the sella is the most common cause of a suprasellar mass in adults. The best diagnostic clue is a sellar mass without separate identifiable pituitary gland. The classic appearance is a "snowman" configuration due to impression on the mass by the diaphragma sella. The tumor is most commonly isodense to gray matter on CT and isointense to gray matter on T1- and T2-weighted MRI. Density or signal may be heterogeneous due to hemorrhage (10%), calcification (1–2%), or cystic change. Almost all macroadenomas enhance, usually heterogeneously. Look for internal carotid artery displacement. With cavernous sinus invasion, there can be carotid artery encasement (>two-thirds typically considered a sign of invasion). Malignant transformation is exceedingly rare, but macroadenomas can appear aggressive with skull base invasion. Peak age of onset is 20 to 40 years of age.

Visual field defects or cranial nerve palsy may occur due to local mass effect. Treatment of choice is resection.
- **Craniopharyngioma.** Craniopharyngiomas are more common in children than adults. The classic pediatric case will present as a suprasellar mass with calcification and cystic change with rim or nodular enhancement. In adults older than 50 years, craniopharyngiomas are of the papillary subtype and present as a solid suprasellar mass without calcification.
- **Aneurysm.** Aneurysm of the parasellar internal carotid artery should always be considered when a suprasellar mass is identified. Aneurysms tend to be eccentric and not directly suprasellar in location. Look for a flow void and pulsation artifact on MRI. Calcification is more common than with pituitary adenomas. The pituitary gland will be seen separate from an aneurysm. CTA, MRA, or DSA can be used to characterize the aneurysm.

■ Additional Differential Diagnoses

- **Meningioma.** Meningiomas arising from the diaphragma sellae can appear similar to a pituitary neoplasm; however, the pituitary gland will be identified separate from the mass. Look for the low MR signal line of the diaphragma sella between the mass (above) and the pituitary gland (below). Dural thickening due to meningioma is more extensive than with a pituitary macroadenoma. Meningiomas more commonly cause internal carotid artery narrowing with encasement than is seen with pituitary macroadenomas. Classically, there is avid, homogenous enhancement with a dural tail. Calcification and adjacent hyperostosis may be seen. They are usually hyperdense on CT with or without calcification.

■ Diagnosis

Aneurysm

✓ Pearls

- Macroadenomas are the most common suprasellar masses in adults; a "snowman" configuration is classic.
- Craniopharyngiomas are solid in adults without calcification; in children, they are commonly cystic and calcified.

- Aneurysms must be considered with a suprasellar mass; look for flow voids and pulsation artifact.
- Meningiomas are commonly hyperdense and avidly enhance; calcification and hyperostosis may be seen.

Suggested Readings

Johnsen DE, Woodruff WW, Allen IS, Cera PJ, Funkhouser GR, Coleman LL. MR imaging of the sellar and juxtasellar regions. Radiographics. 1991; 11(5):727–758

Case 247

Matthew J. Moore

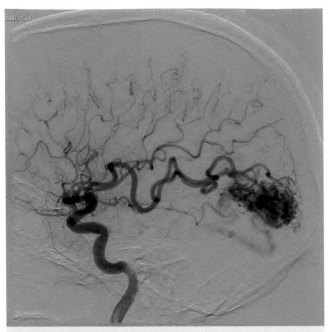

Fig. 247.1 Digital subtraction angiogram of an internal carotid artery injection during late arterial phase demonstrates a large hypervascular mass in the occipital region supplied by enlarged arterial feeders. Notice the early venous opacification just below the mass due to arteriovenous shunting within the lesion.

■ Clinical Presentation

A 40-year-old man with headache for 2 months (▶Fig. 247.1).

■ Key Imaging Finding

Hypervascular cerebral mass/abnormality

■ Top 3 Differential Diagnoses

- **Arteriovenous malformation (AVM)**. AVM is a form of arteriovenous shunting with no intervening capillary network. The peak age of presentation is 20 to 40 years of age. The vast majority become symptomatic during the patient's lifetime with hemorrhage, seizures, and headaches representing the most common presentations. The vast majority are supratentorial and solitary. The best diagnostic clue is a cluster or tangle of flow voids on MRI with minimal or no mass effect. There is little or no intervening brain tissue. FLAIR imaging may show high signal due to gliosis. AVMs demonstrate avid enhancement. Complete characterization is obtained with digital subtraction angiogram, which will define the arterial supply, size of the nidus, and location of venous drainage. The Spetzler–Martin classification determines the operative risk and is based on the AVM's size, location, and venous drainage pattern. Treatment options include transarterial embolization, stereotaxic radiosurgery, and/or microvascular surgery.
- **Hypervascular tumor**. A hypervascular tumor, such as a **glioblastoma multiforme** (GBM) or a **meningioma**, will demonstrate avid enhancement. However, unlike an AVM, a hypervascular tumor will tend to have edema and mass effect. GBM can have MRI flow voids from neovascularity, but will tend to show some brain parenchyma between the flow voids. DSA of a hypervascular tumor will show a prominent tumor blush. GBM may rarely mimic an AVM with early draining veins on DSA due to intralesional shunting. Meningioma on DSA will show a "sunburst" or radial appearance with a prolonged vascular stain. This is termed the "mother-in-law" sign, meaning the enhancement "comes early and stays late."
- **Aneurysm**. A patent intracranial aneurysm can be seen as a well-delineated round, extra-axial mass slightly hyperdense to brain, particularly if partially thrombosed or calcified. Aneurysms show strong enhancement when patent. On MRI, 50% have a flow void and 50% have heterogeneous signal. CTA, MRA, and DSA can be used to identify an aneurysm. A total of 90 to 95% arise from the circle of Willis. The classic clinical profile is a middle age patient with the "worst headache of my life" related to aneurysm rupture with subarachnoid hemorrhage. Cranial neuropathy (especially CN III) and seizure are less common presentations. Treatment options include endovascular coiling or craniotomy with aneurysm clipping.

■ Additional Differential Diagnoses

- **Moyamoya**. Moyamoya refers to an idiopathic, progressive narrowing of the distal internal carotid artery and proximal circle of Willis with secondary formation of multiple collaterals. The moyamoya or "puff of smoke" appearance of cloud-like lenticulostriate and thalamostriate collaterals is seen on MR and angiography. There is a bimodal age distribution with peaks in the first and fourth decades of life.

■ Diagnosis

Arteriovenous malformation

✓ Pearls

- AVMs have an arterial supply, a nidus of vessels, and enlarged draining veins without a capillary network.
- AVMs present with headache or hemorrhage; they are classified by size, location, and venous drainage.

- GBMs and meningiomas may have flow voids from neovascularity, as well as arteriovenous shunting with GBM.
- Moyamoya refers to collateral vessel formation secondary to internal carotid artery occlusion.

Suggested Readings

Geibprasert S, Pongpech S, Jiarakongmun P, Shroff MM, Armstrong DC, Krings T. Radiologic assessment of brain arteriovenous malformations: what clinicians need to know. Radiographics. 2010; 30(2):483–501

Yoon HK, Shin HJ, Chang YW. "Ivy sign" in childhood moyamoya disease: depiction on FLAIR and contrast-enhanced T1-weighted MR images. Radiology. 2002; 223(2):384–389

Case 248

Wayne L. Monsky

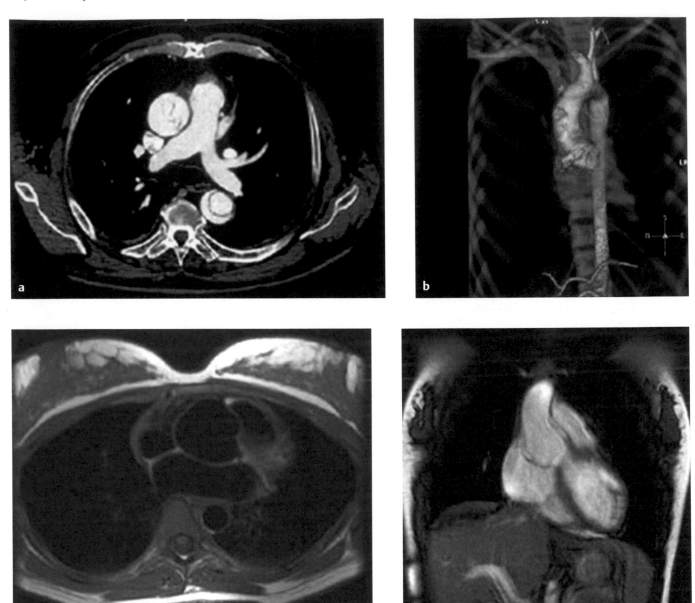

Fig. 248.1 (a) Contrast enhanced axial image through the chest in soft-tissue window demonstrates an intimal flap within both the ascending and descending aorta. (b) Frontal surface rendered CTA image demonstrates enlargement of the aortic root/annulus and proximal ascending aorta. The thorax is elongated and narrowed. (c) Axial T1W spin echo and (d) coronal SPGR show dilation of the aortic annulus and root, measuring up to 47 mm. Slight aortic insufficiency may be seen.

■ Clinical Presentation

Pregnant patient with mild chest pain and early midsystolic blowing, decrescendo, flow murmur auscultated over the right upper sternal border (►Fig. 248.1).

■ Key Imaging Finding

Aortic dissection

■ Top 3 Differential Diagnoses

- **Hypertension**. Hypertension is the most common cause of aortic dissection and typically occurs in men between 50 and 70 years of age. Poorly controlled hypertension results in intimal tearing which may progress to dissection. Patients present acutely with chest pain which radiates to the back. Involvement of the ascending aorta (Stanford A) requires surgical or endovascular intervention; dissections involving only the descending aorta (Stanford B) are treated medically in the absence of end organ ischemia.
- **Trauma**. Thoracic aortic injury from blunt chest trauma typically occurs at the aortic isthmus, just distal to the left subclavian artery, and at the level of the diaphragm. Aortic root injuries are usually fatal. Imaging findings include a widened mediastinum, blurring of the aortic shadow, left apical cap, right tracheal deviation, wide paraspinal lines and right paratracheal stripe, blood in the mediastinum, deformed aortic contour, intimal flaps and debris, and pseudoaneurysm. Frank extravasation is rare.
- **Connective tissue disease**. Connective tissue diseases, such as Ehlers–Danlos, affect the aortic media. Ehlers–Danlos may feature arterial, intestinal, and uterine fragility. Vascular rupture or dissections are common presenting signs in the majority of cases. Arterial rupture may be preceded by aneurysm, arteriovenous fistulae, or dissection, which may be seen with MR, CT, or conventional angiography.

■ Additional Differential Diagnoses

- **Annuloaortic ectasia (cystic medial necrosis)**. Degeneration of the connective tissue of the aortic media results in cystic medial necrosis, leading to dilatation of the ascending aorta and aortic annulus with aortic insufficiency, as seen in Marfan syndrome. Congestive heart failure and aortic dissection are frequent complications. Dissection usually involves the entire length of the aorta, DeBakey type I/Stanford type A. Imaging findings of Marfan include: an elongated narrow thorax; cardiomegaly; enlargement of the sinus of Valsalva, aortic root (>35 mm) and the proximal ascending aorta; and aortic or mitral regurgitation.
- **Bicuspid aortic valve**. Bicuspid aortic valve is a common congenital anomaly which is more common in men. Abnormal valve leaflet morphology results in early degeneration, leading first to stenosis followed in some instances by valve incompetence. Patients with a bicuspid aortic valve are at higher risk of aortic aneurysms and dissection. MR, CT, and conventional angiography can demonstrate the bicuspid valve.
- **Coarctation of the aorta**. Aortic coarctation is a congenital anomaly which results in eccentric narrowing and infolding of the aorta adjacent to the left subclavian artery and stenosis to left ventricular outflow. It may be associated with a bicuspid aortic valve, aortic aneurysms, dissection, and congenital heart disease. Imaging findings include inferior rib notching due to enlarged intercostal arteries providing collateral blood flow. A "figure 3" aortic appearance results from stenosis and dilatation of the aorta.

■ Diagnosis

Annuloaortic ectasia (Marfan syndrome)

✓ Pearls

- Hypertension and trauma are the most common causes of aortic dissection.
- Stanford A (ascending aorta involved) lesions are managed surgically; Stanford B are managed medically.
- Annuloaortic ectasia, bicuspid aortic valve, and aortic coarctation have increased risk of aortic dissection.

Suggested Readings

Kuhlman JE, Pozniak MA, Collins J, Knisely BL. Radiographic and CT findings of blunt chest trauma: aortic injuries and looking beyond them. Radiographics. 1998; 18(5):1085–1106, discussion 1107–1108, quiz 1

Tatli S, Yucel EK, Lipton MJCT. CT and MR imaging of the thoracic aorta: current techniques and clinical applications. Radiol Clin North Am. 2004; 42(3):565–585, vi

Case 249

Charlyne Wu

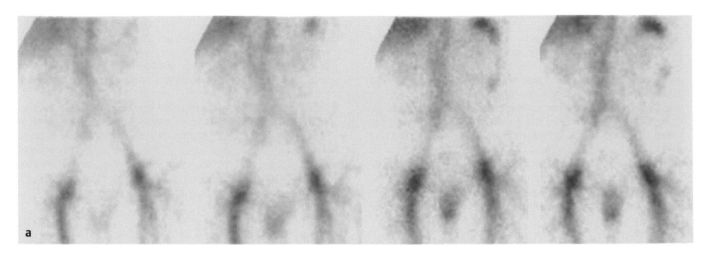

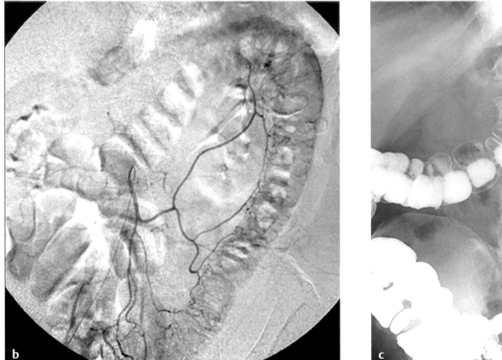
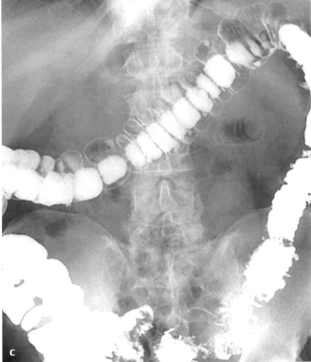

Fig. 249.1 (a) Sequential images from a Tc99m-labeled RBC scan demonstrate extravasated activity within the left upper quadrant. Continued imaging demonstrates transit of intraluminal activity in a pattern consistent with active bleeding from the splenic flexure. (b) Digital subtraction angiography of the inferior mesenteric artery reveals extravasation of contrast at the splenic flexure. (c) Postevacuation barium enema shows en face diverticula with pooling barium (ring shadow) at the splenic flexure and additional diverticula pointing away from the bowel wall ("bowler hat" sign) at the sigmoid colon.

■ Clinical Presentation

A 57-year-old man with intermittent lower gastrointestinal (GI) bleeding over several years now presents with bright red blood per rectum and light headedness (▶Fig. 249.1).

■ Key Imaging Finding

Lower gastrointestinal bleeding (LGIB)

■ Top 3 Differential Diagnoses

- **Diverticulosis**. The most common cause of symptomatic LGIB is diverticulosis (30–50%), which usually presents with hematochezia. Most diverticula are in the left colon; however, most bleeding diverticula are in the right colon. Both scintigraphy (Tc99m RBC and Tc99m sulfur colloid) and angiography demonstrate extravasation of activity or contrast, respectively. On barium enema, a diverticulum may mimic a polyp. En face there is a round barium collection appearing as a ring shadow. The "bowler hat" sign refers to the dome of the hat pointing away from the bowel wall, as opposed to toward the lumen as would be expected in a polyp. Since scintigraphy is more sensitive than angiography at identifying GI bleed (0.1 vs. 1.0 mL/min), it is the initial diagnostic procedure of choice for hemodynamically stable patients. For hemodynamically unstable patients, angiography is best for diagnosis and possibly treatment. Treatment first involves fluid resuscitation and correction of any underlying coagulopathies. Most patients will stop bleeding after conservative management. Colonoscopy and angiography are therapeutic options for hemodynamically stable patients who fail conservative management. For hemodynamically unstable patients, embolization (typically gel foam, coils, or vasopressin infusion) or surgery is considered.

- **Neoplasm**. Both neoplasm, specifically colon carcinoma, and postpolypectomy bleeding account for approximately 20% of cases of LGIB. Once the patient is stabilized and the bleeding has been treated, proper colorectal cancer screening should be verified or performed.

- **Angiodysplasia**. Colonic angiodysplasias are reported to be responsible for approximately 5 to 10% of cases of acute LGIB. These are arteriovenous malformations of mucosa and submucosa, the majority at the cecum and ascending colon, as well as in the small bowel. An association with various systemic diseases has been described; these diseases include aortic stenosis, von Willebrand disease, chronic obstructive pulmonary disease, cirrhosis, chronic renal disease, and collagen vascular disease. On angiography, there is a cluster or tangle of small arteries in the arterial phase with early filling and delayed emptying of dilated veins.

■ Additional Differential Diagnoses

- **Focal colitis**. Focal colitis, typically from inflammatory, infectious, ischemic, or radiation insult, accounts for approximately 20% of cases of LGIB. Treatment is often medical and directed at the underlying cause of the bleeding. If severe, endoscopic, endovascular, or surgical treatment may be necessary.

■ Diagnosis

Diverticulosis

✓ Pearls

- LGIBs are first evaluated by scintigraphy, followed by angiography if positive for active bleed.
- Diverticulosis is the most common cause of LGIB; most bleeding diverticula are on the right.
- Colon carcinoma may present with a LGIB or bleeding may occur due to polypectomy.
- Angiodysplasia involves the right colon and demonstrates early filling of dilated veins during arterial phase.

Suggested Readings

Federle MP, Jeffrey RB, Desser TS, et al. Diagnostic Imaging: Abdomen. Salt Lake City, UT: Amirsys; 2004

Bunker SR, Lull RJ, Tanasescu DE, et al. Scintigraphy of gastrointestinal hemorrhage: superiority of 99mTc red blood cells over 99mTc sulfur colloid. AJR Am J Roentgenol. 1984; 143(3):543–548

Tew K, Davies RP, Jadun CK, Kew J. MDCT of acute lower gastrointestinal bleeding. AJR Am J Roentgenol. 2004; 182(2):427–430

Zuckerman GR, Prakash C. Acute lower intestinal bleeding. Part II: etiology, therapy, and outcomes. Gastrointest Endosc. 1999; 49(2):228–238

Case 250

Wayne L. Monsky

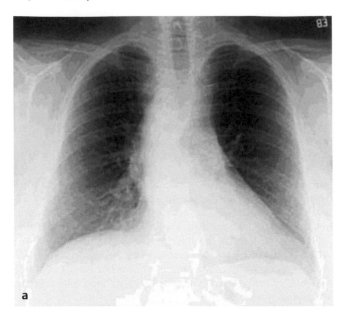

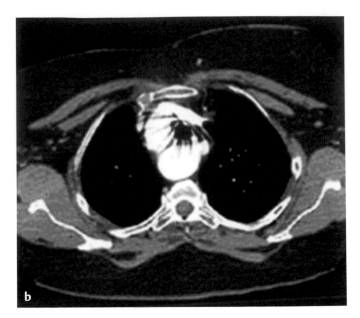

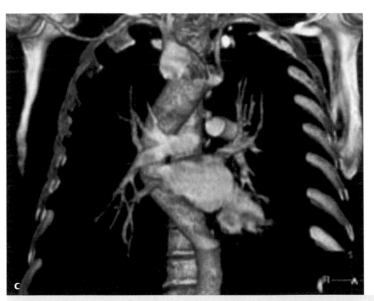

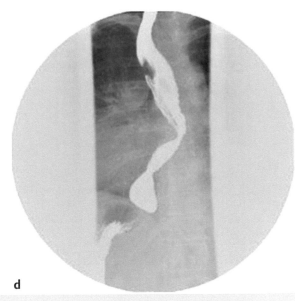

Fig. 250.1 (a) Frontal chest radiograph reveals a right-sided aortic arch with an ectatic tortuous thoracic aorta. (b) Axial enhanced CT image demonstrates the right-sided aortic arch, as well as depicts the origin of the left subclavian artery from a retroesophageal diverticulum (diverticulum of Kommerell). (c) Frontal 3D surface rendered CTA image demonstrates a right-sided aortic arch and the left subclavian artery originating as the last branch of the aortic arch (distal to the right subclavian artery) and arising from the protuberant diverticulum of Kommerell. (d) Frontal esophagram demonstrates the esophagus to be tortuous with distortion and effacement produced by the patient's right- sided aortic arch.

■ Clinical Presentation

Adult patient with worsening dysphasia (▶Fig. 250.1).

■ Key Imaging Finding

Vascular ring/sling

■ Top 3 Differential Diagnoses

- **Aberrant right subclavian artery.** A left aortic arch with aberrant right subclavian artery occurs with a frequency of 0.4 to 2%. It results from involution of embryonic aortic segment between the right subclavian and common carotid arteries. The right subclavian becomes the last aortic branch, reaching the right thorax by passing behind the trachea and esophagus in 85% and between them in 15%. The majority of cases are asymptomatic, although dysphagia (dysphagia lusoria) may occur.

- **Double aortic arch.** A double aortic arch accounts for 40% of all thoracic vascular rings. It is caused by persistence of the right and left fourth branchial arches and is rarely associated with congenital heart disease. The aortic arches pass on both sides of trachea, joining posteriorly behind the esophagus and anteriorly in front of the trachea. The vascular ring produces tracheal and/or esophageal compression with possible airway compromise and dysphagia. Imaging findings include a right arch which is higher and larger than the left. Esophagram shows reverse S pattern, with bilateral esophageal impressions on a frontal views and posterior impression on lateral views. Angiography demonstrates a right arch supplying the right subclavian and right common carotid and the left arch supplying the left common carotid and subclavian arteries.

- **Right arch with aberrant left subclavian artery.** The most frequent branching pattern for a vascular ring with a right aortic arch is an aberrant left subclavian artery originating as the last branch of the aortic arch from a retroesophageal diverticulum of Kommerell. This occurs in 0.05 to 0.1% of the population. The ring is completed by a left-sided ligamentum arteriosum. A right aortic arch occurs when the right dorsal aorta remains patent and the left dorsal aorta regresses abnormally. Vascular rings encircle the trachea and/or esophagus and may cause esophageal compression and dysphagia. Cardiac defects, such as tetralogy of Fallot, occur in 5 to 10%. Radiographic findings include the presence of a right aortic knob, slight leftward deviation of the lower trachea, and posterior indentation of the trachea. Esophagram may show a right-sided indentation of the esophagus and posterior indentation of the esophagus. Cross-sectional imaging and angiography demonstrate the right arch and aberrant left subclavian artery arising from the protuberant diverticulum of Kommerell, which should not be mistaken for a pseudoaneurysm.

■ Additional Differential Diagnoses

- **Pulmonary sling.** Five percent of thoracic vascular rings are due to a pulmonary artery sling. The left pulmonary artery arises from the posterior aspect of the right pulmonary artery and passes between the trachea and esophagus to reach the left hilum. The left pulmonary artery thus forms a sling around the distal trachea and the proximal right main bronchus. There may be associated malformations of the bronchotracheal tree, as well as cardiovascular abnormalities. This may mimic a mediastinal mass on chest radiographs. Computed tomography (CT) or magnetic resonance imaging (MRI) may establish the diagnosis.

■ Diagnosis

Right aortic arch with aberrant left subclavian artery

✓ Pearls

- The majority of aberrant right subclavian arteries pass posterior to the esophagus and are asymptomatic.
- A double aortic arch joins posteriorly behind the esophagus and anteriorly in front of the trachea.

- Right arch with aberrant left subclavian artery is a complete ring, causing tracheal/esophageal compression.
- Pulmonary sling (left pulmonary artery arising from the right) passes between the trachea and esophagus.

Suggested Readings

Castañer E, Gallardo X, Rimola J, et al. Congenital and acquired pulmonary artery anomalies in the adult: radiologic overview. Radiographics. 2006; 26(2):349–371

Case 251

David D. Gover

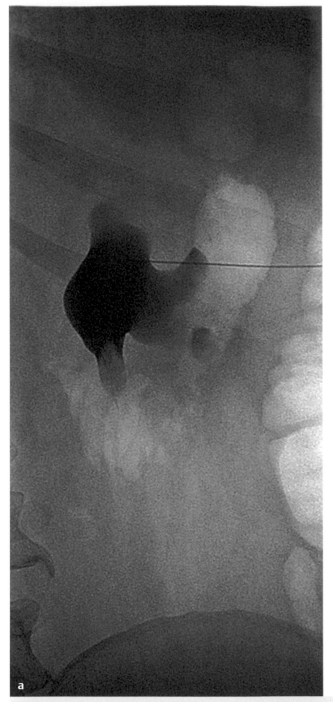 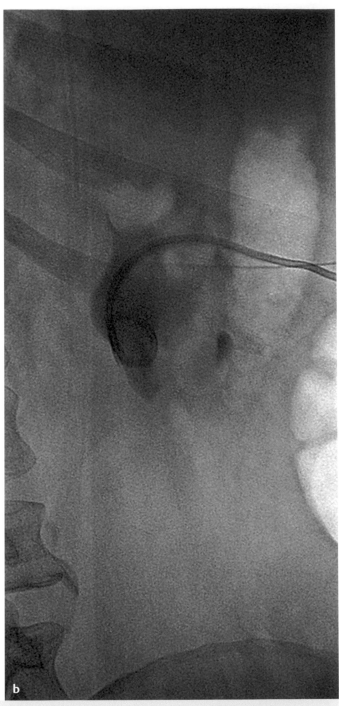

Fig. 251.1 (a) Percutaneous nephrogram demonstrates a large mass obstructing the proximal ureter with contrast within a dilated renal pelvis, consistent with obstruction. **(b)** Post-procedure image reveals placement of a percutaneous nephrostomy tube above the level of obstruction with decompression of the renal pelvis.

■ Clinical Presentation

A 48-year-old man with flank pain and fever (▶Fig. 251.1).

■ Key Imaging Finding

Urinary obstruction

■ Top 3 Differential Diagnoses

- **Nephrolithiasis**. Nephrolithiasis is the most common cause of urinary tract obstruction. Obstruction most often occurs at the ureterovesicular junction (UVJ) or ureteropelvic junction (UPJ). Computed tomography (CT) is useful in identifying the vast majority of stones, which are typically radiopaque. As a general rule, obstructing stones 4 mm or less in size should pass, while stones 8 mm or greater are unlikely to pass. Stones between 4 and 8 mm may or may not pass without intervention. Percutaneous nephrostomy is used to alleviate obstruction in an infected system, which is a medical emergency, or is used in conjunction with treatment of larger stones. This procedure is typically performed with ultrasound (US) guidance. An inferior or middle posterior calyx is accessed via a posterolateral approach to minimize the risk of hemorrhage. A minimal amount of contrast is used to verify positioning, since excess manipulation of an infected system can lead to sepsis.

The tract is then dilated, and a pigtail catheter (most common) is placed.
- **Neoplasm**. Transitional cell carcinoma (TCC) is the most common neoplasm to involve the renal collecting system; it arises from the urothelium. The most commonly involved is the urinary bladder, followed by the renal pelvis, and then the ureters. When identified within the upper urinary tract, a careful evaluation of the bladder should be performed to look for multi-focal disease. Risk factors include smoking, exposure to aromatic amines, and cyclophosphamide. CT urography is useful for evaluation of the kidneys and entire collecting system.
- **Blood clot**. Blood clots may occur within the collecting system due to trauma, stones, or tumors (TCC or renal cell carcinoma [RCC]). Usually, they present as multiple ureteral filling defects which conform to the contour of the collection system. If large, they can cause obstruction. Treatment is directed at the cause of hemorrhage.

■ Additional Differential Diagnoses

- **Fungus ball**. Fungus balls tend to occur in immunocompromised patients or in those with indwelling urinary catheters. Most often, the findings consist of multiple filling defects within the ureter and/or bladder. Occasionally, obstruction may occur when the masses become coalescent. *Candida* is the most common organism.
- **Sloughed papillae**. Papillary necrosis may result from a variety of conditions, including diabetes, analgesic nephropathy, pyelonephritis (especially tuberculosis (TB)), sickle-cell

disease, urinary obstruction, and renal vein thrombosis. The necrotic papillae may become dislodged and result in obstruction of the collecting system. Identification of findings compatible with papillary necrosis in conjunction with filling defects within the collecting system helps suggest the diagnosis. Findings of papillary necrosis include the "lobster claw" and "ball-on-tee" signs, secondary to abnormal contrast collections in the renal pyramids.

■ Diagnosis

Nephrolithiasis (with superimposed infection)

✓ Pearls

- Infection of an obstructed urinary system is a medical emergency requiring emergent decompression.
- Nephrolithiasis is the most common cause of urinary obstruction; the vast majority is radiopaque.

- In general, stones 4 mm or less will pass without intervention, while those 8 mm or greater will not.
- TCC is the most common urothelial neoplasm; be sure to evaluate the entire collecting system.

Suggested Readings

Barbaric ZL. Percutaneous nephrostomy for urinary tract obstruction. AJR Am J Roentgenol . 1984; 143(4):803–809

Dyer RB, Chen MY, Zagoria RJ. Classic signs in uroradiology. Radiographics. 2004; 24(Suppl 1):S247–S280

Case 252

David D. Gover

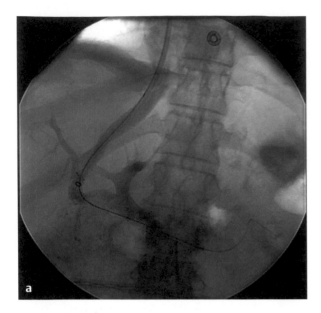

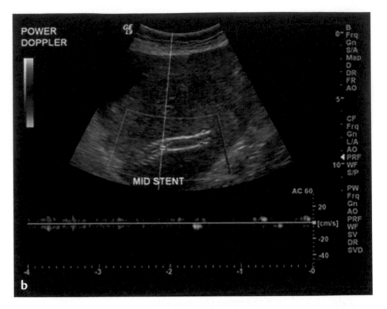

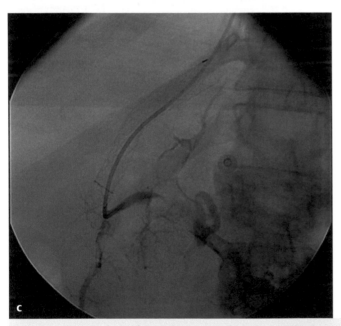

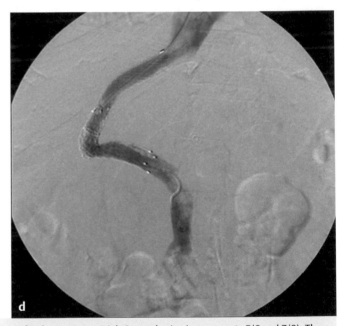

Fig. 252.1 **(a)** Angiogram of the right upper quadrant shows TIPS using a stent-graft. There are two "right" portal veins (to segments 5/6 and 7/8). The stent-graft connects the segment 5/6 portal vein to the right hepatic vein. Note the irregular stenosis of the segment 5/6 portal vein immediately after bifurcation with the main portal vein. **(b)** The initial follow-up ultrasound, done on post-procedure day 5, shows no flow in the TIPS, which is confirmed on **(c)** angiography. Findings are consistent with acute thrombosis of the portal vein and TIPS. **(d)** Digital subtraction angiography after thrombolysis and extension of stent into the portal system shows resumption of flow in the main portal vein and TIPS with resolution of the areas of stenoses.

■ Clinical Presentation

A 71-year-old woman with alcoholic end-stage liver disease and refractory hepatic hydrothorax despite transjugular intrahepatic portosystemic shunt (TIPS) procedure. Image A is from the initial TIPS procedure; images B and C are follow-up studies; and image D is postintervention (▶ Fig. 252.1).

■ Key Imaging Finding

TIPS dysfunction

■ Top 3 Differential Diagnoses

- **Neointimal hyperplasia.** Growth of the intima occurs due to the alterations in blood flow and the presence of a stent, slowly leading to luminal ingrowth and return of the portosystemic gradient (PSG). This effect is somewhat mitigated when stent-grafts are used instead of bare metal stents. At follow-up, recurrence of symptoms (e.g., enlarged varices or recurrent ascites) is the best indicator of TIPS dysfunction. Ultrasonography traditionally has had a role in TIPS surveillance, but is not sensitive. Most institutions perform a baseline ultrasound, then at 1, 3, 6, and 12 months post-TIPS, followed by annual examinations. Doppler interrogation for stent patency and possible stenosis with velocity and waveform analysis (specific for each vascular lab). Proposed ultrasound findings that suggest TIPS dysfunction include filling defects in the stent, velocity gradients across the shunt (with associated turbulence), a marked increase or decrease in shunt velocities (especially relative to the baseline), or changes in portal venous flow direction (relative to baseline). Doppler velocity changes necessitating TIPS venography at our home institution include main portal venous velocity <50 cm/s, shunt velocity <50 or >150 cm/s, or a change in velocity (increase or decrease) from the baseline of >50 cm/s. The presence of new varices or ascites should be noted on these examinations; these findings require a fol-

low-up TIPS venography. Angioplasty or stent placement may be indicated to lessen the PSG to 12 mm Hg or less for bleeding esophageal varices. The target PSG for refractory ascites is less certain; some suggest the target PSG to be 8 mm Hg or less, depending on the degree of hepatic encephalopathy.
- **Thrombosis.** Occlusion of the shunt with clot can occur early after TIPS creation or as a late finding. Early on, thrombosis is most likely attributed to bile leak, while venous stasis in conjunction with neointimal hyperplasia is a later finding. Patients can present with recurrence of symptoms, similar to TIPS stenosis. Alternatively, TIPS ultrasonography may discover the occlusion. Occlusions are treated with catheter-directed or mechanical thrombolysis and stent/stent-graft revision with angioplasty or stent.
- **Technical error.** Early shunt occlusion may occur due to malposition or migration of stents. Injury to the portal system may also lead to occlusion or thrombosis. Careful technique and scrutiny of angiograms during the placement of the shunt help reduce the incidence of technical error. Technical expertise has been shown to be important in the successful placement of TIPS; fatal complications are reduced when greater than 150 shunts have been placed by the interventionalist (3 vs. 1.4%).

■ Diagnosis

Technical error (portal venous injury)

✓ Pearls

- Neointimal hyperplasia is a common cause of TIPS dysfunction; abnormalities on US require venography.
- US evaluation of TIPS should include interrogation of stent patency with velocity and waveform analysis.

- Shunt occlusion may be an early or late finding; patients often present with recurrent symptoms.
- Technical error may be secondary to malposition or migration of stents or due to vessel injury.

Suggested Readings

Boyer TD, Haskal ZJ. American Association for the Study of Liver Diseases Practice Guidelines: the role of transjugular intrahepatic portosystemic shunt creation in the management of portal hypertension. J Vasc Interv Radiol. 2005; 16(5):615–629

Carr CE, Tuite CM, Soulen MC, et al. Role of ultrasound surveillance of transjugular intrahepatic portosystemic shunts in the covered stent era. J Vasc Interv Radiol. 2006; 17(8):1297–1305

Case 253

Charlyne Wu

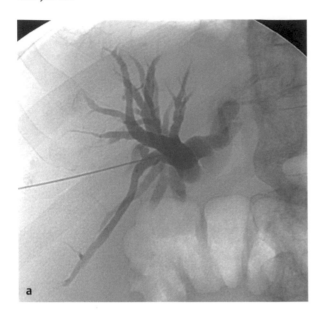

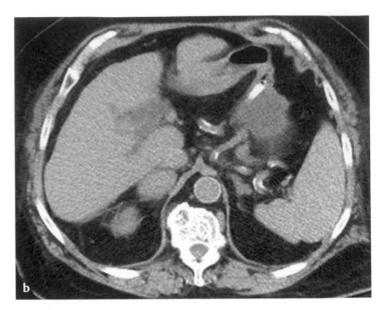

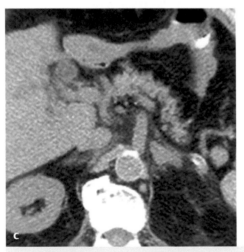

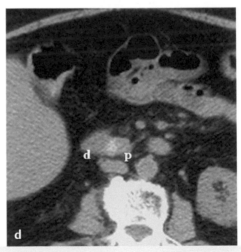

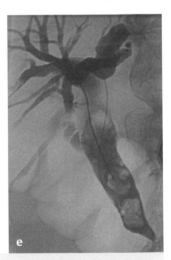

Fig. 253.1 (a) Percutaneous transhepatic cholangiogram (PTC) demonstrates diffusely dilated intrahepatic and extrahepatic biliary ducts with abrupt obstruction at the common bile duct. **(b)** Axial noncontrast CT image reveals "too many tubes" appearance of the dilated intrahepatic ducts. **(c)** Axial noncontrast CT image slightly more inferiorly demonstrates the extrahepatic biliary ductal dilatation without pancreatic ductal dilatation. **(d)** Axial noncontrast CT image through the level of the distal CBD shows a hyperdense focus at the junction of the duodenum, d, and the pancreas, p, in the region of the ampulla of Vater. **(e)** PTC with catheter advanced beyond area of obstruction demonstrates multiple filling defects along the course of the CBD, consistent with choledocholithiasis. *Images courtesy of Bijan Bijan, MD.*

■ Clinical Presentation

An 87-year-old woman with multiple episodes of nausea accompanied by vomiting of gastric contents and decreased oral intake for 4 days (▶ Fig. 253.1).

■ Key Imaging Finding

Biliary duct obstruction

■ Top 3 Differential Diagnoses

- **Choledocholithiasis**. Choledocholithiasis is responsible for 20% of cases of adult obstructive jaundice. Fluoroscopy and magnetic resonance cholangiopancreatography (MRCP) demonstrates filling defects and/or obstruction with dilatation of the more proximal biliary ducts. Ultrasound (US) will reveal ductal dilatation and possibly cholelithiasis or choledocholithiasis, though bowel gas may obscure complete evaluation of the common bile duct (CBD). Computed tomography (CT) may demonstrate intraluminal masses of varying attenuation. A "bull's eye," "target," or "crescent" sign describes a rim of low-attenuation bile surrounding the stone within the bile duct.

- **Cholangiocarcinoma (CCC)**. CCC is the second most common malignant primary hepatic tumor. These malignancies arise from the epithelium of the biliary duct system. There are three main areas in which CCCs occur: intrahepatic, perihi-

lar (Klatskin tumor), and distal extrahepatic. Perihilar are the most common and are seen at the bifurcation of the right and left hepatic ducts. Abrupt stricture and thickening of the duct wall may be the only findings. Prognosis is poor, with fewer than 20% of tumors being resectable.

- **Pancreatic adenocarcinoma**. Pancreatic and ampullary carcinomas are the cause of 20 to 25% of adult biliary obstruction. Tumors arise from pancreatic ducts. The diagnosis is rarely made at an early stage due to late presentation of obstructive symptoms. The role of imaging is to demonstrate the tumor, its relationship to surrounding vasculature, and possibility of curative resection. Imaging demonstrates abrupt obstruction of the common bile and/or pancreatic ducts ("double duct sign"). On CT, a hypovascular mass can be seen associated with the pancreatic head (60%), body (20%), diffusely (15%), or tail (5%).

■ Additional Differential Diagnoses

- **Chronic pancreatitis**. Chronic pancreatitis is responsible for approximately 8% of cases of adult biliary obstruction. Recurrent inflammation, fibrosis, and inflammatory masses cause narrowing and strictures of the bile ducts. Alternating regions of pancreatic ductal narrowing and dilatation lead to the "chain of lakes" appearance. Pancreatic calcifications and atrophy are associated findings.

- **Primary sclerosing cholangitis (PSC)**. PSC is characterized by insidious onset of jaundice with progressive disease, affecting both the intrahepatic and extrahepatic biliary ducts. It is

associated with a history of ulcerative colitis in 50 to 70% of cases. Imaging demonstrates a characteristic beaded pattern of the intrahepatic biliary ducts. On cholangiography, ductal diverticula are pathognomonic. Complications include biliary cirrhosis and cholangiocarcinoma.

- **Parasites**. Ascaris and liver fluke eggs from Clonorchis can lead to biliary obstruction. Opisthorchis should also be considered. Pharmacological treatment is the mainstay. Endoscopic sphincterotomy and extraction of parasites may alleviate symptoms in complex cases with biliary obstruction.

■ Diagnosis

Choledocholithiasis

✓ Pearls

- Choledocholithiasis is a common cause of obstructive jaundice in adults; US, CT, and MRCP are used for diagnosis.
- Cholangiocarcinoma arises from the biliary ductal epithelium; lesions at the hilum are termed Klatskin tumors.

- Pancreatic carcinoma results in the classic "double duct sign" (biliary and pancreatic ductal dilatation).
- PSC is associated with ulcerative colitis; imaging findings include a beaded appearance of biliary ducts.

Suggested Readings

Han JK, Choi BI, Kim AY, et al. Cholangiocarcinoma: pictorial essay of CT and cholangiographic findings. Radiographics . 2002; 22(1):173–187

Yeh BM, Liu PS, Soto JA, et al. MR imaging and CT of the biliary tract. Radiographics . 2009; 29(6):1669–1688

Case 254

Glade E. Roper

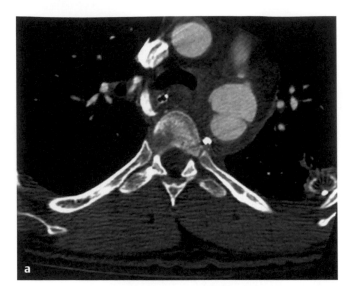

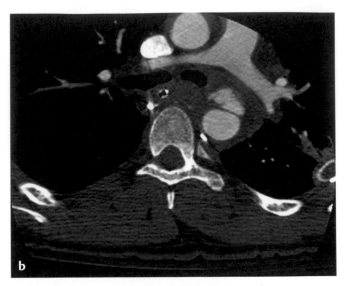

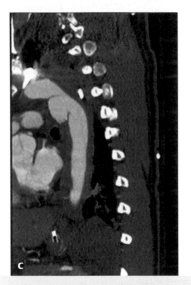

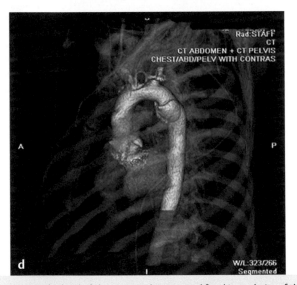

Fig. 254.1 (a,b) Images from a CT aortogram. Coned-down axial images at the level of the aortic isthmus reveal focal irregularity of the aortic wall and a hypodense linear structure within the aortic lumen. **(c)** Sagittal maximum intensity projection (MIP) image through the aorta and **(d)** three-dimensional reconstruction reveal a well-demarcated anterior bulge from the aortic isthmus. The bulge is 3 cm distal to the origin of the left subclavian artery.

■ Clinical Presentation

A 22-year-old restrained passenger in a high-speed automobile accident (▶ Fig. 254.1).

■ **Key Imaging Finding**

Traumatic aortic injury

■ **Top 3 Differential Diagnoses**

- **Pseudoaneurysm**. The aortic wall is composed of three layers of tissue—intima, composed of endothelium and basement membrane; media, composed of elastic and muscular tissue; and adventitia, composed of thin connective tissue. A tear of both the intima and media results in a pseudoaneurysm—a bulge in the lumen of the aorta contained only by the adventitia or other mediastinal tissues. In patients who survive to receive medical attention, such a tear usually involves only a portion of the aortic circumference. Most aortic injuries occur near the ligamentum arteriosum. Radiographs may reveal an enlarged aortic contour and/or widened mediastinum. Contrast-enhanced computed tomography (CECT) or angiography reveals focal irregularity or bulge of the aortic wall without an intimal flap. Often the injured aorta is surrounded by hematoma on CT. Risk of pseudoaneurysm rupture is high, though delayed repair is an option in some patients. Management may include percutaneous stent-graft placement in select patients. Surgical graft placement is often necessary due to proximity of the great vessels.
- **Aortic dissection**. When an injury causes a defect in the intima, blood may enter the media of the artery at arterial pressure. The pressurized blood dissects through the tissue of the media, peeling the intima off the wall of the aorta. Radiographs may reveal enlarged aortic contour. CECT and angiography may reveal irregularity of the aortic lumen, enlarged aorta, and an intimal flap. Aortic intimal calcifications may be displaced. Management depends on a number of factors, including the location of the dissection and its relationship to the great vessels. Some traumatic dissections are amenable to percutaneous stent-graft placement, though dissections of the ascending aorta require urgent surgical management.
- **Intramural hematoma**. The aortic media contains vasa vasorum—blood vessels that supply the tissue of the aorta. Injury to these vessels causes bleeding into the wall of the aorta, resulting in an intramural hematoma. The intima is usually intact. Imaging findings include focal hyperdensity within the wall of the aorta on noncontrast computed tomography (NCCT) and a focally thickened, nonenhancing aortic wall on CECT. Transesophageal echocardiography (TEE) and magnetic resonance imaging (MRI) are more accurate in making the diagnosis, revealing a curvilinear intramural mass with blood products. Angiography often fails to demonstrate the intramural hematoma. Current management is the same as that of aortic dissection, though there is a paucity of clinical trial data.

■ **Additional Differential Diagnoses**

- **Aortic transection**. When all three layers of the aortic wall are circumferentially torn, blood flows freely out of the aorta into the surrounding tissues. Such injuries are nearly always fatal. Eighty-five percent of patients with aortic injuries die before reaching the hospital. Emergent surgical repair is the only treatment option for patients who survive long enough to receive medical care.

■ **Diagnosis**

Aortic pseudoaneurysm

✓ **Pearls**

- Pseudoaneurysms are contained ruptures; prompt treatment (surgical or endovascular) is warranted.
- Dissections result from the intimal injury with true and false lumens; treatment depends on the extent of injury.
- Intramural hematomas are hyperdense (CT) or hyperintense (MRI) collections within the vessel wall.
- Aortic transaction results when all three layers of the aorta are torn; it is nearly always fatal.

Suggested Readings

Koenig TR, West OC. Diagnosing acute traumatic aortic injury with computed tomography angiography: signs and potential pitfalls. Curr Probl Diagn Radiol. 2004; 33(3):97–105

Rousseau H, Dambrin C, Marcheix B, et al. Acute traumatic aortic rupture: a comparison of surgical and stent-graft repair. J Thorac Cardiovasc Surg. 2005; 129(5):1050–1055

Case 255

David D. Gover

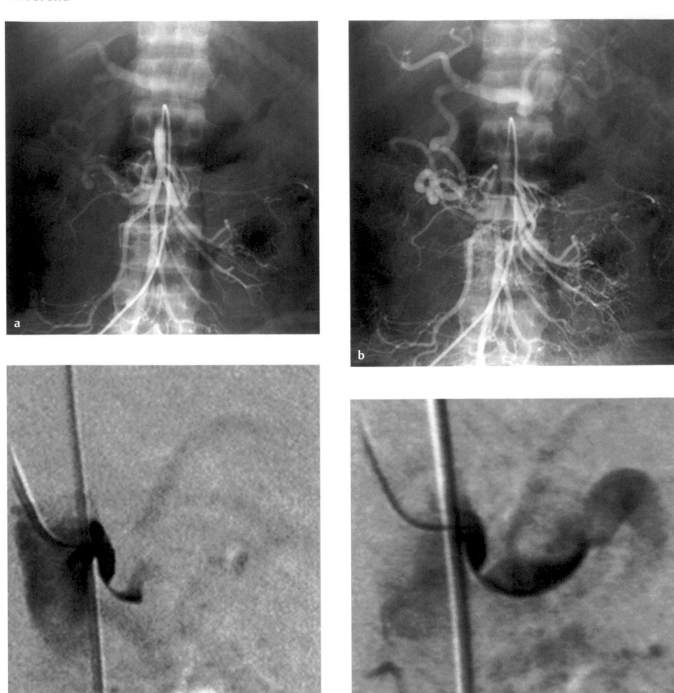

Fig. 255.1 Selective angiogram of the superior mesenteric artery both **(a)** early in the contrast run and **(b)** more delayed shows enlargement of the inferior pancreaticoduodenal and gastroduodenal arteries with retrograde filling of the celiac axis. **(c,d)** Two lateral views from a selective angiogram of the celiac axis confirm a severe origin stenosis with poststenotic dilatation. The stenosis has an extrinsic bandlike appearance.

■ Clinical Presentation

A 33-year-old woman with vague, postprandial abdominal pain and weight loss (▶Fig. 255.1).

■ Key Imaging Finding

Celiac axis stenosis/occlusion

■ Top 3 Differential Diagnoses

- **Atherosclerosis**. Atherosclerosis is the most common cause of narrowing of the mesenteric vessel origins. Patients with atherosclerosis, typically present at an older age, have irregularity of multiple vessels and commonly have associated peripheral vascular disease and/or abdominal aortic aneurysm. Individuals with inadequate collateral circulation usually present with intestinal ischemia (post-prandial pain) and "food fear," leading to weight loss. Management usually involves angioplasty or stent placement over surgery.
- **Thromboembolism**. Thromboembolic disease is usually from a cardiac (atrial fibrillation) or proximal aortic source. The celiac axis is rarely affected in comparison to the superior mesenteric artery, cerebral circulation, or peripheral vessels.

When intra-abdominal vessels are involved, patients usually present with acute mesenteric ischemia. Affected vessels may have a filling defect or be occluded. Treatment options include catheter-directed thrombolysis versus open surgery in cases of bowel infraction.

- **Vasculitis**. Patients with vasculitis present with a multitude of clinical features, including constitutional symptoms. Vasculitis may be a primary syndrome (e.g., Takayasu) or secondary to an underlying infection or malignancy. Treatment centers on corticosteroid administration for primary vasculitides. Catheter-directed treatments may be offered if end-organ involvement in the fibrotic phase of the disease is significant.

■ Additional Differential Diagnoses

- **Median arcuate ligament syndrome**. Median arcuate ligament syndrome typically affects thin women between 20 and 40 years of age who present with vague post-prandial abdominal pain. A low insertion of the median arcuate ligament (a fibrous arch that unites the diaphragmatic crura on either side of the aortic hiatus) causes narrowing of the celiac axis. Angiography reveals an indentation along the superior aspect of the celiac axis, which is worse during expiration. Surgical decompression is the treatment of choice; however, there is controversy regarding this treatment, since many patients have this abnormality without symptoms.

- **Fibromuscular dysplasia (FMD)**. FMD most commonly occurs in younger, mostly female, patients. Characteristic imaging findings include a beaded appearance, secondary to alternating regions of stenosis and dilatation. Angioplasty is the primary treatment option.
- **Radiation**. Radiation changes usually lead to multiple, smooth, long-segment regions of vessel narrowing. Endoluminal treatments (e.g., stent placement) are the norm for symptomatic lesions.

■ Diagnosis

Median arcuate ligament syndrome

✓ Pearls

- Atherosclerotic and embolic disease constitutes most cases of mesenteric vessel stenosis or occlusion.
- Vasculitides (Takayasu arteritis) may cause narrowing of aortic branch vessels; treatment is with steroids.

- Median arcuate ligament syndrome affects young, thin women who present with postprandial pain.

Suggested Readings

Horton KM, Talamini MA, Fishman EK. Median arcuate ligament syndrome: evaluation with CT angiography. Radiographics . 2005; 25(5):1177–1182

White RD, Weir-McCall JR, Sullivan CM, et al. The celiac axis revisited: anatomic variants, pathologic features, and implications for modern endovascular management. Radiographics . 2015; 35(3):879–898

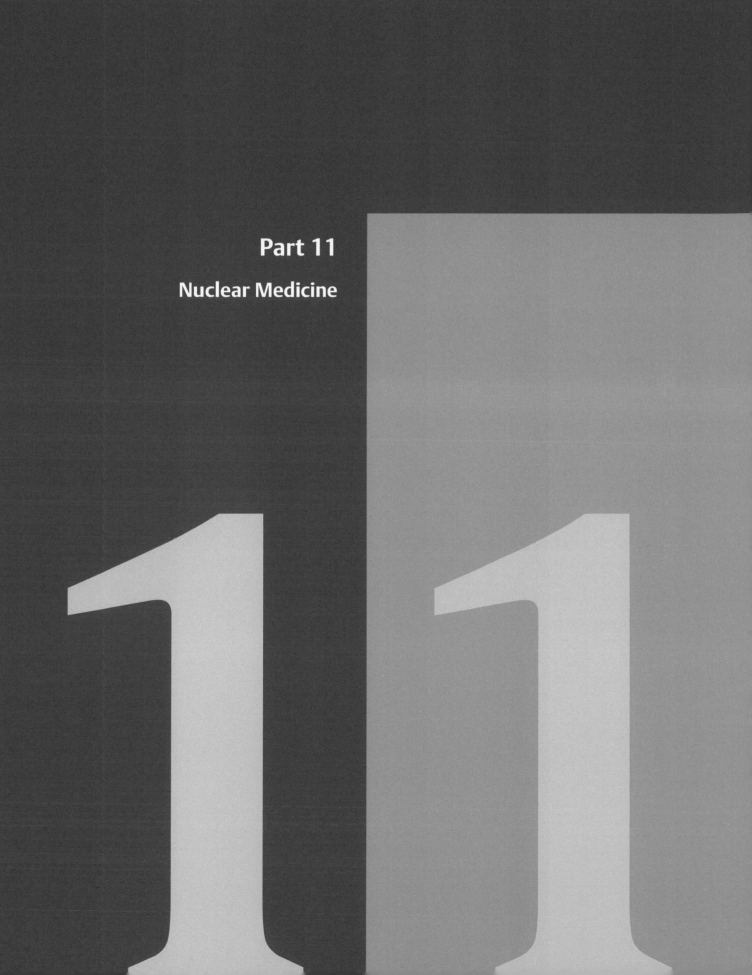

Part 11

Nuclear Medicine

11

Case 256

Ely A. Wolin

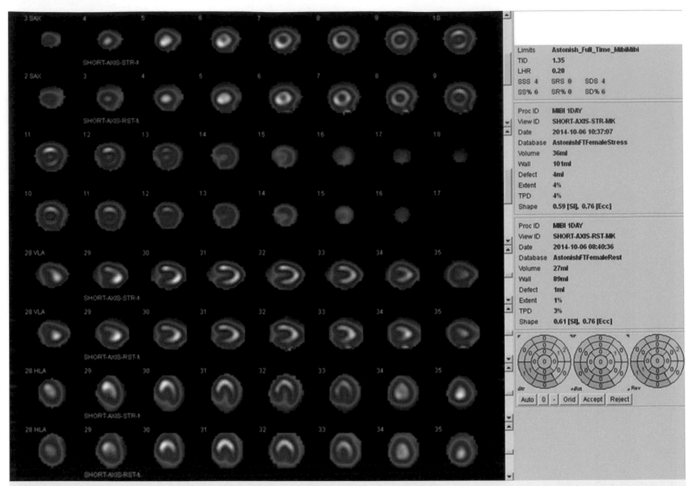

Fig. 256.1 Myocardial perfusion scan with technetium-99m-tetrofosmin demonstrates transient ischemic dilatation (TID) of the left ventricle (TID of 1.35) on stress imaging without apparent perfusion defect.

■ Clinical Presentation

An 80-year-old woman with a history of chronic obstructive pulmonary disease and atrial fibrillation who presents with chest pain (▶Fig. 256.1).

■ Key Imaging Finding

Transient ischemic dilatation (TID)

■ Top 3 Differential Diagnoses

- **Multivessel coronary artery disease**. Myocardial perfusion imaging is designed to detect areas of ischemia which may benefit from reperfusion. Ischemia is diagnosed by noting a reversible defect, decreased activity in a portion of the myocardium on post-stress imaging (exercise or chemical stress) in comparison to rest imaging. With multivessel balanced ischemia, however, focal regions of decreased activity may not be present as the images are normalized to the "hottest" pixels. In these situations, diffuse subendocardial ischemia may cause apparent dilatation of the left ventricular cavity on post-stress imaging. This is an important finding to make, as it may be the only sign of ischemia and can be associated with high-grade stenoses.
- **Hypertensive or hypertrophic heart disease**. Global subendocardial ischemia related to hypertensive heart disease or hypertrophic cardiomyopathy may result in apparent dilation of the left ventricular cavity due to relative photopenia in this region on post-stress imaging. This is likely a multifactorial process; however, delayed diastolic left ventricular relaxation and elevated end-diastolic pressures in the left ventricle are contributory, as they lead to an increased filling pressure of the epicardial coronary vessels. This can cause the appearance of TID without associated coronary artery stenosis.
- **Dilated cardiomyopathy**. TID can be seen in some patients with dilated cardiomyopathy. Although not fully understood, data suggest that this is likely due to a decreased coronary flow reserve in this patient population. As with hypertensive or hypertrophic heart disease, TID may be seen in the absence of coronary artery stenosis.

■ Additional Differential Diagnoses

- **Misaligned single-photon emission computed tomography (SPECT) images:** Misaligned stress and rest images from SPECT analysis may result in apparent TID of the left ventricular cavity. A careful inspection of overall SPECT image alignment at rest and stress, as well as utilization of quantitative analysis, should avoid this post-processing pitfall.

■ Diagnosis

Multivessel coronary artery disease

✓ Pearls

- TID suggests diffuse subendocardial ischemia from balanced multivessel disease.
- In the setting of multivessel balanced ischemia, TID may be the only imaging clue to an underlying pathology.
- Global subendocardial ischemia may result in apparent ventricular cavity dilatation, TID, on stress images.
- Ensure stress and rest SPECT images are appropriately aligned prior to visual interpretation.

Suggested Readings

Abidov A, Bax JJ, Hayes SW, et al. Transient ischemic dilation ratio of the left ventricle is a significant predictor of future cardiac events in patients with otherwise normal myocardial perfusion SPECT. J Am Coll Cardiol . 2003; 42(10):1818–1825

McLaughlin MG, Danias PG. Transient ischemic dilation: a powerful diagnostic and prognostic finding of stress myocardial perfusion imaging. J Nucl Cardiol . 2002; 9(6):663–667

Robinson VJB, Corley JH, Marks DS, et al. Causes of transient dilatation of the left ventricle during myocardial perfusion imaging. AJR Am J Roentgenol . 2000; 174(5):1349–1352

Case 257

Kamal D. Singh

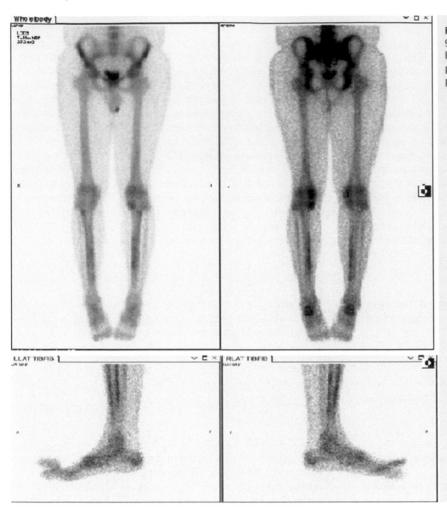

Fig. 257.1 Lower body bone scan with Technetium-99m methylene diphosphonate (MDP) demonstrates linear cortical uptake within the bilateral posteromedial mid-tibial diaphysis in a "tram-track" pattern.

■ Clinical Presentation

A 23-year-old man with bilateral shin pain for over a year, symptoms worsening to the lower tibia (►Fig. 257.1).

■ Key Imaging Finding

Symmetric "tram-track" cortical uptake of long bones

■ Top 3 Differential Diagnoses

- **Hypertrophic osteoarthropathy.** Secondary hypertrophic osteoarthropathy (HOA) is a clinical syndrome of symptomatic periostitis of long bones due to various neoplastic and non-neoplastic pulmonary and extrapulmonary disorders. Common pulmonary causes include bronchogenic carcinoma, fibrous tumor of the pleura, mesothelioma, and chronic pulmonary infection/inflammation; as a result, a chest radiograph should be obtained in patients with scintigraphic evidence of HOA. Extrapulmonary etiologies include inflammatory bowel disease, cyanotic congenital heart disease, and thyroid acropachy. The exact pathophysiology of HOA remains unclear; however, vasoactive agents and hormones secreted by tumors and other inflammatory/infectious processes have been implicated. Scintigraphic findings of bilateral symmetric upper and lower extremity parallel cortical activity in a "tram-track" configuration often precede plain film evidence of undulating periosteal proliferation. There may be associated increased activity within the scapula, mandible/maxilla, and periarticular regions. Patients usually report painful swelling in the affected limb and stiff joints and demonstrate digital clubbing on physical examination. The radiographic and scintigraphic findings usually resolve after treatment of the underlying disease.

- **Shin/quadriceps splints.** Severe bilateral shin and quadriceps splints may produce increased parallel cortical activity within the lower extremities of physically active patients with exertional or overuse lower leg pain. Shin splints (medial tibial stress syndrome) result in unilateral or bilateral posteromedial tibial cortical periostitis. These patients present with *dull-aching leg pain*. Unlike stress fractures which appear as focal regions of increased uptake on all three phases of a bone scan, splints are generalized linear or longitudinal activity along the diaphysis, usually the middle third, detected on delayed phase imaging. While stress fractures may co-exist in a patient with shin or quadriceps splints, there has been no evidence to suggest a progression of splints to stress fracture.

- **Chronic venous stasis.** Chronic venous insufficiency can lead to soft tissue edema, associated skin changes (including stasis ulcers), and thick undulating or nodular periosteal proliferation of the affected extremity due to local hypoxia. Physical examination can help differentiate this entity from other causes of increased parallel long-bone activity within an extremity by noting overlying skin changes. In the setting of cellulitis and chronic venous stasis, it may be difficult to exclude superimposed osteomyelitis.

■ Diagnosis

Bilateral shin splints

✓ Pearls

- Benign and malignant etiologies can lead to HOA; a chest X-ray should be obtained to evaluate underlying tumor.
- Shin and quadriceps splints are common in athletes and result in cortical periostitis with linear activity.

- Chronic venous stasis may lead to undulating periosteal proliferation due to hypoxia.

Suggested Readings

Ali A, Tetalman MR, Fordham EW, et al. Distribution of hypertrophic pulmonary osteoarthropathy. AJR Am J Roentgenol . 1980; 134(4):771–780

Love C, Din AS, Tomas MB, Kalapparambath TP, Palestro CJ. Radionuclide bone imaging: an illustrative review. Radiographics . 2003; 23(2):341–358

Rana RS, Wu JS, Eisenberg RL. Periosteal reaction. AJR Am J Roentgenol . 2009; 193(4):W259–272

Case 258

Kamal D. Singh

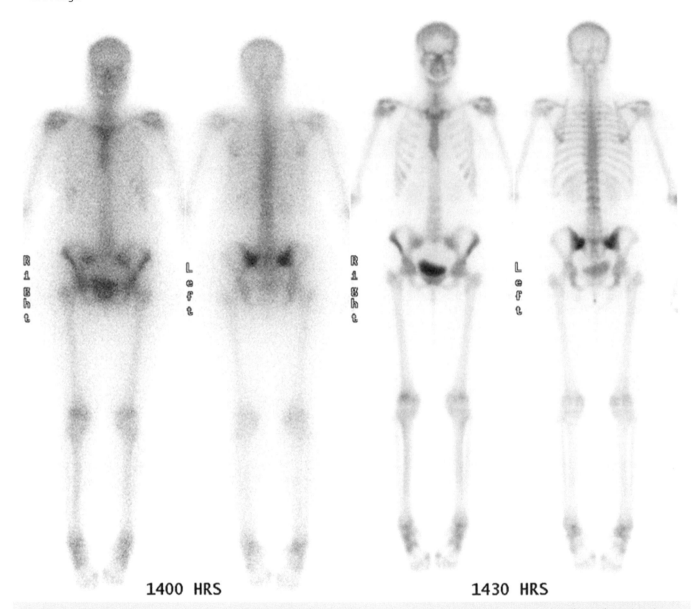

Fig. 258.1 Initial delayed whole body bone scan (left) with Tc99m hydroxydiphosphonate (HDP) demonstrates poor spatial resolution due to imaging acquisition at the wrong photopeak (122 keV for Co57). Repeat imaging (right) at the correct photopeak setting (140 keV for Tc99m) demonstrates improved spatial resolution. Incidentally, the patient had mild bilateral sacroiliitis, which was seen on a prior CT (not shown).

■ Clinical Presentation

A 24-year-old woman with chronic hip pain (▶Fig. 258.1). What is the difference between these two scans performed on the same day?

■ Key Imaging Finding

Poor quality bone scan

■ Top 3 Differential Diagnoses

- **Off-peak gamma camera.** For image acquisition, gamma cameras employ an energy window centered around the photopeak of the desired radioisotope in order to reject scatter radiation. In the case of Technetium-99m (Tc99m), a 20% energy widow is centered around the 140-keV photopeak. Daily morning quality control involves extrinsic field uniformity testing using a Cobalt-57 (Co57) sheet source prior to camera use for clinical studies. The extrinsic field uniformity test requires an energy window for Co57 (122 keV), which is lower than Tc99m. Failure to readjust the window setting for Tc99m prior to clinical use results in a poor resolution scan due to downscatter from 140 keV photons into the 122 keV window. This is referred to as "off-peak" imaging.
- **Poor radiopharmaceutical preparation or infiltrated dose.** Technical errors in radiopharmaceutical preparation can lead to chemical or radionuclidic impurities and poor radiochemical labeling. These errors result in image degradation and, in some cases, an increased dose to the patient. Regulations for radiopharmaceutical quality control have been established by the Nuclear Regulatory Commission (NRC) and the U.S. Pharmacopeia (USP). Examples for Tc99m include less than 0.15 µCi of Molybdenum-99 (Mo99) per 1 mCi of Tc99m (at the time of administration) and a maximum of 10 µg of aluminum breakthrough per 1 mL of Tc99m eluate. Quantum mottle (image noise) may result from inadequate radiotracer accumulation in the organ of interest due to infiltration of the dose at the injection site. This results in decreased counts during image acquisition, resulting in poor target-to-background. If not recognized during the time of injection, the dose infiltration may be confirmed by including the injection site in the imaging field of view.
- **Poor camera positioning.** Ideal image acquisition requires the gamma camera to be as close to the patient as possible. Minimizing the source-to-detector distance allows for optimum performance of the external collimator, the major limitation to resolution. As the detector is moved away from the target, photons with a greater angle of incidence are allowed through the collimator because of the altered geometry. This leads to a blurry image. Using the wrong energy collimator could also similarly affect image quality.

■ Additional Differential Diagnoses

- **Incorrect radiopharmaceutical administration.** Administration of an incorrect radiopharmaceutical, incorrect dose (>20% difference from the prescribed dose), or utilizing an unprescribed route of administration are classified as "misadministration" and may account for unexpected imaging results. A "medical event" is a subset of misadministration where the patient's whole body dose exceeds 5 rem (0.05 Sv) or a single organ dose exceeds 50 rem (0.5 Sv), requiring verbal and written notification to the Nuclear Regulatory Commission.

■ Diagnosis

Off-peak bone scan

✓ Pearls

- Off-peak imaging results in poor resolution imaging from improper radiotracer photopeak selection.
- Poor target-to-background can also result from technical errors in radiotracer preparation or administration.
- Medical events are the misadministration of radiotracer, exceeding the allowable limits of radiation dose.

Suggested Readings

Cecchin D, Poggiali D, Riccardi L, Turco P, Bui F, De Marchi S. Analytical and experimental FWHM of a gamma camera: theoretical and practical issues. Peer J . 2015; 3:e722

Naddaf SY, Collier BD, Elgazzar AH, Khalil MM. Technical errors in planar bone scanning. J Nucl Med Technol . 2004; 32(3):148–153

Zanzonico P. Routine quality control of clinical nuclear medicine instrumentation: a brief review. J Nucl Med . 2008; 49(7):1114–1131

Case 259

Kamal D. Singh

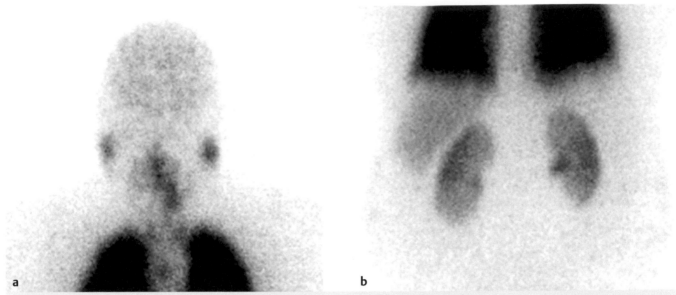

Fig. 259.1 (a,b) Static images from a lung perfusion scan with Tc99m macroaggregated albumin (MAA) demonstrate intracranial (a), thyroid (a), liver (b), and renal (b) activity. There is also activity seen in the salivary glands (a), swallowed activity in the esophagus (a), and expected lung activity (a,b).

■ Clinical Presentation

A 56-year-old man with cirrhosis, alcohol abuse, and hypoxemia (▶ Fig. 259.1).

■ Key Imaging Finding

Extrapulmonary activity on lung perfusion scan

■ Top 3 Differential Diagnoses

• **Free Technetium-99m (Tc99m) pertechnetate**. Free Tc99m pertechnetate is the result of poor labeling of the radiopharmaceutical. The free Tc99m passes through the pulmonary capillary bed and into systemic circulation. Normal biodistribution of Tc99m pertechnetate includes the choroid plexus, salivary glands, thyroid, stomach/intestines, kidneys, urinary collecting system, and bladder. Determination of unbound or free Tc99m within a radiopharmaceutical preparation can be done by thin-layer chromatography (TLC) with acetone solvent. Regulatory standards require at least 95% radiolabeling efficiency.

• **Right-to-left shunt**. Intrapulmonary or intracardiac shunting can be detected on perfusion imaging when Tc99m macroaggregated albumin (MAA) particles bypass the lungs and localize in systemic capillary beds. Cerebral cortical activity distinguishes shunting from other causes of extrapulmonary uptake, such as free Tc99m. Hence, imaging over the brain improves specificity when shunting is suspected. Unlike free Tc99m, the renal uptake in shunting is primarily within the renal cortex; collecting system excretion and bladder activity are absent. Quantification of shunting can be performed by whole body imaging to determine the ratio of systemic counts to whole body counts, which is proportional to the shunt size. Shunting of greater than 5–10% is generally considered significant. A lung perfusion scan is normally accomplished with 2–5 mCi of Tc99m MAA containing 200,000 to 500,000 particles. In cases of known or suspected shunt, the number of particles should be reduced to 100,000. Reduced number of particles also applies to children, pregnant patients, and those with known pulmonary hypertension or a history of pneumonectomy. Superior vena cava obstruction is a much less likely possible cause for shunting to the systemic circulation.

• **Retained activity from a different radiotracer study**. Knowledge of any recent nuclear medicine scans is helpful to avoid interfering activity, which may especially be an issue for radiotracers with long half-lives.

■ Diagnosis

Right-to-left shunt

✓ Pearls

• Extrapulmonary activity on a perfusion scan should be assessed with brain imaging to exclude a shunt.

• Right-to-left shunts can be detected and quantified on lung perfusion scan with Tc99m MAA.

• Reduced particles are used for shunts, pulmonary hypertension, and pregnant/pediatric patients.

Suggested Readings

Esser JP, Oei HY, de Bruin HG, Krenning EP. Liver and vertebral uptake of Tc-99m macroaggregated albumin (MAA). Clin Nucl Med . 2004; 29(12):793–794

Kume N, Suga K, Uchisako H, Matsui M, Shimizu K, Matsunaga N. Abnormal extrapulmonary accumulation of 99mTc-MAA during lung perfusion scanning. Ann Nucl Med . 1995; 9(4):179–184

Parker JA, Coleman RE, Grady E, et al; Society of Nuclear Medicine. SNM practice guideline for lung scintigraphy 4.0. J Nucl Med Technol . 2012; 40(1):57–65

Case 260

John P. Lichtenberger III

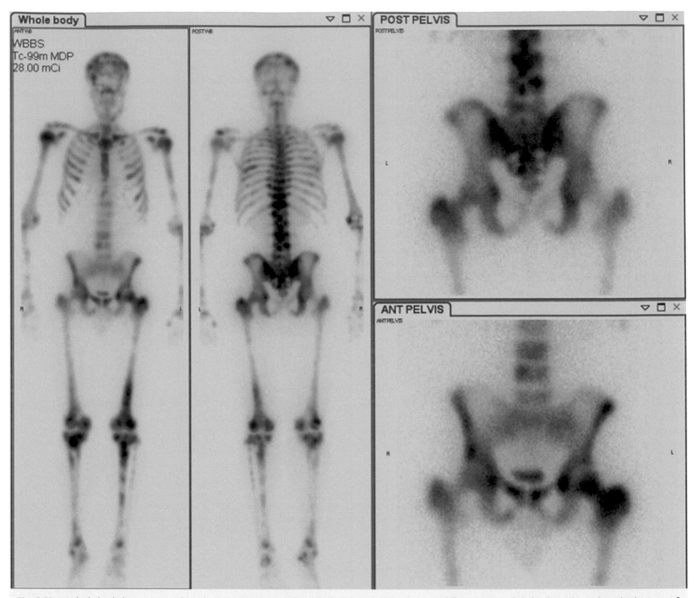

Fig. 260.1 Whole body bone scan with Technetium-99m methylene diphosphonate (MDP) shows diffuse increased skeletal uptake with multiple areas of focally increased activity with no significant soft tissue or renal activity.

■ Clinical Presentation

A 65-year-old man with history otherwise withheld (▶ Fig. 260.1).

■ **Key Imaging Finding**

Superscan

■ **Top 3 Differential Diagnoses**

- **Metastatic disease**. A superscan refers to increased skeletal uptake on bone scan with decreased or absent renal and soft tissue activity. Diffuse osseous metastatic disease is the most common cause of a superscan, most commonly metastatic prostate cancer. With metastatic disease, the skeletal activity is typically inhomogeneous and centered primarily within the axial and proximal appendicular skeletal. Distinct metastatic foci may be discernible.
- **Metabolic bone disease**. Although somewhat varied in scintigraphic appearance, metabolic diseases, such as renal osteodystrophy, hyperparathyroidism, and osteomalacia, may result in generalized increased activity in the skeleton relative to the kidneys and soft tissues (superscan). Features that suggest metabolic disease include uniform distribution of activity, in-

volvement of the appendicular skeleton, and disproportionate increased calvarial uptake. The osseous manifestations of renal osteodystrophy result from altered vitamin D metabolism and secondary hyperparathyroidism. This diagnosis is suggested on bone scan by prominent activity along the costochondral junctions, involvement of distal long bones, "railroad tracking" and bowing of the femurs, and sternal activity. Pseudofractures may be seen in setting of osteomalacia.

- **Paget disease**. Intense activity and expansion of bones are characteristic of Paget disease, most commonly involving the pelvis, femurs, spine, and skull. When multifocal or widespread, concentration of radiopharmaceutical in the skeletal lesions and increased target-to-soft tissue ratio may result in an apparent superscan.

■ **Additional Differential Diagnoses**

- **Myeloproliferative/marrow infiltrative disorder**. A superscan from myeloproliferative diseases, such as lymphoma, mastocytosis, and myelofibrosis, usually manifests as uniform and homogeneous radiotracer uptake within both the axi-

al and appendicular skeleton, similar to metabolic disease. Appropriate history and laboratory values aid in distinguishing between myeloproliferative/marrow infiltrative disorders and metabolic disease.

■ **Diagnosis**

Diffuse osteoblastic metastatic disease (prostate cancer)

✓ **Pearls**

- Superscan refers to increased skeletal and decreased or absent renal and soft tissue activity on bone scan.
- Metastatic disease is the most common cause of a superscan and typically involves the axial skeleton.

- Metabolic bone disease involves both the axial and appendicular skeleton and is usually homogeneous.
- Paget disease may result in a superscan when widespread.

Suggested Readings

Buckley O, O'Keeffe S, Geoghegan T, et al. 99mTc bone scintigraphy superscans: a review. Nucl Med Commun . 2007; 28(7):521–527

Cheng TH, Holman BL. Increased skeletal: renal uptake ratio: etiology and characteristics. Radiology . 1980; 136(2):455–459

Love C, Din AS, Tomas MB, Kalapparambath TP, Palestro CJ. Radionuclide bone imaging: an illustrative review. Radiographics . 2003; 23(2):341–358

Case 261

William T. O'Brien Sr.

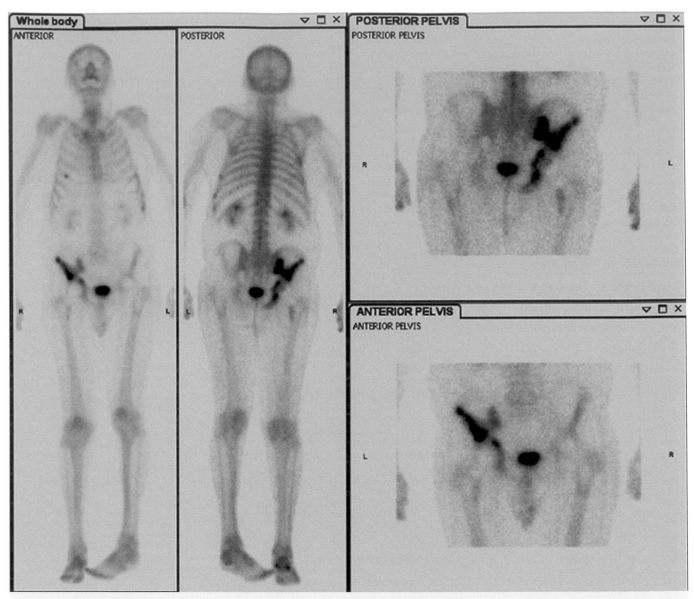

Fig. 261.1 Whole body bone scan with Technetium-99m methylene diphosphonate (MDP) demonstrates confluent areas of increased radiotracer uptake and mild bony expansion involving the right iliac bone, acetabulum, and ischium. Additional foci of increased uptake are noted in the right sixth rib and in the left seventh, ninth, and 10th ribs.

■ Clinical Presentation

A 78-year-old man with hip pain (▶Fig. 261.1).

■ Key Imaging Finding

Increased activity and osseous expansion in the pelvis

■ Top 2 Differential Diagnoses in an Adult

- **Paget disease.** Paget disease most commonly occurs in middle-aged to older men. The cause is unknown. On bone scans, Paget disease exhibits increased activity, often with apparent bony expansion. Distribution is monostotic in 10 to 35%, most commonly affecting the pelvis, spine, sacrum, femur, and cranium. Osteoporosis circumscripta, a classic lytic lesion of the skull, will have uptake at the margins. Paget disease progresses from one end of a long bone to the other with a sharp demarcation from the involved to the uninvolved portion, rendering the classic "blade of grass" appearance. Bone scan uptake is typically increased during all three phases of the disease (lytic, mixed, and sclerotic). Bone scan is more sensitive than radiography, and is useful for identifying polyostotic disease. Sarcomatous degeneration may initially result in increasing focal activity, but may later appear photopenic due to lesional necrosis.

- **Metastases.** Bone scan is the most useful imaging modality to search for osteoblastic metastatic disease. Although usually multifocal, metastases may occasionally be monostotic. The axial skeleton is most commonly involved. Sclerotic metastases are most likely due to prostate cancer in a man and breast carcinoma in a woman. Metastatic disease typically presents as multifocal regions of increased activity on bone scan, with the activity thought to be from the body's reaction to the tumor. The involved bone may be enlarged, secondary to tumor burden. Lesions may demonstrate increased activity within the first 6 months after chemotherapy, referred to as the "flare phenomenon," as a result of a healing osteoblastic response. Increasing activity after 6 months should be considered progression of the disease.

■ Top 3 Differential Diagnoses in a Child

- **Ewing sarcoma.** Ewing sarcoma is the second most common primary bone tumor (after osteosarcoma) in children, most commonly involving the pelvis or femur. Patients typically present with progressive pain. Bone scans demonstrate increased activity; bony expansion may also be seen. Osseous metastases occur in approximately half of the patients; therefore, follow-up imaging is warranted to evaluate for disease progression.
- **Lymphoma.** Lymphoma can mimic Ewing sarcoma clinically and radiographically, but has a more favorable prognosis. Increased activity and bony expansion may be seen on bone

scan. The pelvis is commonly involved in children. Biopsy is warranted to confirm the diagnosis, but should be coordinated with the pediatric surgeon as the tract used for biopsy may alter the surgical approach.
- **Fibrous dysplasia (FD).** FD may be monostotic or polyostotic (McCune-Albright). The lesions may be lucent, have a ground glass matrix, or be sclerotic. Bony expansion is common. Increased uptake is noted in involved bones. Common locations include long bones, pelvis, craniofacial bones, spine, and ribs.

■ Diagnosis

Metastatic prostate cancer

✓ Pearls

- Paget disease most commonly affects the pelvis; bone scans help evaluate sarcomatous degeneration.
- Paget disease and FD can be monostotic or polyostotic. Metastases are usually multifocal.

- Correlation with anatomic imaging can be paramount in distinguishing benign from malignant disease.
- Malignancies in children that lead to increased activity and bony expansion in the pelvis include Ewing sarcoma and lymphoma.

Suggested Readings

Abdelrazek S, Szumowski P, Rogowski F, Kociura-Sawicka A, Mojsak M, Szorc M. Bone scan in metabolic bone diseases. Review. Nucl Med Rev Cent East Eur. 2012; 15(2):124–131

Kumar AA, Kumar P, Prakash M, Tewari V, Sahni H, Dash A. Paget disease diagnosed on bone scintigraphy: Case report and literature review. Indian J Nucl Med. 2013; 28(2):121–123
Orzel JA, Sawaf NW, Richardson ML. Lymphoma of the skeleton: scintigraphic evaluation. AJR Am J Roentgenol. 1988; 150(5):1095–1099

Case 262

Kamal D. Singh

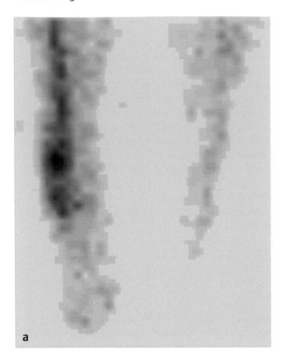

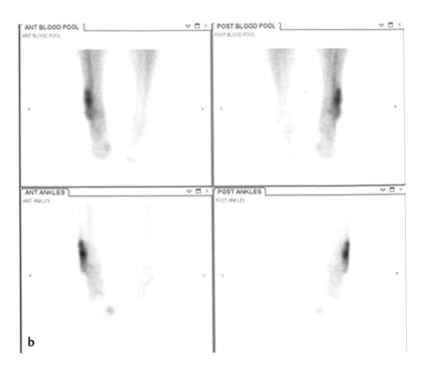

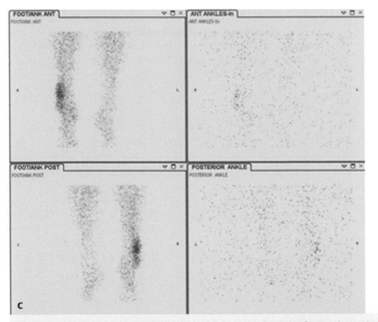

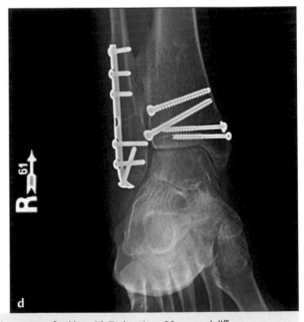

Fig. 262.1 **(a)** Flow image and blood pool and **(b)** delayed images from a three phase bone scan of ankles with Technetium-99m reveal diffuse hyperemia on the right with matched blood pool and delayed uptake in the region of the distal right fibula. **(c)** Images from an indium-111 WBC and Technetium-99m sulfur colloid scan show increased sulfur colloid uptake in the region of the bone scan abnormality, greater than minimal WBC activity. **(d)** Correlative frontal ankle radiograph is shown.

■ Clinical Presentation

A 67-year-old woman with a history of open reduction internal fixation (ORIF) of the right ankle presenting with the right lateral ankle cellulitis, refractory to outpatient treatment, swelling, and tenderness to palpation, with healed scab over later malleolus (▶ Fig. 262.1).

■ Key Imaging Finding

Three-phase positive bone scan

■ Top 3 Differential Diagnoses

- **Trauma**. A three-phase bone scan involves dynamic flow imaging for the first minute after radiopharmaceutical injection, a static blood pool imaging for the next few minutes, and a subsequent static delayed imaging at 2–4 hours. Although a three-phase bone scan is classically performed for the determination of osseous infection, increased uptake on all three phases is a non-specific finding and can be seen in the setting of acute fracture or recent surgery. Approximately 80% of fractures demonstrate increased activity within 24 hours, and more than 95% of fractures demonstrate increased activity by 3 days. A healed extremity fracture may have persistent focal increased activity on the delayed phase of the bone scan for over a year.
- **Osteomyelitis**. Three-phase bone scan not only has a high sensitivity and negative predictive value for acute osteomyelitis, but also may detect abnormalities 1 to 2 weeks earlier than radiographic manifestations. False negative bone scans, however, may be seen in the setting of disrupted blood supply or abscess formation, especially in neonates and infants with hematogenously acquired osteomyelitis. Specificity is decreased in the setting of recent surgery, trauma, or orthopedic hardware. Dual-isotope imaging with indium-111 (In111)-labeled white blood cells (WBC; for infection) and Technetium-99m sulfur colloid (Tc99m-SC; for normal bone marrow mapping) can aide in the assessment of osteomyelitis. Focal uptake on an In111 WBC scan, that is spatially discordant from Tc99m-SC bone marrow scan, is suggestive of infection.
- **Bone tumor**. Primary or secondary malignant bone tumors may demonstrate increased activity on all three phases. Although most benign osseous neoplasms will not demonstrate increased flow or blood pool activity, osteoid osteomas contain a three-phase positive nidus with a "target sign" on delayed imaging.

■ Additional Differential Diagnoses

- **Complex regional pain syndrome (CRPS)**. CRPS typically occurs after trauma or surgery and is characterized by pain, swelling, and vasomotor instability out of proportion to the degree of injury. Periarticular swelling and osteopenia may be seen on plain radiographs. Early or acute CRPS classically demonstrates unilateral increased flow and blood pool activity with periarticular increased radiotracer activity on delayed images. This classic pattern is only seen in two-thirds of affected patients. The flow and blood pool activity may normalize in chronic or long-standing CRPS. Interestingly, CRPS in children commonly demonstrates normal or even decreased activity (so-called cold CRPS).

■ Diagnosis

Reactive bone marrow post-ORIF

✓ Pearls

- Flow, blood pool, and delayed imaging at 2 to 4 hours make up a three-phase bone scan.
- Three-phase positive scans may be seen with acute fractures, osteomyelitis, osteoid osteomas, and CRPS.
- In111 WBC scan with Tc99m-SC scan is highly specific for hardware osteomyelitis.
- CRPS presents with periarticular osteopenia and corresponding increased activity on three-phase bone scan.

Suggested Readings

Kozin F, Soin JS, Ryan LM, Carrera GF, Wortmann RL. Bone scintigraphy in the reflex sympathetic dystrophy syndrome. Radiology . 1981; 138(2):437–443

Love C, Din AS, Tomas MB, Kalapparambath TP, Palestro CJ. Radionuclide bone imaging: an illustrative review. Radiographics . 2003; 23(2):341–358

Case 263

Kamal D. Singh

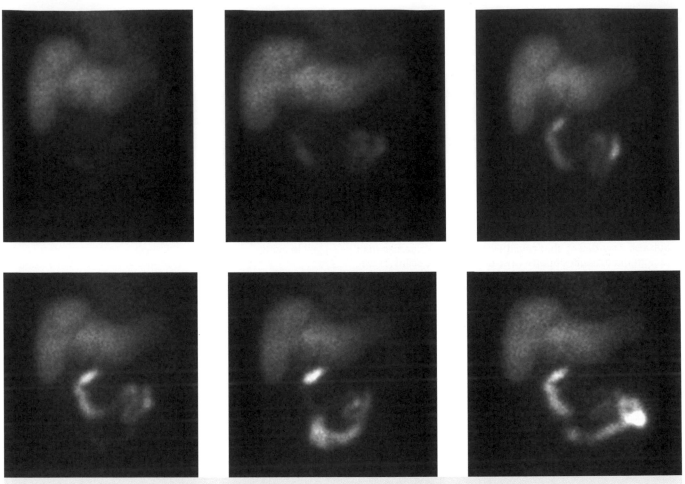

Fig. 263.1 Representative images from anterior 60-minute dynamic imaging after the administration of Technetium-99m Mebrofenin show prompt clearance of the blood pool, normal hepatic transit, and biliary-to-bowel transit, with no activity seen in the gallbladder. There was no evidence of bile leak.

■ Clinical Presentation

A 77-year-old man with known acute cholecystitis post–endoscopic retrograde cholangiopancreatography (ERCP) with concern for bile leak (▶ Fig. 263.1).

■ Key Imaging Finding

Nonvisualization of gallbladder on hepatobiliary imaging

■ Top 3 Differential Diagnoses

- **Acute cholecystitis**. Acute cystic duct obstruction is the hallmark of acute cholecystitis. Hepatobiliary imaging has a high specificity (98%) and negative predictive value (99%) and is very useful in cases where ultrasound findings are equivocal. Under normal circumstances, the gallbladder is visualized within 1 hour of radiotracer administration. Nonvisualization of the gallbladder within 4 hours of radiotracer injection and in the setting of normal visualization of biliary and bowel activity is diagnostic of acute cholecystitis. Alternatively, morphine (0.04 mg/kg intravenously [IV]) may be administered after 1 hour of dynamic imaging. Nonvisualization of the gallbladder within 30 minutes of morphine administration is also diagnostic of acute cholecystitis. The "cystic duct" or "nubbin" sign may be seen as focal activity within the cystic duct to the site of obstruction. Increased pericholecystic hepatic parenchymal activity ("rim sign") can be an ominous sign of complicated/ advanced (gangrenous, necrotic, or perforated) cholecystitis, necessitating immediate surgical intervention.

- **Chronic cholecystitis**. Delayed visualization of the gallbladder between 1 and 4 hours post-injection, or within 30 minutes after morphine augmentation, is suggestive of chronic cholecystitis. A second injection of radiopharmaceutical may be necessary after the initial 60-minute image acquisition if there is insufficient remaining hepatic or biliary activity to permit gallbladder filling.

- **Inadequate patient preparation**. False-positive scans can occur with insufficient (<4 hours) or prolonged (>24 hours) fasting or prolonged hyperalimentation. Pretreatment with cholecystokinin (CCK) 30 minutes prior to injection is usually recommended for prolonged fasting and hyperalimentation to allow the distended gallbladder to drain. Patients with a recent meal are typically imaged after fasting for a minimum of 4 h.

■ Additional Differential Diagnoses

- **Severe hepatocellular disease**. Poor hepatocellular function can result in poor extraction and excretion of the radiotracer, resulting in delayed blood pool clearance (>10 min). False-positive studies occur due to delayed or non-visualization of gallbladder. The key is to note the delayed blood pool clearance.

- **High-grade biliary obstruction**. Prompt hepatic uptake without biliary excretion of radiotracer ("liver scan" sign) suggests biliary duct obstruction. Delayed 4- and 24-hour imaging is generally obtained to evaluate for bowel activity. The gallbladder may or may not fill depending upon the location and duration of obstruction. Computed tomography (CT) scan or magnetic resonance cholangiopancreatography (MRCP) may be helpful not only in establishing the diagnosis but also in determining a possible cause of biliary obstruction.

■ Diagnosis

Acute cholecystitis

✓ Pearls

- Hepatobiliary scan is highly sensitive and specific for acute calculus cholecystitis.
- False positives may be seen with recent meal, extended fasting (>24 hours), and hepatocellular dysfunction.

- The "rim sign" can indicate complicated/advanced (gangrenous, necrotic, or perforated) cholecystitis.

Suggested Readings

Montini KM, Tulchinsky M. Applied hepatobiliary scintigraphy in acute cholecystitis. Appl Radiol . 2015; 44(5):21–30

Tulchinsky M, Ciak BW, Delbeke D, et al; Society of Nuclear Medicine. SNM practice guideline for hepatobiliary scintigraphy 4.0 J Nucl Med Technol . 2010; 38(4):210–218

Uliel L, Mellnick VM, Menias CO, Holz AL, McConathy J. Nuclear medicine in the acute clinical setting: indications, imaging findings, and potential pitfalls. Radiographics . 2013; 33(2):375–396

Case 264

Kamal D. Singh

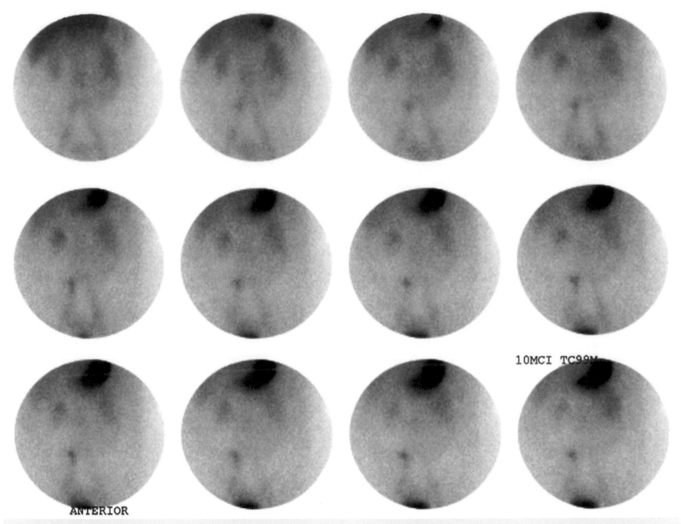

Fig. 264.1 Sequential images from a technetium-99m pertechnetate scan demonstrate focal uptake in the right lower quadrant which appears at the same time as the physiologic gastric mucosal activity and intensifies over time without evidence for peristalsis. The anterior intra-abdominal location of this activity was confirmed on a static lateral projection (not included). Physiologic urinary excretion of radiotracer is also noted.

■ Clinical Presentation

An 8-year-old boy with chronic abdominal discomfort and a history of intermittent lower gastrointestinal bleeding (▶ Fig. 264.1).

■ Key Imaging Finding

Focal intra-abdominal activity on pertechnetate imaging

■ Top 3 Differential Diagnoses

- **Meckel diverticulum**. Meckel diverticulum is a congenital persistence of the omphalomesenteric (vitelline) duct. It occurs in about 2% of the population, has a 2:1 male-to-female ratio, occurs 2 feet from the ileocecal valve, and generally presents within 2 years of age (rule of 2s). Although not all Meckel diverticula have gastric mucosa, the vast majority of symptomatic cases do. Patients may present with bleeding, obstruction, intussusception, or volvulus. Technetium-99m (Tc-99m) pertechnetate is taken up by mucin producing cells and can detect enteric diverticula with ectopic gastric mucosa. Proper patient preparation can improve sensitivity of a Meckel scan, which includes nothing by mouth (NPO) for at least 4 hours with possible pretreatment with cimetidine (blocks radiotracer release from ectopic mucosa), pentagastrin (enhances ectopic mucosal uptake), and glucagon (decreases small bowel peristalsis). Focal activity in the right lower quadrant, which appears at the same time as physiologic gastric uptake, intensifies over time, and is non-peristaltic, is diagnostic of a Meckel diverticulum. Uptake usually appears within 30 minutes, but may take up to 60 minutes depending upon the amount of gastric mucosa present. False-negative studies may be due to the absence of gastric mucosa (no radiotracer uptake mechanism) or diverticular ischemia/necrosis.

- **Focal intra-abdominal infectious or inflammatory process**. False-positive studies may occur in the setting of focal infectious or inflammatory intra-abdominal processes, such as appendicitis or focal enteritis/colitis; heterotopic gastric mucosa, such as gastrointestinal duplication cyst with heterotopic gastric mucosa; and inflammatory bowel disease. Hypervascular masses such as arteriovenous malformations (AVMs) and neoplasms may also be seen as focal regions of increased activity on a Meckel scan. With the exception of duplication cyst with heterotopic gastric mucosa, the remainder of these entities demonstrate increased blood pool that fades over time, rather than focal activity that mirrors physiologic gastric activity. Correlation with cross-sectional imaging may be necessary in some cases to differentiate these conditions from a true Meckel diverticulum.

- **Physiologic renal/urinary activity**. Additional static lateral views can confirm whether focal activity is intra-abdominal or retroperitoneal in location. Upright and post-void imaging can also help in distinguishing physiologic activity within a distended renal pelvis, ureter, ectopic kidney, or bladder diverticulum from a Meckel diverticulum.

■ Diagnosis

Meckel diverticulum

✓ Pearls

- Tc-99m pertechnetate scan detects Meckel diverticulum with ectopic gastric mucosa.
- Focal intra-abdominal activity that intensifies over time without peristalsis suggests a Meckel diverticulum.

- False positives include urinary tracer excretion and intra-abdominal inflammatory/infectious processes.

Suggested Readings

Emamian SA, Shalaby-Rana E, Majd M. The spectrum of heterotopic gastric mucosa in children detected by Tc-99m pertechnetate scintigraphy. Clin Nucl Med . 2001; 26(6):529–535

Lin S, Suhocki PV, Ludwig KA, Shetzline MA. Gastrointestinal bleeding in adult patients with Meckel diverticulum: the role of technetium 99m pertechnetate scan. South Med J . 2002; 95(11):1338–1341

Case 265

Kamal D. Singh

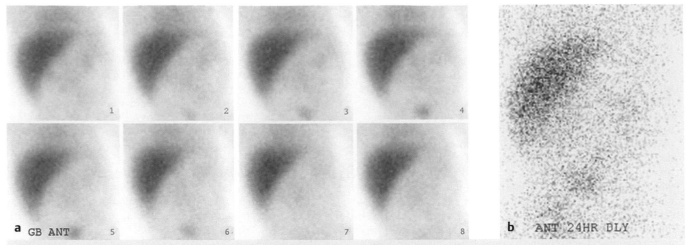

Fig. 265.1 Hepatobiliary scan with technetium-99m mebrofenin. **(a)** Sequential imaging during the first hour demonstrates no biliary excretion of radiotracer or bowel activity. There is mild persistence of cardiac blood pool activity. No significant change was noted on 4-hour delayed imaging (not included). **(b)** A 24-hour delayed anterior static image reveals persistent hepatic parenchymal activity with vicarious genitourinary excretion of radiotracer. There is no evidence of bowel activity.

■ Clinical Presentation

A 2-week-old neonate with jaundice (▶Fig. 265.1).

■ Key Imaging Finding

Persistent hepatogram on neonatal hepatobiliary imaging

■ Top 3 Differential Diagnoses

- **Biliary atresia**. Persistent neonatal conjugated hyperbilirubinemia may be due to biliary atresia or neonatal hepatitis. Biliary atresia involves malformation of extrahepatic ducts, leading to obstructive cholestasis and jaundice. Despite extrahepatic biliary ductal obstruction, intrahepatic biliary ducts are nondilated due to fibrosis. Prompt diagnosis of biliary atresia is essential, since success of the Kasai surgical procedure is greatest if performed within the first 2 months of life. Hepatobiliary imaging can exclude biliary atresia by demonstrating patency of the extrahepatic biliary system. Patients are pretreated with phenobarbital (5 mg/kg PO daily for 5 days) in order to optimize biliary excretion. Good hepatic uptake with poor hepatic clearance (persistent hepatogram) and non-visualization of intestinal activity within 24 hours of radiotracer injection is essentially diagnostic of biliary atresia. Intraoperative cholangiogram, however, remains the gold standard for definitive diagnosis.

- **Neonatal hepatitis**. Neonatal hepatitis may be due to a variety of metabolic, congenital, or infectious causes, as well as idiopathic. Scintigraphic findings include poor hepatic uptake of radiotracer with delayed or decreased biliary excretion, secondary to impaired hepatocyte function. On 24-hour delayed imaging, bowel activity is nearly always present, confirming patency of the biliary system. Lack of bowel activity may rarely be seen in severe hepatic dysfunction or inadequate patient preparation. Hepatic biopsy may further aid in definitive diagnosis prior to medical treatment.

- **Intrahepatic cholestasis from severe parenchymal disease**. Rarely, severe hepatocellular dysfunction or intrahepatic biliary malformation may result in cholestasis with no scintigraphically detectable excretion of radiotracer, resulting in a false positive study for biliary atresia. A repeat study could theoretically help exclude biliary atresia if the patient's hepatic function improves. However, liver biopsy and/or intraoperative cholangiogram may be necessary for definitive diagnosis.

■ Diagnosis

Biliary atresia

✓ Pearls

- Prompt hepatic uptake without biliary excretion into the bowel over 24 hours suggests biliary atresia.
- Pretreatment with phenobarbital increases biliary secretion of tracer, improving examination sensitivity.

- Visualization of radiotracer activity in the bowel essentially excludes biliary atresia.
- Neonatal hepatitis demonstrates poor hepatic uptake with delayed bowel activity.

Suggested Readings

Hartley JL, Davenport M, Kelly DA. Biliary atresia. Lancet . 2009; 374(9702):1704–1713

Kwatra N, Shalaby-Rana E, Narayanan S, Mohan P, Ghelani S, Majd M. Phenobarbital-enhanced hepatobiliary scintigraphy in the diagnosis of biliary atresia: two decades of experience at a tertiary center. Pediatr Radiol . 2013; 43(10):1365–1375

Shah I, Bhatnagar S, Rangarajan V, Patankar N.. Utility of Tc99m-Mebrofenin hepato-biliary scintigraphy (HIDA scan) for the diagnosis of biliary atresia. Trop Gastroenterol . 2012; 33(1):62–64

Case 266

Kamal D. Singh

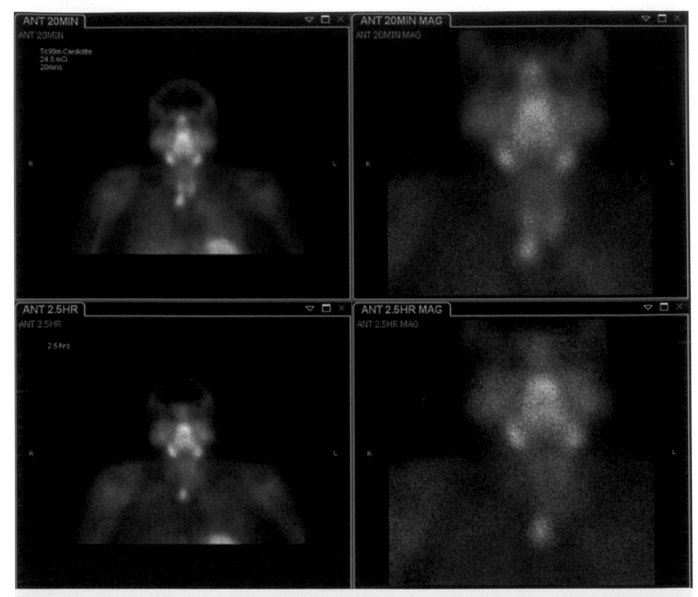

Fig. 266.1 Dual-phase parathyroid scan with technetium-99m sestamibi. Early imaging 20 minutes post injection (top images) demonstrates radiotracer uptake within the thyroid gland, along with a focus of moderately intense uptake inferior to the right lobe of the thyroid gland. Delayed imaging 2.5 hours postinjection (lower images) reveals appropriate washout of thyroid activity with persistent focal uptake inferior to the right thyroid pole. Physiologic activity is seen within salivary glands and myocardium on both early and delayed imaging.

■ Clinical Presentation

A 56-year-old woman with laboratory studies consistent with primary hyperparathyroidism (►Fig. 266.1).

■ Key Imaging Finding

Persistent focal cervical uptake on delayed sestamibi imaging

■ Top 3 Differential Diagnoses

- **Parathyroid adenoma.** Etiologies of primary hyperparathyroidism include parathyroid adenoma (90–94%), hyperplasia (6%), and much less commonly parathyroid carcinoma (<1%). Clinically, patients have manifestations of serum hypercalcemia and hypophosphatasia due to elevated parathyroid hormone (PTH), although more than half of patients may be asymptomatic. Technetium-99m (Tc99m) sestamibi initially localizes within both the thyroid gland and hyperfunctioning parathyroid adenoma with normal washout of thyroid activity on delayed imaging. Dual-phase (early and delayed) parathyroid scan utilizes this differential washout between thyroid gland and hyperfunctioning parathyroid tissue to localize an adenoma. While the majority of parathyroid adenomas are solitary and located adjacent to the thyroid tissue, they can be multiple in number and/or ectopic in location (10–15%); hence, the mediastinum is included in the field of view. Single-photon emission computed tomography (SPECT) imaging can improve contrast resolution for detection and localization of adenomas. Frequently, parathyroid adenomas may demonstrate rapid washout of radiotracer (similar to thyroid tissue), resulting in a false-negative study since no discrete focus persists on delayed imaging. In such cases, either iodine-123 (I123, oral) or Tc99m pertechnetate (IV) scan can be performed to outline normal thyroid tissue, and this image may be subtracted from the early Tc99m sestamibi image, making the parathyroid adenoma more conspicuous.

- **Thyroid adenoma or carcinoma.** Tc99m sestamibi demonstrates nonspecific localization in tumors via passive transport across cell membranes and active transport into mitochondria. False-positive studies include thyroid adenoma (most common), thyroid carcinoma, and parathyroid carcinoma. Dual isotope imaging (Tc99m sestamibi plus either I123 or Tc99m pertechnetate) with or without subtraction can improve sensitivity and avoid some of these pitfalls. Also, correlation with ultrasound or cross-sectional imaging (computed tomography [CT] or magnetic resonance imaging [MRI]) can be helpful.

- **Metastatic lymphadenopathy.** Tc99m sestamibi is a nonspecific tumor localization agent. Focal cervical activity may be seen within metastatic lymph nodes from any primary malignancy (including thyroid, head/neck, and breast cancers). Correlation with a clinical history and cross-sectional imaging is helpful in these cases.

■ Diagnosis

Parathyroid adenoma

✓ Pearls

- Parathyroid scan is performed as a localizing procedure prior to surgical exploration.
- Parathyroid adenoma is seen as focal persistent activity on delayed Tc99m sestamibi scan.
- False-positive studies may occur with thyroid adenoma, thyroid carcinoma, and parathyroid carcinoma.
- Thyroid imaging with either I123 or Tc99m pertechnetate can be used for problem solving.

Suggested Readings

Eslamy HK, Ziessman HA. Parathyroid scintigraphy in patients with primary hyperparathyroidism: 99mTc sestamibi SPECT and SPECT/CT. Radiographics . 2008; 28(5):1461–1476

Johnson NA, Tublin ME, Ogilvie JB. Parathyroid imaging: technique and role in the preoperative evaluation of primary hyperparathyroidism. AJR Am J Roentgenol . 2007; 188(6):1706–1715

Lavely WC, Goetze S, Friedman KP, et al. Comparison of SPECT/CT, SPECT, and planar imaging with single- and dual-phase (99m)Tc-sestamibi parathyroid scintigraphy. J Nucl Med . 2007; 48(7):1084–1089

Case 267

Kamal D. Singh

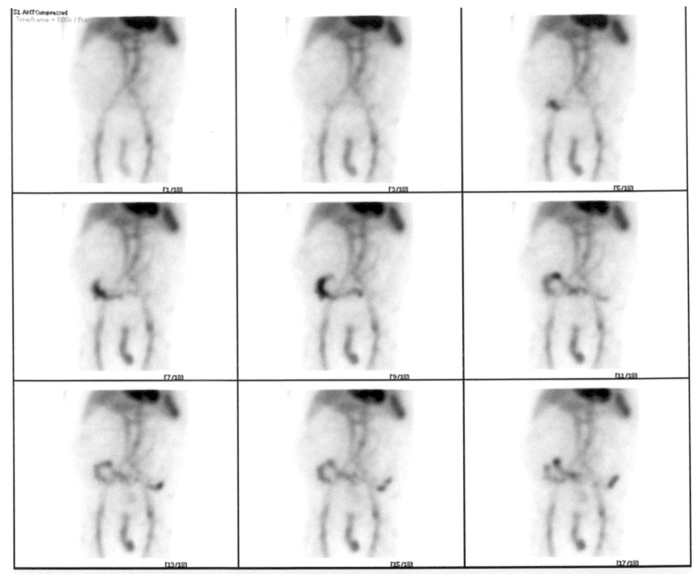

Fig. 267.1 Representative images from dynamic imaging performed for 90 minutes after technetium-99m-labeled red blood cell administration show the appearance of extravascular activity in the right lower quadrant which appears to conform to the bowel, progresses in intensity, and demonstrates both retrograde and antegrade movement.

■ Clinical Presentation

An 89-year-old man with lower gastrointestinal (GI) bleed
(▶ Fig. 267.1).

■ Key Imaging Finding

Intra-abdominal activity on technetium-99m (Tc99m)-labeled red blood cell (RBC) scan

■ Top 3 Differential Diagnoses

- **Active GI bleed**. Tc99m RBC scan is obtained for confirmation and localization of an active lower gastrointestinal bleed (hematochezia or bright red blood per rectum) prior to angiographic intervention. In contrast, patients with hematemesis from an upper GI bleed (proximal to ligament of Treitz) typically undergo endoscopy for diagnosis and management. Common causes of lower GI bleed include diverticulosis, angiodysplasia, inflammatory bowel disease, and neoplasm. After intravenous (IV) administration of the Tc-labeled RBC, dynamic imaging is performed for 60 to 90 minutes. Classic findings for active GI bleed include a focus of activity which appears and conforms to bowel anatomy, increases in activity over time, and demonstrates peristalsis (intraluminal antegrade or retrograde transit). Scintigraphy is highly sensitive and can detect bleeding rates as low as 0.1 mL/min, compared to 1 mL/min for angiography. Given the intermittent nature of most GI bleeds, Tc-RBC allows for delayed imaging up to 24 hours from the time of the initial injection. However, if bleeding is only detected on the delayed static imaging, precise localization is not possible due to bowel transit from the time of bleeding to the time of imaging.

- **Neoplasm or inflammatory bowel disease**. Hypervascular intestinal tumors or inflammatory bowel disease may be detected on a Tc-99m-labeled RBC scan as focal or segmental static activity that does not change in position over time. Cross-sectional imaging or colonoscopy aid in definitive diagnosis.

- **Genitourinary activity**. An area of activity that is fixed in location is not typical of an active GI bleed. Common causes of fixed activity include urinary tract activity—especially within the bladder—due to renal excretion of Tc-RBC. Additionally, penile activity in a man and uterine activity in a menstruating woman can mimic rectosigmoid bleeding. Static lateral views are useful in distinguishing these entities from an active GI bleed.

■ Additional Differential Diagnoses

- **Free technetium**. The in vitro technique for Tc-RBC allows for higher labeling efficiency (98%) compared to the modified in vivo (90%) or the in vivo (80%) methods. A higher labeling efficiency results in less free or unbound technetium in the blood-stream. Excess free technetium accumulates in the gastric mucosa and may enter the small bowel through peristalsis, simulating an active GI bleed. Imaging over the neck to detect thyroid activity can confirm the presence of free technetium.

■ Diagnosis

Active lower gastrointestinal bleed

✓ Pearls

- In vitro labeling of RBC has high labeling efficiency and is the preferred method for GI bleed scan.
- Active GI bleed presents with focal activity that increases with time and demonstrates peristalsis.

- If bleeding is not detected on the initial dynamic imaging, delayed images can be obtained up to 24 hours.
- Etiologies of false-positive scans usually present as focal activity without peristalsis.

Suggested Readings

Currie GM, Kiat H, Wheat JM. Scintigraphic evaluation of acute lower gastrointestinal hemorrhage: current status and future directions. J Clin Gastroenterol . 2011; 45(2):92–99

Mariani G, Pauwels EK, AlSharif A, et al. Radionuclide evaluation of the lower gastrointestinal tract. J Nucl Med . 2008; 49(5):776–787

Uliel L, Mellnick VM, Menias CO, Holz AL, McConathy J. Nuclear medicine in the acute clinical setting: indications, imaging findings, and potential pitfalls. Radiographics . 2013; 33(2):375–396

Case 268

Cameron C. Foster

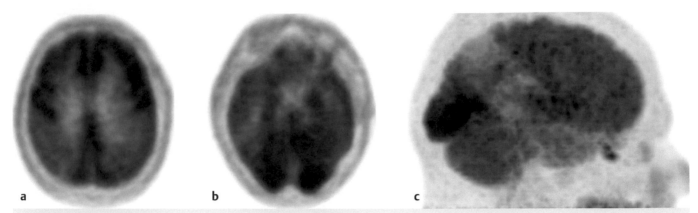

Fig. 268.1 (a, b) Attenuation-corrected axial FDG-PET images of the brain demonstrate decreased activity within the bilateral parietal **(a)** and temporal lobes **(b)** with intact normal activity within the bilateral frontal and occipital lobes. **(c)** Attenuation-corrected FDG-PET maximum intensity projection (MIP) image, in sagittal projection, demonstrates decreased activity in both the parietal and temporal lobes with intact normal activity within the cerebellum and the frontal and occipital lobes.

■ Clinical Presentation

A 62-year-old man with a 6-year history of cognitive decline (▶Fig. 268.1).

■ Key Imaging Finding

Decreased cortical fluorodeoxyglucose (FDG) activity in the setting of dementia

■ Top 3 Differential Diagnoses

- **Alzheimer disease (AD)**. AD is the most common dementing disorder affecting adults. Presentation is usually after the age of 65 years, and prevalence increases with age. The initial imaging findings are of decreased metabolism (FDG-positron emission tomography [PET]) and blood flow (single-photon emission computed tomography [SPECT]) in the bilateral temporoparietal areas with relative sparing of the primary motor, somatosensory, and visual cortices. One of the earliest findings includes hypometabolic posterior cingulate gyri. Early-stage AD may show hemispheric asymmetry. Later stage AD will also begin to show metabolic decline in the frontal lobes at a faster rate than normal aging dementia. In general, the amount of decreased metabolism correlates with the degree of symptoms.
- **Pick disease**. Pick disease is the classic, although rare, member of the frontotemporal dementia (FTD) family. It is characterized by decreased metabolism in the bilateral frontal lobes and anterior temporal lobes on FDG-PET imaging. Differentiation

from other disorders, such as AD, is based on symptoms, as Pick disease has memory impairment as a secondary or absent feature rather than a primary symptom as is seen in AD. Differential considerations for isolated decreased metabolism in the frontotemporal regions include entities such as depression, schizophrenia, cocaine abuse, and amyotrophic lateral sclerosis (ALS). This distribution is rarely seen in AD.
- **Multi-infarct dementia (MID)**. MID is the most common cause of vascular dementia and is the second most common cause of all dementias for adults older than 65 years (behind AD). While MID is usually identified via computed tomography (CT) or magnetic resonance imaging (MRI), FDG-PET and SPECT imaging show similar patterns of decreased activity in a diffuse or multi-focal distribution that progresses over time. Frontotemporal distribution can be seen in MID and can be difficult to differentiate from other FTDs; diffuse distribution of MID can also be difficult to differentiate from severe AD.

■ Additional Differential Diagnoses

- **Parkinson disease (PD) and Lewy body dementia (LBD)**. PD is largely a clinical diagnosis that has normal appearance on FDG-PET in early stages (striatum may be mildly increased). In later stages, decreased activity will be seen in the cortices and will progress along with the disease. Use of serial FDOPA-PET scans in patients with PD will initially show decreased activity within the posterior putamen with sparing of the caudate that, over time, will involve more of the putamen and eventually

include the posterior aspect of the caudate. Patients with PD may develop dementia. LBD is related to PD with patients initially presenting with dementia and occasional visual hallucinations, followed by development of movement abnormalities with rigidity and tremors similar to PD. LBD may have a similar imaging appearance to AD on FDG-PET with less sparing of the occipital lobes.

■ Diagnosis

Alzheimer disease

✓ Pearls

- AD shows bilateral temporoparietal hypometabolism with sparing of the occipital lobes (visual cortices).
- Frontal lobe hypometabolism can be seen in FTD (e.g., Pick disease), depression, schizophrenia, and ALS.

- MID presents as multifocal regions of decreased activity.
- Dementia with Lewy bodies has similar appearance to AD with less sparing of occipital lobe.

Suggested Readings

Herholz K, Herscovitch P, Heiss WD. NeuroPET. Berlin, Germany: Springer-Verlag; 2004

Hoffman JM, Welsh-Bohmer KA, Hanson M, et al. FDG PET imaging in patients with pathologically verified dementia. J Nucl Med . 2000; 41(11):1920–1928

Van Heertum RL, Tikofsky RS. Positron emission tomography and single-photon emission computed tomography brain imaging in the evaluation of dementia. Semin Nucl Med . 2003; 33(1):77–85

Case 269

Cameron C. Foster

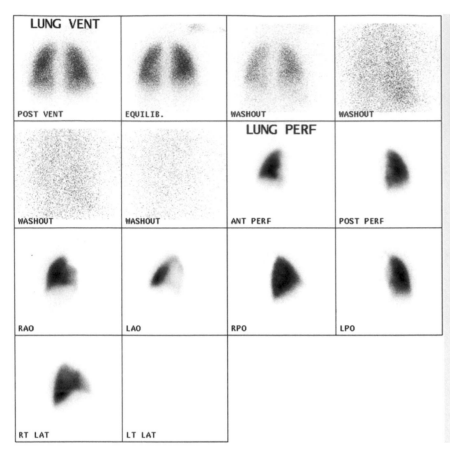

Fig. 269.1 Ventilation-Perfusion scintigraphy (V/Q scan) demonstrates normal inspiratory and equilibrium ventilation images in posterior projection without evidence of tracer (Xe-133 gas) retention on washout images. Perfusion imaging in multiple obliquities demonstrates unilateral absence of tracer (Technetium-99m microaggregated albumin [Tc99m MAA]) in the left lung with normal distribution of tracer within the right lung.

■ Clinical Presentation

A 54-year-old man with shortness of breath (▶Fig. 269.1).

■ Key Imaging Finding

Unilateral diffusely decreased lung perfusion

■ Top 3 Differential Diagnoses for Perfusion Worse than Ventilation

- **External compression (tumor, fibrosing mediastinitis).** Unilateral absence of lung perfusion is a rare finding. A ventilation/perfusion (V/Q) scan cannot determine the cause on its own. However, extrinsic compression of the pulmonary artery is the most common cause of a perfusion defect which is worse than ventilation. Typically it is from a central lung tumor. Fibrosing mediastinitis is another entity which could lead to pulmonary artery occlusion and absence of perfusion. Cross-sectional imaging is essential to determine the presence of external compression.
- **Pulmonary artery anomalies or corrected congenital heart disease.** Pulmonary artery atresia, severe pulmonary artery stenosis, or pulmonary webs may cause unilateral absence of perfusion with perfusion defect worse than ventilation. Additionally, corrected congenital heart disease may produce similar findings on V/Q scan. Dedicated contrast enhanced cross-sectional imaging via computed tomography (CT) or magnetic resonance imaging/magnetic resonance angiography (MRI/MRA) can greatly improve detection, as well as correlation for prior surgical history.
- **Massive unilateral pulmonary embolism (PE).** Pulmonary emboli typically present with wedge-shaped, peripheral, segmental mismatched perfusion defects. While massive unilateral PE can produce unilateral absent perfusion, it is less likely in comparison to other causes. Massive PE of this magnitude will often have more than one V/Q mismatch affecting both lungs. As per the Prospective Investigation of Pulmonary Embolism Diagnosis II (PIOPED II) criteria, absent perfusion of an entire lung is low probability of PE.

■ Top 3 Differential Diagnoses for Ventilation Worse than Perfusion

- **Mucus plug.** A mucous plug may obstruct ventilation with compensatory vasoconstriction of the pulmonary arteries. The degree of accompanying perfusion abnormality will increase with time with continued obstruction due to arteriolar constriction induced by local hypoxia. As this is primarily an airway abnormality, the ventilation defect will be larger than the perfusion defect.
- **Endobronchial lesion (mass or foreign body).** Endobronchial lesions can cause a ventilation defect which is larger than perfusion. Central lesions can cause diminished activity within an entire lung. The relative decrease in ventilation to perfusion is an indicator of the extent of luminal involvement.
- **Unilateral diffuse parenchymal disease.** Diffuse air-space disease, atelectasis, or large pneumothorax involving an entire lung will result in decreased or absent ventilation with compensatory vasoconstriction of the pulmonary arteries. The degree of lung involvement will determine the degree of perfusion and ventilation defects.

■ Diagnosis

Extrinsic compression (left hilar malignancy)

✓ Pearls

- Ventilation scan may be performed with Xe133 gas or Tc99m DTPA aerosol.
- Extrinsic pulmonary artery compression is the most common cause of unilateral absent perfusion.
- Central airway obstruction is the most common cause of unilateral ventilation > perfusion defect.
- Wedge-shaped (peripheral), segmental mismatched perfusion defects are concerning for pulmonary emboli.

Suggested Readings

Pickhardt PJ, Fischer KC. Unilateral hypoperfusion or absent perfusion on pulmonary scintigraphy: differential diagnosis. AJR Am J Roentgenol . 1998; 171(1):145–150

Slonim SM, Molgaard CP, Khawaja IT, Seldin DW. Unilateral absence of right-lung perfusion with normal ventilation on radionuclide lung scan as a sign of aortic dissection. J Nucl Med . 1994; 35(6):1044–1047

White RI , Jr, James AE , Jr, Wagner HN , Jr. The significance of unilateral absence of pulmonary artery perfusion by lung scanning. Am J Roentgenol Radium Ther Nucl Med . 1971; 111(3):501–509

Case 270

Cameron C. Foster

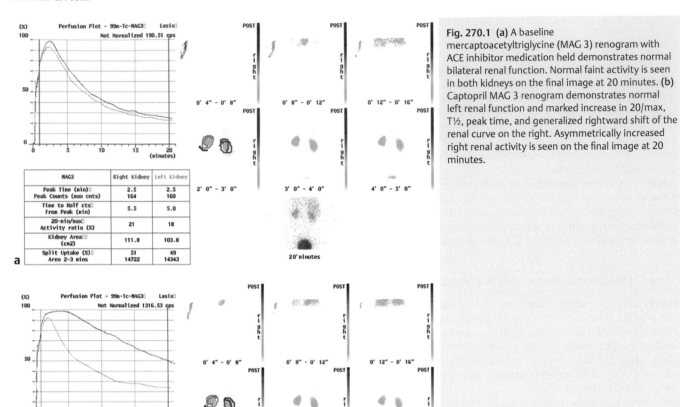

Fig. 270.1 (a) A baseline mercaptoacetyltriglycine (MAG 3) renogram with ACE inhibitor medication held demonstrates normal bilateral renal function. Normal faint activity is seen in both kidneys on the final image at 20 minutes. **(b)** Captopril MAG 3 renogram demonstrates normal left renal function and marked increase in 20/max, T½, peak time, and generalized rightward shift of the renal curve on the right. Asymmetrically increased right renal activity is seen on the final image at 20 minutes.

■ Clinical Presentation

A 61-year-old woman with hypertension (▶Fig. 270.1).

■ Key Imaging Finding

Worsening renal function on (mercaptoacetyltriglycine [MAG] 3) renal scan following Captopril administration

■ Top 3 Differential Diagnoses

- **Renal artery stenosis (RAS).** Renovascular hypertension accounts for approximately 1–4% of all hypertension cases. It is most commonly due to atherosclerosis or fibromuscular dysplasia. Although other modalities such as magnetic resonance angiography (MRA) may be better at detecting an actual stenosis, angiotensin-converting enzyme (ACE) inhibition renography is very specific for functional renovascular hypertension. Narrowing of the afferent renal artery greater than 60% typically is the low-end cutoff for causing renovascular hypertension via the renin angiotensin cascade. ACE inhibitor is administered before radiotracer injection, and the patient is monitored hemodynamically during imaging. MAG 3 imaging is considered positive by curvilinear changes due to cortical retention (increase in time to peak cortical activity and 20/max, decreased split function, rightward shift of the curve, etc.) when compared to a baseline scan. When appropriately performed, the test approaches 90% sensitivity and 95% specificity. A positive study generally predicts improvement in hypertension upon revascularization.

- **Unilateral urinary obstruction.** Differentiation between unilateral urinary obstruction and RAS by MAG 3 renography is usually done by appearance of an obstructive curve (poor/delayed excretion) on the baseline scan that does not improve with Lasix administration. If the affected kidney is already demonstrating significant renal impairment, the response to Lasix as well as to the ACE inhibitor challenge may be diminished, which results in reduced sensitivity and specificity for both entities.

- **False-positive scan in patients on calcium channel blocker.** False-positive renal impairment on a MAG 3 renogram with ACE inhibitor challenge study can be seen in patients who are on chronic calcium channel blockers. This effect should be bilateral and symmetric (except in cases of existing unilateral renal impairment or nephrectomy). In the setting of bilateral renal decline on a renogram in the presence of calcium channel blocking medication, the study should be repeated after discontinuance of these medications.

■ Diagnosis

Renal artery stenosis (right-sided)

✓ Pearls

- Adequate fluid hydration prior to and blood pressure monitoring during Captopril scan are important.
- A positive scan suggests hemodynamically significant RAS and predicts benefit from revascularization.

- The baseline renal scan with MAG 3 is compared to a post-Captopril renal scan with MAG 3 for diagnosis.
- False positives can result from dehydration, obstruction, hypotension, and calcium channel blockers.

Suggested Readings

Ludwig V, Martin WH, Delbeke D. Calcium channel blockers: a potential cause of false-positive Captopril renography. Clin Nucl Med . 2003; 28(2):108–112

Soulez G, Oliva VL, Turpin S, Lambert R, Nicolet V, Therasse E. Imaging of renovascular hypertension: respective values of renal scintigraphy, renal Doppler US, and MR angiography. Radiographics . 2000; 20(5):1355–1368, discussion 1368–1372

Taylor AT , Jr, Fletcher JW, Nally JV , Jr, et al; Society of Nuclear Medicine. Procedure guideline for diagnosis of renovascular hypertension. J Nucl Med . 1998; 39(7):1297–1302

Case 271

Kamal D. Singh

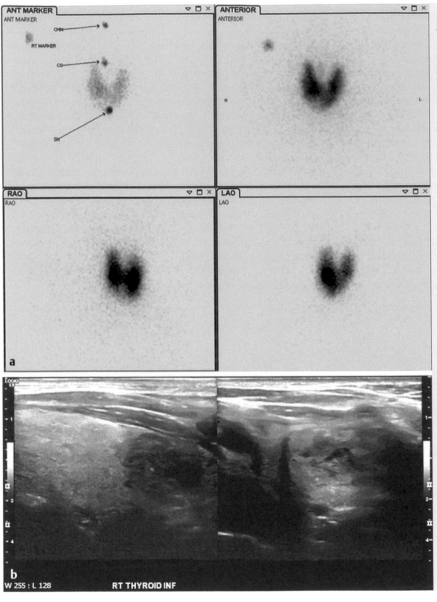

Fig. 271.1 (a) Planar imaging of the thyroid with iodine-123 performed at 24 hours after oral radioiodine administration demonstrates photopenia in the inferior right thyroid lobe. Both 4- and 24-hour uptake measurements were normal, and TSH was normal at the time of the examination. **(b)** Sonographic images show a correlative nodule.

■ Clinical Presentation

A 63-year-old man with solitary 2-cm right thyroid nodule and a long history of laboratory values consistent with subclinical hyperthyroidism (►Fig. 271.1).

■ Key Imaging Finding

Cold nodule on iodine-123 (I123) thyroid scan

■ Top 3 Differential Diagnoses

• **Thyroid carcinoma.** Ultrasound (US) and fine needle aspiration (FNA) are the primary diagnostic procedures for thyroid nodules in a euthyroid patient. Nuclear medicine thyroid imaging for nodule characterization should be reserved for patients with hyperthyroidism (suppressed thyroid-stimulating hormone (TSH)) or an indeterminate biopsy. Cold or nonfunctioning nodules on I123 thyroid scans are nonspecific and may represent colloid cyst (40%), nonfunctioning adenoma (40%), or thyroid carcinoma (15–20%). The incidence of cancer is lower (<5%) in the setting of multinodular goiter. Hot or hyperfunctioning nodules on I123 scan, defined as uptake in the nodule suppressing the rest of the thyroid gland, are essentially always benign. However, a hot nodule on Technetium (Tc) pertechnetate scan requires further evaluation with I123 scan to exclude a discordant nodule, which requires FNA to exclude thyroid carcinoma. Risk factors for thyroid malignancy include age <20 or >60 years, male patient, family history, prior radiation therapy to the head/neck, and/or a dominant nodule with concerning US features (solid, hypoechoic, and hypervascular nodule with microcalcifications). Papillary carcinoma is the most common subtype, followed by follicular. Medullary and anaplastic carcinomas are less common and are highly aggressive. Treatment of localized thyroid carcinoma typically consists of total thyroidectomy, followed by I131 ablation therapy.

Patients are followed up with thyroglobulin levels, as well as whole body I131 imaging, for at least 2 years after radioiodine ablation.

• **Colloid cyst.** Colloid cysts are benign localized follicles filled with gelatinous colloid. They usually originate from cystic degeneration of thyroid adenomas and are hyperintense on T1-weighted magnetic resonance imaging (MRI) due to high protein content. US characteristics include a cystic lesion with inspissated colloid, which is hyperechoic and demonstrates ring-down or comet tail artifact.

• **Nonfunctioning adenoma.** Thyroid adenomas are benign lesions that may be functioning (hot nodule) or nonfunctioning (cold nodule). They can be multiple in the setting of multinodular goiter. On US, benign adenomas are typically encapsulated well with a hypoechoic halo. Interval growth is not unusual. A dominant hyperfunctioning adenoma with suppression of the remainder of the gland in the setting of hyperthyroidism is called an autonomous nodule (produces thyroid hormones independent of TSH). Hyperthyroid patients with multinodular goiter or autonomous nodules are generally more resistant to ablation therapy than patients with Graves' disease; hence, these patients are treated with higher doses of I131 (about 30 mCi).

■ Diagnosis

Nonfunctioning adenoma

✓ Pearls

• I123 thyroid scan is indicated in hyperthyroidism or nodule evaluation after an indeterminate biopsy.
• A cold nodule may be a colloid cyst (40%), nonfunctioning adenoma (40%), or thyroid cancer (15–20%).

• A hot nodule on Tc pertechnetate may be cold or "discordant" on I123 (trapping without organification).
• Papillary and follicular cancers are amenable to I131 ablation; medullary and anaplastic carcinomas are not.

Suggested Readings

Intenzo CM, Dam HQ, Manzone TA, Kim SM. Imaging of the thyroid in benign and malignant disease. Semin Nucl Med . 2012; 42(1):49–61

Nachiappan AC, Metwalli ZA, Hailey BS, Patel RA, Ostrowski ML, Wynne DM. The thyroid: review of imaging features and biopsy techniques with radiologic-pathologic correlation. Radiographics . 2014; 34(2):276–293

Yeung MJ, Serpell JW. Management of the solitary thyroid nodule. Oncologist . 2008; 13(2):105–112

Case 272

Vicki Nagano

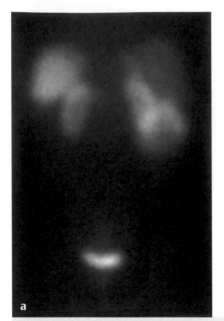
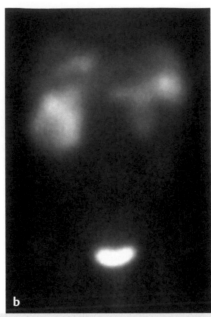
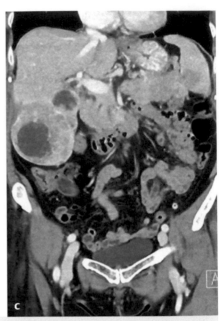

Fig. 272.1 (a, b) Twenty-four-hour delayed indium-111 (I-111) pentetreotide images show several regions of abnormal uptake within the liver and pancreatic tail with **(c)** heterogeneous masses seen on corresponding coronal reformatted contrast-enhanced CT.

■ Clinical Presentation

A 73-year-old woman with right liver mass in the setting of pancreatic tail masses and smaller liver lesions (▶ Fig. 272.1).

■ Key Imaging Finding

Focal abdominal uptake on indium-111 (In111) pentetreotide scan (OctreoScan)

■ Top 3 Differential Diagnoses

- **Neuroendocrine tumor.** Somatostatin is a peptide that inhibits the release of anterior pituitary hormones and certain intestinal and pancreatic peptides, such as insulin, gastrin, glucagon, and cholecystokinin (CCK). In111 pentetreotide (OctreoScan) contains an amino acid analog of somatostatin and is frequently used for the evaluation of neuroendocrine tumors. Normal radiopharmaceutical distribution includes intense splenic uptake with slightly less prominent uptake in the kidneys, followed by the liver. Physiologic uptake is also seen within the thyroid gland, gallbladder, bowel, and bladder. Planar imaging surveys the entire body; single-photon emission computed tomography (SPECT) imaging is essential in the chest and abdomen. OctreoScan is most commonly used for islet cell and carcinoid tumors. The sensitivity for islet cell tumors varies based upon the subtype: insulinoma (50%), gastrinoma (75–93%), glucagonoma (73%), and VIPoma (88%). Sensitivity for various other neuroendocrine tumors is as follows: carcinoid (80–90%), neuroblastoma (over 85%), medullary thyroid carcinoma (54%), malignant pheochromocytoma (87%), paraganglioma (93%), and small cell carcinoma of the lung (100%). Neuroblastoma and pheochromocytoma are more commonly imaged with iodine-123 meta-iodobenzylguanidine (MIBG), as physiologic renal uptake with OctreoScan may obscure an adrenal lesion.

- **Metastatic disease.** Non-neuroendocrine tumors that contain somatostatin receptors and can metastasize to the mesentery include non-small cell lung cancer, breast cancer, and lymphoma (sensitivity of ~70% each). Lymphoma is the most common malignant neoplasm affecting the mesentery. Approximately 30–50% of patients with non-Hodgkin lymphoma will have disease in mesenteric lymph nodes.

- **Granulomatous disease.** Somatostatin receptors are also present in granulomatous diseases, such as sarcoidosis and tuberculosis (TB). Intra-abdominal TB lymphadenopathy has most commonly been reported in the lesser omental, mesenteric, and upper para-aortic regions. Contrast computed tomography (CT) typically demonstrates rim enhancement in the peripheral inflammatory reaction and a low-attenuation center representing the caseous necrosis. In contrast, malignant and reactive lymph nodes generally demonstrate homogeneous enhancement on contrast-enhanced CT. Enlarged mesenteric nodes can also be seen in some non-infectious, inflammatory conditions such as sarcoidosis.

■ Diagnosis

Metastatic pancreatic neuroendocrine tumor (gastrinoma)

✓ Pearls

- In111 pentetreotide (OctreoScan) is useful for imaging metastatic neuroendocrine tumors.
- Physiologic activity is seen within spleen, liver, gallbladder, kidneys, bowel, bladder, and faint thyroid.

- In111 uptake is also seen in granulomatous disease, lymphoma, meningioma, astrocytoma, and breast cancer.
- Neuroblastoma and pheochromocytoma are more commonly imaged with MIBG.

Suggested Readings

Balon HR, Brown TL, Goldsmith SJ, et al; Society of Nuclear Medicine. The SNM practice guideline for somatostatin receptor scintigraphy 2.0. J Nucl Med Technol . 2011; 39(4):317–324

Intenzo CM, Jabbour S, Lin HC, et al. Scintigraphic imaging of body neuroendocrine tumors. Radiographics . 2007; 27(5):1355–1369

Lucey BC, Stuhlfaut JW, Soto JA. Mesenteric lymph nodes seen at imaging: causes and significance. Radiographics . 2005; 25(2):351–365

Sheth S, Horton KM, Garland MR, Fishman EK. Mesenteric neoplasms: CT appearances of primary and secondary tumors and differential diagnosis. Radiographics . 2003; 23(2):457–473, quiz 535–536

Case 273

Kamal D. Singh

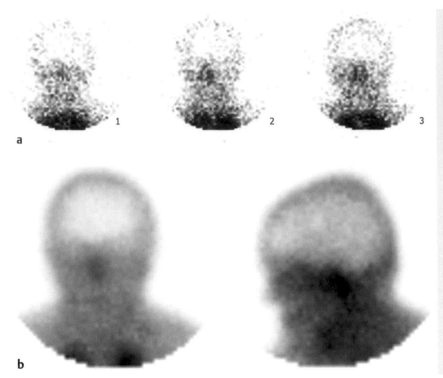

Fig. 273.1 Brain death study with technetium-99m hexamethylpropyleneamine (HMPAO). **(a)** Selected images from dynamic flow (1 second per frame for 1 minute) demonstrate absence of intracranial flow. **(b)** Blood pool imaging in anterior and lateral projections reveals absent cerebral or cerebellar uptake and physiologic faint scalp activity, along with increased activity in the nasal region ("hot nose" sign). These findings were confirmed on delayed SPECT imaging of the head (not included).

■ Clinical Presentation

A 57-year-old man unresponsive after a motor vehicle accident (▶Fig. 273.1).

■ Key Imaging Finding

Absent intracranial activity on a technetium-99m hexamethyl-propyleneamine oxime (Tc99m HMPAO) scan

■ Top 3 Differential Diagnoses

- **Brain death**. Brain death is a clinical diagnosis utilizing a combination of physical examination, electroencephalography, and imaging findings. A brain death scan has high specificity as a confirmatory study for absent intracranial perfusion. Scintigraphic imaging can be performed at the patient's bedside with a portable gamma camera. Imaging may be performed with a non-specific flow agent (Tc99m diethylenetriamine pentaacetic acid [DTPA]), or with lipophilic brain perfusion agents (Tc99m HMPAO or Tc99m ethyl cysteinate dimer [ECD]) which cross the blood–brain barrier and are extracted by viable brain tissue proportional to cerebral flow. A scalp band or tourniquet may be placed around the head to avoid interfering activity from extracranial vessels. The scalp band, however, is contraindicated in pediatric patients due to increased intracranial pressure. First-minute dynamic flow imaging is performed in an anterior projection, with the subsequent static blood pool images in both anterior and lateral projections. Delayed single-photon emission computed tomography (SPECT) imaging may improve sensitivity in cases where lipophilic agents are utilized. Normal imaging reveals symmetric flow within the anterior and middle cerebral arteries ("trident" sign) on the anterior view, with visualization of dural venous sinuses on blood pool imaging. In brain death, there is termination of carotid activity at the skull base due to increased intracranial pressure overcoming the perfusion pressure, thereby shunting blood through the external carotid artery branches projecting over nasal region ("hot nose" sign).

- **Injection error.** Peripheral intravenous injection of the radiotracer is performed as a rapid/tight bolus. A proper bolus is confirmed by visualizing distinct activity within the proximal common carotid arteries. Dose infiltration, slow radiotracer injection, or missed bolus can result in false-positive studies, especially when flow agents (like Tc99m DTPA, which does not cross the blood–brain barrier) are used. Tc99m DTPA is rapidly cleared through renal excretion which allows for reinjection and reimaging in the setting of equivocal or technically limited studies.

- **Poor radiopharmaceutical labeling/quality control.** Quality control is essential with lipophilic brain-specific agents. Poor labeling and instability can result in a false-positive examination. HMPAO should be labeled with fresh eluate, within 2 hours of elution. If it is stabilized, it has a shelf life of 4 hours after labeling.

■ Diagnosis

Brain death

✓ Pearls

- Absent intracranial flow and no cerebral/cerebellar uptake of Tc99m HMPAO confirm brain death in the appropriate clinical setting.
- Brain parenchymal uptake of radiotracer is not seen with flow agents like Tc99m DTPA.
- Scintigraphic evaluation is unaffected by drug intoxication, hypothermia, or metabolic derangements.
- Besides brain death, Tc99m HMPAO can image cerebral ischemia, seizure focus, and dementia.

Suggested Readings

Conrad GR, Sinha P. Scintigraphy as a confirmatory test of brain death. Semin Nucl Med . 2003; 33(4):312–323

Donohoe KJ, Agrawal G, Frey KA, et al. SNM practice guideline for brain death scintigraphy 2.0. J Nucl Med Technol . 2012; 40(3):198–203

Sinha P, Conrad GR. Scintigraphic confirmation of brain death. Semin Nucl Med . 2012; 42(1):27–32

Case 274

Ely A. Wolin

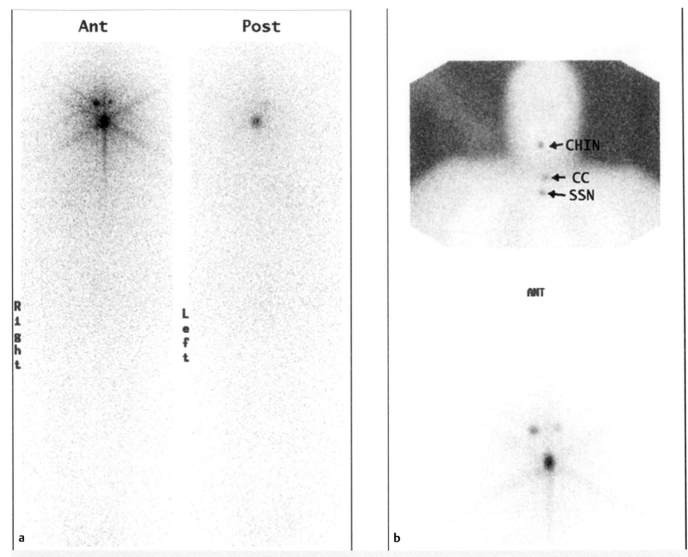

Fig. 274.1 (a,b) Postablation I131 whole body scan. (a) Anterior and posterior whole body images and (b) spot views of the neck with and without markers demonstrate midline cervical uptake in the expected region of the thyroid bed with "star artifact."

■ Clinical Presentation

A 37-year-old woman with a history of papillary thyroid carcinoma post total thyroidectomy and 107 mCi iodine-131 (I131) therapy (►Fig. 274.1).

■ Key Imaging Finding

Focal neck uptake on I131 postablation scan

■ Top 3 Differential Diagnoses

- **Residual thyroid tissue.** Patients with differentiated thyroid carcinoma are typically treated surgically with postoperative radioiodine (I131) ablation. The goals of postoperative radioiodine therapy are to ablate residual thyroid tissue to facilitate surveillance, provide adjuvant therapy for microscopic iodine avid disease, and further evaluate for metastases with posttreatment scan. The I131 dose is determined by risk of recurrence, typically falling between 75 and 200 mCi. Limiting factors generally include no more than 200 rads to bone marrow and a 1 Curie (Ci) lifetime limit. Limiting the dose to the lungs with known pulmonary metastases is also important to avoid pulmonary fibrosis. There has been a push to decrease to a 30 mCi remnant ablation dose in low-risk patients, but this approach has not been completely validated, as pre-ablation staging is limited. In preparation for ablation, the patient should discontinue thyroid hormone replacement therapy (6 weeks for T4 and 2 weeks for T3) and should be on a low iodine diet for at least 10–14 days. As an alternative to hormone withdrawal, recombinant thyroid-stimulating hormone (TSH) may be administered 48 and 24 hours prior to dose administration. If there is concern for a significant thyroid remnant, a preablation scan can be performed with 1–2 mCi I123 or <5 mCi I131, although with I131 specifically, there is a concern for thyroid stunning, which will limit effectiveness of the therapy dose. Postablation imaging is usually performed 7 to 10 days after therapy as a baseline for future surveillance scans and to provide more accurate staging information. On any I131 imaging study, a high degree of functional thyroid tissue (residual thyroid tissue or metastatic disease) may result in septal penetration due to the high energy of the I131 photons (364 keV), which may result in the "star artifact."
- **Cervical nodal metastases.** Thyroid carcinoma may have local (cervical nodes) or distant (mediastinal, pulmonary, or osseous) metastases, which requires a larger I131 ablation dose than does ablation of normal thyroid gland remnant. Papillary carcinoma typically spreads via lymphatics to local cervical lymph nodes, whereas follicular carcinoma spreads hematogenously to distant sites. After the initial radioiodine therapy, surveillance includes serum thyroglobulin levels, and if indicated, a diagnostic I131 whole body metascan. I131 cancer treatment may be repeated in event of recurrent disease with a 6-month to 1-year interval between ablation doses.
- **Physiologic pharyngeal/esophageal activity.** On all I131 or I123 scans, physiologic uptake is expected within the salivary glands, stomach, intestines, and urinary bladder. Non-focal hepatic uptake is also seen in cases where there is residual functioning thyroid tissue, since thyroid hormone is metabolized by the liver. Focal increased activity, however, is more suggestive of metastases. In addition to primary renal excretion, radioiodine is excreted in saliva. Therefore, transient swallowed activity within the pharynx or esophagus may mimic cervical or mediastinal metastases. Physiologic activity can be confirmed by re-imaging after the patient drinks water.

■ Diagnosis

Residual or remnant thyroid bed activity

✓ Pearls

- Pretherapy I123 or I131 diagnostic metascan can identify residual thyroid tissue and detect metastases.
- Using I131 for pretherapy scan comes with risk of thyroid "stunning" prior to therapy.
- Postablation I131 whole body scan provides additional staging information and establishes a baseline.
- Positron emission tomography is recommended if thyroglobulin is elevated, and I131 scan is negative.

Suggested Readings

Blumhardt R, Wolin EA, Phillips WT, et al. Current controversies in the initial post-surgical radioactive iodine therapy for thyroid cancer: a narrative review. Endocr Relat Cancer . 2014; 21(6):R473–R484

Haugen BR, Alexander EK, Bible KC, et al. 2015 American Thyroid Association management guidelines for adult patients with thyroid nodules and differentiated thyroid cancer: The American Thyroid Association Guidelines Task Force on Thyroid Nodules and Differentiated Thyroid Cancer. Thyroid . 2016; 26(1):1–133

Mazzaferri EL. Managing thyroid microcarcinomas. Yonsei Med J . 2012; 53(1):1–14

Case 275

Kamal D. Singh

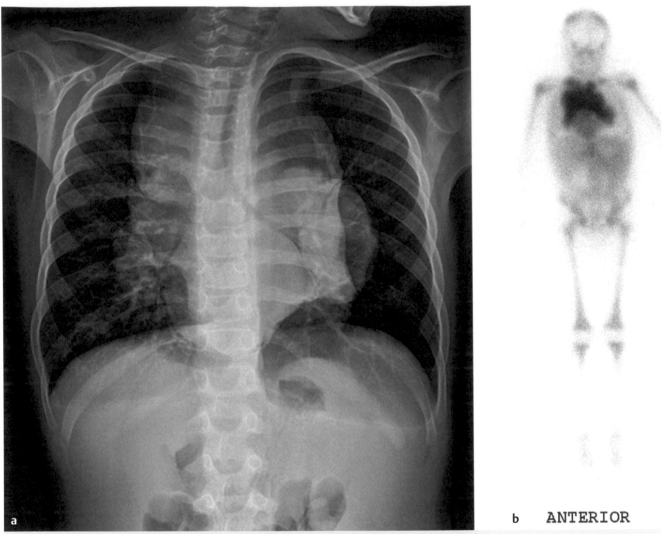

Fig. 275.1 **(a)** Frontal chest radiograph demonstrates mediastinal widening with bilateral hilar enlargement. **(b)** Anterior whole body Ga-67 scan performed 48 hours postinjection demonstrates corresponding intense mediastinal and hilar uptake. Physiologic uptake is seen within the lacrimal glands, salivary glands, liver, spleen, intestines, bone, and bone marrow.

■ Clinical Presentation

A 10-year-old boy with cough and weight loss (▶Fig. 275.1).

■ Key Imaging Finding

Increased mediastinal uptake on gallium (Ga) scan

■ Top 3 Differential Diagnoses

- **Malignancy.** Ga-avid neoplasms include lymphoma, hepatoma, lung cancer, sarcoma (except Kaposi sarcoma which is thallium avid, but Ga negative), and melanoma. Typical dose for tumor imaging is 10 mCi with whole body imaging performed at 48–72 hours postinjection. Physiologic activity includes lacrimal and salivary glands, liver > spleen, breast, cortical bone, and bone marrow, with primarily renal excretion during first 24 hours and gastrointestinal excretion thereafter. Ga67 has a physical half-life of 78 hours and multiple photopeaks (only 93, 184, and 296 keV are acquired for clinical imaging). Its primary mode of localization includes resemblance to ferric ion and as a calcium analog. Sensitivity for detection of lymphoma is based upon the size of the lesion (higher if >1 cm) and tumor grade (lower detection rate for low grade). Ga67 is especially useful for defining complete response and for early detection of viable tumor recurrence/relapse after chemoradiation therapy. Baseline Ga67 scan prior to the therapy initiation can help for future follow-up. Evaluation of the abdomen is limited due to interfering physiologic intestinal activity. PET-CT with its higher resolution has now largely replaced Ga67 for malignancy (lymphoma) workup.
- **Granulomatous disease.** Active pulmonary or mediastinal sarcoidosis is Ga-avid, and the degree of uptake typically corresponds to the severity of disease. Right paratracheal and bilateral hilar lymphadenopathy uptake is seen as the "lambda sign," while prominent bilateral lacrimal and parotid activity represents the "panda sign." Ga67 scan is only positive in the setting of active parenchymal disease and is negative while in remission. Ga uptake is also seen with other pulmonary granulomatous processes, to include TB and fungal disease.
- **Nonspecific inflammatory/infectious process**. Ga67 citrate accumulates within sites of inflammation or infection. Infection imaging is generally performed with 5 mCi, starting at 24 hours postinjection. Ga67 is especially useful for workup of a fever of an unknown origin, detection of opportunistic pulmonary infections in immunocompromised patients, and for osteomyelitis (especially vertebral). Diffuse lung activity can be seen with pneumocystis pneumonia in patients with acquired immunodeficiency syndrome (AIDS). Ga67 may have non-specific uptake within areas of inflammation, such as reactive lymphadenopathy in setting of pneumonia, hyperplastic thymic tissue, postsurgical bed, or recent radiation therapy. Indium-111 labeled white blood cells (WBCs) is a more specific agent for acute pyogenic infections.

■ Diagnosis

Malignancy (Hodgkin lymphoma)

✓ Pearls

- Focal uptake on Ga scan is nonspecific and may represent inflammation, infection, or neoplasm.
- Diffuse lung activity can be seen with pneumocystis pneumonia in patients with AIDS.
- Renal excretion of radiotracer is seen during the first 24 hours with primarily gastrointestinal excretion thereafter.

Suggested Readings

Hussain R, Christie DR, Gebski V, Barton MB, Gruenewald SM. The role of the gallium scan in primary extranodal lymphoma. J Nucl Med . 1998; 39(1):95–98

Liu FY, Shiau YC, Yen RF, Wang JJ, Ho ST, Kao CH. Comparison of gallium-67 citrate and technetium-99m tetrofosmin scan to detect Hodgkin disease. Ann Nucl Med . 2003; 17(6):439–442

Love C, Palestro CJ. Radionuclide imaging of infection. J Nucl Med Technol . 2004; 32(2):47–57, quiz 58–59

Case 276

Vicki Nagano

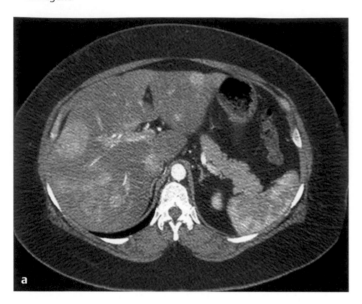
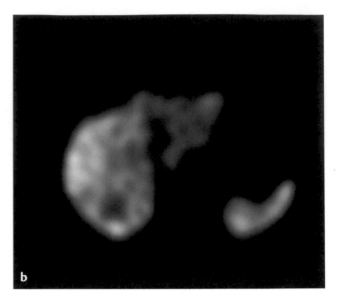
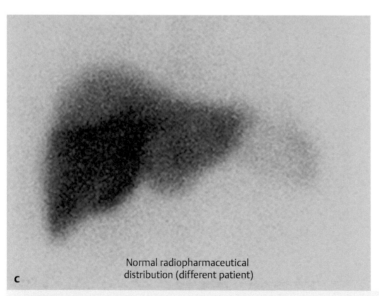

Normal radiopharmaceutical
distribution (different patient)

Fig. 276.1 (a) Contrast-enhanced axial CT image through the liver shows multiple hyperdense enhancing lesions in both lobes of the liver. The heterogeneous appearance of the spleen is due to the phase of contrast. **(b)** Tc99m sulfur colloid SPECT image shows mildly increased uptake in the lateral right lobe and lateral left lobe which is compatible with focal nodular hyperplasia. The large cold defect in the posterior right lobe was diagnosed as a hemangioma on the subsequent Tc99m red blood cell scintigraphy (not shown). **(c)** Planar image demonstrating the normal radiopharmaceutical distribution of Tc-SC predominantly within the liver with faint activity within the spleen. Breast attenuation creates geographic decreased counts overlying hepatic dome.

■ Clinical Presentation

A 35-year-old woman not on birth-control pills (▶ Fig. 276.1).

■ Key Imaging Finding

Uptake in a hepatic lesion on sulfur colloid (SC) scan

■ Top 3 Differential Diagnoses

- **Focal nodular hyperplasia (FNH)**. FNH is a benign hepatic tumor which is found most commonly (80%) in women. It typically appears as a solitary solid mass consisting of hepatocytes, bile ducts, and Kupffer cells. Most lesions are 2 to 5 cm in diameter, 20% are multiple, and they are more common (70%) in the right lobe of the liver. Computed tomography (CT) often demonstrates a contrast-enhancing lesion with a central area of scarring; the central scar of FNH fills in with delayed imaging and is T2 hyperintense on magnetic resonance imaging (MRI). Due to the presence of Kupffer cells, two-thirds of FNH nodules have normal or increased SC uptake. One-third have decreased uptake, which may be related to the existence of a large number of fibrotic cells. If the nodule does not accumulate SC, FNH is not ruled out, and the remaining broad differential includes hepatic adenoma, hepatocellular carcinoma (HCC; including the fibrolamellar variant), and metastases.

For radionuclide studies, the practical limits of resolution are 1 to 2 cm for single-photon emission computed tomography (SPECT) imaging and 2 to 3 cm for planar imaging.

- **Regenerating nodular cirrhosis**. Decreased hepatic uptake of SC occurs in cirrhosis due to alteration of the liver's microcirculation. Regenerating nodules are composed primarily of hepatocytes that are surrounded by course fibrous septations. They have normal SC uptake and, thus, appear as relative hot spots surrounded by a region of diminished uptake.
- **Budd–Chiari syndrome**. In Budd–Chiari syndrome, obstruction of the hepatic veins results in congestion, hemorrhage, and necrosis of the liver parenchyma. However, the caudate lobe retains its function due to direct venous drainage into the inferior vena cava. On SC imaging, it appears as a hot spot in the caudate lobe of the liver, surrounded by an area of diminished uptake.

■ Additional Differential Diagnoses

- **Superior vena cava (SVC) syndrome**. In obstruction of the superior vena cava, collateral vessels return blood via the left internal mammary and left umbilical veins into the quadrate lobe, resulting in a focal hot spot when SC is injected into the upper extremity. Injection in the lower extremity results in a normal scan.

■ Diagnosis

Focal nodular hyperplasia

✓ Pearls

- Two-thirds of FNH demonstrate uptake on Technetium-9mm (Tc99m) SC scan.
- Regenerating nodules, Budd-Chiari, and SVC syndrome produce focal hepatic uptake on Tc99m SC scans.

- Hepatic adenomas, hemangiomas, HCC, metastases, and abscesses are photopenic on Tc99m SC scan.
- Hemangiomas are cold on Tc99m SC and hepatobiliary scan with uptake on delayed Tc99m RBC scan.

Suggested Readings

Boulahdour H, Cherqui D, Charlotte F, et al. The hot spot hepatobiliary scan in focal nodular hyperplasia. J Nucl Med . 1993; 34(12):2105–2110

Huynh LT, Kim SY, Murphy TF. The typical appearance of focal nodular hyperplasia in triple-phase CT scan, hepatobiliary scan, and Tc-99m sulfur colloid scan with SPECT. Clin Nucl Med . 2005; 30(11):736–739

Ziessman HA, O'Malley JP, Thrall JH. Nuclear Medicine: The Requisites. 4th ed. Philadelphia, PA: Elsevier; 2014

Case 277

Kamal D. Singh

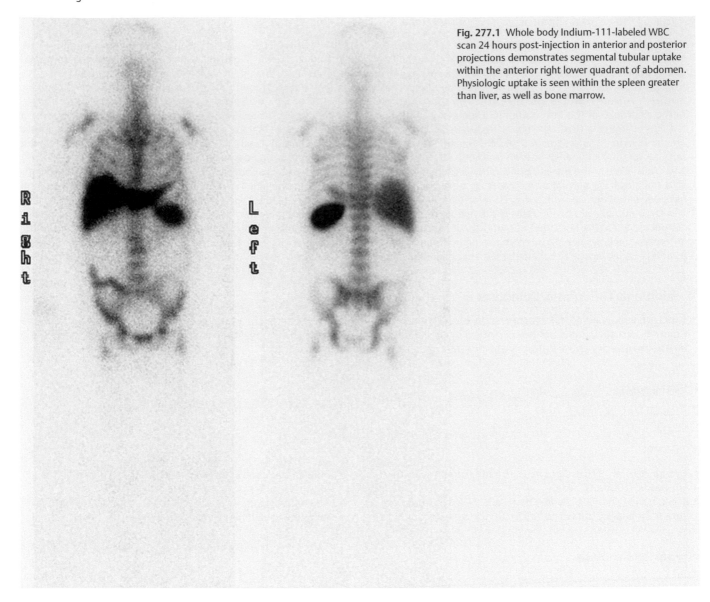

Fig. 277.1 Whole body Indium-111-labeled WBC scan 24 hours post-injection in anterior and posterior projections demonstrates segmental tubular uptake within the anterior right lower quadrant of abdomen. Physiologic uptake is seen within the spleen greater than liver, as well as bone marrow.

■ Clinical Presentation

A 39-year-old man with vague abdominal pain, fever, and elevated WBC (▶Fig. 277.1).

■ Key Imaging Finding

Focal bowel uptake on Indium-111 (In111)-labeled white blood cell (WBC) scan

■ Top 3 Differential Diagnoses

• **Infectious enteritis/colitis.** Indications for In111 labeled WBC scan include detection and localization of abdominopelvic abscesses, acute osteomyelitis (including orthopedic hardware), infected vascular grafts, and for work-up of a fever of an unknown origin. Approximately 50 mL of blood is drawn from the patient, and In111 oxine is labeled to leukocytes (predominantly neutrophils). Imaging is generally performed starting 24 hours after the injection. In111-labeled WBCs localize to the sites of infection by chemotaxis and increased vascular permeability. Donor WBCs (ABO matched) may be used in neutropenic patients with WBC <2,000 cells/mL. Physiologic activity is seen within spleen, liver, and bone marrow. Early transient and non-focal pulmonary activity is physiologic and normally decreases over time. The lack of significant gastrointestinal (GI) uptake or hepatobiliary/renal excretion makes In111-labeled WBCs preferable over gallium for abdominopelvic infectious processes, such as abscesses, enteritis/colitis, and appendicitis. There is lower sensitivity for detection of chronic nonpyogenic processes and vertebral osteomyelitis. False-positive studies may be secondary to an accessory spleen, or abdominal wall inflammation from surgical wounds, percutaneous tubes, or catheters.

• **Inflammatory bowel disease (IBD).** Segmental bowel activity may be seen in active IBD due to WBCs within sloughed mucosa at the site of inflammation. Localization and extent of active disease is best depicted on early imaging (1–6 hour postinjection) before migration of activity distal to the site of origin due to peristalsis. Technetium 99m (Tc99m) hexylmethylpropyleneamine (HMPAO)-labeled WBCs are typically used in pediatric patients instead of indium to reduce radiation dose to the spleen. When Tc99m HMPAO is used, early imaging (before 4 hours) is paramount to avoid interfering physiologic colonic activity.

• **GI bleed.** Active GI bleeding causes passage of WBCs (along with red blood cells [RBCs] and platelets) into the bowel lumen, resulting in activity which may simulate active intestinal infection or inflammation. Careful patient history and correlation with Tc99m-labeled RBCs (more sensitive and specific for active GI bleeding) can aid in establishing the correct diagnosis. Acute hematomas can also accumulate labeled WBCs.

■ Additional Differential Diagnoses

• **Swallowed activity from sinusitis/pharyngitis.** Focal infection from a more proximal source, such as sinusitis, pharyngitis, or esophagitis may have mucosal shedding of WBCs, resulting in poorly localized transient bowel activity. This can also be seen in the setting of inflammation around indwelling endotracheal or nasogastric tubes.

■ Diagnosis

Inflammatory bowel disease (Crohn disease)

✓ Pearls

• In111-labeled WBC scan is more specific than bone scan and gallium scan for acute pyogenic infection.
• Sensitivity of the In111 WBC scan is generally not affected by antibiotic therapy for acute infection.

• False-negative scans are seen in chronic nonpyogenic infections and vertebral osteomyelitis.
• False-positive scans are seen in operative wounds, GI bleeding, focal inflammation, and reactive marrow.

Suggested Readings

Becker W, Meller J. The role of nuclear medicine in infection and inflammation. Lancet Infect Dis . 2001; 1(5):326–333

Hughes DK. Nuclear medicine and infection detection: the relative effectiveness of imaging with 111In-oxine-, 99mTc-HMPAO-, and 99mTc-stannous fluoride colloid-labeled leukocytes and with 67Ga-citrate. J Nucl Med Technol . 2003; 31(4):196–201, quiz 203–204

Navab F, Boyd CM. Clinical utility of In-111 leukocyte imaging in Crohn disease. Clin Nucl Med . 1995; 20(12):1065–1069

Case 278

Vicki Nagano

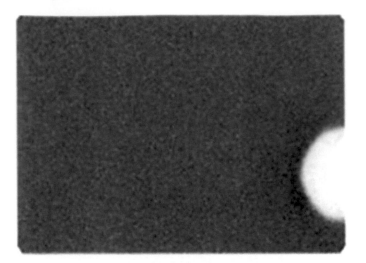

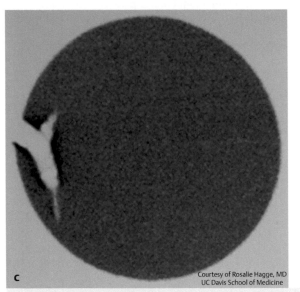

Courtesy of Rosalie Hagge, MD
UC Davis School of Medicine

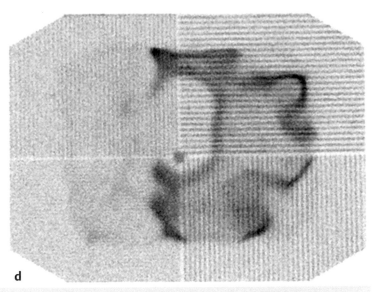

Fig. 278.1 Multiple field uniformity flood images show **(a)** a defective photomultiplier tube, **(b)** two subtle photopenic defects due to dented lead in the collimator, **(c)** a crack in the sodium iodide crystal, and **(d)** an electronic problem affecting the main circuitry behind the photomultiplier tubes. *Images provided courtesy of Rosalie Hagge, MD, UC Davis School of Medicine.*

■ Clinical Presentation

A technician presents flood field images for quality control (▶Fig. 278.1).

■ Key Imaging Finding

Focal defect on quality control (QC) images

■ Top 3 Differential Diagnoses

- **Photomultiplier tube (PMT) failure**. An array of PMTs behind the sodium iodide crystal converts the light pulse from the scintillation event into an electrical signal. Malfunction of the PMTs can be caused by a damaged tube, decoupling of the gel between the crystal and the PMT, or a loose electrical connection. Scintillation events occurring under the defective PMT will not result in a measurable electrical signal. A round defect will be seen in the field uniformity image, corresponding to the position of the malfunctioning PMT. A similar focal defect can also be caused by an overlying attenuating structure on the camera head or by an air bubble in the liquid flood phantom.
- **Crystal defect**. Gamma ray photons produce a scintillation event within the sodium iodide crystal. A crack in the sodium iodide crystal on a flood field image results in a branching white pattern due to lack of scintillations in this region. The surrounding dark edges are due to the edge-packing phenomenon.
- **Collimator defect**. The collimator helps in localizing the radionuclide in the patient by allowing only those photons traveling in an appropriate direction to interact with the crystal. The soft lead in the collimators can be dented, resulting in bending and distorting of the septa. The defect appears as a focal area of decreased activity on the flood field image. Repeating the flood image with the collimator removed will show resolution of the defect.

■ Additional Differential Diagnoses

- **Electronic artifact**. Complex computer circuitry mounted along each PMT calculates the position and strength of the scintillation event. Electronic malfunctions can result in various artifacts, depending upon which electronic system is involved. The findings on flood imaging are less characteristic than are seen with other flood field artifacts.

■ Diagnosis

PMT failure (a); dented collimator (b); cracked crystal (c); and electronic artifact (d)

✓ Pearls

- Daily QC includes extrinsic flood with cobalt 57 (Co57) sheet source placed on the camera with collimator.
- Daily flood QC images should be reviewed if there is concern for external artifact on any diagnostic study.
- Weekly spatial resolution/linearity is tested with a bar phantom between the Co57 sheet and collimator.
- Intrinsic flood (no collimator) and single-photon emission computed tomography QC are done monthly.

Suggested Readings

Mettler FA, Guiberteau MJ. Essentials of Nuclear Medicine Imaging. 6th ed. Philadelphia, PA: Elsevier; 2012

Zanzonico P. Routine quality control of clinical nuclear medicine instrumentation: a brief review. J Nucl Med . 2008; 49(7):1114–1131

Ziessman HA, O'Malley JP, Thrall JH. Nuclear Medicine: The Requisites. 4th ed. Philadelphia, PA: Elsevier; 2014

Case 279

Kamal D. Singh

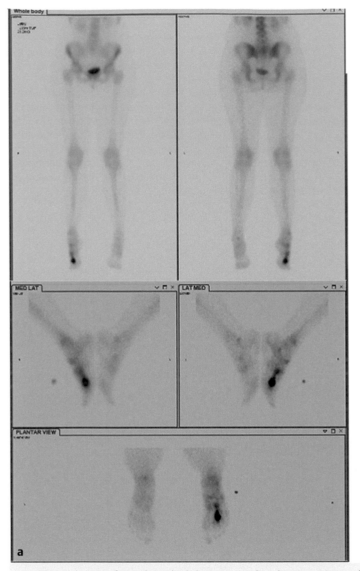

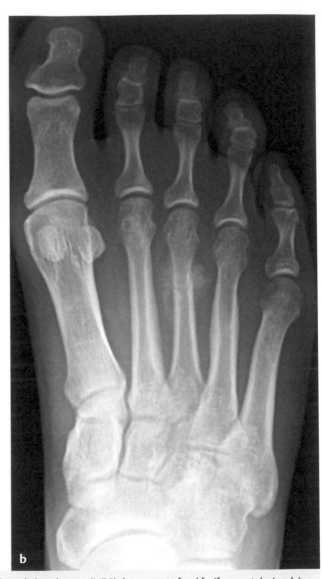

Fig. 279.1 (a) Images from a lower body bone scan with technetium-99m methylene diphosphonate (MDP) demonstrate focal fusiform uptake involving the mid left third metatarsal. **(b)** Correlative radiograph shows nondisplaced fracture with surrounding periosteal healing.

■ **Clinical Presentation**

A 24 year-old woman with right fourth metatarsal pain and tenderness (▶Fig. 279.1).

■ Key Imaging Finding

Focal increased activity within an extremity on bone scan

■ Top 3 Differential Diagnoses

• **Stress fracture**. Technetium-99m hydroxydiphosphate (Tc99m HDP) or methylene diphosphonate (MDP) localizes to areas of increased osteoblastic activity. More than 80% of fractures are detected within the first 24 hours, and nearly 95% by 72 hours. Stress fractures are classified as fatigue fractures, fractures in normal bone exposed to abnormal stress, or insufficiency fractures, fractures in abnormal bone exposed to normal stress. Repetitive stress can lead to microfractures, which may progress to overt fracture if unrecognized or untreated. Typical sites for fatigue-type stress fractures include the tibia, fibula, medial femoral neck, inferior pubic ramus, metatarsals, and calcaneus. Stress fractures are seen as intense focal, fusiform activity on bone scan, typically greater in intensity than the anterior superior iliac spine on the anterior image or sacroiliac joints on the posterior image. Stress fractures within long bones can be graded based on their extent of corticomedullary involvement. Single-photon emission computed tomography (SPECT) should be performed if concern is for femoral neck stress fracture, as up to 50% of cases can be missed on planar images. Treatment includes rest and modification of activity.

• **Osteomyelitis**. Osteomyelitis may occur due to extension from adjacent soft tissue cellulitis, direct inoculation from open wound, or by hematogenous spread. Three-phase bone scan has high negative predictive value for osteomyelitis. Cellulitis demonstrates hyperemia and soft tissue uptake on early phases, but no abnormal bone activity on delayed imaging. Osteomyelitis, in contrast, is positive on all three phases. Specificity for osteomyelitis is lower in the setting of recent trauma, surgery, or orthopedic hardware, necessitating correlation with In111 WBC and Tc99m sulfur colloid scans.

• **Neoplasm (benign and malignant)**. Primary bone malignancies (e.g., osteosarcoma and Ewing) and osteoblastic metastases generally demonstrate avid uptake on bone scan. Sensitivity is lower for predominantly lytic lesions (multiple myeloma, renal cell, and thyroid cancer). Benign bone tumors have a variable appearance on bone scan, but generally do not demonstrate significant hyperemia, with the exception of osteoid osteoma. Osteoid osteoma has focal intense uptake within a central vascular nidus with comparatively less uptake in the surrounding reactive sclerosis, described as the "double-density" or "target" sign. Clinically, patients present with dull, achy night pain that is relieved by nonsteroidal anti-inflammatory drugs (NSAIDs). Solitary bone cysts are generally photopenic, while bone islands and osseous hemangiomas are rarely detectable on bone scan. Benign, uncomplicated exostoses and enchondromas are usually warm on bone scan.

■ Additional Differential Diagnoses

• **Fibrous dysplasia**. Fibrous dysplasia is a congenital, non-hereditary skeletal dysplasia that generally demonstrates intense uptake on bone scan. Common areas of involvement include the ribs, tibia, femur, and craniofacial bones. The skeletal lesions demonstrate the classic expanded, ground-glass matrix on plain film. Bone scan is helpful in detecting polyostotic involvement.

■ Diagnosis

Completed stress fracture

✓ Pearls

• Stress fractures (fatigue or insufficiency) present as focal uptake in characteristic locations.
• Osteoid osteoma is positive on all three phases of a bone scan with a characteristic "target" sign.

• Primary bone malignancies and osteoblastic metastases generally demonstrate avid uptake on bone scan.

Suggested Readings

Bryant LR, Song WS, Banks KP, Bui-Mansfield LT, Bradley YC. Comparison of planar scintigraphy alone and with SPECT for the initial evaluation of femoral neck stress fracture. AJR Am J Roentgenol . 2008; 191(4):1010–1015

Love C, Din AS, Tomas MB, Kalapparambath TP, Palestro CJ. Radionuclide bone imaging: an illustrative review. Radiographics . 2003; 23(2):341–358

Case 280

Kamal D. Singh

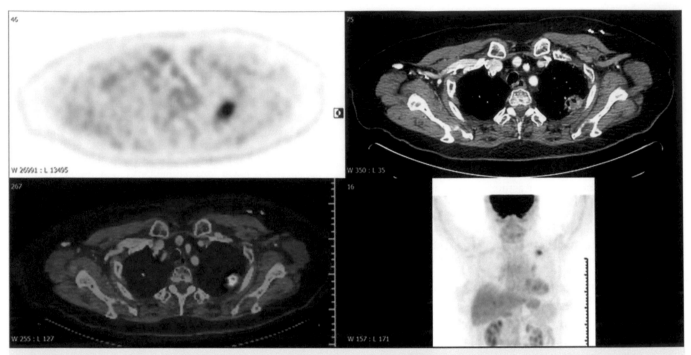

Fig. 280.1 Multiple images from a positron emission tomography (PET) scan with fluorine-18 FDG demonstrate a hypermetabolic left upper lobe cavitary lesion. Physiologic uptake is seen within the brain, liver, spleen, kidneys, bladder, and bone marrow.

■ Clinical Presentation

An 84-year-old woman with left upper nodule (▶Fig. 280.1).

■ Key Imaging Finding

Solitary hypermetabolic pulmonary lesion on positron emission tomography (PET) scan

■ Top 3 Differential Diagnoses

- **Malignancy.** Fluorodeoxyglucose (FDG) is a glucose analog that enters cells via glucose transporters and is phosphorylated. Unlike glucose, FDG is trapped in cells and does not undergo glycolysis. Fluorine-18 (F-18) is a cyclotron-produced positron emitter which simultaneously generates two 511 keV gamma photons at approximately 180 degrees through an annihilation reaction. Standard PET imaging is performed from the skull base to proximal thighs 45 to 90 minutes after injection of 15 mCi of F-18 FDG. Corresponding low-dose computed tomography (CT) is performed for attenuation correction and anatomic localization. Malignant cells have increased metabolic activity. PET/CT is indicated for detection and staging of malignancies, including post-therapy response. PET/CT has sensitivity of 95% and specificity of 80% for determining whether a solitary pulmonary nodule (>1 cm in size) is benign or malignant. Negative findings on PET are less helpful in the setting of high pretest likelihood of malignancy. Standardized uptake value (SUV) is a semi-quantitative index for tumor metabolism, and a maximum SUV of 2.5 is generally regarded as cutoff for malignancy. However, any uptake within a pulmonary nodule greater than mediastinal background activity is suspicious. False negatives may occur due to the partial-volume effect in sub-centimeter nodules and low-grade or well-differentiated malignancies.
- **Active granulomatous disease.** FDG uptake is nonspecific and can be seen within active non-neoplastic processes, including granulomatous diseases such as sarcoidosis, fungal infection, and tuberculosis (TB). Increased glycolysis within activated macrophages is likely responsible for FDG uptake. SUV may be high (>2.5) within these benign lesions. A biopsy or close follow-up may be the next appropriate step for definitive diagnosis. Dual-time point imaging in some instances may improve accuracy, since non-neoplastic lesions generally do not demonstrate increasing FDG accumulation on delayed scan.
- **Pulmonary infection/inflammation.** Increased FDG activity is also seen within sites of active infection or inflammation, likely due to inflammatory cell metabolism and mediators. Focal pulmonary infection, abscesses, radiation pneumonitis, active fibrosis, and postsurgical changes can demonstrate increased FDG uptake, simulating malignancy. Correlation with the patient's history and corresponding anatomical imaging (i.e., CT scan) can aid in making the appropriate diagnosis.

■ Diagnosis

Acute inflammation/fibrosis (no evidence of malignancy on pathology)

✓ Pearls

- Patient preparation prior to PET includes 4-hour fasting, no recent regular Insulin, and serum glucose <200.
- FDG uptake is nonspecific and is seen in the setting of neoplasm and active infection or inflammation.
- An SUV ≥2.5 is generally considered as the cutoff for malignancy, but is not reliable in small lesions.
- Bronchoalveolar carcinoma or mucinous metastases to the lung may be falsely negative on PET scan.

Suggested Readings

Bunyaviroch T, Coleman RE. PET evaluation of lung cancer. J Nucl Med . 2006; 47(3):451–469

Choromańska A, Macura KJ. Evaluation of solitary pulmonary nodule detected during computed tomography examination. Pol J Radiol . 2012; 77(2):22–34

Truong MT, Ko JP, Rossi SE, et al. Update in the evaluation of the solitary pulmonary nodule. Radiographics . 2014; 34(6):1658–1679

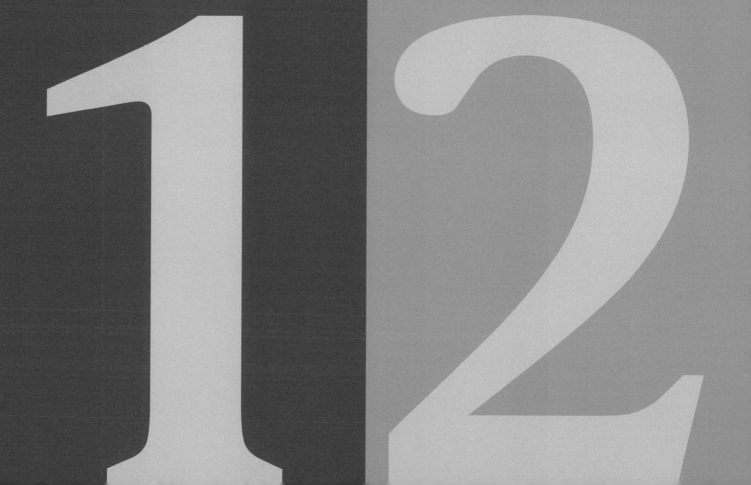

Part 12

Breast Imaging

Case 281

Matthew R. Denny and Jessica W. T. Leung

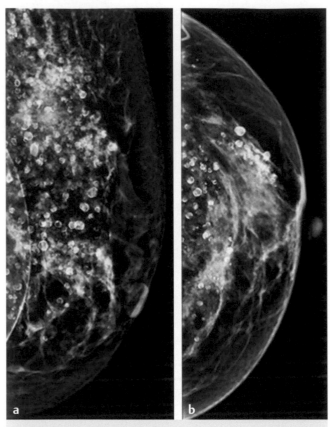

Fig. 281.1 Anterior aspects of a left diagnostic mammogram in **(a)** the mediolateral oblique (MLO) and **(b)** craniocaudal (CC) projections show a diffuse distribution of calcifications with rim, punctuate, and round forms.

■ Clinical Presentation

A 63-year-old woman with saline breast implants who presents for diagnostic mammography due to localized lateral left breast pain (▶Fig. 281.1).

■ Key Imaging Finding

Benign-appearing calcifications: rim, punctuate, and round forms

■ Top 3 Differential Diagnoses

- **Calcified oil cyst**. Oil cysts form as a result of fat necrosis in the breast. Various etiologies may result in fat necrosis and oil cyst formation, including surgery, trauma, or ischemia. Oil cysts are round or oval radiolucent structures which calcify over time. Most commonly, the calcifications occur along the periphery. Occasionally, the entire oil cyst may become calcified, so that the calcifications appear round or punctuate. Rim, punctuate, and round calcifications are benign and do not need to be biopsied.
- **Dystrophic calcifications**. Dystrophic calcifications form in the breast as part of fat necrosis. As with oil cysts, dystrophic calcifications may result from various etiologies, including surgery, trauma, or ischemia. Such calcifications are dense and coarse; they may increase over time. Dystrophic calcifications are benign and do not need to be biopsied.
- **Dermal calcifications**. Dermal calcifications are of geometric or polygonal shape, often with lucent centers. They are most commonly found in the upper inner breast in a regional distribution, but may also be diffuse. Dermal calcifications are diagnosed when they display the classic morphology or when they project over the skin. When there is uncertainty regarding the diagnosis of dermal calcifications, tangential mammographic views may be performed for confirmation or exclusion of dermal calcifications. Dermal calcifications are benign and do not need to be biopsied.

■ Additional Differential Diagnoses

- **Fibrocystic change**. Fibrocystic change is a normal spectrum of breast physiology, likely related to hormonal influences. It most commonly occurs in the premenopausal woman and may give rise to calcifications with various appearances. Some calcifications of fibrocystic change are characteristically benign in morphology (e.g., round or punctuate) or distribution (e.g., bilateral and diffuse), while others are indeterminate (e.g., clustered or amorphous) and require biopsy to exclude malignancy.
- **Hyalinized fibroadenoma calcifications**. As a fibroadenoma involutes or degenerates with time, its stromal components become hyalinized. Coarse, curvilinear, "popcorn" calcifications may appear. Such characteristic calcifications are pathognomonic for a degenerating fibroadenoma. Calcifications associated with a hyalinized fibroadenoma are benign and do not need to be biopsied.

■ Diagnosis

Calcified oil cysts

✓ Pearls

- Benign oil cyst calcifications may be rim, punctuate, or round; they should not be biopsied.
- Dystrophic calcifications may result from surgery, trauma, or ischemia; they should not be biopsied.
- Tangential views are useful in confirming dermal origin of calcifications on mammography.
- Calcifications associated with fibrocystic change vary from classically benign to indeterminate.

Suggested Readings

American College of Radiology. ACR Breast Imaging Reporting and Data System (BI-RADS). 5th ed. Reston, VA: American College of Radiology; 2013

Berg WA, Arnoldus CL, Teferra E, Bhargavan M. Biopsy of amorphous breast calcifications: pathologic outcome and yield at stereotactic biopsy. Radiology. 2001; 221(2):495–503

Ikeda DM. Breast Imaging: The Requisites. 2nd ed. Philadelphia, PA: Elsevier; 2010

Sickles EA. Breast calcifications: mammographic evaluation. Radiology . 1986; 160(2):289–293

Case 282

Jessica W. T. Leung

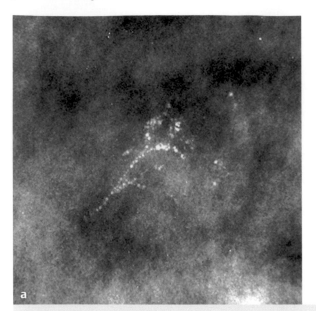 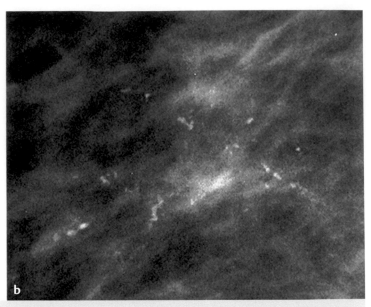

Fig. 282.1 Spot compression magnification mammograms in **(a)** the lateromedial (LM) and **(b)** CC projections show calcifications with linear distribution and linear and branching forms.

▪ Clinical Presentation

A 78-year-old woman recalled from screening mammography for new breast calcifications (▶Fig. 282.1).

■ Key Imaging Finding

Malignant-appearing calcifications: linear and branching forms

■ Top 3 Differential Diagnoses

- **Ductal carcinoma in situ (DCIS)/invasive carcinoma**. DCIS is most commonly diagnosed by calcifications at screening mammography. The calcifications result from ischemic necrosis as the devascularized tumor sheds into the duct and outgrows its blood supply. Malignant calcifications display a variety of appearances: some are classic for cancer, while others are indeterminate and cannot be distinguished from benign calcifications without biopsy. While analyzing calcifications, it is important to consider both the morphology (shape or form) and distribution (how the calcifications are arranged in space). Linear distribution and linear and branching morphology are highly suggestive of malignancy. Spot compression magnification views better portray the morphology and distribution of calcifications. Malignant calcifications may represent DCIS with invasive carcinoma.
- **Vascular calcifications**. Calcifications deposit in arterial walls as a result of aging, atherosclerosis, or hypercalcemic state.

When the vessel is seen in cross-section, vascular calcifications may appear curvilinear or rim-like. "Tram-track" calcifications are seen in profile when both walls of the vessel are calcified. Vascular calcifications may increase over time. They may be identified with confidence by recognizing their typical morphology and distribution; biopsy should be avoided.
- **Secretory calcifications**. Secretory calcifications, also known as plasma cell mastitis, are benign and form in large or intermediate-sized ducts. They are more common in elderly women and appear as coarse linear (sometimes branching) calcifications, located in the retroareolar breast and radiating to the nipple. They are usually unilateral or asymmetric if bilateral. Secretory calcifications may increase over time. Classic imaging features are diagnostic; when present, biopsy should be avoided.

■ Additional Differential Diagnoses

- **Milk-of-calcium**. Milk-of-calcium is liquid calcium sediment in tiny benign cysts. Because of its fluid nature, its morphology varies depending upon the position of the cysts. When viewed in the lateral projection, the milk-of-calcium within the cysts appears linear, discoid, layering, or meniscoid. When viewed in the craniocaudal projection, the milk-of-calcium appears round, amorphous, or smudgy.

- **Fibrocystic change**. Fibrocystic change is a normal spectrum of breast physiology, likely related to hormonal influences. It commonly occurs in premenopausal women and can give rise to calcifications with various appearances. Some calcifications of fibrocystic change are characteristically benign in morphology (e.g., round or punctuate) or distribution (e.g., bilateral and diffuse), while others are indeterminate (e.g., clustered amorphous) and require biopsy to exclude malignancy.

■ Diagnosis

Ductal carcinoma in situ, high grade

✓ Pearls

- Spot compression magnification views are used to evaluate the morphology and distribution of calcifications.
- Calcifications with linear distribution and linear and branching morphology are suspicious for cancer.

- Indeterminate calcifications require biopsy to determine whether they are malignant or benign.

Suggested Readings

Al-Attar MA, Michell MJ, Ralleigh G, et al. The impact of image guided needle biopsy on the outcome of mammographically detected indeterminate microcalcification. Breast. 2006; 15(5):635–639

American College of Radiology. ACR Breast Imaging Reporting and Data System (BI-RADS). 5th ed. Reston, VA: American College of Radiology; 2013

Ikeda DM. Breast Imaging: The Requisites. 2nd ed. Philadelphia, PA: Elsevier; 2010

Case 283

Jessica W. T. Leung

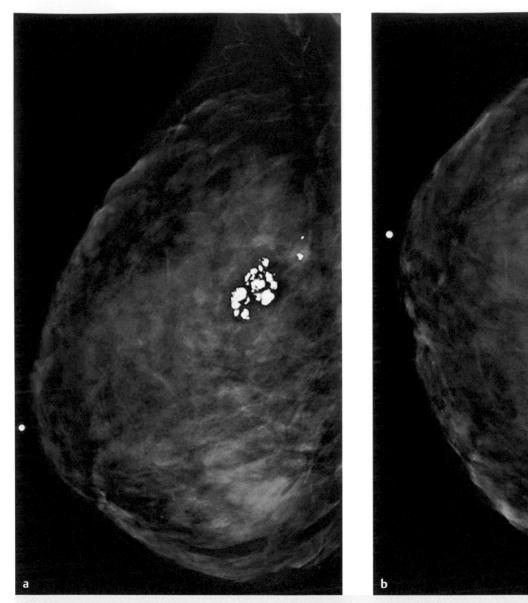

Fig. 283.1 Screening mammograms of the right breast in **(a)** the mediolateral oblique (MLO) and **(b)** craniocaudal (CC) projections show a partially circumscribed mass containing coarse curvilinear calcifications in the posterior-superior right breast.

■ Clinical Presentation

A 56-year-old woman who presented for screening mammography (▶ Fig. 283.1).

■ Key Imaging Finding

Coarse calcifications in a partially circumscribed mass

■ Top 3 Differential Diagnoses

- **Degenerating fibroadenoma**. Fibroadenoma is a solid benign mass. It is the most common mass in young women and the most common palpable mass in women in their thirties. It may be seen at mammography as a circumscribed or lobulated, round, or oval mass. As a fibroadenoma involutes or degenerates with time, its stromal components become hyalinized. Coarse, curvilinear, "popcorn" calcifications may appear. Such characteristic calcifications are pathognomonic for a degenerating fibroadenoma, provided the mass margins are circumscribed. Biopsy is not needed.

- **Fat necrosis**. Trauma to the breast, including post-surgical changes and ischemia, results in fat necrosis and the formation of dystrophic calcifications. Such calcifications are dense and coarse and may be associated with a mass. Dystrophic calcifications may increase over time. They are benign and do not need to be biopsied.
- **Oil cyst**. Oil cyst formation is a dystrophic reaction of the breast. It appears as a round or oval lucent mass. Curvilinear rim calcifications are often present at the periphery of the lucent mass. This is a benign lesion that does not need to be biopsied.

■ Additional Differential Diagnoses

- **Hematoma**. A hematoma appears as a high-density mass at mammography. It is usually preceded by a history of trauma or in the setting of anticoagulation. As a hematoma evolves and becomes organized, dense dystrophic calcifications may appear. Clinical history contributes in making the correct diagnosis. This is a benign mass that does not need to be biopsied.
- **Abscess**. An abscess appears as an irregular or circumscribed mass, often associated with signs of mastitis (e.g., skin thick-

ening and edema). Over time, calcifications may form as part of a dystrophic reaction. These calcifications are usually dense and coarse. As with hematomas, a clinical history contributes in making the correct diagnosis. This is a benign mass that does not need to be biopsied; however, percutaneous drainage may be necessary for treatment, along with antibiotic therapy.

■ Diagnosis

Degenerating fibroadenoma

✓ Pearls

- Fibroadenomas are the most common benign solid mass in premenopausal women.
- "Popcorn" calcifications are pathognomonic for a degenerating fibroadenoma; biopsy is not necessary.

- A lucent mass with curvilinear rim calcifications is a benign oil cyst.
- Diagnoses of hematoma and abscess are primarily based upon clinical findings.

Suggested Readings

Ikeda DM. Breast Imaging: The Requisites. 2nd ed. Philadelphia, PA: Elsevier; 2010

Kopans DB. Breast Imaging. 3rd ed. Philadelphia, PA: Lippincott Williams & Wilkins; 2007

Tse GM, Tan PH, Pang AL, Tang AP, Cheung HS. Calcification in breast lesions: pathologists' perspective. J Clin Pathol. 2008; 61(2):145–151

Case 284

Chloe M. Chhor

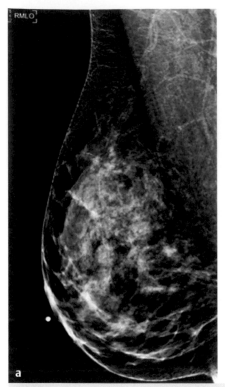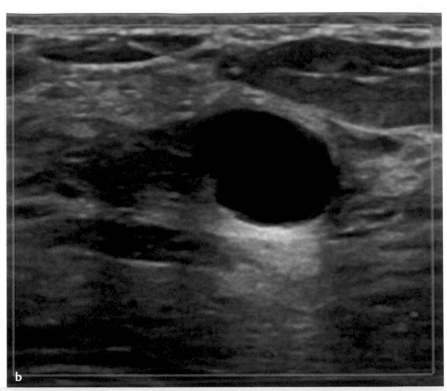

Fig. 284.1 (a) Screening mammogram of the right breast in the mediolateral oblique (MLO) projection shows a circumscribed mass in the mid-depth right breast slightly above the posterior nipple line. **(b)** Targeted Doppler ultrasound shows a corresponding anechoic mass with posterior acoustic enhancement, thin imperceptible walls, and no internal color Doppler flow.

■ Clinical Presentation

A 44-year-old woman recalled from screening mammography for a mass in the central retroareolar right breast (▶ Fig. 284.1).

■ Key Imaging Finding

Circumscribed non-palpable mass in a premenopausal woman

■ Top 3 Differential Diagnoses

- **Cyst**. A cyst is the most common breast mass in women older than 35 years. It is benign and not associated with an increased risk of breast cancer. At mammography, cysts may appear as asymmetries or masses. Ultrasound is used to distinguish a simple cyst from a complicated cyst or solid mass. A simple cyst appears as an anechoic mass with posterior acoustic enhancement and thin, imperceptible walls. A complicated cyst contains hypoechoic debris with homogeneous diffuse internal echoes. A complicated cyst is also benign; however, aspiration may be necessary to distinguish it from a hypoechoic solid mass. Most cysts are asymptomatic. Symptomatic cysts often present with pain correlating to menstrual cycles; they can be treated with aspiration.
- **Fibroadenoma**. A fibroadenoma is the most common benign solid mass in young women. It can have a variable appearance at ultrasound, but classically appears as a circumscribed or gently lobulated, mildly hypoechoic, thinly encapsulated, ovoid mass which is oriented parallel to the chest wall (wider-than-tall). A fibroadenoma can be mistaken for a complicated cyst when it is homogeneously hypoechoic with posterior acoustic enhancement. If there is significant fibrosis or calcifications associated with the fibroadenoma, posterior acoustic shadowing may be seen at ultrasound, and suspicion for malignancy may be erroneously raised. Correlation with mammography may reveal dystrophic calcifications and contribute to the correct diagnosis of a benign fibroadenoma.
- **Intramammary lymph node**. An intramammary lymph node usually is seen as a non-palpable mammographic finding. At mammography, an intramammary lymph node classically appears as a well-circumscribed, ovoid, reniform mass with a fatty hilum. At sonography, it is an ovoid or gently lobulated hypoechoic reniform mass with an echogenic fatty hilum that contains a vascular pedicle, best seen on Doppler imaging. If an intramammary lymph node maintains its characteristic shape and does not reach pathologic size criteria, no further follow-up is required.

■ Additional Differential Diagnoses

- **Breast carcinoma**. The majority of newly diagnosed well-circumscribed, round, or oval masses in the breast are benign, but 2 to 5% of such masses are new cancers. Breast carcinomas can have variable appearances at mammography and ultrasound, which make it difficult to distinguish a benign solid mass from cancer. Medullary carcinoma is a classic example of an invasive carcinoma mimicking a cyst at ultrasound. If there is any uncertainty, percutaneous core biopsy is recommended to exclude malignancy.
- **Papilloma**. Papilloma is a benign fibroepithelial tumor of the breast that can be detected at screening mammography or present with a palpable lump or nipple discharge. Ultrasound and ductography are used to further evaluate nipple discharge and to assess the presence and extent of papillomas. At sonography, papilloma may appear as an intraductal, intracystic, or solid mass. Papilloma is often surgically excised because of the difficulty in differentiating it from papillary carcinoma.

■ Diagnosis

Simple cyst

✓ Pearls

- Ultrasound is used to evaluate a palpable lump and to distinguish a simple cyst from a solid mass.
- Fibroadenoma is the most common solid mass in young women; a cyst is the most common breast mass in women older than 35 years.

- Lymph nodes are classically reniform in shape with a fatty hilum, which contains a vascular pedicle.

Suggested Readings

Ikeda DM. Breast Imaging: The Requisites. 2nd ed. Philadelphia, PA: Elsevier; 2010

Stavros AT. Breast Ultrasound. Philadelphia, PA: Lippincott Williams & Wilkins; 2004

Case 285

Natasha Brasic and Robert A. Jesinger

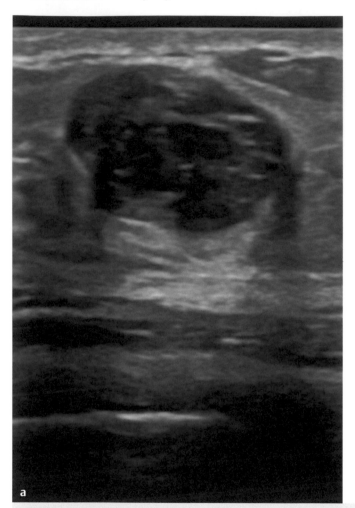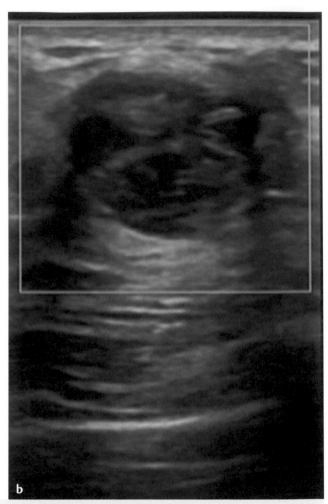

Fig. 285.1 **(a)** Sonogram in the transverse plane with **(b)** color Doppler analysis shows a palpable oval, mildly lobulated, hypoechoic mass with variable internal echoes and posterior acoustic enhancement.

■ Clinical Presentation

A 35-year-old woman who presented for evaluation of a palpable mobile breast mass (▶Fig. 285.1).

■ **Key Imaging Finding**

Palpable circumscribed solid breast mass

■ **Top 3 Differential Diagnoses**

- **Fibroadenoma.** Fibroadenoma is a solid benign mass and is the most common breast mass in young women and the most common palpable breast mass in women in their thirties. Fibroadenoma is the result of idiopathic overgrowth of connective tissue. Most studies suggest that fibroadenoma carries no significant risk for the subsequent development of breast cancer, though cancer can occur in fibroadenoma, just as in any other breast epithelium. At mammography, this mass appears as a circumscribed or lobulated round or oval mass possibly associated with dystrophic "popcorn" calcifications. At sonography, it is classically hypoechoic, well-circumscribed, gently lobulated, round or oval, and oriented parallel to the chest wall (wider-than-tall). Posterior sound transmission is variable.

- **Circumscribed breast carcinoma.** There are a small number of palpable cancers that are round, oval, or lobulated with circumscribed margins. The most common cancer that grows as a circumscribed mass is infiltrating ductal carcinoma, not otherwise specified. The medullary subtype of breast carcinoma is often circumscribed, although indistinct margins may be seen. Lymphoma, colloid carcinoma, and papillary carcinoma can occasionally appear as round, smoothly marginated masses. Metastases to the breast are often well circumscribed, but they are also usually multiple and bilateral, and the presence of an extramammary primary is often known.

- **Papilloma.** While occurring in the major (retroaerolar) ducts, a solitary benign papilloma can grow large and be palpable. A papilloma consists of epithelial proliferations on a fibrovascular stalk. It is typically sub- or periareolar in location and may produce serous or sanguineous nipple discharge. An intraductal papilloma may be associated with solitary duct enlargement due to duct obstruction or as an isolated solid mass. At sonography, a palpable solid ovoid vascularized mass may be seen.

■ **Additional Differential Diagnoses**

- **Hamartoma (fibroadenolipoma).** Hamartoma is a benign mass of normal, but disorganized ducts and lobules admixed with stroma and adipose tissue. It presents as a circumscribed, smoothly marginated fat-containing mass. At mammography, various mixtures of fat and soft tissue are seen within a fibrous capsule. Sonography of these lesions is often confounding: fibrous elements produce specular reflections, while adenomatous elements appear heterogeneously hypoechoic.

■ **Diagnosis**

Fibroadenoma

✓ **Pearls**

- Fibroadenoma is a common benign solid mass that is characteristically circumscribed and wider-than-tall.
- Common circumscribed carcinomas include invasive ductal, not-otherwise-specified (NOS); mucinous; medullary; and papillary.

- Hamartoma is a palpable circumscribed, smoothly marginated fat-containing mass with a fibrous capsule.
- Hamartomas are best diagnosed at mammography; sonographic evaluation may confound the workup.

Suggested Readings

Ikeda DM. Breast Imaging: The Requisites. 2nd ed. Philadelphia, PA: Elsevier; 2010.

Sklair-Levy M, Sella T, Alweiss T, Craciun I, Libson E, Mally B. Incidence and management of complex fibroadenomas. AJR Am J Roentgenol . 2008; 190(1):214–218

Case 286

Frederick R. Margolin

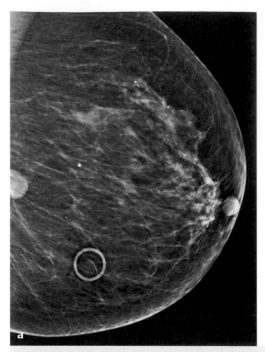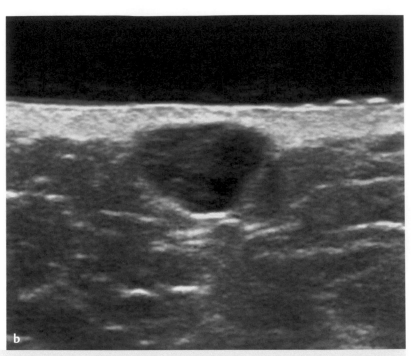

Fig. 286.1 **(a)** Mammogram of the left breast in the mediolateral oblique (MLO) projection shows a partially imaged circumscribed mass posteriorly. **(b)** Sonogram in the radial plane shows a corresponding circumscribed oval hypoechoic mass, contiguous with the skin, with subtle posterior acoustic enhancement.

▪ Clinical Presentation

A 47-year-old woman with a small palpable lump in her medial left breast, close to the skin surface (▶Fig. 286.1).

■ Key Imaging Finding

Superficial breast mass

■ Top 3 Differential Diagnoses

- **Sebaceous cyst**. A sebaceous cyst is a benign self-limiting condition created by the blockage of a sebaceous gland. Unless infected, it is usually nontender. Tomosynthesis imaging and/or tangential views with a skin marker placed on the lesion will demonstrate that the finding is in or closely related to the skin. As a result, breast cancer would be unlikely, as breast cancer arises from breast tissue deep to the skin. Sonography employing a high-frequency transducer and/or stand-off pad will allow optimal imaging of the skin and subcutaneous tissues. A sebaceous cyst will be seen as a circumscribed, near anechoic or hypoechoic oval mass, contiguous with or causing interruption of the subdermal skin layer. Extension to the skin surface may be demonstrated. Posterior acoustic enhancement is often present. Clinical examination is important to corroborate the imaging findings, as a sebaceous cyst is usually evident at clinical examination.

- **Epidermal inclusion cyst**. Epidermal inclusion cyst is the result of inclusion of keratinizing squamous epithelium within the dermis. A cyst filled with lamellated keratin is seen, which may give rise to an "onion-ring" appearance of alternating concentric echogenic and hypoechoic rings at sonography, representing a layered appearance of keratin. An epidermal inclusion cyst may resemble a sebaceous cyst at mammography and sonography. The diagnosis of an epidermal inclusion cyst can be made if there is an antecedent history of surgery or percutaneous core biopsy at the affected site.
- **Focal infection**. Mastitis may result in a focal inflammatory collection near the skin, which may present as a tender, palpable lump. The imaging appearance often resembles a sebaceous or epidermal inclusion cyst, except that the margins are more likely to be irregular or ill defined. Additionally, inflammatory changes are present in the adjacent skin and subcutaneous tissues, particularly at clinical examination.

■ Additional Differential Diagnoses

- **Steatocystoma multiplex**. Steatocystoma multiplex is a rare autosomal dominant disorder involving the pilosebaceous unit, resulting in numerous dermal cysts that contain sebum. Multiple circumscribed lucent masses are seen bilaterally. The torso and upper extremities are also commonly involved.
- **Breast carcinoma**. Breast carcinoma uncommonly presents near the skin surface. When it occurs in this location, the mammographic or sonographic appearance will be similar to

breast cancer elsewhere in the breast. The diagnosis can be made via core biopsy.
- **Lymphoma**. Lymphoma of the breast is generally of the non-Hodgkin subtype and may present as diffuse breast enlargement or as partially circumscribed mass(es) in the breast. Uncommonly, focal deposits of lymphoma can be seen in the skin or in the subcutaneous tissues of the breast.

■ Diagnosis

Sebaceous cyst

✓ Pearls

- A sebaceous cyst occurs within the skin and is best diagnosed with targeted sonography.
- Epidermal inclusion cyst may have an "onion-ring" appearance at sonography.

- Focal infection is characterized by concomitant inflammatory changes.

Suggested Readings

Crystal P, Shaco-Levy R. Concentric rings within a breast mass on sonography: lamellated keratin in an epidermal inclusion cyst. AJR Am J Roentgenol . 2005; 184(3, Suppl):S47–S48

Giess CS, Raza S, Birdwell RL. Distinguishing breast skin lesions from superficial breast parenchymal lesions: diagnostic criteria, imaging characteristics, and pitfalls. Radiographics . 2011; 31(7):1959–1972

Case 287

Boon Chye Ching

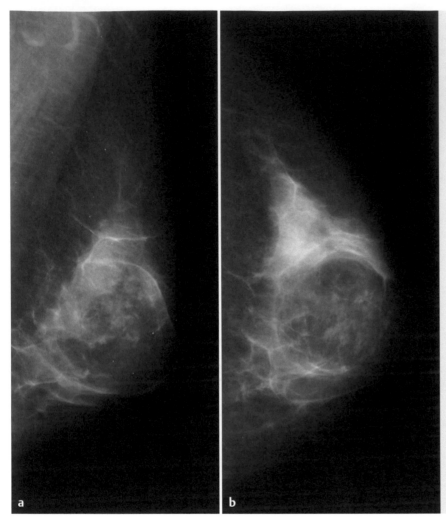

Fig. 287.1 **(a)** Mammograms in the mediolateral oblique (MLO) and **(b)** craniocaudal (CC) projections show an oval circumscribed mass with pseudocapsule in the retroareolar breast. The mass is primarily radiolucent (fatty) at mammography, but also contains a few soft-tissue densities. (These images are provided courtesy of Jill S L, Wong, MB, ChB, FACR (UK), National Cancer Centre, Singapore.)

■ Clinical Presentation

A 45-year-old woman who presented for screening mammography (▶ Fig. 287.1).

■ Key Imaging Finding

Fatty breast lesion

■ Top 3 Differential Diagnoses

- **Lipoma**. Lipoma is a fatty, radiolucent mass that may or may not have a thin discrete rim separating it from the surrounding glandular tissue. Lipoma can present as a palpable lump. Unlike fat necrosis, it does not calcify. Ultrasound shows a well-circumscribed mass that is nearly isoechoic or slightly hyperechoic to the subcutaneous fat.
- **Hamartoma (fibroadenolipoma)**. Hamartoma is an uncommon (incidence of <1%) circumscribed benign mass composed of variable amounts of glandular tissue, fat, and fibrous connective tissue. It is usually asymptomatic, but can sometimes present as a palpable mass. Distinct mammographic features include circumscribed margins and a combination of fatty and soft tissue densities surrounded by a thin radiopaque capsule or pseudocapsule (which may be complete or partial). On ultrasound, it typically appears as a circumscribed oval mass with heterogeneous internal echoes. It is usually diagnostic at

mammography with a "breast within a breast" appearance. A classical hamartoma is benign and does not need to be biopsied. However, as it contains breast elements and ducts, carcinoma can develop within a hamartoma; therefore, any suspicious mass or microcalcifications arising within a hamartoma should be biopsied.
- **Galactocele**. Galactocele is a benign cyst containing thick, inspissated milk caused by ductal obstruction in patients with a history of lactation. Patients usually present with a painless mobile palpable lump. Mammography will show single or multiple masses with density similar or less than the surrounding fibroglandular tissue. However, if the fat content is very high, galactocele can be completely radiolucent and simulate a lipoma. When in doubt, the diagnosis can be made by aspirating milk-like fluid with resolution of the lesion.

■ Additional Differential Diagnoses

- **Fat necrosis**. Fat necrosis occurs when intracellular fat escapes the damaged cells into the surrounding tissue and causes the body to react by forming granulation tissue. As there are different stages of this process, the manifestations of fat necrosis are varied. Fat necrosis can present with very benign-appearing to very worrisome imaging features. Fat necrosis can present as a lipid cyst, microcalcifications, coarse calcifications, spiculated areas of increased asymmetry, or focal masses. As a lipid cyst, it would be radiolucent at mammography, and dystrophic cal-

cifications would appear over time. There may or may not be a history of trauma or surgery.
- **Oil cyst**. Oil cyst is a focal form of fat necrosis. The causes are varied, and the patient may not recall a history of trauma or surgery. It is usually clinically occult. Fat necrosis is commonly seen at sites of reduction mammoplasty or lumpectomy post radiation and presents as round or oval lesions with peripheral calcification.

■ Diagnosis

Hamartoma (fibroadenolipoma)

✓ Pearls

- Hamartoma presents as a circumscribed fatty and soft tissue mass with a thin capsule or pseudocapsule.
- The mammographic appearance of a hamartoma is classically referred to as "breast within a breast."

- Lipomas are fatty, radiolucent masses that may or may not have a thin discrete rim; they do not calcify.
- Clinical history of lactation is crucial in the diagnosis of galactocele.

Suggested Readings

Freer PE, Wang JL, Rafferty EA. Digital breast tomosynthesis in the analysis of fat-containing lesions. Radiographics . 2014; 34(2):343–358

Wahner-Roedler DL, Sebo TJ, Gisvold JJ. Hamartomas of the breast: clinical, radiologic, and pathologic manifestations. Breast J . 2001; 7(2):101–105

Case 288

Natasha Brasic

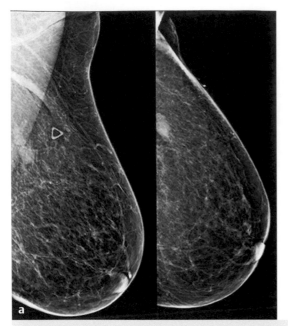 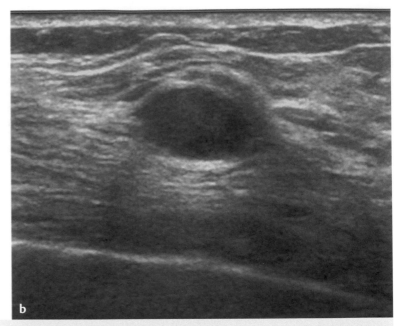

Fig. 288.1 Mammograms of the left breast in **(a)** the mediolateral oblique (MLO) and exaggerated craniocaudal lateral (XCCL) and **(b)** targeted breast ultrasound show a circumscribed, mass in the upper outer posterior left breast.

■ Clinical Presentation

A 61-year-old woman with known breast carcinoma within the left breast (▶ Fig. 288.1).

■ Key Imaging Finding

Circumscribed breast cancer

■ Top 3 Differential Diagnoses

- **Invasive ductal carcinoma, not-otherwise-specified (NOS).** The majority of invasive breast cancers are non-specific forms that originate in the ductal epithelium, likely in the terminal duct at its junction with the lobule. The majority (65%) of ductal malignancies fall into the general category of undifferentiated lesions that have no particular distinguishing histologic features. Invasive ductal carcinoma, NOS, elicits a fairly vigorous desmoplastic response with resultant fibrosis, producing a spiculated mass at mammography and a palpable hard mass. However, it may, at times, present as a well-circumscribed mass, particularly if it is rapidly growing. Given that invasive ductal carcinoma, NOS, is the majority of breast cancers, a well-circumscribed cancer is most likely of invasive ductal carcinoma, NOS, histology.
- **Mucinous carcinoma.** Mucinous carcinoma, also known as colloid carcinoma, accounts for 2–3% of all invasive breast cancers. The abundant production of mucin by this cancer is felt to reflect its high degree of differentiation, which likely accounts for the better prognosis. There are no mammographic features distinguishing mucinous carcinoma from other breast cancers. At sonography, these lesions may be difficult to identify as they may be isoechoic to fat. They may also have a hypoechoic appearance with posterior acoustic enhancement. At magnetic resonance imaging (MRI), mucinous carcinoma is characterized by intrinsically hyperintense T2-signal, reflecting the mucin content, that could simulate a fibroadenoma, and progressive enhancement kinetics are common.
- **Medullary carcinoma.** Medullary carcinoma constitutes approximately 3% of all breast cancers. It is distinctive in that it frequently grows quite large before it is detected. Classically, medullary carcinoma is described as circumscribed round or oval mass at mammography. Although these lesions frequently exhibit necrosis, calcification is an uncommon feature. At sonography, medullary carcinoma usually appears as a circumscribed hypoechoic mass with homogeneous echotexture. Posterior acoustic enhancement may be present. At MRI, medullary carcinomas enhance diffusely with plateau kinetics.

■ Additional Differential Diagnoses

- **Papillary carcinoma.** Papillary cancer is primarily an intraductal malignancy and represents less than 1% of invasive cancers. Its incidence increases with age. When mammographically visible, papillary carcinoma may appear as a well-circumscribed mass. At sonography, a solid mass possibly with cystic spaces may be seen. On MRI, washout kinetics is typical in the solid portion of the mass.
- **Ductal carcinoma in situ (DCIS).** DCIS is most commonly detected as calcifications at mammography. However, DCIS may also present as a mammographic or sonographic mass (which is often well circumscribed), giving rise to the nodular form of DCIS.

■ Diagnosis

Papillary carcinoma

✓ Pearls

- Most well-circumscribed breast cancers are invasive ductal carcinoma, NOS.
- Mucinous carcinoma has circumscribed margins and is intrinsically hyperintense on T2 MR sequences.
- Medullary carcinoma is typically large with circumscribed margins and round or ovoid shape.

Suggested Readings

Ikeda DM, Andersson I. Ductal carcinoma in situ: atypical mammographic appearances. Radiology . 1989; 172(3):661–666

Okafuji T, Yabuuchi H, Sakai S, et al. MR imaging features of pure mucinous carcinoma of the breast. Eur J Radiol . 2006; 60(3):405–413

Yoo JL, Woo OH, Kim YK, et al. Can MR Imaging contribute in characterizing well-circumscribed breast carcinomas? Radiographics. 2010; 30(6):1689–1702

Case 289

Frederick R. Margolin

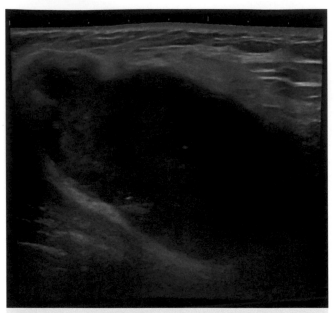

Fig. 289.1 Sonogram in the transverse plane shows a complex cystic and solid mass with hypoechoic debris and a thick wall.

■ Clinical Presentation

A 34-year-old lactating woman with erythema, warmth, swelling, and tenderness of the breast of 9 days duration (▶ Fig. 289.1).

Key Imaging Finding

Complex cystic and solid mass

Top 3 Differential Diagnoses

- **Abscess**. A breast abscess is most commonly seen in post-partum and lactating women as a complication of mastitis. At sonography, a complex fluid collection is present, consisting of echogenic fluid/debris, internal septations, and thick surrounding walls. Hypoechoic debris may be adherent to the walls of the collection, resembling solid mural nodules, and internal echoes that may "float" during real-time examination. The diagnosis of abscess is made in the proper clinical setting of mastitis and in conjunction with the signs of infection and inflammation. Ultrasound may be used to guide percutaneous aspiration for cytologic analysis, as well as abscess drainage.
- **Hematoma**. A hematoma may closely resemble an abscess at sonography, but the clinical presentation distinguishes the two entities. The clinical signs of infection and inflammation are usually absent, and a history of trauma, surgery, or antico-

agulation may be elicited. Hematomas should be followed up to resolution to exclude an underlying malignant lesion.
- **Cystic neoplasm**. A tumor arising within a cyst (i.e., intracystic papillary carcinoma) or a solid cancer that has undergone necrosis may exhibit similar sonographic features to an abscess. However, the clinical signs of infection and inflammation are absent, which is helpful in distinguishing a cystic neoplasm from an abscess. Typically, a poorly differentiated invasive carcinoma grows so rapidly that it outgrows its blood supply and undergoes ischemic necrosis, resulting in a complex cystic and solid mass that is seen at sonography. The presence of Doppler signal representing blood flow distinguishes the solid component in a cystic neoplasm from pus or blood clot present in an abscess or hematoma, respectively.

Additional Differential Diagnoses

- **Fat necrosis**. Fat necrosis results from various injuries to the breast, including ischemia and trauma, and has various appearances, including that of a complex cystic and solid mass. Correlation with mammography is important to identify classic benign mammographic features of fat necrosis that may be present, such as internal fat, oil cyst formation, and coarse dystrophic calcification. In the absence of classic mammographic signs, ultrasound-guided core biopsy may be needed to exclude malignancy.

- **Cyst with debris (complicated cyst)**. A complicated cyst is a benign mass most commonly seen in premenopausal women. Hemorrhage, protein, and cholesterol deposits may be present within the cyst, resulting in a complex appearing mass at sonography. The debris may be differentiated from a solid tissue based upon mobility and also by ultrasound-guided cyst aspiration.

Diagnosis

Abscess

✓ Pearls

- A breast abscess is usually seen in post-partum and lactating women as a complication of mastitis.
- Hematomas often occur in the setting of trauma or anticoagulation; they should be followed up to resolution.

- Tumors arising within a cyst or large tumors undergoing necrosis can resemble benign cystic lesions.
- Benign cysts with debris (complicated cysts) can be differentiated from carcinomas through aspiration.

Suggested Readings

Doshi DJ, March DE, Crisi GM, Coughlin BF. Complex cystic breast masses: diagnostic approach and imaging-pathologic correlation. Radiographics . 2007; 27(Suppl 1):S53–S64

Case 290

Jessica W. T. Leung

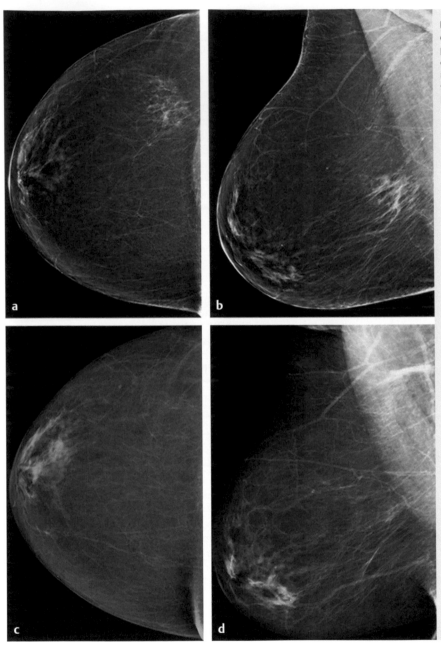

Fig. 290.1 Screening mammograms in **(a)** the craniocaudal (CC) and **(b)** mediolateral oblique (MLO) projections show a focal asymmetry in the lower outer right breast. When compared with prior mammograms in **(c)** the CC and **(d)** MLO projections, the focal asymmetry has shown interval increase. Hence, it is a developing asymmetry.

■ Clinical Presentation

A 64-year-old woman who presented for screening mammography (▶ Fig. 290.1).

■ Key Imaging Finding

Developing asymmetry

■ Top 3 Differential Diagnoses

- **Invasive ductal carcinoma**. Albeit uncommon, a developing asymmetry is a mammographic sign of malignancy. A developing asymmetry is new or increasing when compared with a prior examination. In contrast to an enlarging mass, a developing asymmetry lacks a central density, and its margins are not necessarily convex. One study showed that the probability of malignancy in a developing asymmetry is 13% at screening and 27% at diagnostic mammography. Since the probability is higher than 2% (threshold for BIRADS that can be safely followed up), biopsy is indicated, regardless of whether there is a sonographic correlate. Among those in whom malignancy is identified, invasive ductal carcinoma is the most common type.
- **Invasive lobular carcinoma**. Invasive lobular carcinoma constitutes approximately 10% of invasive cancers. However, in one study of a developing asymmetry, invasive lobular carcinoma constituted approximately 16% of the cancers identified.

Hence, invasive lobular carcinoma is disproportionately represented in a developing asymmetry, which corresponds to its "single-file" growth pattern (rather than forming a central tumor mass). Stage-for-stage, invasive lobular carcinoma carries the same prognosis as invasive ductal carcinoma. However, invasive lobular carcinoma tends to be diagnosed at a later, more advanced stage. Targeted sonography and magnetic resonance imaging (MRI) are helpful in diagnosing invasive lobular carcinoma.
- **Pseudoangiomatous stromal hyperplasia (PASH)**. PASH is a benign proliferative stromal lesion which consists of fibroblasts. It responds to hormonal stimulus and is usually found in premenopausal women or postmenopausal women on hormone replacement therapy. PASH may present as a mass or developing asymmetry. PASH is considered a benign concordant diagnosis in core biopsy of a developing asymmetry.

■ Additional Differential Diagnoses

- **Asymmetric breast tissue**. Benign breast tissue may develop over time, particularly in response to hormonal stimulation. Increase in breast density is usually diffuse, but it may also be focal. If the increase in density is focal, malignancy needs to be considered. Biopsy may be needed to exclude cancer.
- **Stromal fibrosis**. Stromal fibrosis is a benign condition that may present as a developing asymmetry. When a sonographic correlate is present, posterior acoustic shadowing may be seen and mimic malignancy. Core biopsy is helpful in making this diagnosis when the imaging findings are nonspecific. Stromal

fibrosis is considered a benign concordant diagnosis in core biopsy of a developing asymmetry.
- **Fat necrosis**. Fat necrosis has varied imaging appearances, including a developing asymmetry. Correlation with mammography is helpful, particularly when classic mammographic features of fat necrosis are present (e.g., coarse calcifications and oil cysts). Sonographic features are nonspecific and may mimic malignancy. Fat necrosis is considered a benign concordant diagnosis in core biopsy of a developing asymmetry.

■ Diagnosis

Invasive lobular carcinoma

✓ Pearls

- Biopsy is indicated for a developing asymmetry, since the chance of malignancy is greater than 2%.
- Invasive lobular carcinoma presents as a developing asymmetry because of its "single-file" growth pattern.

- PASH is a benign stromal lesion which responds to hormonal stimulus.

Suggested Readings

Leung JW, Sickles EA. Developing asymmetry identified on mammography: correlation with imaging outcome and pathologic findings. AJR Am J Roentgenol. 2007; 188(3):667–675

Price ER, Joe BN, Sickles EA. The developing asymmetry: revisiting a perceptual and diagnostic challenge. Radiology . 2015; 274(3):642–651

Case 291

Boon Chye Ching

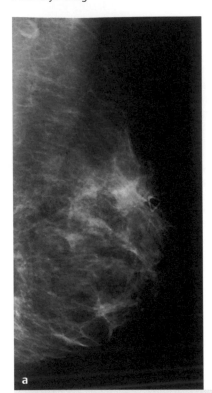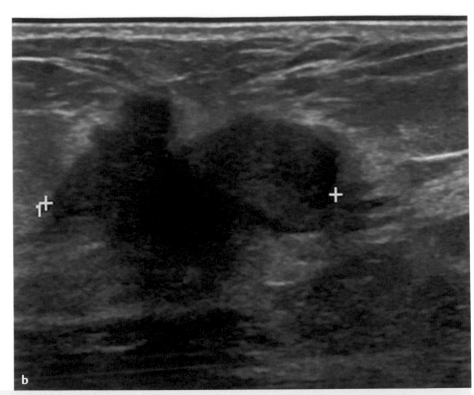

Fig. 291.1 (a) Left breast mammogram in the mediolateral oblique (MLO) projection shows an ill-defined mass deep to a triangular-shaped skin marker. **(b)** Sonogram shows a corresponding ill-defined hypoechoic mass with hyperechoic margin, corresponding to the palpable mammographic mass.

■ Clinical Presentation

A 54-year-old woman with a palpable mass in the lateral left breast of 6 weeks duration (▶Fig. 291.1).

■ Key Imaging Finding

Ill-defined, infiltrative breast mass

■ Top 3 Differential Diagnoses

• **Invasive ductal carcinoma.** Invasive ductal carcinoma is the most common invasive breast cancer, accounting for more than 90% of all invasive breast cancers. Invasive ductal carcinoma arises from the ductal epithelium and typically presents as an irregular mass with spiculated margins. These imaging features reflect the infiltrative growth of invasive cancers. There may be associated malignant microcalcifications, representing concomitant cellular necrosis. At sonography, it usually manifests as an irregular hypoechoic mass with posterior acoustic shadowing. However, approximately one-third of invasive ductal carcinomas may be associated with posterior acoustic enhancement, which reflects that the cancer is composed of uniform cells and likely poorly differentiated. A hyperechoic margin may be present, representing infiltrative tumor reaction in the adjacent tissues.

• **Invasive lobular carcinoma.** Invasive lobular carcinoma arises from the breast lobules. The cancer cells grow in a single-file; thus, they are difficult to detect at imaging or physical examination. Invasive lobular carcinoma may be seen at mammography as a developing asymmetry, architectural distortion, mass, or calcifications. Sonographic findings range from subtle tissue distortion to an obvious spiculated mass. In general, the extent of invasive lobular carcinoma is underestimated at mammography and ultrasound because of its infiltrative nature which is obscured by fibroglandular tissue. When compared with invasive ductal carcinoma, it has a higher rate of having multiple and bilateral disease. Magnetic resonance imaging (MRI) is a useful diagnostic tool in determining the extent of disease in cases of invasive lobular carcinoma.

• **Post-surgical scar.** For the diagnosis of post-surgical scar to be made, a history of prior surgery is needed. It may be seen at mammography or sonography as architectural distortion extending to the overlying skin. It may also present as an irregular spiculated mass. Posterior acoustic shadowing is often present at sonography in scar. It is often useful to put a scar marker on the skin to confirm that the imaging finding corresponds to the site of the surgery. Temporal change is vital in diagnosing or excluding malignancy at post-surgical sites, as scars should remain stable or decrease over time. While an increasing scar may be the result of benign fat necrosis, biopsy is needed to exclude recurrent cancer. Most scars will not enhance at MRI after 18 months, though some may enhance for a longer period of time.

■ Additional Differential Diagnoses

• **Fibrosis.** Fibrosis is a common incidentally detected benign finding which may have suspicious features at mammography and sonography. It may present as an irregular mass or a developing asymmetry at mammography and may appear hypoechoic or echogenic at sonography. Core biopsy is helpful in making this diagnosis.

■ Diagnosis

Invasive ductal carcinoma (poorly differentiated)

✓ Pearls

• Invasive ductal carcinoma (>90% of breast cancers) classically presents as an irregular spiculated mass.
• Imaging underestimates the extent of invasive lobular carcinoma because it grows in a "single file."

• Comparison with prior imaging studies and temporal assessment are crucial in assessing post-surgical scar.

Suggested Readings

Lopez JK, Bassett LW. Invasive lobular carcinoma of the breast: spectrum of mammographic, US, and MR imaging findings. Radiographics. 2009; 29(1):165–176.

Stavros AT. Breast Ultrasound. 1st ed. Philadelphia, PA: Lippincott Williams & Wilkins; 2007

Case 292

Boon Chye Ching

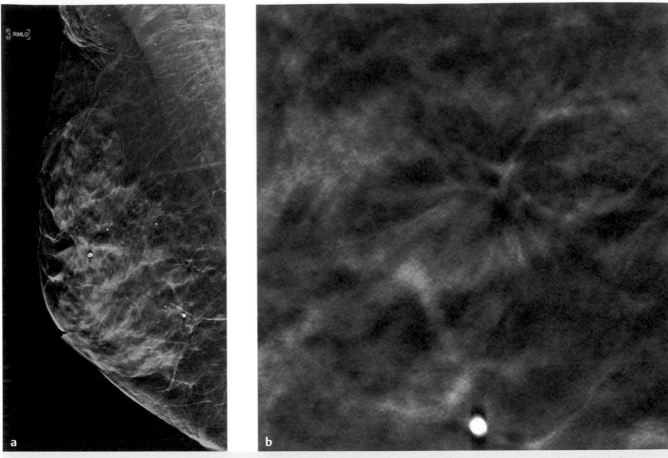

Fig. 292.1 **(a)** Screening right breast mammogram in the mediolateral oblique (MLO) projection, augmented by **(b)** an image from the right breast tomosynthesis in the MLO projection demonstrates an area of architectural distortion with areas of central lucency in the posterior right breast along the posterior nipple line.

■ Clinical Presentation

A 45-year-old woman who presented for screening mammography (▶Fig. 292.1).

■ Key Imaging Finding

Architectural distortion with central lucency

■ Top 3 Differential Diagnoses

- **Radial scar**. A radial scar, also known as complex sclerosing lesion when larger than 1 cm, is a benign but high-risk lesion; about 33% of radial scars are associated with atypical or malignant conditions. The term radial scar is a misnomer because it is not a scar and is not related to prior surgery or trauma. It is usually nonpalpable. A radial scar at mammography and tomosynthesis appears as an area of architectural distortion with central radiolucent areas representing fat. It has long, thin radiating spicules against a backdrop of radiolucent fat ("black star" appearance). Radial scar is usually better seen on tomosynthesis. At sonography, it usually appears as an area of architectural distortion, but may also range from sonographically occult to an obvious hypoechoic mass. Sometimes radial scar has to be completely excised for accurate diagnosis.
- **Invasive carcinoma**. Invasive ductal and lobular carcinoma can present at mammography as an architectural distortion with central lucency. The architectural distortion is usually the result of a desmoplastic reaction, though in some cases, it is the result of tumor infiltration. Invasive carcinoma may present as a palpable lump, while a radial scar is usually nonpalpable. At sonography, invasive carcinoma can present as an irregular hypoechoic mass with posterior acoustic shadowing and spiculated margins.
- **Tubular carcinoma**. Tubular carcinoma is usually seen as a small central mass with long spicules extending from its margins. The mass component is typically less than 1 cm in diameter and is very slow growing. There is a bilateral incidence of 12 to 40%. Pure tubular carcinoma is extremely well-differentiated. Less pure tubular carcinomas are known as mixed tubular carcinoma, while those with lobular elements are known as tubulolobular carcinoma. These histologic distinctions are clinically important because there is a higher chance of multifocality and metastatic spread as the non-tubular elements increase. Prognosis of pure tubular carcinoma is excellent.

■ Additional Differential Diagnoses

- **Fat necrosis**. Fat necrosis occurs when intracellular fat escapes the damaged cells into the surrounding tissues and causes the body to react by forming granulation tissue. The imaging manifestations are varied based upon the stage of fat necrosis, ranging from very benign to very malignant features. There may or may not be an identifiable history of trauma or surgery.
- **Postsurgical scar**. Postsurgical scar mimics breast carcinoma in which a spiculated mass or architectural distortion may be present. At sonography, postsurgical scar may manifest as an irregular hypoechoic mass with posterior acoustic shadowing. There should be distortion of the subcutaneous tissue extending from the skin overlying the scar in the plane of incision down to the spiculated mass. Comparison with previous studies and imaging follow-up are helpful. Biopsy may be needed to differentiate from malignancy.

■ Diagnosis

Radial scar

✓ Pearls

- Long radiating spicules with intervening lucency and absent central mass are suggestive of a radial scar.
- Invasive ductal carcinoma classically presents as a dense mass with spiculated margins and short spicules.
- Tubular carcinoma is a very slow growing cancer with excellent prognosis.

Suggested Readings

Alleva DQ, Smetherman DH, Farr GH, Jr, Cederbom GJ. Radial scar of the breast: radiologic-pathologic correlation in 22 cases. Radiographics. 1999; 19(Spec No):S27–S35, discussion S36–S37

Cooper HS, Patchefsky AS, Krall RA. Tubular carcinoma of the breast. Cancer. 1978; 42(5):2334–2342

Gaur S, Dialani V, Slanetz PJ, Eisenberg RL. Architectural distortion of the breast. AJR Am J Roentgenol. 2013; 201(5):W662–70

Case 293

Jessica W. T. Leung

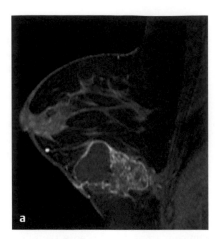
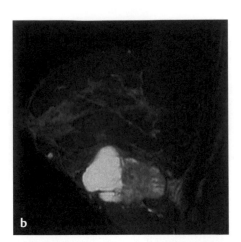

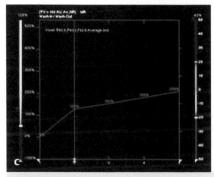
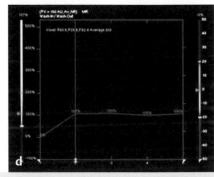
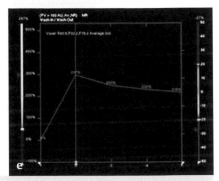

Fig. 293.1 **(a)** Contrast-enhanced 3D-gradient-recalled-echo MR image with fat saturation in the sagittal plane shows a large, irregular, heterogeneous, rim-enhancing mass in the lower breast. Cystic necrosis is present in much of the mass, especially the anterior portion, as indicated by relative lack of enhancement **(a)** and intrinsic T2-hyperintensity **(b)** on fast-spin-echo MR image with fat saturation in the sagittal plane. Kinetic analysis shows that the mass is composed of **(c)** type 1 persistent, **(d)** type 2 plateau, and **(e)** type 3 washout curves. Of note, all three curves show fast (>100%) initial enhancement.

■ Clinical Presentation

A 49-year-old woman with a large palpable lump in the lower breast of unknown duration (▶Fig. 293.1).

■ Key Imaging Finding

MRI enhancement patterns

■ Top 3 Differential Diagnoses

- **Type 1 persistent kinetics**. In type 1 persistent kinetics, the degree of contrast enhancement continues to increase over the duration of the magnetic resonance (MR) scan in the delayed phase. Type 1 persistent kinetics is consistent with the biology of benign lesions such as fibrocystic change or fibroadenoma. However, many cancers may also display type 1 persistent kinetics. Kinetic analysis cannot be used alone to establish or exclude malignancy.
- **Type 2 plateau kinetics**. In type 2 plateau kinetics, the degree of contrast enhancement levels over the duration of the MR scan in the delayed phase. Type 2 plateau kinetics is indeterminate and seen in both benign and malignant conditions. Kinetic analysis cannot be used alone to establish or exclude malignancy.
- **Type 3 washout kinetics**. In type 3 washout kinetics, the degree of contrast enhancement decreases over the duration of the MR scan in the delayed phase. Type 3 washout kinetics is consistent with the principle of angiogenesis and the biology of malignancy. Neovessels form in cancers, which are characterized by increased vascular permeability. Hence, cancers enhance strongly and rapidly in the initial phase, but demonstrate washout of contrast in the delayed phase. However, not all cancers demonstrate type 3 washout kinetics, and some benign entities (lymph node) display type 3 washout kinetics. Hence, kinetic analysis cannot be used in isolation to establish or exclude malignancy.

■ Additional Differential Diagnoses

- **Initial phase**. The initial phase of contrast enhancement may be more predictive for malignancy than the delayed phase. There are three patterns of contrast enhancement in the initial phase: slow, medium, and fast (rapid). Cancers generally enhance rapidly in the initial phase.

■ Diagnosis

Poorly differentiated invasive ductal carcinoma with rapid initial enhancement and types 1, 2, and 3 kinetics curves

✓ Pearls

- Kinetic analysis of breast MRI enhancement consists of both initial and delayed phase assessments.
- Proper interpretation of breast MR images requires consideration of both morphology and kinetic data.
- Classically, cancers show rapid initial enhancement and washout of contrast in the delayed phase.

Suggested Readings

American College of Radiology. ACR Breast Imaging Reporting and Data System (BI-RADS). 5th ed. Reston, VA: American College of Radiology; 2013

Ikeda DM. Breast Imaging: The Requisites. 2nd ed. Philadelphia, PA: Elsevier; 2010

Kuhl CK, Schild HH, Morakkabati N. Dynamic bilateral contrast-enhanced MR imaging of the breast: trade-off between spatial and temporal resolution. Radiology. 2005; 236(3):789–800

Case 294

Robert A. Jesinger

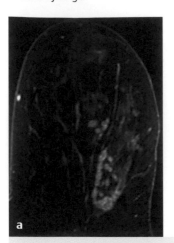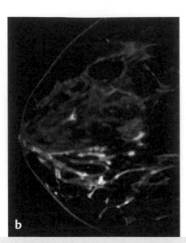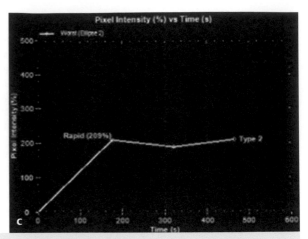

Fig. 294.1 Contrast-enhanced 3D-gradient-recalled-echo MR image with fat saturation in **(a)** the axial plane and **(b)** sagittal plane of the left breast shows a segmental distribution of ductal enhancement with a "clustered ring" appearance. **(c)** Kinetic analysis shows that the non–mass enhancement (NME) is composed of rapid initial enhancement (>100%) with a type 2 delayed plateau curve (±10% of peak enhancement).

■ Clinical Presentation

A 40-year-old woman with recently diagnosed BRCA1 mutation undergoing high-risk screening breast magnetic resonance imaging (MRI) (▶Fig. 294.1).

■ Key Imaging Finding

Suspicious non-mass enhancement (NME)

■ Top 3 Differential Diagnoses

- **Ductal carcinoma in situ (DCIS).** At MRI, DCIS is classically seen as suspicious NME in a linear or segmental distribution with clumped or clustered ring enhancement. The enhancement results from neovessels that supply cancer cells in the inner ductal lining and within tumor-distended breast ducts. Focal heterogeneous or homogeneous enhancement is less specific for DCIS. While kinetic analysis may help identify suspicious areas of NME, morphology takes precedence in interpretation. For example, a suspicious distribution of NME may represent DCIS, in spite of type 1 persistent kinetics. Note that a multimodality approach correlating any suspicious findings on mammography (calcifications), ultrasound (stacked ducts), and MRI is important in breast MRI interpretation, especially since low-grade DCIS may be occult on MRI.

- **Atypical ductal/lobular hyperplasia (ADH/ALH).** Atypical hyperplastic lesions are considered high-risk lesions, and when encountered on breast biopsy, follow-up surgical excision is required as up to one-third of cases may be upstaged to malignancy, such as DCIS. On MRI, these lesions are usually found in suspicious areas of NME (usually focal linear enhancement). When performing breast MRI-guided biopsy, up to 6% of cases may find ADH on core biopsy, of which 38% of cases underestimate underlying DCIS.
- **Fibrocystic change.** Fibrocystic (fibroproliferative) changes are most often seen on breast MRI as NME with initial slow or medium enhancement with type 1 delayed progressive enhancement. Careful review of the T2 images may help identify small hyperintense cysts, and the contrast-enhanced images may show rim enhancement of the small cysts.

■ Additional Differential Diagnoses

- **Papillomatosis.** Multiple intraductal papillomas may produce an appearance of suspicious NME. A papilloma usually appears as an ovoid intraductal mass which often appears as linear NME on MRI with rapid enhancement and type 3 washout kinetics. Pathologically, a papilloma is characterized by complex architecture consisting of infolding and redundancy of epithelium, which is often associated with atypia. It may be difficult to distinguish benign papilloma from papillary carcinoma at percutaneous core biopsy; surgical excision may be needed.

- **Sclerosing adenosis.** Sclerosing adenosis is a known reported pathologic finding associated with NME, accounting for 1 to 2% of all cases in a large published series. Correlation with mammography may be helpful in identifying the classic punctate and round calcifications within an asymmetry.
- **Pseudoangiomatous stromal hyperplasia (PASH).** PASH is a known reported pathologic finding associated with NME, accounting for 1 to 2% of all cases in a large published series. Focal or segmental clumped NME with variable enhancement kinetics may be seen.

■ Diagnosis

Ductal carcinoma in situ

✓ Pearls

- When interpreting breast MRI, morphology of NME takes precedence in interpretation over kinetics.
- Linear or segmentally distributed clumped or clustered ring enhancement is quite worrisome for DCIS.

- Benign causes for suspicious NME include fibrocystic change, papilloma, sclerosing adenosis, and PASH.

Suggested Readings

American College of Radiology. ACR Breast Imaging Reporting and Data System (BI-RADS). 5th ed. Reston, VA: American College of Radiology; 2013

Raza S, Vallejo M, Chikarmane SA, Birdwell RL. Pure ductal carcinoma in situ: a range of MRI features. AJR Am J Roentgenol. 2008; 191(3):689–699

Case 295

Robert A. Jesinger

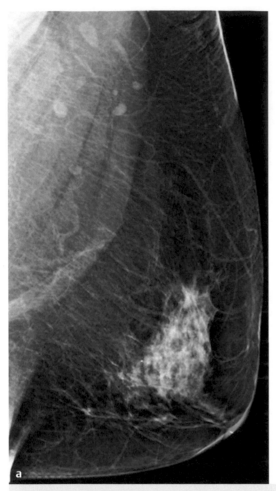
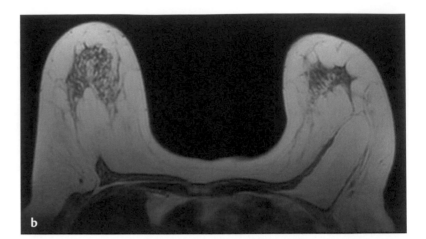
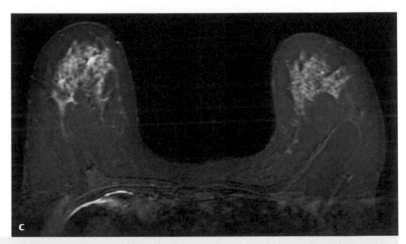

Fig. 295.1 (a) Mammogram in the mediolateral oblique (MLO) projection in the left breast shows an enlarged appearance of the left pectoralis major muscle with associated diffusely decreased density. Sonogram of the left breast (not shown) was normal. The subsequent breast MRI utilizing **(b)** T1- and **(c)** fat-suppressed T2-weighted imaging shows a large left chest wall mass arising between the pectoralis major and the pectoralis minor muscles.

■ Clinical Presentation

A 50-year-old woman presents for diagnostic mammography and breast ultrasound for a slowly enlarging self-palpated mass deep in her left breast (▶ Fig. 295.1).

■ Key Imaging Finding

Palpable chest wall mass

■ Top 3 Differential Diagnoses

- **Lipoma.** The chest wall is composed of fat and soft tissue, including nerves, blood vessels, lymphatic vessels, muscle, bone, cartilage, and fibrous connective tissue. Chest wall lesions can arise from any of these component tissues. Of the myriad of possibilities, lipoma is seen with some frequency. On mammogram, an expanded appearance of the pectoralis muscle may be seen in association with decreased density of the muscle. This may be erroneously interpreted as muscular laxity and/ or atrophy (evoking diagnoses such as Poland syndrome and muscular dystrophy). On sonogram, no obvious abnormality may be seen if unilateral imaging is performed, whereas bilateral chest wall ultrasound may increase the conspicuity of the fatty mass. On magnetic resonance imaging (MRI), a homogeneously T1 hyperintense encapsulated mass is seen, which appears hypointense with fat saturation techniques.
- **Cavernous Hemangioma.** A chest wall hemangioma may be occasionally seen on both mammogram and ultrasound and is usually of the cavernous subtype, which may contain a substantial amount of fat. Calcifications are associated with cavernous hemangiomas in approximately 50% of cases and may be seen mammographically. Sonography can reveal a complex mass containing dilated vascular channels. If calcifications are abundant, acoustic shadowing may also be documented. Doppler evaluation may show hypervascularity and low-resistance arterial flow. If contrast-enhanced mammography is performed, heterogeneous contrast uptake may be seen. On MRI, these lesions characteristically show intermediate T1 signal intensity and marked T2 hyperintensity, indicating the central angiomatous core of the neoplasm. Signal intensity voids, caused by rapidly flowing blood, can also be seen. Cavernous hemangiomas do not spontaneously involute and, therefore, may require surgical intervention.
- **Lymphadenopathy.** Potential causes for abnormal lymph nodes between the pectoralis major and pectoralis minor (Rotter lymph nodes) include reactive causes and metastatic involvement, with breast cancer and systemic lymphoma being primary considerations. Other considerations would be metastatic spread from head and neck cancer and spread of abdominal malignancy via the thoracic duct, particularly for left anterior chest wall involvement. Systemic diseases, including rheumatoid arthritis and sarcoidosis, are considerations, but usually these conditions result in bilateral adenopathy. Reactive adenopathy is most often unilateral and can resolve with time and treatment.

■ Additional Differential Diagnoses

- **Normal rib.** Women with chest wall pain or self-palpation of a hard lump may present for diagnostic breast imaging, and when targeted ultrasound is performed, a normal-appearing rib may be identified. Potential causal scenarios could include developmental chest wall deformity recently self-recognized by the patient, costochondritis, and rib fracture/hematoma resulting in pain referenced to a rib. Reassuring the patient, when a corresponding normal-appearing rib is seen, is important to alleviate a concern for breast cancer.
- **Soft-tissue sarcomas.** Fibrosarcoma and malignant fibrous histiocytoma are the most common malignant tumors arising from the soft tissues of the chest wall in adult patients. Rhabdomyosarcoma, malignant schwannoma, and synovial sarcoma are less common. All these tumors have similar imaging appearances, including potential central necrosis and tumor calcification.

■ Diagnosis

Intermuscular lipoma

✓ Pearls

- Bilateral anterior chest wall ultrasound may assist in the diagnosis of an anterior chest wall lipoma.
- A cavernous hemangioma may have calcifications and internal flow on sonographic evaluation.
- Metastatic lymphadenopathy in the anterior chest wall should be considered in all chest wall mass cases.

Suggested Readings

Ikeda DM. Breast Imaging: The Requisites. 2nd ed. Philadelphia, PA: Elsevier; 2010

Jeung MY, Gangi A, Gasser B, et al. Imaging of chest wall disorders. Radiographics. 1999; 19(3):617–637

Youk JH, Kim EK, Kim MJ, Oh KK. Imaging findings of chest wall lesions on breast sonography. J Ultrasound Med. 2008; 27(1):125–138

Case 296

Frederick R. Margolin

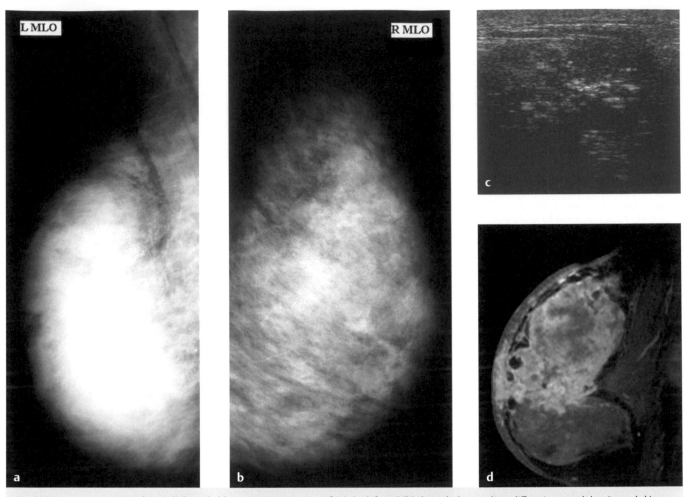

Fig. 296.1 Mammograms in the mediolateral oblique (MLO) projection of **(a)** the left and **(b)** the right breast show diffuse increased density and skin thickening involving the left breast. Amorphous microcalcifications were seen with magnification (not shown). The right breast is unremarkable. **(c)** Sonogram of the left breast in the transverse plane demonstrates marked skin thickening and an underlying hypoechoic irregular mass with echogenic foci consistent with calcifications. **(d)** Contrast-enhanced 3D gradient-recalled-echo magnetic resonance (MR) image with fat saturation of the left breast in the sagittal plane reveals heterogeneous irregular non-mass enhancement. The skin is diffusely thickened and demonstrates nodular enhancing foci, consistent with involvement of the dermal lymphatics.

■ Clinical Presentation

A 38-year-old woman with erythema and tenderness of the left breast of 2 weeks duration. Upon physical examination, findings consistent with "peau d'orange" are seen. The contralateral breast was normal (▶Fig. 296.1).

■ Key Imaging Finding

Unilateral breast skin thickening

■ Top 3 Differential Diagnoses

- **Inflammatory breast cancer.** Inflammatory breast carcinoma refers to breast cancer (ductal or lobular) with invasion of the dermal lymphatics, resulting in skin thickening, erythema, pain, and swelling. The skin of the affected breast resembles the thick rind of an orange, giving rise to the description "peau d'orange." Inflammatory breast cancer is biologically aggressive; metastasis to axillary lymph nodes at the time of diagnosis is often present. Bacterial superinfection is also common, such that affected patients may present with signs of mastitis. The diagnosis is made through punch biopsy of the skin, demonstrating tumor invasion of the dermal lymphatics. Imaging findings include diffuse skin thickening and increased density. An underlying malignancy (such as a spiculated mass or pleomorphic microcalcifications) may be seen. Overall, the prognosis is poor. Neoadjuvant (preoperative) chemotherapy is the usual treatment.

- **Mastitis.** Mastitis is an infection of the breast, usually caused by bacterial organisms such as *Staphylococcus*. Patients often present with fever, elevated white blood cell count, swelling, erythema, warmth, and tenderness. Patients should be followed up to resolution, since mastitis may be clinically indistinguishable from inflammatory breast cancer. At imaging, diffuse skin thickening and increased density may be seen. Abscess formation often requires percutaneous drainage in addition to antibiotic therapy.

- **Invasive breast cancer.** Invasive breast cancer (ductal or lobular) may involve the skin by local extension, resulting in focal skin thickening, erythema, and warmth. In contrast to inflammatory breast cancer, this is a focal rather than diffuse process. At imaging, the underlying cancer is seen with adjacent skin involvement. Local invasion of the skin carries a better prognosis than dermal lymphatic invasion.

■ Additional Differential Diagnoses

- **Post-surgical or post-radiation changes.** Skin thickening may be seen after surgery or (more commonly) after radiation. This is a unilateral finding affecting the treated breast. Post-surgical skin thickening is usually focal, while radiation results in diffuse skin thickening. Skin thickening may decrease over time.

- **Subclavian vein thrombosis.** Unilateral subclavian vein or brachiocephalic vein thrombosis can result from external compression, indwelling catheter, or in the setting of throm-

botic states. Increased venous pressure can result in stasis of fluids and breast edema, manifesting as unilateral skin thickening. Thickening of the breast trabeculae may also be present. Bilateral breast skin thickening can be seen in the setting of superior vena cava (SVC) syndrome.

- **Lymphedema.** Axillary lymph node dissection may be complicated by disruption of the lymphatic drainage of the ipsilateral breast. This results in edema, manifesting as skin and trabeculae thickening.

■ Diagnosis

Inflammatory breast carcinoma

✓ Pearls

- Inflammatory breast carcinoma is diffuse with clinical and imaging findings involving the entire breast.
- Skin involvement by local tumor extension has a better prognosis than inflammatory breast cancer.

- Mastitis may be indistinguishable from inflammatory breast cancer based on clinical and imaging findings.
- Post-surgical skin thickening is usually focal, while post-radiation skin thickening is often diffuse.

Suggested Readings

Ikeda DM. Breast Imaging: The Requisites. 2nd ed. Philadelphia, PA: Elsevier; 2010

Merajver SD, Sabel MS. Inflammatory breast cancer. In: Harris JR, Lippman ME, Morrow M, Osborne CK, eds. Diseases of the Breast. 5th ed. Philadelphia, PA: Lippincott Williams and Wilkins; 2014

Yeh ED, Jacene HA, Bellon JR, et al. What radiologists need to know about diagnosis and treatment of inflammatory breast cancer: a multidisciplinary approach. Radiographics. 2013; 33(7):2003–2017

Case 297

Chloe M. Chhor

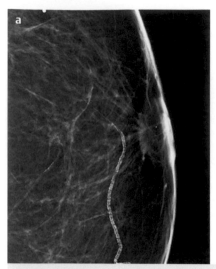 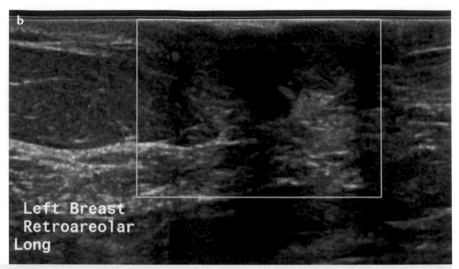

Fig. 297.1 **(a)** Spot compression magnification mammogram of the retroareolar left breast reveals architectural distortion. **(b)** Doppler ultrasound shows a hypoechoic vascularized mass inseparable from the nipple.

■ Clinical Presentation

A 67-year-old woman who presented with erythema and crusting of the nipple of 3 months duration (▶Fig. 297.1).

■ Key Imaging Finding

Unilateral nipple/skin changes

■ Top 3 Differential Diagnoses

- **Paget disease of the nipple**. Paget disease of the nipple refers to breast cancer involving the nipple-areolar complex. Cancer cells extend into the large ducts and lymphatics and out into the skin of the nipple, manifesting as an eczematous, crusty nipple. Paget disease typically occurs in older women. Most commonly, ductal carcinoma in situ (DCIS) is the underlying malignancy, although an invasive component may be present. Clinically, patients present with bloody nipple discharge and crusting of the nipple. Malignant calcifications representing DCIS may be seen at mammography. At magnetic resonance imaging (MRI), either mass or non-mass enhancement may be present with extension to the nipple-areolar complex. MRI is also helpful in identifying an invasive component of the disease that is otherwise occult. Mastectomy is the usual treatment.

- **Mastitis**. Mastitis is usually infectious (bacterial) in origin. Common bacterial agents include *Streptococcus* and *Staphylococcus*. The affected breast is erythematous, swollen, warm, and tender. Predisposing factors include lactation and trauma.

Mammography may show increased density and skin thickening. Sonography may show skin thickening and edema and is useful in evaluating for abscess formation. If symptoms do not resolve following antibiotic treatment, carcinoma (especially inflammatory breast carcinoma) must be excluded (usually with skin punch biopsy).

- **Inflammatory breast carcinoma**. Inflammatory breast carcinoma is a relatively infrequent, but very aggressive form of breast carcinoma that invades the dermal lymphatics. It may be of ductal or lobular histology. Patients present with rapid onset of a warm, erythematous breast. The skin can have a pitted, thickened appearance similar to an orange skin (hence known as peau d'orange). Inflammatory breast carcinoma is primarily a clinical diagnosis, though skin punch biopsy is often diagnostic. Mammography, ultrasound (US), or MRI may reveal signs of cancer diffusely. Alternatively, the underlying cancer may be occult at imaging, and only skin thickening is identified. This disease has a poor prognosis.

■ Additional Differential Diagnoses

- **Nipple adenoma**. Nipple adenoma, also known as florid papillomatosis or papillary adenoma, is a benign tumor of the lactiferous ducts that develops in the superficial portion of the nipple and can present as a well-circumscribed, non-encapsulated mass. Symptoms may resemble those of Paget disease with serosanguinous nipple discharge, skin ulceration, erythema, and nipple enlargement.

- **Eczema of the breast**. Eczema of the breast may mimic Paget disease; it is characterized by an erythematous, crusty nipple with pruritic patches. This diagnosis is made when the signs and symptoms resolve with treatment, such as with topical steroids.

■ Diagnosis

Paget disease of the nipple

✓ Pearls

- Paget disease can be associated with DCIS or an invasive underlying cancer.
- Cellulitis and inflammatory carcinoma can have similar clinical manifestations.

- If mastitis or eczema of the breast does not resolve with treatment, malignancy should be considered.

Suggested Readings

Kushwaha AC, Whitman GJ, Stelling CB, Cristofanilli M, Buzdar AU. Primary inflammatory carcinoma of the breast: retrospective review of mammographic findings. AJR Am J Roentgenol. 2000; 174(2):535–538

Lim HS, Jeong SJ, Lee JS, et al. Paget disease of the breast: mammographic, US, and MR imaging findings with pathologic correlation. Radiographics. 2011; 31(7):1973–1987

Case 298

Frederick R. Margolin

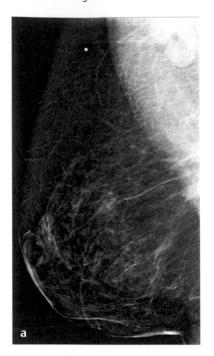
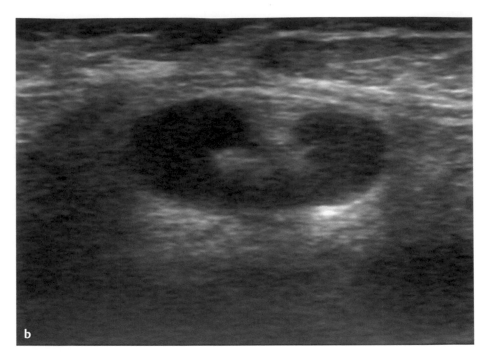
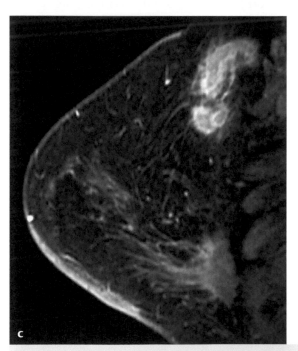

Fig. 298.1 **(a)** Mammogram in the mediolateral oblique (MLO) projection reveals enlarged axillary lymph nodes with thickened cortices, corresponding to the clinical symptom of palpable axillary lump. **(b)** Sonogram in the transverse plane shows an enlarged (>2 cm) reniform mass with thickened hypoechoic cortex and relative effacement of the fatty hilum, consistent with lymphadenopathy. **(c)** Contrast-enhanced 3D gradient-recalled-echo MR image with fat saturation in the sagittal plane not only confirms the presence of axillary lymphadenopathy but also shows an underlying heterogeneous irregular enhancing mass in the lower breast near the pectoralis muscle, consistent with a primary breast carcinoma.

■ Clinical Presentation

A 73-year-old woman with palpable lump in the left axilla of 2 months duration (▶ Fig. 298.1).

■ **Key Imaging Finding**

Axillary lymphadenopathy

■ **Top 3 Differential Diagnoses**

- **Breast cancer with lymph node spread**. When breast cancer spreads to the ipsilateral axillary node(s), this is considered a locoregional disease and not a systemic metastatic disease. Depending upon staging, prognosis is still relatively good, and the patient can potentially be cured. When sufficiently large, lymphadenopathy may be seen at mammography, ultrasound (US), or magnetic resonance imaging (MRI). However, imaging cannot exclude disease in nodes that are not enlarged, and that retain their normal morphology. Sentinel node biopsy is the standard-of-care in evaluating for axillary node involvement. If the sentinel node(s) are normal, axillary nodal dissection would not be indicated. In women with adenocarcinoma of the axillary nodes, but without identifiable primary cancer, the ipsilateral breast is the likely source. MRI has been shown to be a useful tool in identifying breast malignancies which are otherwise occult at mammography and US.

- **Lymphoma**. Systemic lymphoma (either Hodgkin or non-Hodgkin lymphoma) may present with axillary lymphadenopathy. Patients most often have lymphadenopathy elsewhere in the body as well. Patients may report systemic symptoms, such as weight loss and malaise. Diagnosis is made through correlation with clinical history, identification of lymphadenopathy elsewhere in the body, and biopsy.
- **Reactive lymphadenopathy**. Reactive lymphadenopathy in the axilla is generally due to an infection of the upper extremity. The involved nodes may be tender. Cat scratch fever is one cause of painful regional lymphadenopathy. Correlation with clinical history and physical examination is important in making the diagnosis. Reactive lymphadenopathy is generally unilateral and should resolve with time. Human immunodeficiency virus (HIV) may cause bilateral reactive axillary lymphadenopathy.

■ **Additional Differential Diagnoses**

- **Metastases from remote primary**. Metastases from a remote primary cancer may present in the axilla. Reported primary cancers include thyroid, ovarian, pancreatic, and head and neck region. Lymphadenopathy may be unilateral or bilateral. Patients with such nodal disease have a poor prognosis. Diagnosis is often made with a clinical and imaging workup for malignancy, as well as biopsy.
- **Connective tissue and granulomatous disorders**. Systemic diseases, including rheumatoid arthritis or sarcoidosis, may result in axillary lymphadenopathy. When this occurs, the

lymphadenopathy is usually bilateral. Sarcoidosis classically manifests with concomitant mediastinal and hilar lymphadenopathy.
- **Castleman disease**. Castleman disease is a rare inflammatory lymphoproliferative disorder of unknown etiology. It most commonly presents as mediastinal lymphadenopathy, but may rarely present as axillary lymphadenopathy (bilateral or unilateral), usually with hypervascular (hyperenhancing) adenopathy.

■ **Diagnosis**

Breast cancer with axillary lymph node spread

✓ **Pearls**

- MRI is useful in demonstrating occult breast malignancies in the setting of axillary lymphadenopathy.
- Patients with lymphoma often have systemic symptoms, bilateral involvement, and involvement elsewhere.

- Reactive lymphadenopathy secondary to infection is most often unilateral and often resolves with time.

Suggested Readings

Chang YW, Noh HJ, Hong SS, Hwang JH, Lee DW, Moon JH. Castleman disease of the axilla mimicking metastasis. Clin Imaging. 2007; 31(6):425–427

Ecanow JS, Abe H, Newstead GM, Ecanow DB, Jeske JM. Axillary staging of breast cancer: what the radiologist should know. Radiographics. 2013; 33(6):1589–1612

Ikeda DM. Breast Imaging: The Requisites. 2nd ed. Philadelphia, PA: Elsevier; 2010

Ko EY, Han BK, Shin JH, Kang SS. Breast MRI for evaluating patients with metastatic axillary lymph node and initially negative mammography and sonography. Korean J Radiol. 2007; 8(5):382–389

Case 299

Natasha Brasic

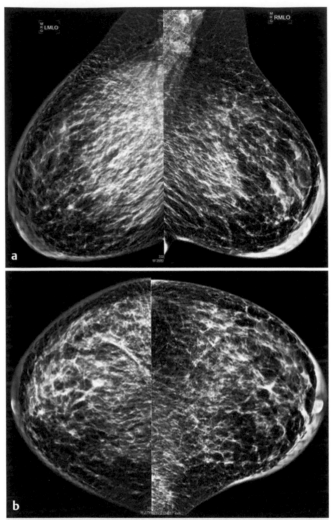

Fig. 299.1 Bilateral (a) mediolateral oblique (MLO) and (b) cranial-caudal (CC) mammograms demonstrate bilateral diffuse skin thickening and thickened trabeculae, more pronounced on the right.

■ Clinical Presentation

A 67-year-old woman undergoing screening mammography (►Fig. 299.1).

■ Key Imaging Finding

Bilateral skin thickening

■ Top 3 Differential Diagnoses

- **Congestive heart failure**. With elevated intracardiac pressures and impaired venous drainage in congestive heart failure, edema most commonly occurs in the lower extremities, but it may also occur in the breasts. Impaired venous return results in increased capillary hydrostatic pressures, resulting in soft tissue edema. This is seen as skin thickening at mammography (normal skin thickness measures up to approximately 2 mm). Trabecular thickening in the breast parenchyma may also be present.

- **Superior vena cava (SVC) obstruction**. Obstruction of the SVC is usually due to a thoracic tumor such as lung cancer. External compression coupled with thrombosis results in obstruction of the SVC. Subsequently, venous return to the heart is impaired, and increased venous pressure with elevated intracapillary hydrostatic pressure occurs. This results in edema of the

breasts, visualized as skin thickening. If long-standing, collateral vessels will form, resulting in multiple dilated veins which may be visualized at mammography.

- **Bilateral lymphedema**. Lymphatic drainage of the skin is contiguous with the lymphatics that pass through the breasts. In up to 50% of axillary lymph node dissections, the lymphatic drainage is disrupted enough to result in lymphatic congestion of the skin. Often, there may be subtle or pronounced thickening of the breast trabeculae as defined by Cooper's ligaments. Lymphedema may result in significant morbidity. This complication has significantly decreased with the advent of sentinel node biopsy techniques. In breast cancer cases where the sentinel node is free of cancer, full axillary lymph node dissection may be safely obviated, thus reducing patient morbidity.

■ Additional Differential Diagnoses

- **Renal failure and volume overload**. Renal failure, whether acute or chronic, leads to volume overload and increased capillary hydrostatic pressures. The end result is skin and trabecular thickening caused by the same mechanism as congestive heart failure.

- **Psoriasis**. Psoriasis is a chronic disease of unknown etiology which leads to dry scaly plaques and skin thickening. Patients

are affected to varying degrees. Although a relatively uncommon cause of skin thickening of the breasts, psoriasis should be considered when skin thickening occurs in both breasts. Other systemic diseases with skin involvement include scleroderma, dermatomyositis, and congenital absence of the lymphatics. These conditions rarely affect the breasts.

■ Diagnosis

Congestive heart failure

✓ Pearls

- Normal skin overlying the breast measures up to 2 mm in thickness.
- Volume overload or venous drainage obstruction leads to elevated hydrostatic pressure and edema.

- Disruption of lymphatic drainage from bilateral axillary lymph node dissection may cause skin thickening.
- Psoriasis may present with bilateral dry scaly plaques and skin thickening.

Suggested Readings

Jesinger RA, Lattin GE, Jr, Ballard EA, Zelasko SM, Glassman LM. Vascular abnormalities of the breast: arterial and venous disorders, vascular masses, and mimic lesions with radiologic-pathologic correlation. Radiographics. 2011; 31(7):E117–E136

Oraedu CO, Pinnapureddy P, Alrawi S, Acinapura AJ, Raju R. Congestive heart failure mimicking inflammatory breast carcinoma: a case report and review of the literature. Breast J. 2001; 7(2):117–119

Rönkä RH, Pamilo MS, von Smitten KA, Leidenius MH. Breast lymphedema after breast conserving treatment. Acta Oncol. 2004; 43(6):551–557

Case 300

Matthew R. Denny and Jessica W. T. Leung

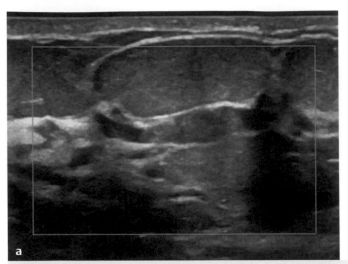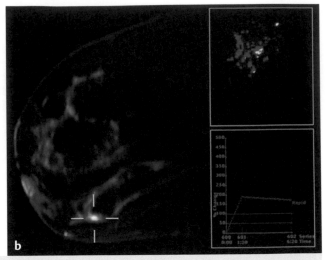

Fig. 300.1 (a) Targeted Doppler ultrasound in the inferior right breast shows an intraductal mass. (b) Breast magnetic resonance imaging (MRI) with kinetic mapping shows rapid enhancement and washout of the mass in the inferior right breast.

■ Clinical Presentation

A 45-year-old woman who presented with spontaneous clear nipple discharge (▶Fig. 300.1).

■ Key Imaging Finding

Breast lesion with unilateral nipple discharge

■ Top 3 Differential Diagnoses

- **Intraductal papilloma.** Papilloma is a benign breast mass that grows on a fibrovascular stalk. It may secrete fluid and form a surrounding cyst, resulting in intracystic papilloma with an appearance of a circumscribed cystic mass. It may also undergo necrosis with bloody nipple discharge. Pathologically, papilloma is often associated with atypia. Hence, it may be difficult to distinguish benign papilloma from papillary carcinoma with core biopsy, and surgical excision may be needed. Intracystic papillary carcinoma is similar in its biologic behavior as in situ carcinoma. Invasive papillary carcinoma is rare. At mammography, papillary lesions may appear as circumscribed masses. At sonography, hypoechoic solid and cystic components may be present. Doppler signal may be present within the solid component, distinguishing it from cystic debris. Percutaneous core biopsy should include the solid component. A marker clip should be placed, as the lesion may be difficult to identify after biopsy if the cystic fluid component ruptures (the lesion may then appear isoechoic and difficult to identify).

- **Mammary duct ectasia.** Mammary duct ectasia results when a duct in the retroareolar breast becomes inflamed, dilated, or obstructed. Whitish, greenish, or blackish nipple discharge may result. Etiologies include hormonal changes, smoking, or a newly inverted nipple. This condition is benign and usually self-limiting. Mammography is usually negative. Non-specific dilated duct(s) may be seen at ultrasound.

- **Breast carcinoma (ductal or papillary).** Nipple discharge that is the result of a malignancy is usually bloody and originates from a single duct. The underlying malignancy is most often intraductal carcinoma, such as ductal carcinoma in situ (DCIS). Other malignancies that can give rise to bloody nipple discharge include intracystic papillary carcinoma or invasive carcinomas (of either ductal or lobular histology). Mammography and ultrasound may show signs of malignancy, such as a mass or calcifications. Paget disease of the breast, or DCIS affecting the nipple-areolar complex, classically presents with bloody nipple discharge and crusting of the nipple. Calcifications may be seen in Paget disease.

■ Additional Differential Diagnoses

- **Fibrocystic change.** Fibrocystic change is within the spectrum of normal physiologic changes in the breast. At clinical examination, lumpy, tender breasts are found. A clear, yellow, or light green discharge may be expressed from both breasts. This is benign and usually self-limiting. Imaging is usually negative.

- **Galactorrhea.** Galactorrhea is a benign condition in which there is milky nipple discharge, usually from multiple ducts in both breasts. It may be a result of medication or disorders of the hypothalamus or pituitary gland, such as a prolactinoma. Mammography and ultrasound are usually negative.

■ Diagnosis

Intraductal papilloma

✓ Pearls

- Bloody nipple discharge may be benign (papilloma) or malignant (Paget disease and breast carcinoma).
- Imaging is often negative in the setting of nipple discharge due to fibrocystic change or galactorrhea.

- Patients with Paget disease present with bloody nipple discharge and nipple crusting.

Suggested Readings

Doshi DJ, March DE, Crisi GM, Coughlin BF. Complex cystic breast masses: diagnostic approach and imaging-pathologic correlation. Radiographics. 2007; 27(Suppl 1):S53–S64

Ferris-James DM, Iuanow E, Mehta TS, Shaheen RM, Slanetz PJ. Imaging approaches to diagnosis and management of common ductal abnormalities. Radiographics. 2012; 32(4):1009–1030

Ganesan S, Karthik G, Joshi M, Damodaran V. Ultrasound spectrum in intraductal papillary neoplasms of breast. Br J Radiol. 2006; 79(946):843–849

Case 301

Chloe M. Chhor

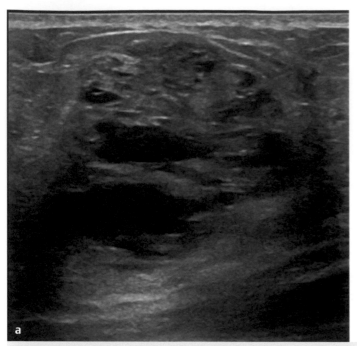
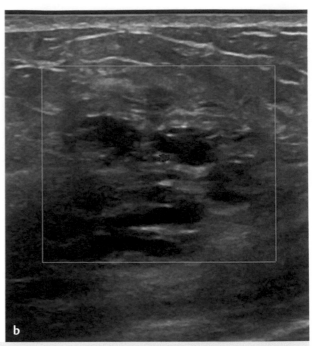

Fig. 301.1 (a) Sonogram in the transverse plane of the palpable lump demonstrates an ovoid mass of mixed echotexture with cystic spaces. **(b)** Doppler sonogram reveals no significant internal vascular flow.

■ Clinical Presentation

A 28-year-old lactating woman with a large palpable breast lump of 3-week duration (▶Fig. 301.1).

■ Key Imaging Finding

Complex cystic mass in a lactating woman

■ Top 3 Differential Diagnoses

- **Galactocele**. Galactocele is the most common of the several benign breast masses found in a lactating woman. It is a cystic mass that forms as a result of duct dilatation and contains fluid that resembles milk. Diagnosis and therapy can be achieved with percutaneous aspiration. Mammographic and sonographic appearance depends on the stage of development and on varying proportions of fat and proteinaceous material present, as well as on the density and viscosity of the fluid.
- **Abscess**. Infection is relatively common during lactation due to disruption of the epithelial interface of the nipple-areola complex with retrograde dissemination of bacteria. On ultrasound, abscesses usually appear as irregular hypoechoic or anechoic masses, sometimes with fluid–debris levels and posterior acoustic enhancement. Treatment consists of antibiotic

therapy, as well as surgical incision and drainage or percutaneous aspiration in some cases. If patients do not respond, biopsy is indicated to exclude malignancy.

- **Fibroadenoma**. Fibroadenoma is the most common benign solid mass in young women. It has a variable appearance at ultrasound, but classically appears as a circumscribed or gently lobulated, mildly hypoechoic, thinly encapsulated, elliptically shaped mass which is oriented parallel to the chest wall. During pregnancy, fibroadenoma may grow to a very large size because of hormonal influences and undergo infarction because it has outgrown its blood supply. It may also develop secretory hyperplasia. These changes may result in varying sonographic appearances, including a complex cystic appearance.

■ Additional Differential Diagnoses

- **Hematoma**. Hematoma is usually preceded by trauma or anticoagulation use. It may appear well-defined or ill-defined at mammography. The ultrasound appearance varies based upon the age of the hematoma. It is often anechoic in its hyperacute stage, mimicking a cyst. As it evolves, it may become hyperechoic and heterogeneous as the clotting process proceeds. Hematomas should be followed to resolution.
- **Lactating adenoma**. Lactating adenoma is a benign solid and cystic breast mass that occurs in response to the physiologic changes that characterize pregnancy and lactation. Its sonographic appearance closely resembles that of a fibroadenoma.

Hyperechoic areas represent the fat content of milk due to lactational hyperplasia. Lactating adenoma occasionally displays suspicious features for malignancy, some of which may be attributed to infarction. It usually regresses spontaneously after pregnancy and lactation.

- **Fibrocystic change**. Fibrocystic change is a physiologic finding consisting of varying degrees of cystic dilatation and cystic enlargement. The ultrasound features of fibrocystic change will vary depending on the predominating tissue component: cystic and/or solid proliferative.

■ Diagnosis

Lactating adenoma

✓ Pearls

- Galactocele is the most common benign cystic mass in a lactating female; the fluid resembles milk.
- In patients with suspected breast abscesses unresponsive to treatment, malignancy needs to be excluded.

- Lactating adenoma is a solid and cystic mass occurring with pregnancy/lactation; it spontaneously regresses.
- Fibroadenoma can grow, undergo infarction, or develop secretory hyperplasia during pregnancy.

Suggested Readings

Sabate JM, Clotet M, Torrubia S, et al. Radiologic evaluation of breast disorders related to pregnancy and lactation. Radiographics. 2007; 27(Suppl 1):S101–S124

Stavros AT. Breast Ultrasound. Philadelphia, PA: Lippincott Williams & Wilkins; 2004

Case 302

Boon Chye Ching

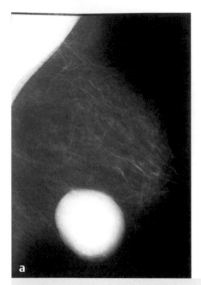 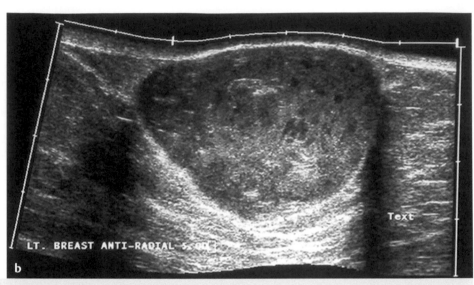

Fig. 302.1 **(a)** Mammogram in the mediolateral oblique (MLO) projection shows a large circumscribed dense mass in the lower left breast. **(b)** Sonogram in the anti-radial plane demonstrates a corresponding hypoechoic solid mass.

■ Clinical Presentation

A 45-year-old woman with a palpable lump that has increased in size over several months (▶Fig. 302.1).

■ **Key Imaging Finding**

Large solid breast mass

■ **Top 3 Differential Diagnoses**

• **Phyllodes tumor**. The term *phyllodes* comes from a Greek word meaning "leaf-like," as its tumor microscopy exhibits papillary protuberances of epithelial lined stroma. The spectrum of phyllodes tumor ranges from low to high grade, with high-grade tumors tending to have intramural cystic spaces. Like fibroadenoma, phyllodes tumor is a fibroepithelial lesion, and cellular fibroadenoma is difficult to distinguish from phyllodes tumor on pathologic analysis. Phyllodes tumor appears as a dense circumscribed mass on mammography and as a hypoechoic mass on sonography. It is seldom associated with calcifications. These tumors can be locally aggressive, necessitating wide surgical margins. Imaging is not reliable in differentiating fibroadenoma from phyllodes tumor, and phyllodes tumor should be expected with a history of a rapidly enlarging circumscribed mass.

• **Fibroadenoma**. Fibroadenoma is a solid benign mass and is the most common breast mass in young women and the most common palpable breast mass in women in their thirties. At mammography, this mass appears as a circumscribed or lobulated round or oval mass possibly associated with dystrophic calcifications. At sonography, it appears as a circumscribed hypoechoic mass with homogeneous internal echoes. There may be two or three gentle lobulations. Fibroadenoma may increase in size with hormonal stimulation, such as pregnancy. If increased to a large size, it may undergo necrosis and develop cystic areas.

• **Circumscribed breast carcinoma**. Because of aggressive growth of cancers across tissue planes and because cancers may elicit desmoplastic reaction, cancers are generally irregular in shape with spiculated margins. Hence, less than 10% of breast carcinomas are circumscribed. The most common circumscribed breast carcinoma is invasive ductal carcinoma, not-otherwise-specified (NOS). Other circumscribed breast carcinomas can include mucinous, medullary, and papillary carcinomas.

■ **Additional Differential Diagnoses**

• **Hematoma**. A breast hematoma most often occurs in the setting of trauma, surgery, or anticoagulation. Its imaging appearance varies depending on early or late presentation. At sonography, a hematoma may present as a hypoechoic mass with heterogeneous internal echoes (especially as clots develop) or a cystic lesion with fluid–debris levels. Hematomas should decrease in size and resolve over time without intervention.

• **Abscess**: Breast abscess typically presents as a tender palpable mass near the subareolar region. It is usually associated with lactation or recent surgical intervention. A breast abscess is painful and, thus, better imaged with ultrasound than mammography. Sonographic findings include a hypoechoic mass with internal heterogeneous echoes and possibly containing cystic regions, septations, or gas. Edema may be seen in adjacent breast tissue. When superficial, skin thickening may be seen. Hyperemia can also be detected at Doppler imaging. Abscesses should be followed up to resolution to exclude necrotic malignancy.

■ **Diagnosis**

Phyllodes tumor

✓ **Pearls**

• Phyllodes tumor is a fibroepithelial lesion which is typically large; wide surgical margins are necessary.
• Imaging findings alone are not reliable in differentiating fibroadenoma from phyllodes tumor.

• Common circumscribed carcinomas include invasive ductal, NOS; mucinous; medullary; and papillary.
• Clinical history is helpful in diagnosing hematomas and abscesses; these should be followed up to resolution.

Suggested Readings

Goel NB, Knight TE, Pandey S, Riddick-Young M, de Paredes ES, Trivedi A. Fibrous lesions of the breast: imaging-pathologic correlation. Radiographics. 2005; 25(6):1547–1559

Ikeda DM. Breast Imaging: The Requisites. 2nd ed. Philadelphia, PA: Elsevier; 2010

Case 303

Boon Chye Ching

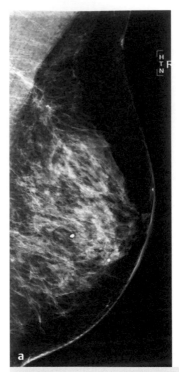
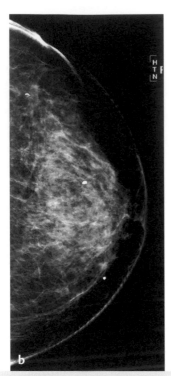
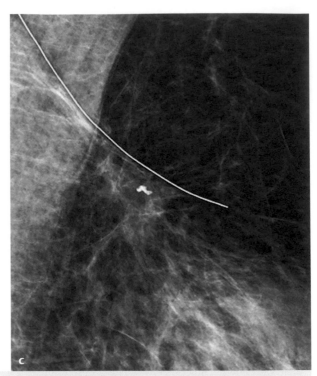

Fig. 303.1 Mammograms in **(a)** the mediolateral oblique (MLO) and **(b)** craniocaudal (CC) projections show an area of architectural distortion in the posterior upper outer breast. This area is better seen on the MLO than on the CC projection. The CC view shows overlying skin thickening. **(c)** Spot compression magnification mammography with a scar marker confirms that the scar seen on the skin of the patient corresponds to the architectural distortion identified at mammography. Spot compression magnification mammography demonstrates the coarse morphology of the associated calcifications.

■ Clinical Presentation

A 46-year-old woman with a previous history of lumpectomy (►Fig. 303.1).

■ Key Imaging Finding

Postoperative changes

■ Top 3 Differential Diagnoses

- **Postsurgical architectural distortion**. An established history of prior surgery is crucial for the diagnosis of architectural distortion as a result of postsurgical scarring. Tissue distortion can be seen at mammography or sonography with the distortion extending all the way to the overlying skin. A marker placed on the scar is often helpful to confirm that the architectural distortion corresponds to the site of surgery. The initial postsurgical changes at sonography may include a complex cystic mass. The cystic portion may be subsequently resorbed, leaving a nonspecific irregular hypoechoic mass which may mimic cancer. Postoperative changes will stabilize or decrease over time. At mammography, dystrophic calcifications may develop. Sonography is somewhat limited in evaluating the postsurgical sites, as scarring often results in intense posterior acoustic shadowing. Most scars will not enhance at magnetic resonance imaging (MRI) after 18 months, though some may enhance for a longer period.

- **Recurrent cancer**. Recurrent cancer usually occurs at or adjacent to the surgical site. There may be new suspicious microcalcifications (fine linear or pleomorphic microcalcifications in clustered, linear, or segmental distribution), a developing asymmetry, a new mass, or an increasing architectural distortion. Except for dystrophic calcifications, imaging findings that increase over time require immediate biopsy to exclude recurrent cancer.
- **Fat necrosis**. Fat necrosis occurs when intracellular fat escapes from damaged cells into the surrounding tissue, causing the body to react by forming granulation tissue. It is often due to surgery or trauma. As there are different stages, the imaging manifestations of fat necrosis range from benign-appearing to suspicious. It may present as lipid cysts, microcalcifications, coarse calcifications, focal asymmetries, or focal masses. Initially, the calcifications of fat necrosis may appear suspicious, but they coarsen over time.

■ Additional Differential Diagnoses

- **Radial scar**. Radial scar is a benign proliferative lesion, but may be associated with atypical and malignant conditions. Classically, radial scar appears at mammography as an area of architectural distortion with central lucent areas representing fat. There is no central mass. Radial scar is usually better seen on one of the two standard mammographic projections (usually better seen on craniocaudal projection) and can have varying appearances on orthogonal imaging. At sonography, radial scar usually appears as an area of architectural distortion, but a hypoechoic mass or posterior acoustic shadowing may be seen.

- **Tubular carcinoma**. At mammography, tubular carcinoma classically appears as a central mass with spiculated margins and, hence, simulates architectural distortion. It is generally less than 1 cm in diameter. It is usually very slow growing. It can be associated with amorphous or pleomorphic microcalcifications in up to 50% of cases. At sonography, tubular carcinoma typically presents as an irregular hypoechoic mass with spiculated or indistinct margins. Pure tubular carcinoma has a very good prognosis.

■ Diagnosis

Post-surgical architectural distortion

✓ Pearls

- Post-surgical architectural distortion stabilizes or decreases in size and/or conspicuity over time.
- Recurrent cancer often presents as increasing mass, architectural distortion, or suspicious calcifications.

- Microcalcifications seen in fat necrosis should coarsen over time; asymmetries should decrease with time.

Suggested Readings

Berg WA, Birdwell RL. Diagnostic Imaging. Breast. 1st ed. Salt Lake City, UT: Amirsys; 2006

Ikeda DM. Breast Imaging: The Requisites. Philadelphia, PA: Elsevier; 2004

Mendelson EB. Evaluation of the postoperative breast. Radiol Clin North Am. 1992; 30(1):107–138

Case 304

Chloe M. Chhor

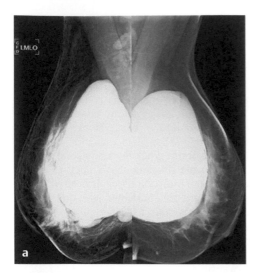
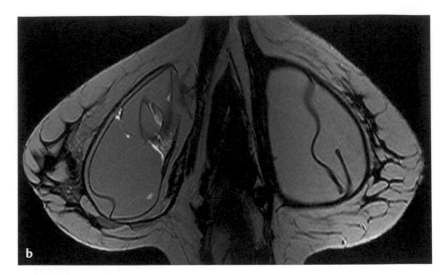
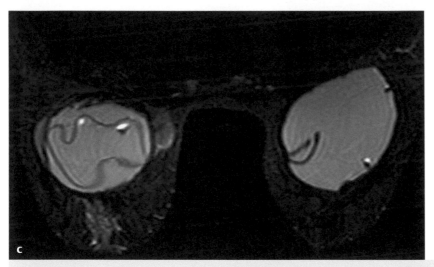

Fig. 304.1 (a) Mammograms in the mediolateral oblique (MLO) projection demonstrate bilateral prepectoral silicone implants. Extravasated silicone and implant discontinuity are present in the left breast. The right breast silicone implant appears intact. (b) Sagittal spin echo and (c) axial short tau inversion recovery (STIR) MR images show multiple curvilinear hypointense lines within high-signal silicone and free silicone within the breast parenchyma on the left. On the right, there are long hypointense curvilinear folds inferiorly, superiorly, and medially within the implant, which end blindly within the silicone gel.

■ Clinical Presentation

A 54-year-old woman with a history of bilateral breast augmentation with a change in contour of the left implant (▶ Fig. 304.1).

■ Key Imaging Finding

Implant defect

■ Top 3 Differential Diagnoses

- **Intracapsular rupture**. Silicone implant is a foreign body. The breast forms a fibrous capsule around the implant as a foreign body response, thus walling off the implant from the breast. Intracapsular rupture occurs when the shell of the implant ruptures, but the fibrous capsule formed by the breast remains intact. Silicone remains encapsulated and, therefore, does not freely extravasate. The contour of the implant remains largely intact; hence, this diagnosis is difficult to make on clinical examination or mammography. Magnetic resonance imaging (MRI) is the best method to diagnose intracapsular rupture. When the implant shell collapses within the fibrous capsule, curvilinear hypointense lines within high-signal silicone are seen, giving rise to the "linguine sign" of intracapsular rupture. The high signal silicone is seen on both sides of the collapsed shell.

- **Extracapsular rupture**. If the fibrous capsule ruptures in addition to the implant shell, extracapsular rupture occurs, allowing free silicone to extrude into the breast parenchyma. By definition, intracapsular rupture is also present when there is extracapsular rupture. Extracapsular rupture can lead to a change in the implant contour and, thus, may be detected on clinical examination or mammography.
- **Radial fold**. Radial folds represent infolding of an intact implant shell and may be confused with subtle intracapsular rupture. Radial folds appear thicker than the lines associated with a collapsed implant shell, because radial folds consist of two adjacent shell layers. On a single image, they may be confused with intracapsular rupture. Careful and detailed evaluation of serial images can usually distinguish between radial folds and an intracapsular rupture. Radial folds are characteristically blind-ending within the implant.

■ Additional Differential Diagnoses

- **Gel bleed**. Gel bleed can occur when silicone molecules diffuse through an intact implant shell. If enough silicone molecules diffuse through the shell, "gross" gel bleed can be seen as a visible layer of silicone coating the outer surface of the implant. This may appear as if there is extracapsular rupture, even when the implant shell is intact. Separation of the intact shell from the fibrous capsule can also be seen when gross gel bleed occurs, giving the appearance of an intracapsular rup-

ture. Rupture is more common than gross gel bleed and should be considered first.
- **Herniation**. Herniation refers to bulging of the implant with an intact shell. Herniation can occur through a defect in the surrounding fibrous capsule before it fully envelops the entire implant shell. Herniation can be confused with rupture and capsular contraction. Unlike rupture or capsular contraction, the deformity from herniation remains stable with time, and no extravasated silicone is seen elsewhere.

■ Diagnosis

Left breast: intra- and extracapsular rupture; Right breast: radial folds

✓ Pearls

- Intracapsular rupture is best detected at MRI; the "linguine sign" is characteristic.
- Free silicone in the breast or in axillary lymph nodes implies extracapsular rupture.

- Radial folds are thicker than a collapsed implant shell; they are typically blind-ending within the implant.
- Gel bleed mimics extravasated silicone, but occurs with an intact implant shell.

Suggested Readings

Hölmich LR, Vejborg I, Conrad C, Sletting S, McLaughlin JK. The diagnosis of breast implant rupture: MRI findings compared with findings at explantation. Eur J Radiol. 2005; 53(2):213–225

Soo MS, Kornguth PJ, Walsh R, Elenberger CD, Georgiade GS. Complex radial folds versus subtle signs of intracapsular rupture of breast implants: MR findings with surgical correlation. AJR Am J Roentgenol. 1996; 166(6):1421–1427
Yang N, Muradali D. The augmented breast: a pictorial review of the abnormal and unusual. AJR Am J Roentgenol. 2011; 196(4):W451–W460

Case 305

Matthew R. Denny and Jessica W. T. Leung

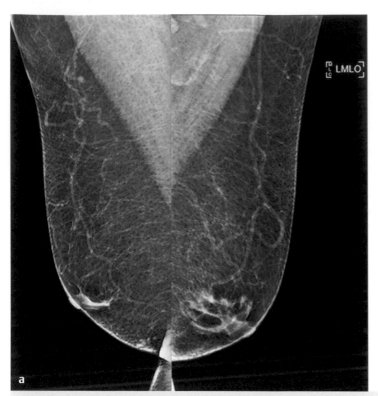

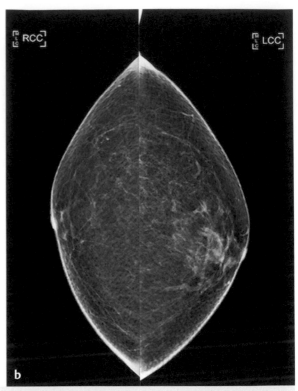

Fig. 305.1 Mammograms of both breasts in **(a)** the mediolateral oblique (MLO) and **(b)** craniocaudal (CC) projections reveal asymmetric breast tissue with a "flame-shaped" appearance in the retroareolar region of the left breast. No mass or calcifications are identified. The remainder of the left breast and the entire right breast are fatty, but otherwise unremarkable.

■ Clinical Presentation

A 47-year-old man with painful palpable lump in left retroareolar breast of 2 months duration (►Fig. 305.1).

■ Key Imaging Finding

Breast lesion in a man

■ Top 3 Differential Diagnoses

- **Gynecomastia**. Gynecomastia is a benign condition in men in which breast tissue is stimulated and becomes prominent. Etiologies include hormonal stimulation, either exogenous (antiandrogens or gonadotropin-releasing hormone (GnRH) agonists for treatment of prostate cancer) or endogenous (testicular and adrenal tumors), medication use (e.g., marijuana, cimetidine, omeprazole, and spironolactone), and idiopathic causes. Physiological gynecomastia may occur in newborns, during puberty, or in elderly or obese men. Men may present with a painful palpable lump in the retroareolar region. At mammography, gynecomastia appears as "flame-shaped" tissue in the retroareolar region without an associated mass or calcification. Tissue is usually unilateral, but may be bilateral and asymmetric. In the absence of a mass at mammography, sonography need not be performed. In point, ultrasound findings may be confusing and lead to unnecessary follow-up or biopsy.

- **Breast cancer**. Male breast cancer constitutes approximately 1% of all breast cancers. Because of the typical lack of lobular differentiation, almost all male breast cancers are of ductal (not lobular) histology. Male breast cancer usually presents with a palpable lump, hard/fixed breast tissue, skin/nipple changes, and/or lymphadenopathy. A history of gynecomastia has been noted in up to 40% of male breast cancer patients. At mammography, male breast cancer usually manifests as a mass. Calcifications are less common than in female breast cancer, but may be present. Ultrasound findings consist of a hypoechoic solid mass. Treatment is similar to that for female breast cancer; however, men tend to present at a later stage.

- **Lipoma**. Lipoma is a fat-containing mass. It appears lucent and circumscribed at mammography. The sonographic appearance may be variable, ranging from a hypoechoic solid mass to a mass of mixed echotexture. This benign diagnosis is often made at mammography, and biopsy is generally not needed.

■ Additional Differential Diagnoses

- **Hematoma**. A hematoma appears as a high-density mass at mammography. It is usually preceded by a history of trauma or anticoagulation use. Upon visual inspection, ecchymosis of the overlying soft tissues is often present. Hematomas are benign, but should be followed up to resolution.

- **Abscess**. An abscess appears as an irregular or circumscribed mass, often associated with signs of mastitis (e.g., skin thickening and edema). Focal or diffuse pain is often present. Clini-

cal history contributes to making this diagnosis. Percutaneous or surgical drainage may be necessary, along with antibiotic therapy.

- **Metastases**. Metastases to male breasts are rare. When present, they usually present as multiple bilateral round or oval partially circumscribed masses (as opposed to multicentric primary breast cancer which is often irregular or spiculated). Melanoma and lymphoma are the most common metastases.

■ Diagnosis

Gynecomastia

✓ Pearls

- Gynecomastia presents as unilateral or bilateral asymmetric "flame-shaped" retroareolar breast tissue.
- Male breast cancer is usually of ductal (not lobular) origin; treatment is similar to that for breast cancer in women.

- Hematomas and abscesses are suggested by clinical history; they should be followed up to resolution.

Suggested Readings

Lattin GE, Jr, Jesinger RA, Mattu R, Glassman LM. From the radiologic pathology archives: diseases of the male breast: radiologic-pathologic correlation. Radiographics. 2013; 33(2):461–489

Nguyen C, Kettler MD, Swirsky ME, et al. Male breast disease: pictorial review with radiologic-pathologic correlation. Radiographics. 2013; 33(3):763–779

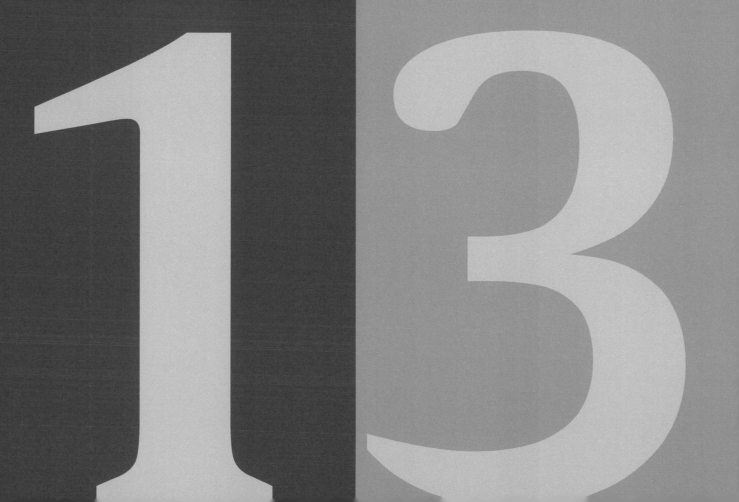

Part 13

Roentgen Classics

Case 306

Brady S. Davis

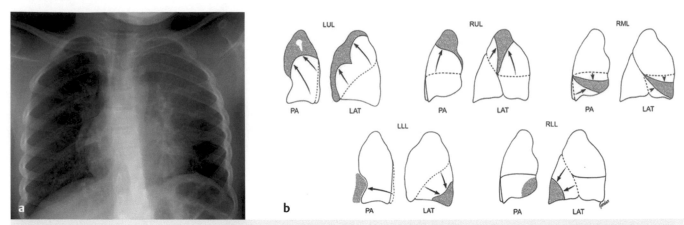

Fig. 306.1 (a) Frontal chest radiograph demonstrates veil-like opacification of the left lung with an elevated hilum, volume loss and left diaphragmatic juxtaphrenic peak. Increased lucency adjacent to the aortic knob is consistent with a Luftsichel (air crescent) sign. (b) Characteristic patterns of lobar collapse. LAT, lateral; LLL, left lower lobe; LUL, left upper lobe; PA, posteroanterior; RLL, right lower lobe; RML, right middle lobe; RUL, right upper lobe.

■ Clinical Presentation

A 7-year-old boy with difficulty breathing (▶Fig. 306.1).

■ Key Imaging Finding

Veil-like opacification and volume loss of the left upper lobe

■ Diagnosis

- **Left upper lobe collapse.** Lobar collapse (atelectasis) results from decreased aeration of the lung that may result from various underlying etiologies, including an obstructing endobronchial lesion (obstructive atelectasis), extrinsic compression from an adjacent neoplastic process (compressive atelectasis), a pleural effusion or pneumothorax (passive atelectasis), reduced lung compliance seen with loss of surfactant (adhesive atelectasis), or lung fibrosis (cicatrization atelectasis).
- The radiographic features of lobar collapse are fairly predictable based on the lobe involved and pattern of collapse (▶Fig. 306.1B). A specific pattern includes the Luftsichel sign (German for "air sickle") associated with left upper lobe (LUL) collapse. This sign refers to a sickle-shaped lucency interposed between the aortic arch and the atelectatic LUL due to compensatory hyperexpansion of the left lower lobe (LLL). LUL collapse may result in a juxtaphrenic peak along the insertion site of an inferior accessory fissure.
- A central hilar mass can lead to obstructive upper lobe collapse, resulting in the characteristic "S sign of Golden." The S- or reverse S-shape refers to the configuration of the minor fissure due to superomedial collapse of the right (RUL) with a superimposed central mass. This sign should prompt more advanced imaging, such as computed tomography, to exclude a hilar, central lung, or endobronchial (e.g., bronchogenic carcinoma, carcinoid, lymphoma, and salivary gland tumors) malignancy.

✓ Pearls

- Patterns of lobar collapse should be recognized by their characteristic features.
- Evaluation for a central endobronchial lesion is necessary when there is unexplained lobar collapse.
- Imaging findings include volume loss, hilar retraction, and fissure displacement.
- LUL collapse results in the Luftsichel sign; (reverse) "S sign of Golden" may be seen with RUL or LUL collapse.

Suggested Readings

Ashizawa K, Hayashi K, Aso N, Minami K. Lobar atelectasis: diagnostic pitfalls on chest radiography. Br J Radiol . 2001; 74(877):89–97

Blankenbaker DG. The Luftsichel sign. Radiology . 1998; 208(2):319–320
Gupta P. The Golden S sign. Radiology . 2004; 233(3):790–791

Case 307

Brady S. Davis

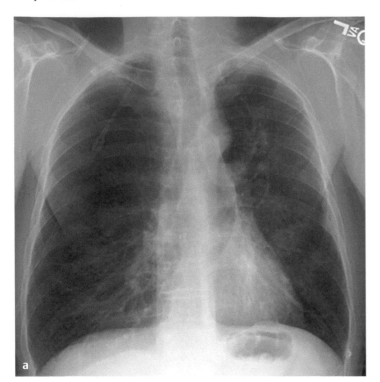
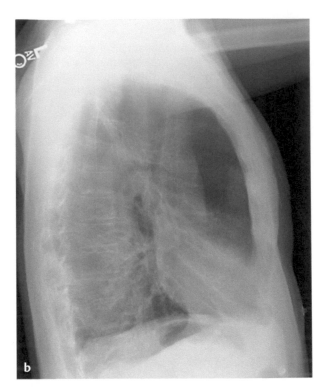
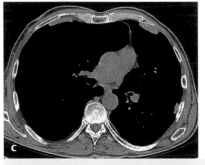
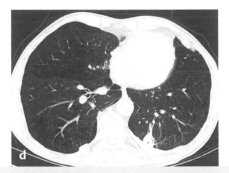
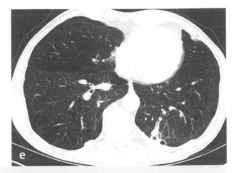

Fig. 307.1 **(a)** Posteroanterior (PA) and **(b)** lateral chest radiographs demonstrate multiple peripheral pleural based lesions. **(c)** Axial CT image in soft tissue window reveals bilateral pleural plaques with and without regions of calcification. **(d,e)** Axial CT images in lung window reveal a peripheral oval-shaped nodular density with adjacent pleural thickening in contiguity with the bronchovascular bundle, which has a curvilinear or "comet tail" configuration leading into the mass.

■ Clinical Presentation

A 63-year-old man with shortness of breath (▶Fig. 307.1).

◼ Key Imaging Finding

Pleural-based rounded opacity adjacent to pleural thickening

◼ Diagnosis

- **Round atelectasis.** Rounded atelectasis is a focal region of collapsed peripheral lung associated with adjacent pleural disease, such as pleural thickening or pleural effusion. The posterior aspects of the lower lobes are the most common site of involvement with the remaining lung fields being involved less frequently. The region of involvement most often ranges from 1 to 10 cm in size. There is an increased incidence in patients with asbestos-related pleural disease.
- The focally atelectatic lung takes on a rounded, oval, or wedge shape, hence the aptly descriptive name. The supplying bronchovascular bundle typically has a swirling or curvilinear appearance as it converges along the edge of the rounded atelec-

tatic lung, resulting in a characteristic "comet tail" sign. Other computed tomography (CT) features include angular margins, localized volume loss, and the presence of air bronchograms.

- Rounded atelectasis is a benign entity and is usually asymptomatic. If characteristic features are not present, however, follow-up imaging or further evaluation with 18-fluorodeoxyglucose positron emission tomography (FDG PET) should be considered, since tumors will persist or enlarge and demonstrate increased metabolic activity, whereas rounded atelectasis may decrease in size or resolve and lack increased metabolic activity.

✓ Pearls

- Round atelectasis occurs adjacent to the underlying pleural disease and has angular margins and volume loss.
- A curvilinear bronchovascular bundle leading into the mass is referred to as the "comet tail" sign.

- Round atelectasis is most commonly associated with asbestos-related pleural disease.
- 18-FDG PET may be useful in evaluating for underlying neoplasm in equivocal cases.

Suggested Readings

Hansell DM, Armstrong P, Lynch DA, et al. Imaging of the Diseases of the Chest. 4th ed. Philadelphia, PA:Elsevier-Mosby; 2005

Hansell DM, Bankier AA, MacMahon H, McLoud TC, Müller NL, Remy J. Fleischner Society: glossary of terms for thoracic imaging. Radiology . 2008; 246(3):697–722

Stathopoulos GT, Karamessini MT, Sotiriadi AE, Pastromas VG. Rounded atelectasis of the lung. Respir Med . 2005; 99(5):615–623

Case 308

Brady S. Davis

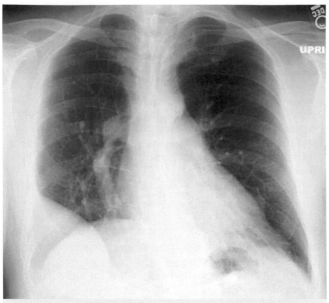

Fig. 308.1 Posteroanterior (PA) chest radiograph demonstrates right lung volume loss with a curvilinear opacity coursing inferiorly from the right hilum below the diaphragm. Incidentally, there is a right-sided pleural based lesion, consistent with a known lipoma.

■ Cl inical Presentation

A 42-year-old man with cough (▶ Fig. 308.1).

■ Key Imaging Finding

Right lung volume loss with a curvilinear opacity descending below the diaphragm

■ Diagnosis

- **Scimitar syndrome**. Scimitar syndrome, also known as hypogenetic lung syndrome or congenital pulmonary venolobar syndrome, is characterized by right-sided pulmonary hypoplasia with partial anomalous pulmonary venous return, resulting in a left-to-right shunt. The anomalous pulmonary vein most often drains below the diaphragm into the inferior vena cava. Less common sites of drainage include the right atrium, portal vein, hepatic veins, and azygos vein. Drainage into the left atrium, which is rare, is referred to as a "meandering" pulmonary vein. The course of the anomalous pulmonary vein typically results in a curvilinear opacity adjacent to the right heart border, resembling a Turkish sword or scimitar.

- Although most patients remain asymptomatic, symptoms can manifest during childhood with right heart failure, pulmonary hypertension, and recurrent pneumonia in the affected lung. Contrast-enhanced computed tomography (CT) or magnetic resonance imaging (MRI) remain the best modalities for complete evaluation of the anomalous vein. Cross-sectional imaging may also demonstrate associated anomalies often linked to scimitar syndrome, including congenital heart abnormalities, tracheobronchial abnormalities, diaphragmatic malformations or hernias, vertebral anomalies, and/or horseshoe lung—a rare associated anomaly in which the posterior portion of the lungs is fused by an isthmus of lung tissue.

✓ Pearls

- Scimitar syndrome is characterized by a hypoplastic lung and partial anomalous pulmonary venous return.
- Patients are usually asymptomatic, except with associated anomalies or a significant left-to-right shunt.

- CT or MRI can be utilized for evaluating associated cardiac, pulmonary, and vascular anomalies.

Suggested Readings

Gavazzi E, Ravanelli M, Farina D, Chiari ME, Maroldi R. Scimitar syndrome: comprehensive, noninvasive assessment with cardiovascular magnetic resonance imaging. Circulation . 2008; 118(3):e63–e64

Holt PD, Berdon WE, Marans Z, Griffiths S, Hsu D. Scimitar vein draining to the left atrium and a historical review of the scimitar syndrome. Pediatr Radiol . 2004; 34(5):409–413

Woodring JH, Howard TA, Kanga JF. Congenital pulmonary venolobar syndrome revisited. Radiographics . 1994; 14(2):349–369

Case 309

Grant E. Lattin Jr.

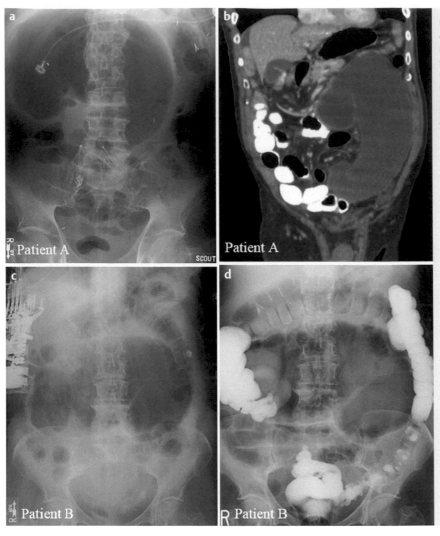

Fig. 309.1 (a) Plain radiograph of the abdomen demonstrates a coffee bean-shaped, dilated, loop of bowel which points toward the left upper quadrant. (b) Reformatted coronal CT image confirms a dilated cecum that has twisted on the axis of the right colon. (c) Plain radiograph and (d) barium enema in another patient with the same disease process displays a gas-filled, dilated cecum with "beaking" of contrast within the mid-ascending colon.

■ Clinical Presentation

A 63-year-old man with severe abdominal pain (▶ Fig. 309.1).

■ Key Imaging Finding

Dilated, gas-filled cecum pointing toward the left upper quadrant (LUQ) of the abdomen

■ Diagnosis

- **Cecal volvulus.** Cecal volvulus occurs less commonly than sigmoid volvulus, but has increased in incidence, now accounting for approximately one-third of all cases of colonic volvulus. Seen usually in younger women, cecal volvulus is due to rotation about the axis of the right colon, often due to a redundant mesentery with narrow fixation, related to incomplete fusion of the right colon to the posterior parietal peritoneum
- Plain film radiographs demonstrate a dilated, gas-filled cecum directed toward the LUQ of the abdomen. Often referred to as having a "kidney bean" or "coffee bean" appearance, cecal volvulus may contain only one air–fluid level, rather than two, as can be observed in sigmoid volvulus. Contrast enema will show "beaking" of the contrast column at the mid-ascending colon. Computed tomography (CT) will show tapering of the ends of the dilated cecum with "whirling" of the adjacent mesenteric vessels.

- Although cecal volvulus may present classically with an acute abdomen, an initial differential diagnosis may include cecal bascule, acute ileus, Ogilvie syndrome (mechanical pseudo-obstruction), or toxic megacolon, in addition to sigmoid volvulus. Anatomic distribution of the dilated bowel, as well as patient history, may assist in making the diagnosis.
- Treatment options may include reduction via colonoscopy or surgery, depending upon the patient's condition, with surgical management occurring in the majority of cases. Mortality rates for isolated cecal volvulus are reported at 6-7%. Delayed diagnosis and treatment may lead to bowel necrosis, sepsis, bowel perforation, and subsequent death. Prognosis, therefore, depends upon the degree of complications associated with the volvulus.

✓ Pearls

- Cecal volvulus appears as a "coffee bean" configuration of a dilated cecum oriented in the LUQ.
- On barium enema, there is "beaking" of the contrast column within the mid-ascending colon.

- On CT, there is tapering of the ends of the dilated cecum with "whirling" of the adjacent mesenteric vessels.

Suggested Readings

Delabrousse E, Sarliève P, Sailley N, Aubry S, Kastler BA. Cecal volvulus: CT findings and correlation with pathophysiology. Emerg Radiol . 2007; 14(6):411–415

Feldman D. The coffee bean sign. Radiology . 2000; 216(1):178–179

Halabi WJ, Jafari MD, Kang CY, et al. Colonic volvulus in the United States: trends, outcomes, and predictors of mortality. Ann Surg . 2014; 259(2):293–301

Case 310

Grant E. Lattin Jr.

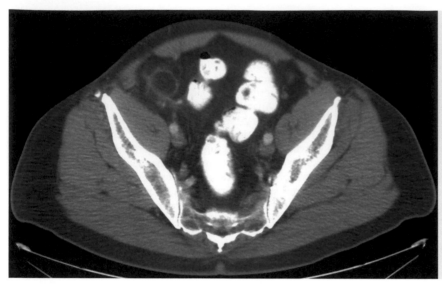

Fig. 310.1 Contrast-enhanced axial CT image through the pelvis demonstrates inflammatory change around a focus of fat attenuation, located along the right colon. The appendix (not shown) was normal in appearance.

■ Clinical Presentation

A 53-year-old man with the right lower quadrant pain (►Fig. 310.1).

■ Key Imaging Finding

Inflammatory fatty focus within the right lower quadrant of the abdomen

■ Diagnosis

- **Epiploic appendagitis.** Epiploic appendagitis is a condition characterized by inflammatory change surrounding an epiploic appendage of the colon. These appendages are peritoneal outpouchings which arise from the colonic serosa and consist of fat and vessels. Venous occlusion or torsion may contribute to the localized abdominal pain experienced by patients.
- Computed tomography (CT) characteristics include an oval fatty lesion along the serosa of the colon with a hyperdense ring of inflammatory change, seen most commonly along the anterior sigmoid colon. Care should be taken to identify a normal appendix and exclude any adjacent inflamed diverticula. Other intra-abdominal, inflammatory, fat-containing lesions to be initially considered in the differential diagnosis would include omental infarction, mesenteric panniculitis, trauma, or neoplasm, such as liposarcoma. Thickening of the colonic wall is generally mild as compared to that of other mimickers of epiploic appendagitis with more impressive mural thickening.
- Location and appearance by CT allow for differentiation of epiploic appendagitis from omental infarction. Omental infarction typically occurs deep to the anterior abdominal musculature within the right abdomen and may lack the hyperdense ring of inflammatory change surrounding the central fat attenuation. Omental infarction may occur in pediatric patients (15%), as compared to epiploic appendagitis, which is typically seen in adults.
- Treatment for epiploic appendagitis is conservative with pain medication, typically resolving spontaneously within 1 week, but inflammatory change may evolve and persist for as long as 6 months.

✓ Pearls

- Epiploic appendagitis occurs most commonly along the anterior sigmoid colon.
- CT appearance is an ovoid fatty lesion with surrounding inflammatory change.
- Treatment of epiploic appendagitis is conservative pain management.

Suggested Readings

Almeida AT, Melão L, Viamonte B, Cunha R, Pereira JM. Epiploic appendagitis: an entity frequently unknown to clinicians--diagnostic imaging, pitfalls, and look-alikes. AJR Am J Roentgenol . 2009; 193(5):1243–1251

Sandrasegaran K, Maglinte DD, Rajesh A, Akisik FM. Primary epiploic appendagitis: CT diagnosis. Emerg Radiol . 2004; 11(1):9–14

Singh AK, Gervais DA, Hahn PF, Rhea J, Mueller PR. CT appearance of acute appendagitis. AJR Am J Roentgenol . 2004; 183(5):1303–1307

Case 311

Cam Chau and Rebecca Stein-Wexler

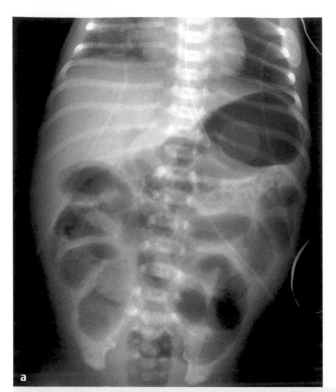 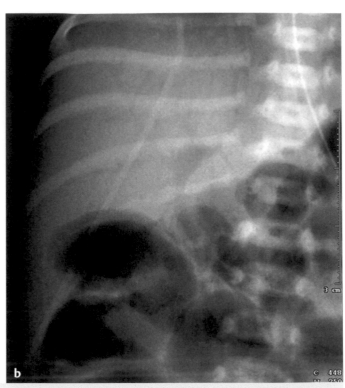

Fig. 311.1 (a) Supine abdominal radiograph demonstrates generalized bowel distention, along with linear and rounded lucencies along the bowel wall. Branching lucencies are also seen over the liver. **(b)** A coned-down view over the right upper quadrant better depicts the pneumatosis within gas-distended loops of bowel, as well as the portal venous gas over the liver.

■ Clinical Prese ntation

A 7-day-old premature infant with respiratory distress, abdominal distention, and bloody diarrhea (▶Fig. 311.1).

■ Key Imaging Finding

Pneumatosis and portal venous gas in a premature infant

■ Diagnosis

- **Necrotizing enterocolitis** (NEC). NEC is the most common gastrointestinal emergency in premature infants. It usually occurs in infants in the neonatal intensive care unit weighing less than 1,000 g at birth, although about 10% of neonates with NEC are born at term (cardiac disease or maternal cocaine use is often present). The peak incidence is during the first or second week of life, although NEC may occur later in extremely premature infants. The etiology of NEC is multifactorial and is associated with prematurity, intestinal ischemia/mucosal damage caused by bacterial colonization, inflammatory mediators, and early feeding. The end result is bowel wall coagulative and hemorrhagic necrosis and inflammation.
- NEC may occur anywhere in the gastrointestinal tract, but is found most often in the right colon and terminal ileum. Clinical symptoms include feeding intolerance, vomiting, diarrhea, bloody stools, and abdominal distention. Respiratory distress, acidosis, sepsis, shock, and temperature instability are associated sequela.
- Infants with clinical suspicion of NEC are followed up with serial supine and often also with left lateral decubitus radiographs of the abdomen. The earliest finding is fixed bowel distension. Bowel wall pneumatosis constitutes definitive radiographic evidence of NEC and is seen in 50 to 70% of patients with this disease. The pneumatosis appears as bubbly or curvilinear lucencies within the bowel wall, depending on whether the gas is submucosal or subserosal. Portal venous gas may be seen as branching lucencies over the liver, with more peripheral extension than occurs with biliary gas. Free intraperitoneal air most often occurs due to perforation of the distal ileum or proximal colon and is the only universally accepted indication for surgical intervention. Radiographic findings of free air include increased lucency over the liver, gas outlining the falciform ligament, and gas on both sides of the bowel wall (Rigler sign) on supine radiographs; additional findings on the left lateral decubitus views include triangular lucencies at the non-dependent portion of the abdomen, along with larger collections of extraluminal gas.
- When there is strong clinical suspicion of NEC, or if the diagnosis has been established radiographically, infants are monitored with serial abdominal radiographs. Treatment includes bowel rest and decompression, broad spectrum antibiotics, parenteral nutrition, oxygen, and intravenous fluids. Long-term sequelae include intestinal strictures, malabsorption, fistulae formation, and short gut syndrome. Overall mortality for NEC is approximately 20 to 30%.

✓ Pearls

- NEC most commonly occurs in premature infants weighing <1,000 g at birth.
- Pneumatosis most commonly occurs in the right lower quadrant.
- Portal venous gas is depicted as linear branching lucencies over the peripheral margin of the liver.
- Free intraperitoneal air necessitates surgical intervention.

Suggested Readings

Donnelly LF. Diagnostic Imaging Pediatrics. Salt Lake City, Utah: Amirsys; 2005

Epelman M, Daneman A, Navarro OM, et al. Necrotizing enterocolitis: review of state-of-the-art imaging findings with pathologic correlation. Radiographics. 2007; 27(2):285–305

Moss RL, Dimmitt RA, Barnhart DC, et al. Laparotomy versus peritoneal drainage for necrotizing enterocolitis and perforation. N Engl J Med. 2006; 354(21):2225–2234

Case 312

Cam Chau and Rebecca Stein-Wexler

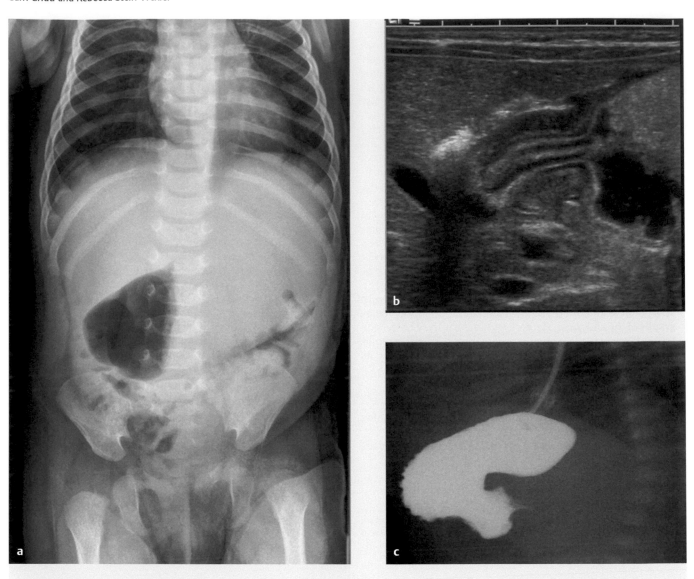

Fig. 312.1 **(a)** Left lateral decubitus radiograph of the abdomen demonstrates a distended stomach and minimal distal bowel gas. **(b)** Axial oblique ultrasound image shows elongation of the pyloric channel and thickening of the hypoechoic muscular wall. **(c)** A lateral view from an upper gastrointestinal examination shows shouldering of the gastric antrum and partial visualization of the elongated and narrowed pyloric channel resulting in the "string sign."

■ Clinical Presentation

A 6-week-old infant with a 4-day history of nonbilious vomiting after feeds (▶ Fig. 312.1).

■ Key Imaging Finding

Gastric outlet obstruction with enlarged pyloris

■ Diagnosis

- **Hypertrophic pyloric stenosis** (HPS). HPS develops in early infancy, presenting in infants between 2 and 12 weeks of age. It occurs in 2 to 5 per 1,000 births per year, and the male to female ratio is 4:1 to 5:1. Most common among first-born Caucasians, HPS is not truly inherited, but does have a familial link. Its true etiology remains unclear.
- Clinical symptoms include non-bilious vomiting that begins as occasional regurgitation, but may progress to projectile vomiting after most feedings. Examiners may palpate an olive-shaped mass in the midepigastrium; if found, this sign is 97% specific. Other presentations include hypochloremic, hypokalemic metabolic alkalosis and weight loss, though this is encountered infrequently due to relatively early diagnosis.
- Ultrasound is the examination of choice when HPS is suspected. The patient is positioned supine or right lateral decubitus, and glucose water may be administered to facilitate identification of the pylorus and to assess gastric emptying. Peristaltic waves are absent from the thickened, elongated circular pyloric muscle, and the pyloric channel does not open to allow passage of gastric contents. When the pylorus is viewed in cross-section, single wall thickness of greater than 3 mm is generally considered abnormal, as is length greater than 14 mm (these standards do vary slightly among researchers). Pylorospasm may mimic HPS and is diagnosed when the configuration of the pylorus alters, allowing fluid to traverse the channel. Occasionally, HPS is identified on an upper gastrointestinal (UGI) examination. Exaggerated gastric motility results in a "caterpillar" appearance of the stomach. Barium within the elongated and narrowed pyloric channel results in the "string sign." Mass effect from the hypertrophied muscle causes "shouldering" of the antrum and a "mushroom" appearance of the duodenum.
- Non-surgical treatment of HPS includes administration of atropine and frequent small feedings. Pyloromyotomy is the surgical management of choice, whether open or laparoscopic. The thickened muscle is split longitudinally and the edges closed transversely, relieving the stricture.

✓ Pearls

- HPS is most common among first-born Caucasian males and occurs between 2 and 12 weeks of age.
- Ultrasound demonstrates a thickened and elongated pyloris (≥3 mm single wall thickness and ≥ 14 mm length).
- UGI examination demonstrates the "string sign" and shouldering at the gastric antrum.

Suggested Readings

Donnelly LF. Diagnostic Imaging Pediatrics. Salt Lake City, UT: Amirsys; 2005

Hernanz-Schulman M. Infantile hypertrophic pyloric stenosis. Radiology . 2003; 227(2):319–331

Hernanz-Schulman M, Lowe LH, Johnson J, et al. In vivo visualization of pyloric mucosal hypertrophy in infants with hypertrophic pyloric stenosis: is there an etiologic role? AJR Am J Roentgenol . 2001; 177(4):843–848

van der Bilt JD, Kramer WL, van der Zee DC, Bax NM. Laparoscopic pyloromyotomy for hypertrophic pyloric stenosis: impact of experience on the results in 182 cases. Surg Endosc . 2004; 18(6):907–909

Case 313

Cam Chau and Rebecca Stein-Wexler

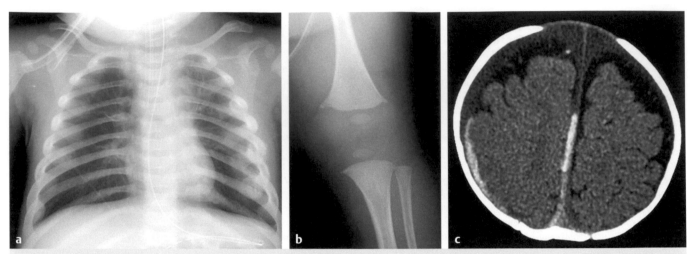

Fig. 313.1 **(a)** Frontal radiograph of the chest demonstrates multiple bilateral healing posterior and lateral rib fractures. **(b)** There are endotracheal and enteric tubes. Frontal radiograph of the left knee reveals a metaphyseal corner fracture of the distal femur. **(c)** Noncontrast head CT demonstrates acute extra-axial hemorrhages along the parafalcine region and right posterior convexity, as well as older bilateral frontoparietal subdural hematomas/hygromas.

■ Clinical Presentation

A 6-month-old infant brought to the emergency room (ER) by her mother, having lost consciousness after rolling off the bed (▶ Fig. 313.1).

■ Key Imaging Finding

Multiple high specificity fractures and injuries of varying ages

■ Diagnosis

- **Non-accidental trauma (NAT).** Suspicion for NAT must arise when characteristic fractures are encountered in infants, older children present with injuries that are not consistent with their clinical history, multiple injuries are noted in various stages of healing, or there are multiple types of coexisting injuries.
- Rib fractures are common in abused infants, representing as many as 48% of bony injuries. Infants' ribs are pliable and do not readily fracture from a direct blow; such fractures in abused infants occur when the child is held by the chest and shaken. Posterior rib fractures, which overlie the adjacent transverse process, are high-specificity fractures for NAT due to the nature of the fracture, although anterior and lateral fractures are also common. Acute fractures are difficult to visualize, while callous formation results in increased conspicuity. Follow-up views at 2 weeks can be helpful.
- Corner metaphyseal lesions (CML) are also highly specific for child abuse. Also known as "corner" or "bucket-handle" fractures, they result from torsional stress and shear, when an infant is shaken and the limbs flail, or when an extremity is twisted or pulled. The most immature and, thus, vulnerable region in a growing bone is the paraphyseal metaphysis; this fractures to form the CML. Viewed tangentially, the bone fragment resembles a "corner"; viewed obliquely, the larger curved fragment resembles a "bucket handle." Sternal, scapular, and spinous process fractures also suggest NAT in infants.
- Intracranial injury is also common in abused infants and may be lethal. Subdural hematomas are suggestive, as are hemorrhages of varying ages. Parenchymal hemorrhage is usually relatively mild, but hypoxic-ischemic injury may be significant. Retinal hemorrhages provide a clinical clue for "shaken baby syndrome."
- The skeletal survey is the study of choice for assessing suspected child abuse. Up to the age of 2 years, all bones are radiographed; in older children, a more selective survey is performed. Follow-up radiographs after 2 weeks may reveal additional fractures.
- It is important that if a radiologist suspects child abuse, the findings must be promptly reported to the referring clinician and, when necessary, to the appropriate governmental body.

✓ Pearls

- Posterior rib and metaphyseal corner fractures are common high-specificity fractures in NAT.
- Multiple fractures of different ages or discordant clinical history should raise suspicion for NAT.

- Workup for NAT typically includes a skeletal survey and noncontrast head computed tomography.

Suggested Readings

Kemp AM, Butler A, Morris S, et al. Which radiological investigations should be performed to identify fractures in suspected child abuse? Clin Radiol . 2006; 61(9):723–736

Kocher MS, Kasser JR. Orthopaedic aspects of child abuse. J Am Acad Orthop Surg. 2000; 8(1):10–20

Jenny C; Committee on Child Abuse and Neglect. Evaluating infants and young children with multiple fractures. Pediatrics . 2006; 118(3):1299–1303

Donnelly LF. Diagnostic Imaging Pediatrics. Salt Lake City, UT: Amirsys; 2005

Case 314

William T. O'Brien Sr.

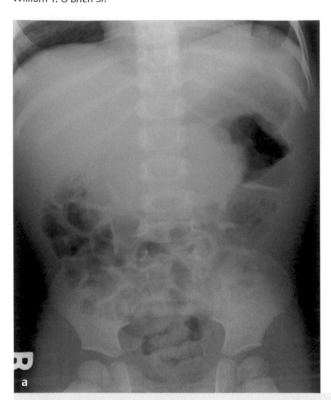

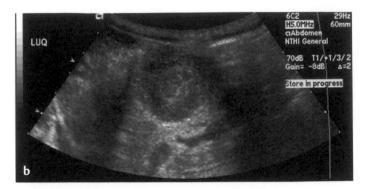

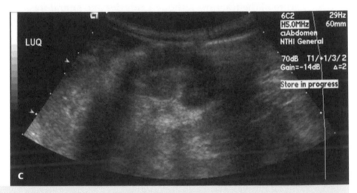

Fig. 314.1 **(a)** Plain radiograph of the abdomen demonstrates a meniscus of soft tissue projecting distally into the bowel lumen of the transverse colon within the left upper abdomen. **(b)** Sonographic evaluation through this region in the transverse plane reveals the bowel wall signature with central concentric rings of increased and decreased echotexture. **(c)** Longitudinal sonographic evaluation reveals circumferential hypoechoic bowel wall with a central region of increased echotexture and distal bowel wall shadowing, an appearance referred to as the "pseudokidney" sign.

■ Clinical Presentation

A 3-year-old boy with severe intermittent abdominal pain and diarrhea (▶Fig. 314.1).

■ Key Imaging Finding

Intraluminal mass with bowel signature on ultrasound (US)

■ Diagnosis

- **Intussusception**. Intussusception is a common and important cause of intestinal obstruction in children. The peak incidence occurs between 5 and 9 months of age, while nearly all idiopathic cases occur before 3 years of age. More than 90% of cases are idiopathic with an antecedent viral infection. If intussusception occurs in a child older than 3 years of age, a pathologic lead point from entities such as lymphoma, Meckel diverticulum, bowel hemorrhage (Henoch–Schonlein Purpura), etc. should be investigated.
- With regard to location, 90% of cases of intussusception are ileocolic, with the remainder either ileoileal or colocolic. The clinical symptoms include abdominal pain, vomiting, blood per rectum, palpable abdominal mass, fever, and "currant jelly" stools. Differential diagnosis includes appendicitis and Meckel diverticulum.
- Plain radiographs demonstrate a meniscus of soft tissue protruding into the distal bowel lumen with the location dependent upon the type of intussusception. Most cases involve the cecum or ascending colon. On US, transverse images demonstrate alternating concentric rings of increased and decreased echotexture in a typical target appearance. Longitudinal scanning reveals peripheral hypoechoic bowel wall with a central region of increased echotexture referred to as the "pseudokidney" sign.
- When intussusception is suspected based upon imaging findings, a diagnostic and therapeutic examination, such as an air enema, may be performed. Air insufflation is performed via the rectum with a tight seal under fluoroscopic guidance, maintaining a pressure of less than 120 mm of mercury. Once reduced, air will reflux into the small bowel through the ileocecal valve. A follow-up film should demonstrate intraluminal bowel gas without free intraperitoneal air. Similarly, hydrostatic enema under fluoroscopic or US guidance is another technique used with success. Pediatric surgery should be readily available in the event of an adverse outcome during reduction, such as perforation, which occurs in less than 0.5% of cases. Contraindications to reduction include peritoneal signs on physical examination or free intraperitoneal air on imaging studies.

✓ Pearls

- More than 90% of cases of intussusception occur before 3 years of age and are idiopathic in nature.
- A pathologic lead point should be suspected in patients older than 3 years of age.
- Imaging findings include a meniscus of soft tissue on plain films and target and pseudokidney sign on US.
- When using air reduction technique, pressures should not exceed 120 mm of mercury.

Suggested Readings

Applegate KE. Clinically suspected intussusception in children: evidence-based review and self-assessment module. AJR Am J Roentgenol. 2005; 185(3, Suppl):S175–S183

Bouali O, Mouttalib S, Vial J, Galinier P. Intussusception in infancy and childhood: Radiological and surgical management [in French] Arch Pediatr. 2015; 22(12):1312–1317

Donnelly LF. Fundamentals of Pediatric Radiology. Philadelphia, PA: WB Saunders; 2001

Case 315

Grant E. Lattin Jr.

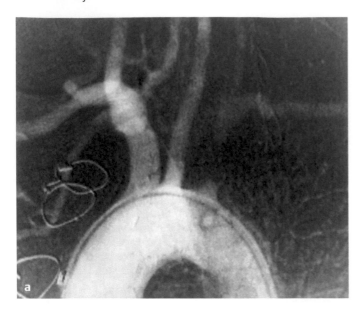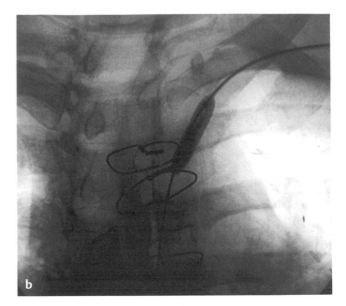

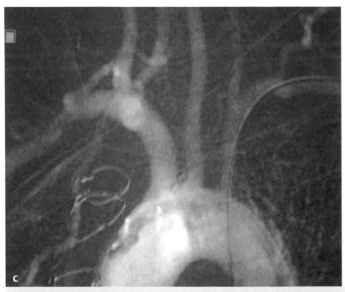

Fig. 315.1 (a) Aortic arch digital subtraction angiogram demonstrates cutoff of the more central left subclavian artery with delayed filling of the peripheral left subclavian artery via retrograde flow through the vertebral artery. (b) Balloon angioplasty of the left subclavian artery occlusion was performed with (c) satisfactory angiographic result.

■ Clinical Presentation

A 60-year-old man experiencing vertebrobasilar symptoms with exercise (▶Fig. 315.1).

■ Key Imaging Finding

Left subclavian artery occlusion with retrograde filling distally from the vertebral artery

■ Diagnosis

- **Subclavian steal**. Subclavian steal is a phenomenon that occurs secondary to subclavian artery stenosis or occlusion central to the origin of the vertebral artery with greater than 80% of cases occurring on the left side. The distal subclavian arterial supply comes from retrograde flow via the vertebral artery. Subclavian steal most commonly occurs secondary to atherosclerotic disease in elderly men, although other congenital and acquired etiologies do exist. Patients may be asymptomatic, have decreased blood pressure or a weak pulse in the affected arm, or experience vertebrobasilar symptoms, often associated with exercise of the upper extremity.
- Conventional angiography shows cutoff or stenosis of the subclavian artery with lack of antegrade opacification within the vertebral artery, followed by delayed retrograde filling of the distal subclavian artery via the vertebral artery. Computed tomography (CT) may show an area of stenosis, but associated calcification may be obscured by contrast or streak artifact.

Magnetic resonance (MR) phase contrast imaging will display flow reversal in the vertebral artery. Two-dimensional (2D) time-of-flight imaging, however, will not, as it is not sensitive to the direction of flow. Gadolinium magnetic resonance angiogram (MRA) will also demonstrate the area of stenosis. Duplex ultrasound of the ipsilateral vertebral artery may show complete reversal of flow, although diminished peak systolic velocities may be an early sign. Additionally, markedly increased contralateral vertebral artery peak systolic flow or a parvus-tardus waveform in the peripheral ipsilateral subclavian artery may support the diagnosis, especially following exercise of the upper extremity.

- Treatment options include endovascular balloon angioplasty with possible stent placement and surgery. Surgical options include a common carotid or innominate artery to subclavian artery bypass, depending on the anatomic location of the lesion.

✓ Pearls

- Subclavian steal is characterized by proximal stenosis/occlusion and distal filling via the vertebral artery.
- Patients commonly present with vertebrobasilar insufficiency when exercising the affected arm.

- MR phase contrast imaging will show flow reversal within the ipsilateral vertebral arterial.
- Treatment options include angioplasty with possible stent placement versus surgical bypass procedures.

Suggested Readings

Henry M, Amor M, Henry I, Ethevenot G, Tzvetanov K, Chati Z. Percutaneous transluminal angioplasty of the subclavian arteries. J Endovasc Surg. 1999; 6(1):33–41

Kliewer MA, Hertzberg BS, Kim DH, Bowie JD, Courneya DL, Carroll BA. Vertebral artery Doppler waveform changes indicating subclavian steal physiology. AJR Am J Roentgenol. 2000; 174(3):815–819

Labropoulos N, Nandivada P, Bekelis K. Prevalence and impact of the subclavian steal syndrome. Ann Surg. 2010; 252(1):166–170

Sueoka BL. Percutaneous transluminal stent placement to treat subclavian steal syndrome. J Vasc Interv Radiol. 1996; 7(3):351–356

Case 316

Jeffrey P. Tan

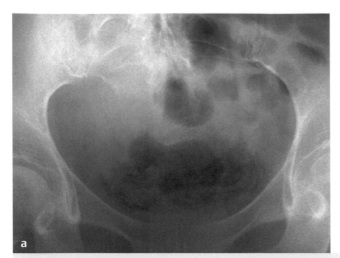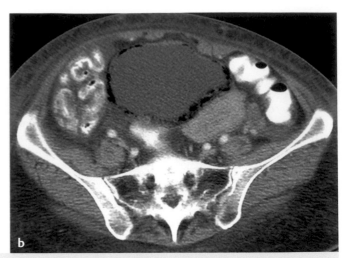

Fig. 316.1 **(a)** Anteroposterior(AP) radiograph of the pelvis reveals several small linear areas of lucency projecting over the bladder, distinct from gas within the rectum. **(b)** Contrast-enhanced axial CT image through the pelvis reveals multiple foci of gas within the bladder wall.

■ Clinical Presentation

A 63-year-old woman with dysuria and pelvic pain (▶ Fig. 316.1).

■ Key Imaging Finding

Gas within the bladder wall

■ Diagnosis

- **Emphysematous cystitis**. Emphysematous cystitis is an inflammatory condition characterized by gas in the bladder mucosa and underlying muscular tissue. This condition is most commonly identified in middle-aged diabetic women. Other predisposing conditions include neurogenic bladder, recurrent urinary tract infections, and urinary stasis from bladder outlet obstruction.
- Clinical presentation is variable, ranging from asymptomatic to dysuria, pneumaturia, or abdominal pain with sepsis. The infection is usually caused by a gas-forming organism. The most common bacterial infection is *Escherichia coli* followed by *Klebsiella pneumoniae*, *Pseudomonas aeruginosa*, and *Prote-*

us mirabilis. Noninfectious causes may include bladder instrumentation, vesicocolic or vesicovaginal fistulas, and trauma.
- Management of emphysematous cystitis is primarily medical. Therapy may include antibiotics, bladder drainage, and correction of hyperglycemia and any other comorbid conditions. Evaluation with computed tomography (CT) is useful to assess for perforation, fistula, abscess, or emphysematous pyelonephritis. The latter condition is an important entity to exclude, as the mortality for emphysematous pyelonephritis has been reported to be 21% as opposed to 7% for emphysematous cystitis. Management of emphysematous pyelonephritis typically requires percutaneous drainage with some cases requiring nephrectomy.

✓ Pearls

- Emphysematous cystitis is characterized by gas within the bladder wall and is typically managed medically.
- Emphysematous cystitis most commonly occurs in older diabetic females.

- *E. coli* is the most common infectious organism.
- CT is useful to evaluate for potential complications, such as perforation or emphysematous pyelonephritis.

Suggested Readings

Grayson DE, Abbott RM, Levy AD, Sherman PM. Emphysematous infections of the abdomen and pelvis: a pictorial review. Radiographics. 2002; 22(3):543–561

Lu YC, Chiang BJ, Pong YH, et al. Emphysematous pyelonephritis: clinical characteristics and prognostic factors. Int J Urol. 2014; 21(3):277–282

Thomas AA, Lane BR, Thomas AZ, Remer EM, Campbell SC, Shoskes DA. Emphysematous cystitis: a review of 135 cases. BJU Int. 2007; 100(1):17–20

Case 317

Grant E. Lattin Jr.

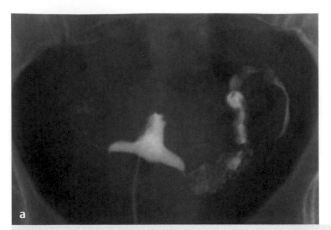 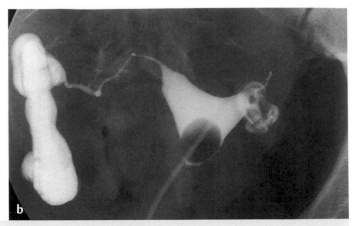

Fig. 317.1 **(a)** Early image from a hysterosalpingogram (HSG) demonstrates multiple small diverticula confined to the isthmic portion of the left fallopian tube and occlusion of the right fallopian tube. **(b)** HSG image from a different patient with the same disease process reveals fallopian tube diverticula, as well as resultant right hydrosalpinx.

■ Clinical Presentation

Two young women with infertility (▶Fig. 317.1).

■ Key Imaging Finding

Multiple small diverticula affecting the proximal portion of the fallopian tube

■ Diagnosis

- **Salpingitis isthmica nodosa (SIN).** SIN or tubal diverticulosis is a condition that affects the proximal fallopian tubes and is observed in 0.6 to 11% of healthy, fertile women. Its etiology is unknown, but may be related to prior inflammation and/or pelvic infection in many patients. This condition is characterized by multiple small diverticula seen extending from the lumen of the fallopian tube into its wall, most commonly affecting the isthmus. Infertility and ectopic pregnancy are known associations. Hydrosalpinx is a common secondary finding.
- Hysterosalpingography is the imaging modality of choice which will assist in making this diagnosis, although SIN has also been described via ultrasound and magnetic resonance imaging (MRI). Often, SIN is diagnosed while the patient is undergoing a comprehensive work-up for infertility. Although classic imaging findings are diagnostic of SIN, tubal endometriosis, salpingitis, or tuberculosis may have thickening or irregularity of the isthmus as well. Usually, tubal endometriosis will have isthmic thickening with a somewhat honeycombed appearance, whereas tuberculous salpingitis may have calcifications within the wall. MRI may be of benefit in the identification of tubal blood products in suspected cases of endometriosis.
- Treatments for infertility associated with SIN such as fallopian tube microcatheter recanalization or microsurgery have not documented increased pregnancy rates as successfully as other advanced reproductive technology. As a result, typical first line therapy for SIN is now in vitro fertilization and embryo transfer.

✓ Pearls

- SIN is characterized by multiple small diverticula confined to the proximal portion of the fallopian tube.
- Associations may include previous pelvic infection, infertility, and tubal pregnancy.

- Advanced reproductive technology may assist in reversing the patient's infertility.

Suggested Readings

Allahbadia GN, Merchant R. Fallopian tube recanalization: lessons learnt and future challenges. Womens Health (Lond). 2010; 6(4):531–548, quiz 548–549

Creasy JL, Clark RL, Cuttino JT, Groff TR. Salpingitis isthmica nodosa: radiologic and clinical correlates. Radiology. 1985; 154(3):597–600

Thurmond AS, Burry KA, Novy MJ. Salpingitis isthmica nodosa: results of transcervical fluoroscopic catheter recanalization. Fertil Steril. 1995; 63(4):715–722

Yaranal PJ, Hegde V. Salpingitis isthmica nodosa: a case report. J Clin Diagn Res. 2013; 7(11):2581–2582

Case 318

Grant E. Lattin Jr.

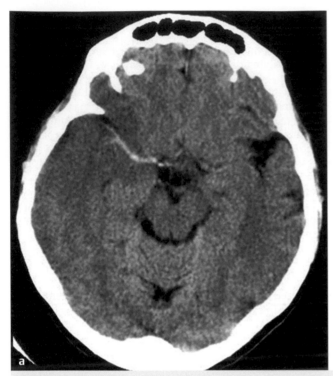 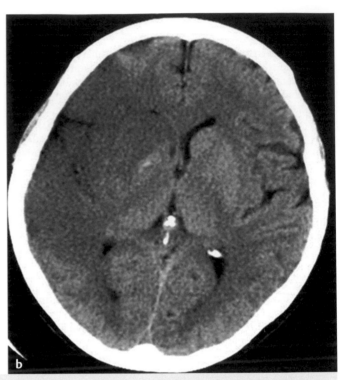

Fig. 318.1 (a,b) Axial CT images of the head without contrast demonstrate a hyperdense right middle cerebral artery (MCA) **(a)** with a region of hypoattenuation affecting portions of the right frontal, parietal, and temporal lobes, as well as the basal ganglia, insula, and deep white matter tracts. Sulcal effacement, loss of the grey-white matter differentiation, and mass effect on the right lateral ventricle are also present **(b)**.

■ Clinical Presentation

A 62-year-old man with left-sided weakness (▶Fig. 318.1).

■ Key Imaging Finding

Hyperdense middle cerebral artery (MCA; with additional findings consistent with infarction)

■ Diagnosis

- **MCA distribution cerebral infarction.** Cerebral infarction is the result of loss of blood flow to the brain parenchyma, often associated with atherosclerosis or thromboembolic disease in older adults. An early sign on unenhanced computed tomography (CT) of brain ischemia/evolving infarction, which has high specificity but low sensitivity, is a hyperdense vessel, commonly the M1 segment of the MCA, also referred to as the "dense MCA" sign. More peripheral branches may display a focus of hyperattenuation described as the "dot" sign when imaged in cross-section.
- CT findings of stroke also include loss of the cortical ribbon (grey-white matter junction) within the first 3 hours, subsequent parenchymal hypoattenuation, and sulcal effacement with gyral swelling within 12 to 24 hours. Hemorrhagic transformation may also occur, typically during the subacute phase with increased blood flow into injured brain parenchyma, or more acutely if thrombolytics are administered. Acute strokes are hyperintense on diffusion-weighted imaging (DWI) with

corresponding low signal on the apparent diffusion coefficient (ADC) map. This pattern remains from minutes after the infarction to approximately 10 days following the ischemic insult. DWI sequences can be obtained very quickly, in less than a minute.

- Acute treatment may include intravenous (IV) or catheter-directed intra-arterial (IA) thrombolytic therapy within 4.5 or 6 hours of the symptom onset, respectively, in nonhemorrhagic acute strokes without contraindications to therapy. Mechanical clot retrieval devices may also be a treatment option. Perfusion CT and computed tomography angiography (CTA) of the brain are helpful in identifying patients that can benefit from revascularization and guiding management. Both prior and recent studies have shown that IV thrombolytic therapy is most effective when given early, ideally within 3 hours of the symptom onset; however, more recent studies show efficacy of IV thrombolytic therapy up to 4.5 hours from the symptom onset in select candidates.

✓ Pearls

- The "dense MCA" sign or MCA "dot" is an early, highly specific marker of acute ischemia.
- MRI with DWI and ADC map confirms an acute ischemic event.

- IV or catheter-directed IA thrombolysis are possible treatment options in specific clinical settings.

Suggested Readings

Barber PA, Demchuk AM, Hudon ME, Pexman JH, Hill MD, Buchan AM. Hyperdense sylvian fissure MCA "dot" sign: a CT marker of acute ischemia. Stroke. 2001; 32(1):84–88

Bourekas EC, Slivka AP, Shah R, Sunshine J, Suarez JI. Intraarterial thrombolytic therapy within 3 hours of the onset of stroke. Neurosurgery. 2004; 54(1):39–44, discussion 44–46

Broome LJ, Battle CE, Lawrence M, Evans PA, Dennis MS. Cognitive outcomes following thrombolysis in acute ischemic stroke: a systematic review. J Stroke Cerebrovasc Dis. 2016; 25(12):2868–2875

Leary MC, Kidwell CS, Villablanca JP, et al. Validation of computed tomographic middle cerebral artery "dot" sign: an angiographic correlation study. Stroke. 2003; 34(11):2636–2640

Case 319

William T. O'Brien Sr.

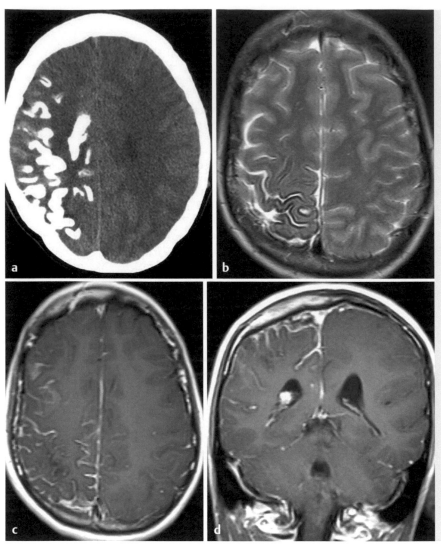

Fig. 319.1 **(a)** Axial noncontrast CT image of the head demonstrates "tram-track" cortical calcifications and underlying parenchymal atrophy primarily along the right frontal and parietal lobes. **(b)** Axial T2-weighted (T2W) image shows linear hypointensity in a similar distribution. **(c)** Axial and **(d)** coronal post-gadolinium T1W images demonstrate pial enhancement involving predominantly the right parietal and frontal lobes with underlying parenchymal atrophy and enlargement of the ipsilateral choroid plexus **(d)**. There is also compensatory thickening of the overlying calvarium.

■ Clinical Presentation

A pediatric patient with seizures (▶Fig. 319.1).

■ Key Imaging Finding

"Tram-track" calcifications, pial angiomatosis, and cerebral parenchymal atrophy

■ Diagnosis

- **Sturge-Weber syndrome (SWS).** SWS, also known as encephalotrigeminal angiomatosis, is typically a sporadic neurocutaneous disorder, but has been linked to the guanine nucleotide-binding protein G(q) (GNAQ) somatic mutation. It is characterized by a cutaneous facial angioma (port wine stain or nevus plexus flammeus) that is associated with ipsilateral pial angiomatosis and seizures. The port wine stain typically occurs in the ophthalmic distribution, followed by the maxillary distribution, of the trigeminal nerve (fifth cranial nerve [CN V]). Rarely, the pial angiomatosis may be bilateral or contralateral to the facial angioma. Clinically, patients present with seizures (most common), hemiplegia, visual disturbances, and/or developmental delay.
- The primary cause of the central nervous system (CNS) malformation is failure to form normal cortical venous drainage in the involved portion(s) of the brain with either development or persistence of a leptomeningeal vascular plexus. Although any portion of the brain may be involved, the occipital and parietal lobes are most frequently involved. The overlying vascular plexus consists of thin-walled, dilated veins and capillaries.

There is also an increase in the number and size of collateral medullary and subependymal veins on the affected side. The increased flow leads to hypertrophy and increased enhancement of the ipsilateral choroid plexus. Venous congestion results in underlying chronic venous ischemia and hypoxic parenchymal injury.

- Imaging findings parallel the pathophysiology of the malformation. Enhanced studies reveal leptomeningeal enhancement of the pial angiomatosis, enhancement of the enlarged ipsilateral collateral medullary and subependymal veins, and hypertrophy and increased enhancement of the ipsilateral choroid plexus. Chronic venous ischemia underlying the angiomatosis results in parenchymal atrophy, decreased subcortical T2 signal intensity, and "tram-track" cortical calcifications. Late findings include compensatory ipsilateral calvarial thickening and enlargement of the paranasal sinuses (Dyke–Davidoff–Mason syndrome) as a result of the underlying parenchymal volume loss. Orbital findings include choroidal angiomas, which may lead to glaucoma.

✓ Pearls

- SWS is characterized by a facial angioma, pial angiomatosis, cortical atrophy, and seizures.
- Imaging findings include cortical "tram track" calcifications, atrophy, and leptomeningeal enhancement.

- Increased collateral deep venous drainage results in increased size and enhancement of the choroid plexus.

Suggested Readings

Akpinar E. The tram-track sign: cortical calcifications. Radiology. 2004; 231(2):515–516

Nakashima M, Miyajima M, Sugano H, et al. The somatic GNAQ mutation c.548G>A (p.R183Q) is consistently found in Sturge-Weber syndrome. J Hum Genet. 2014; 59(12):691–693

Smirniotopoulos JG, Murphy FM. The phakomatoses. AJNR Am J Neuroradiol. 1992; 13(2):725–746

Case 320

Grant E. Lattin Jr.

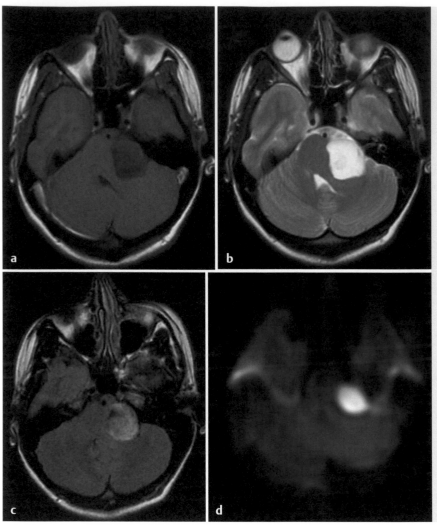

Fig. 320.1 **(a)** Axial T1- and **(b)** T2-weighted images demonstrate a left cerebellopontine angle mass, which is isointense to slightly hyperintense to cerebrospinal fluid signal. **(c)** Fluid attenuation inversion recovery (FLAIR) imaging demonstrates mixed signal intensity without complete signal loss. **(d)** On diffusion-weighted imaging, there is restricted diffusion characterized by increased signal.

■ Clinical Presentation

A 23-year-old woman with headache (▶Fig. 320.1).

■ Key Imaging Finding

Left cerebellopontine angle (CPA) mass with similar signal to cerebrospinal fluid(CSF) and restricted diffusion on diffusion-weighted imaging (DWI)

■ Diagnosis

- **Epidermoid**. Epidermoid is the third most common CPA cisternal mass, with vestibular schwannomas and meningiomas being the two most common. They contain ectodermal elements due to inclusion during neural tube closure. When discussed under the heading of tumors, epidermoids account for 1% of all intracranial lesions and occur most frequently between the ages of 20 and 40 with an equal distribution between men and women. Symptoms are usually minor.
- Classically, epidermoids occur in the posterior fossa, most commonly at the CPA with an insinuating appearance. Unlike other CPA masses, to include arachnoid cysts, epidermoids engulf cranial nerves and vessels rather than displacing them. Their margins are scalloped and irregular, and occasionally, they may be invasive. On computed tomography (CT), epidermoids are isodense to CSF. Peripheral enhancement may occur. Calcification is seen in approximately 20% of cases.

- On T1-weighted image (T1WI), epidermoids are isointense to slightly hyperintense to CSF, resulting in the descriptor "dirty CSF." On T2WI, they are isointense to hyperintense to CSF. Peripheral enhancement can sometimes be seen. Mixed signal on fluid attenuation inversion recovery (FLAIR) images and diffusion restriction (hyperintense on DWI) essentially confirms the diagnosis of epidermoid.
- Considering only the T1- and T2-weighted signal characteristics, an arachnoid cyst would still be within the differential diagnosis. However, an arachnoid cyst will follow CSF on all pulse sequences with low signal on T1WI and high signal on T2WI. Also, FLAIR images of an arachnoid cyst will show signal isointense to CSF, and there is no restricted diffusion on DWI.
- Complete removal is the surgical goal with smaller lesions having better postoperative results.

✓ Pearls

- Epidermoids most commonly occur at the CPA—they are the third most common CPA mass.
- Epidermoids have similar signal to CSF, but increased signal on DWI, confirming the diagnosis.

- Epidermoids engulf vessels rather than displace them, contrary to arachnoid cysts.

Suggested Readings

Bonneville F, Sarrazin JI, Marsot-Dupuch K, et al. Unusual lesions of the cerebellopontine angle: a segmental approach. Radiographics. 2001; 21(2):419–438

Dutt SN, Mirza S, Chavda SV, Irving RM. Radiologic differentiation of intracranial epidermoids from arachnoid cysts. Otol Neurotol. 2002; 23(1):84–92

Pikis S, Margolin E. Malignant transformation of a residual cerebellopontine angle epidermoid cyst. J Clin Neurosci. 2016; 33:59–62

Case 321

William T. O'Brien Sr.

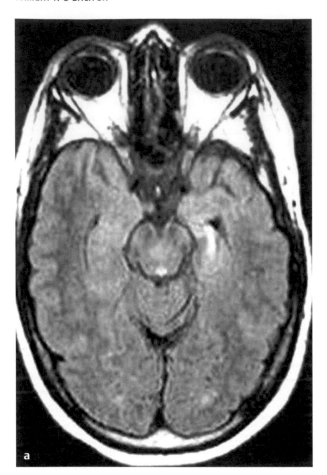

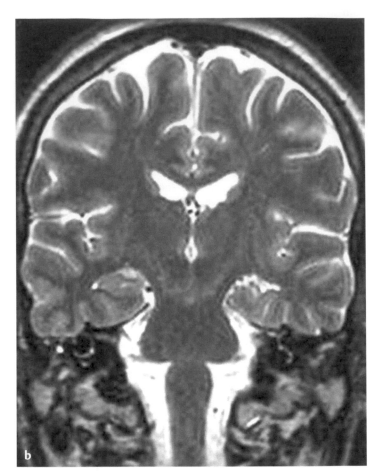

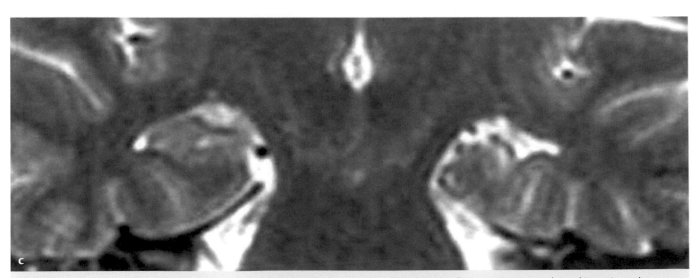

Fig. 321.1 **(a)** Axial fluid attenuation inversion recovery (FLAIR) and **(b)** coronal T2-weighted images demonstrate increased signal intensity and associated atrophy within the left mesial temporal lobe. **(c)** Magnified coronal T2-weighted image through the medial temporal lobes confirms volume loss on the left.

■ Clinical Presentation

A 14-year-old boy with complex partial seizures (▶Fig. 321.1).

■ Key Imaging Finding

Atrophy and increased T2-weighted image (T2WI) signal intensity of the mesial temporal lobe

■ Diagnosis

- **Mesial temporal sclerosis (MTS)**. Temporal lobe epilepsy is relatively common in adolescents and young adults and typically manifests as complex partial seizures. Within this patient population, MTS is thought to represent the most common identifiable cause of temporal lobe seizures. Debate exists as to whether MTS is acquired or a developmental abnormality. Some studies show an increased incidence in patients with a history of infant febrile seizures.
- MRI is the mainstay in the work-up of seizure disorders, since computed tomography (CT) is often normal. Seizure protocols for children and young adults typically include high-resolution coronal sequences through the mesial temporal lobes/hippocampal formations. Imaging findings of MTS include hippocampal atrophy with associated dilatation of the ipsilateral temporal horn of the lateral ventricle. Increased T2/fluid attenuation inversion recovery (FLAIR) signal intensity is also commonly seen and increases the specificity in terms of suggesting the diagnosis. Magnetic resonance spectroscopy (MRS) shows decreased N-acetyl-aspartate(NAA) in the affected temporal lobe and may be helpful in localizing certain cases. Interictal fluorodeoxyglucose-positron emission tomography (FDG-PET) imaging demonstrates hypometabolism with decreased uptake within the affected mesial temporal lobe.
- Medical treatment is typically the first-line therapy with surgical resection reserved for patients with persistent seizures or inability to tolerate medical therapy. Alternative therapy may include options such as neuromodulation. Ultimately, a comprehensive therapeutic approach, including rehabilitation, is necessary to optimize the patient's quality of life.

✓ Pearls

- Temporal lobe epilepsy is common in adolescents and young adults with complex partial seizures.
- MTS is characterized by atrophy and increased T2/FLAIR signal intensity within the involved hippocampus.
- Interictal FDG-PET shows hypometabolism with decreased uptake in the affected mesial temporal lobe.

Suggested Readings

Bocti C, Robitaille Y, Diadori P, et al. The pathological basis of temporal lobe epilepsy in childhood. Neurology. 2003; 60(2):191–195

Castillo M, Smith JK, Kwock L. Proton MR spectroscopy in patients with acute temporal lobe seizures. AJNR Am J Neuroradiol. 2001; 22(1):152–157

Usui N. Current topics in epilepsy surgery. Neurol Med Chir (Tokyo). 2016; 56(5):228–235

Case 322

Grant E. Lattin Jr.

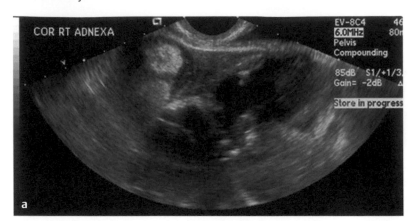
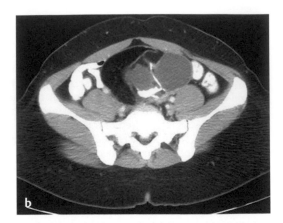
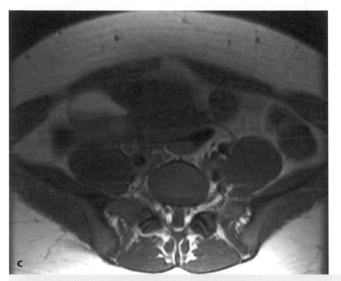
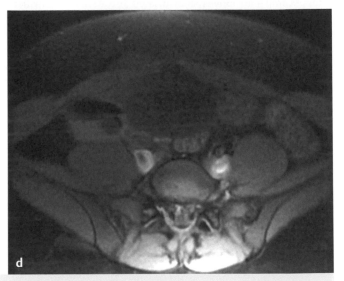

Fig. 322.1 **(a)** Endovaginal ultrasound image through the pelvis demonstrates a partially hyperechoic cystic mass that has posterior shadowing and adjacent specular reflectors, consistent with the "tip of the iceberg" sign. **(b)** Axial CT image through the pelvis confirms a multiloculated cystic midline mass, which contains calcium and macroscopic fat. Findings are consistent with an ovarian teratoma (dermoid) originating from the left ovary. **(c)** Axial T1 and **(d)** T2 fat-suppressed images in the same patient demonstrate a smaller right ovarian cystic mass with macroscopic fat, also consistent with an ovarian teratoma.

■ Clinical Presentation

A 25-year-old woman with pelvic fullness (▶ Fig. 322.1).

■ Key Imaging Finding

Ovarian cystic mass with "tip of the iceberg" sign and macroscopic fat

■ Diagnosis

- **Ovarian teratoma (dermoid)**. Ovarian teratoma typically refers to a mature cystic teratoma and may also be described as a dermoid or dermoid cyst. Uncommon subtypes include immature and monodermal ovarian teratomas. Mature cystic teratoma is the most common benign ovarian tumor in young women. Occasionally, they may be bilateral, which is an extremely important finding if surgical excision is contemplated. Often, these tumors may be incidentally found, but they may become more symptomatic, especially as they increase in size.
- Classically, ovarian teratoma appears as a cystic adnexal mass with a shadowing hyperechoic component by ultrasound (US). A hyperechoic nodule which projects into the lumen of the mass is known as a Rokitansky or dermoid plug. An echogenic component with posterior shadowing is known as the "tip of the iceberg" sign. However, if central linear or dotlike echogenic reflectors are present, the term "dermoid mesh" is ap-

plicable. Based on the US findings alone, the initial differential diagnosis may include an endometrioma, hemorrhagic cyst, bowel, or a pedunculated lipoleiomyoma.
- Noncontrast computed tomography (CT) or magnetic resonance imaging (MRI) confirms the diagnosis by identifying the presence of macroscopic fat within the lesion. Commonly, teeth or calcifications may also be present, allowing the diagnosis to be suggested on radiographs. T1-weighted fat-saturation techniques confirm the presence of fat as opposed to hemorrhage which may also be hyperintense on T1WI, but will not suppress.
- Treatment for smaller teratomas is often nonsurgical given their slow growth. Larger lesions (>4–6 cm) may be excised due to increased risk of ovarian torsion. Rarer complications may include rupture, peritonitis, and malignant transformation.

✓ Pearls

- Dermoids are the most common benign ovarian tumor in young females.
- Characteristic US findings include the Rokitansky plug and "tip of the iceberg" sign.

- The presence of fat on CT or MR confirms the diagnosis of ovarian dermoid.
- Larger dermoids are excised due to increased risk of ovarian torsion.

Suggested Readings

Hurwitz JL, Fenton A, McCluggage WG, McKenna S. Squamous cell carcinoma arising in a dermoid cyst of the ovary: a case series. BJOG. 2007; 114(10):1283–1287

Jung SE, Lee JM, Rha SE, Byun JY, Jung JI, Hahn ST. CT and MR imaging of ovarian tumors with emphasis on differential diagnosis. Radiographics. 2002; 22(6):1305–1325

Lee KH, Song MJ, Jung IC, Lee YS, Park EK. Autoamputation of an ovarian mature cystic teratoma: a case report and a review of the literature. World J Surg Oncol. 2016; 14(1):217

Rim SY, Kim SM, Choi HS. Malignant transformation of ovarian mature cystic teratoma. Int J Gynecol Cancer. 2006; 16(1):140–144

Case 323

Grant E. Lattin Jr.

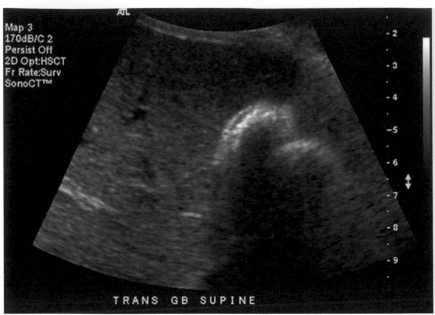

Fig. 323.1 Sonographic image of the gallbladder demonstrates the gallbladder wall (linear hyperechoic focus) with a second thin curvilinear hyperechoic focus just deep to this and posterior acoustic shadowing. This appearance of two curvilinear echogenic lines with an intervening area of decreased echotexture is commonly described as the "wall-echo-shadow" sign.

■ Clinical Presentation

A 47-year-old woman with right upper quadrant pain (▸Fig. 323.1).

■ Key Image Finding

Wall-echo-shadow (WES) sign.

■ Diagnosis

- **Cholelithiasis.** The WES sign is characterized by two curvilinear echogenic lines created by the gallbladder wall and a gallbladder lumen filled with stones. These hyperechoic foci are separated by an intervening sonolucent region of bile within the gallbladder lumen. The gallstones cause posterior acoustic shadowing.
- Gallstones commonly present in women in their 40s with right upper quadrant discomfort, following a fatty meal. The evaluation of gallstones is best performed by ultrasound (US). Decubitus imaging should be performed to look for mobility, as impacted stones may result in concurrent cholecystitis. Likewise, the common bile duct should be imaged as well to exclude choledocholithiasis. US findings which may indicate associated cholecystitis include pericholecystic fluid, a gallbladder wall measuring greater than 3 mm in diameter, and a sonographic Murphy sign.
- Computed tomography (CT) is less sensitive than US in the evaluation of gallstones. T2-weighted image (T2WI) on magnetic resonance imaging (MRI) will show the stones as areas of signal void surrounded by hyperintense bile. Hepatobiliary scintigraphy may be of benefit if concern exists for an obstructing stone, and US findings are equivocal for cholecystitis.
- Although the WES sign is classic for cholelithiasis, care should be taken to exclude potential mimickers, such as emphysematous cholecystitis or porcelain gallbladder. Emphysematous cholecystitis presents with gas within the gallbladder wall and associated "dirty" posterior shadowing, as opposed to the "clean" shadowing seen with calcifications. Porcelain gallbladder is characterized by calcification within the gallbladder wall with posterior shadowing. Since the calcification is within the wall and not within the gallbladder lumen, there is absence of the second hyperechoic focus which makes up the WES sign. If uncertain, CT will help evaluate for gas or calcifications within the gallbladder wall.
- Treatment of cholelithiasis may be conservative if asymptomatic. If symptomatic, surgical removal of the gallbladder is usually performed.

✓ Pearls

- The WES sign is caused by a gallbladder lumen full of gallstones.
- US is more sensitive than CT in the evaluation of gallbladder pathology.
- Exclude mimickers of the WES sign, such as emphysematous cholecystitis and porcelain gallbladder.

Suggested Readings

Bortoff GA, Chen MY, Ott DJ, Wolfman NT, Routh WD. Gallbladder stones: imaging and intervention. Radiographics. 2000; 20(3):751–766

Duncan CB, Riall TS. Evidence-based current surgical practice: calculous gallbladder disease. J Gastrointest Surg. 2012; 16(11):2011–2025

Rosenthal SJ, Cox GG, Wetzel LH, Batnitzky S. Pitfalls and differential diagnosis in biliary sonography. Radiographics. 1990; 10(2):285–311

Case 324

Grant E. Lattin Jr.

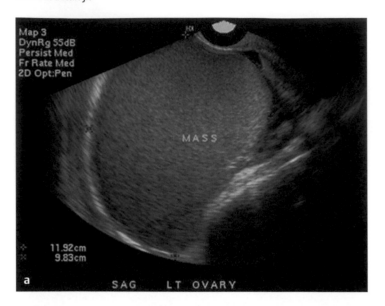
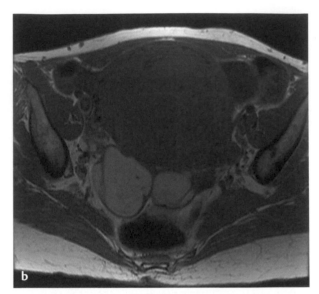
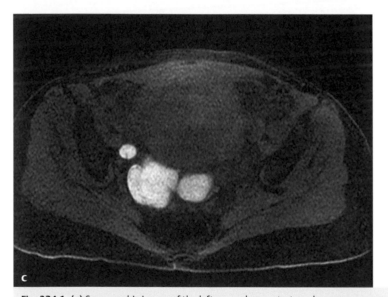
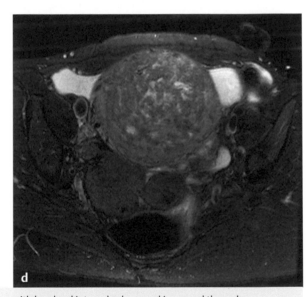

Fig. 324.1 (a) Sonographic image of the left ovary demonstrates a homogeneous mass with low-level internal echoes and increased through transmission, suggestive of a ground-glass appearance. Another patient with the same diagnosis has **(b, c)** a T1W image of the pelvis that shows T1 hyperintense masses posterior to the uterus, which remain hyperintense with fat suppression. **(d)** These same masses demonstrate T2 "shading" or hypointensity on T2W imaging. Secondary findings of adenomyosis are noted in the second patient.

■ **Clinical Presentation**

Two young adult women with pelvic pain. The first image is for the first patient, and the remaining images are of the second patient (▸Fig. 324.1).

■ Key Imaging Finding

Adnexal mass with increased through transmission and homogeneous low-level echoes

■ Diagnosis

- **Endometrioma**. Endometriomas are cysts which contain functioning endometrium outside of the uterus, resulting in contained cyclical hemorrhage. Endometriomas are seen within the spectrum of endometriosis and are associated with infertility and pelvic pain. Commonly, endometriomas may be multiple and can be found in the ovaries and throughout the pelvis.
- When unilocular with homogenous low-level echoes centrally, ultrasound (US) findings are essentially diagnostic. Peripheral echogenic foci within the wall of such a mass are also suggestive of endometrioma. However, endometriomas with features such as true nodularity, fluid-fluid levels, or dense calcifications may be less clear. Magnetic resonance imaging (MRI) may then be useful in differentiating between an endometrioma and other ovarian masses, such as hemorrhagic cysts, teratomas (dermoids), or ovarian cystic neoplasms.

- On MRI, endometriomas appear T1 hyperintense (secondary to hemorrhage) which may increase in conspicuity with fat suppression. Conversely, a teratoma (dermoid) would decrease in signal intensity with fat suppression. On T2-weighted image (T2WI), endometriomas will appear hypointense, an appearance sometimes referred to as T2 "shading" which can vary in degree of decreased intensity. Thick septations and nodularity should raise the suspicion for an ovarian cystic neoplasm, especially if unilateral.
- Treatment options include medical management or varying degrees of surgery depending on the patient's desire for fertility. With time, the symptoms associated with endometriosis will often dissipate with menopause. Although, a small minority of patients may be at increased risk for the subsequent development of ovarian tumors.

✓ Pearls

- Endometriomas are a form of endometriosis and commonly present with pain and occasionally with infertility.
- Classic US findings of endometrioma include homogeneous low-level echoes and through transmission.

- MRI findings include T1 hyperintensity (secondary to hemorrhage) and T2 shading.

Suggested Readings

Alborzi S, Zarei A, Alborzi S, Alborzi M. Management of ovarian endometrioma. Clin Obstet Gynecol. 2006; 49(3):480–491

Haraguchi H, Koga K, Takamura M, et al. Development of ovarian cancer after excision of endometrioma. Fertil Steril. 2016; 106(6):1432–1437.e2

Woodward PJ, Sohaey R, Mezzetti TP, Jr. Endometriosis: radiologic-pathologic correlation. Radiographics. 2001; 21(1):193–216, 288–294

Case 325

Michael A. Mahlon

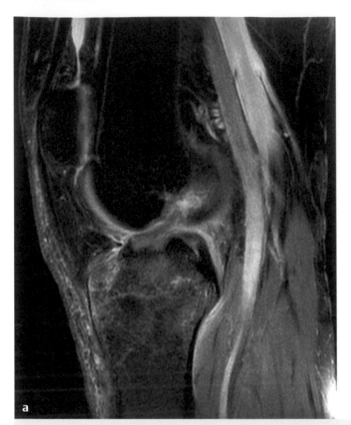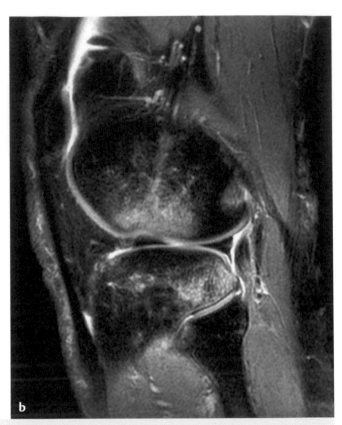

Fig. 325.1 (a) Fat-saturated sagittal T2-weighted image of the knee reveals high signal intensity within and disruption of the anterior cruciate ligament. (b) Another image from the same sequence demonstrates "kissing contusions" of the lateral femoral condyle and proximal tibia. A deep lateral femoral sulcus, anterior translation of the tibia, and a small suprapatellar effusion are also seen.

■ Clinical Presentation

A 26-year-old man with knee pain following loud pop while exercising (▶ Fig. 325.1).

■ Key Imaging Finding

Disruption of the anterior cruciate ligament (ACL) with "kissing contusions"

■ Diagnosis

- **ACL tear**. The ACL attaches to the inner aspect of the lateral femoral condyle proximally and fans out to attach to the anterior aspect of the intercondylar eminence of the tibia distally. It runs from the femur to the tibia anteriorly, medially, and inferiorly within the intercondylar notch. It is intra-articular and extrasynovial throughout its course. The primary role of the ACL is to provide stability to the knee joint. It resists anterior translocation and internal rotation of the tibia over the femur. The ACL also limits hyperextension and both valgus and varus forces on the knee.
- Most ACL tears (~70%) occur in the middle aspect of the ligament, 20% occur proximally near its origin, and only 10% occur distally at the tibial attachment. Primary signs of an ACL tear include nonvisualization, focal or diffuse increased T2 signal intensity within the ligament, focal discontinuity, acute angulation, and a wavy contour of the ligament.
- Secondary signs of an ACL tear include a joint effusion, "kissing contusions" involving the lateral femoral condyle and lateral tibia, an angle between the lateral tibial plateau and ACL less than 45 degrees, posterior displacement of lateral meniscus more than 3.5 mm, anterior displacement of tibia more than 7 mm, and a lateral femoral sulcus deeper than 1.5 mm. Co-existing internal derangements of the knee, which may occur with ACL tears, include medial collateral ligament tears, posterolateral corner injuries, meniscal tears, cartilage damage, lateral tibial plateau fractures (Segond fracture), posterior cruciate ligament tears, and extensor mechanism injuries.

✓ Pearls

- ACL tears present as increased signal, abnormal contour, or discontinuity of the ligament.
- "Kissing contusions," anterior tibial displacement, and deep sulcus sign are secondary signs of ACL injury.
- ACL tears are associated with internal derangement of other ligaments, menisci, cartilage, and fractures.

Suggested Readings

Gentili A, Seeger LL, Yao L, Do HM. Anterior cruciate ligament tear: indirect signs at MR imaging. Radiology. 1994; 193(3):835–840

Tung GA, Davis LM, Wiggins ME, Fadale PD. Tears of the anterior cruciate ligament: primary and secondary signs at MR imaging. Radiology. 1993; 188(3):661–667

Hall FM. Radiographic features of anterior cruciate ligament tear. Radiology. 2002; 222(2):576

Case 326

Michael A. Mahlon

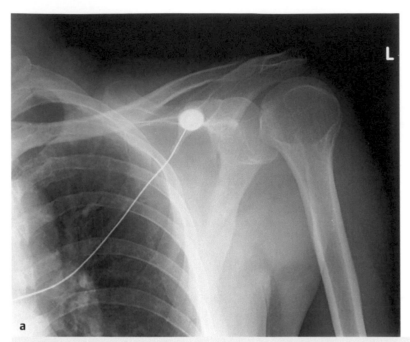
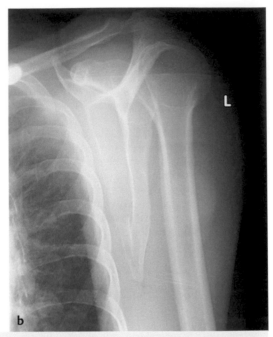

Fig. 326.1 **(a)** AP view of the shoulder reveals a high riding humeral head in relation to the glenoid with linear sclerosis and a cortical cleft of the medial humeral head, consistent with a "trough line" sign. **(b)** Scapular Y view shows posterior displacement of the humeral head in relation to the glenoid. On both views, the humeral head is fixed in internal rotation, referred to as the "light bulb" sign.

■ Clinical Presentation

A 35-year-old man with left shoulder pain (▶Fig. 326.1).

■ Key Imaging Finding

Posterior displacement and fixed internal rotation of the humeral head

■ Diagnosis

- **Posterior dislocation of the shoulder.** Posterior shoulder dislocation accounts for less than 5% of all shoulder dislocations. Acute traumatic posterior shoulder dislocation most commonly results from axial loading of the adducted internally rotated arm, as can be seen in convulsive seizures, violent muscle contraction, or electric shock. Posterior dislocations are clinically apparent approximately 95% of the time.
- Radiographically, the anteroposterior (AP) view may show a focus of linear sclerosis paralleling the medial border of the humeral head known as the "trough line" sign. In a patient without a dislocation, the humeral head should overlap the glenoid on the AP view, forming what has been described as a "crescent" or "half moon" sign. In patients with posterior shoulder dislocations, this overlap is usually absent. A "rim" sign may also be identified on the AP view. This sign is present when the distance from the anterior glenoid rim to the medial humeral head measures more than 6 mm. To diagnose a posterior dislocation, a scapular Y or axillary view of the shoulder should be obtained, although the axillary view may be difficult to obtain as patients may experience pain with abduction. On all views, the humeral head is commonly fixed in internal rotation, resulting in a "light bulb" appearance of the humeral head.
- Associated injuries of the shoulder include reverse Hill–Sachs lesions, reverse Bankart lesions, avulsed posterior labrum injuries with periosteal sleeve avulsion (POLPSA), rotator cuff tears, dislocation of the biceps tendon, intra-articular loose bodies, and impaction fractures of the humerus and glenoid. These injuries are often better appreciated on magnetic resonance imaging.

✓ Pearls

- Findings of posterior dislocation include the "trough line" sign, "rim" sign, and loss of the "crescent" sign.
- The humeral head is fixed in internal rotation with posterior dislocation, referred to as the "light bulb" sign.
- Scapular Y and axillary views are helpful in confirming the posterior dislocation radiographically.
- MRI is useful in evaluating for associated injuries of the shoulder.

Suggested Readings

Brant WE, Helms CA. Fundamentals of Diagnostic Radiology. Philadelphia, PA: Lippincott Williams and Wilkins; 1999

Saupe N, White LM, Bleakney R, et al. Acute traumatic posterior shoulder dislocation: MR findings. Radiology. 2008; 248(1):185–193

Case 327

Michael A. Mahlon

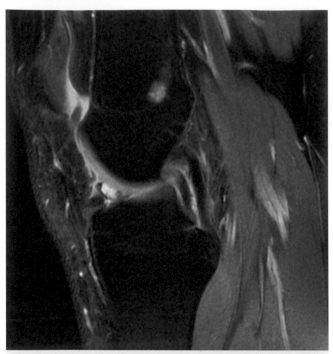

Fig. 327.1 Sagittal fat-saturated T2-weighted image reveals a crescent shaped, linear low-signal structure anterior to and paralleling the posterior cruciate ligament, referred to as the double PCL sign, along with a small joint effusion.

■ Clinical Presentation

A 31-year-old woman with knee pain after injury (▶ Fig. 327.1).

◼ Key Imaging Finding

Double posterior cruciate ligament (PCL) sign

◼ Diagnosis

- **Bucket-handle tear of the medial meniscus**. The double PCL sign is associated with a bucket-handle tear of the medial meniscus that occurs in the presence of an intact anterior cruciate ligament (ACL). A bucket-handle tear is a longitudinal tear of a meniscus that results in a displaced, but attached meniscal fragment. The fragment may become displaced into the notch between the PCL and the medial tibial eminence along the midline, with the fragment oriented parallel to the PCL. The intact ACL serves as a barrier that prevents further lateral displacement of the meniscal fragment.
- As ligaments and menisci demonstrate a hypointense signal on all pulse sequences, the displaced fragment will mimic a second PCL that is anterior and inferior to the true ligament, hence the name double PCL sign. The double PCL sign remains a highly specific indicator of a bucket-handle tear, with a specificity range of 98 to 100% and a positive predictive value of approximately 93%. A potential pitfall of the double PCL sign is the presence of an anterior meniscofemoral ligament which is known as the ligament of Humphrey and the oblique meniscomeniscal ligament, a normal variant.
- Bucket-handle tears involve the medial meniscus more commonly than the lateral meniscus by a ratio of approximately 2:1. Displaced bucket-handle tears can cause substantial symptoms, including knee locking or a lack of full extension. Arthroscopy is required to excise or reattach the free fragment.

✓ Pearls

- Double PCL sign occurs when there is a bucket-handle medial meniscal tear with an intact ACL.
- Potential mimickers include the ligament of Humphrey and the oblique meniscomeniscal ligament.

Suggested Readings

Boody BS, Omar IM, Hill JA. Displaced medial and lateral bucket handle meniscal tears with intact ACL and PCL. Orthopedics. 2015; 38(8):e738–e741

Camacho MA. The double posterior cruciate ligament sign. Radiology. 2004; 233(2):503–504

Watt AJ, Halliday T, Raby N. The value of the absent bow tie sign in MRI of bucket-handle tears. Clin Radiol. 2000; 55(8):622–626

Weiss KL, Morehouse HT, Levy IM. Sagittal MR images of the knee: a low-signal band parallel to the posterior cruciate ligament caused by a displaced bucket-handle tear. AJR Am J Roentgenol. 1991; 156(1):117–119

Wright DH, De Smet AA, Norris M. Bucket-handle tears of the medial and lateral menisci of the knee: value of MR imaging in detecting displaced fragments. AJR Am J Roentgenol. 1995; 165(3):621–625

Case 328

Jeffrey P. Tan

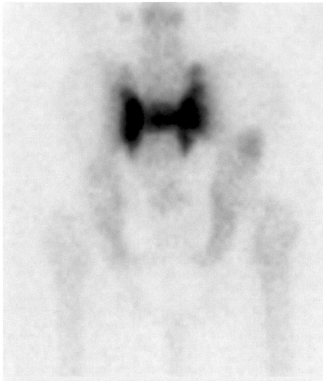

Fig. 328.1 Planar image over the pelvis from a Technetium 99m-hydroxydiphosphonate (Tc-99m-HDP) bone scan reveals intense uptake within the sacrum in an H-shaped configuration.

■ Clinical Presentation

A 64-year-old woman with low back pain (▶Fig. 328.1).

■ Key Imaging Finding

Intense sacral uptake in an H-shaped configuration on bone scan

■ Diagnosis

- **Sacral insufficiency fracture**. Sacral insufficiency fractures are due to normal stresses on weakened bone. Most commonly, these occur in elderly females with osteoporosis. Other predisposing factors include rheumatoid arthritis, chronic corticosteroid use, and pelvic radiation therapy. Clinical symptoms typically include low back pain, which is exacerbated by movement, with radiation to the hip or groin. There may be point tenderness over the sacrum.
- On nuclear medicine imaging, the classic findings include uptake vertically along the sacral ala bilaterally with a transverse line in between in an "H" configuration, which resembles the Honda symbol. It is therefore referred to as the "Honda sign." Other variants of the Honda sign include the half butterfly pattern where the superior aspects of the vertical lines are absent, the bar pattern where the transverse line is thickened, and the tramline pattern where the transverse component of the "H" is absent.

- Evaluation with conventional radiography may demonstrate the lucent fracture line, cortical disruption, or sclerotic bands; however, it is usually limited by the overlying bowel gas. Computed tomography (CT) may demonstrate the fracture lines or sclerosis with greater sensitivity. Magnetic resonance imaging (MRI) may reveal a T1 hypointense fracture line with increased T2 signal intensity in the marrow from the underlying edema from the sacral insufficiency fracture. In addition, MRI is useful in evaluating for an underlying neoplastic process.
- Management of sacral insufficiency fractures consists of rest, pain control, and treatment of the underlying cause. Analgesia and medical management of osteoporosis are common with avoidance of nonsteroidal anti-inflammatory drugs (NSAIDs) which may delay fracture healing due their blockage of prostaglandin activity. Other therapies may include pulsed electromagnetic fields, low-intensity pulsed ultrasound, extracorporeal shock wave therapy, sacroplasty, and surgery.

✓ Pearls

- Sacral insufficiency fractures are usually due to osteoporosis.
- On bone scan, there is a typical H-shaped configuration, known as the "Honda sign."

- It is important to consider MRI for the evaluation of an underlying neoplastic process.

Suggested Readings

Blake SP, Connors AM. Sacral insufficiency fracture. Br J Radiol. 2004; 77(922):891–896

Fujii M, Abe K, Hayashi K, et al. Honda sign and variants in patients suspected of having a sacral insufficiency fracture. Clin Nucl Med. 2005; 30(3):165–169

Longhino V, Bonora C, Sansone V. The management of sacral stress fractures: current concepts. Clin Cases Miner Bone Metab. 2011; 8(3):19–23

White JH, Hague C, Nicolaou S, Gee R, Marchinkow LO, Munk PL. Imaging of sacral fractures. Clin Radiol. 2003; 58(12):914–921

Case 329

Jeffrey P. Tan

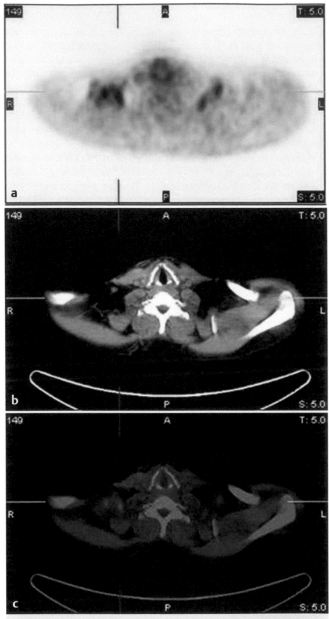

Fig. 329.1 (a) ^{18}F-FDG PET image demonstrates bilateral symmetric uptake in the supraclavicular soft tissues. (b) Noncontrast axial CT scan of the same region reveals primarily fat attenuation within the supraclavicular soft tissues. (c) PET/CT fusion image confirms uptake in regions of fat tissue.

■ Clinical Presentation

A 52-year-old woman with history of lymphoma (▶Fig. 329.1).

■ Key Imaging Finding

18F-fludeoxyglucose (FDG) uptake in supraclavicular fat

■ Diagnosis

- **Brown fat**. There are two types of adipose tissue in the human body, white adipose and brown adipose. White adipose or white fat is the primary type of adipose tissue which is utilized as energy storage. In contrast, brown adipose or brown fat is metabolically active and is used to generate heat. Brown fat is found in abundance in newborns and decreases with aging. The most common location of brown fat is within the supraclavicular soft tissues. Other typical locations include the neck, axilla, perivascular regions in the chest, perinephric spaces, intercostal spaces, along the spine, and in the para-aortic regions.
- Brown fat contains a mitochondrial protein which causes the uncoupling of oxidative phosphorylation. This results in heat generation instead of the production of adenosine triphosphate (ATP). Brown fat is active primarily in cold conditions or during food ingestion. Although glucose is not the primary source of energy for brown fat, during cold conditions, there

is increased uptake of glucose in brown fat. When 18F-FDG PET imaging is used, brown fat may increase its glucose metabolism which results in uptake of 18F-FDG. With the advent of combined positron emission tomography/computed tomography (PET/CT) scanners, fusion imaging can demonstrate that regions of uptake correlate to fat tissue. It is important to exclude other causes of uptake, such as metastatic lymph nodes, primary neoplasms such as lymphoma, or inflammatory lesions.

- Research interests are ongoing regarding brown fat and its benefits. Current evidence suggest an inverse relationship between active supraclavicular brown fat and arterial inflammation and possibly resulting in fewer cardiac events. Identification and quantification of brown fat can be made using imaging techniques within PET/CT and magnetic resonance imaging (MRI) scans via CT Hounsfield units, MRI-derived fat signal fraction, and MRI R2* values.

✓ Pearls

- Brown fat is metabolically active with 18F-FDG PET imaging.
- The most common location of brown fat includes the supraclavicular soft tissues.

- PET/CT fusion images can confirm uptake within fat rather than a suspicious underlying lesion.

Suggested Readings

Cohade C, Osman M, Pannu HK, Wahl RL. Uptake in supraclavicular area fat ("USA-Fat"): description on 18F-FDG PET/CT. J Nucl Med. 2003; 44(2):170–176

Gifford A, Towse TF, Walker RC, Avison MJ, Welch EB. Characterizing active and inactive brown adipose tissue in adult humans using PET-CT and MR imaging. Am J Physiol Endocrinol Metab. 2016; 311(1):E95–E104

Takx RA, Ishai A, Truong QA, MacNabb MH, Scherrer-Crosbie M, Tawakol A. Supraclavicular brown adipose tissue 18F-FDG uptake and cardiovascular disease. J Nucl Med. 2016; 57(8):1221–1225

Yeung HW, Grewal RK, Gonen M, Schöder H, Larson SM. Patterns of (18)F-FDG uptake in adipose tissue and muscle: a potential source of false-positives for PET. J Nucl Med. 2003; 44(11):1789–1796

Case 330

Grant E. Lattin Jr.

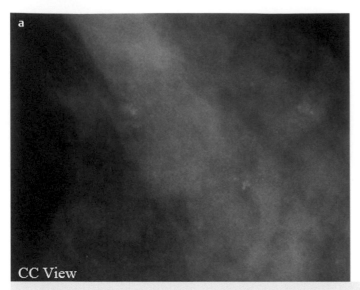

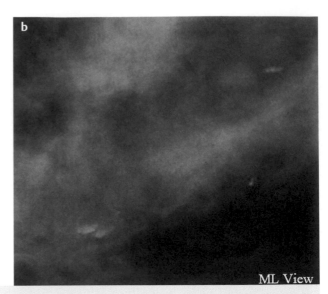

Fig. 330.1 **(a)** Magnified craniocaudal mammographic view reveals calcifications with a somewhat amorphous appearance. **(b)** A subsequent horizontal beam magnification view shows that these calcifications are now more linear or crescentic in configuration, suggestive of a "tea cup" appearance.

■ Clinical Presentation

A 43-year-old woman with amorphous calcifications on mammogram (▶ Fig. 330.1).

■ Key Imaging Finding

Amorphous calcifications on craniocaudal (CC) view which appear crescentic on lateral view

■ Diagnosis

- **Milk of calcium**. Milk of calcium is a descriptor used when calcium accumulates in benign microcysts and is identified in 4 to 6% of women obtaining a mammogram. The calcium, also referred to as sedimented calcium, appears smudgy or amorphous on CC mammographic views. Horizontal beam views will show these calcifications to have a crescentic or linear appearance secondary to the layering within the cysts. This appearance is commonly referred to as a "tea cup" configuration.
- Often, on the true lateral view, not all of the amorphous calcifications will change in morphology. In these cases, a prone pendent view can be obtained and may help in making the diagnosis. As the patient leans forward, gravity and patient positioning will help the sedimented calcium to change in morphology. This change in appearance will confirm the diagnosis of milk of calcium.
- Milk of calcium is a benign finding and requires no further work-up. However, care should be taken to identify any other suspicious calcifications which may exist adjacent to milk of calcium.

✓ Pearls

- Amorphous calcifications on CC views should be evaluated with horizontal beam magnification views.
- "Tea cup" appearance on mediolateral oblique (MLO) or lateral views is diagnostic of milk of calcium, a benign finding.
- Prone pendent view may be helpful in identifying of milk of calcium if unclear on traditional views.

Suggested Readings

American College of Radiology. Breast Imaging Reporting and Data System: BI-RADS, Mammography. 4th ed. Reston, VA: American College of Radiology; 2003

Gomes FV, Almeida MJR, Marques JC. 'Milk of calcium' in the breast. BMJ Case Rep. 2012

Moy L, Slanetz PJ, Yeh ED, et al. The pendent view: an additional projection to confirm the diagnosis of milk of calcium. AJR Am J Roentgenol. 2001; 177(1):173–175

Index by Differential Diagnosis

Index of Key Findings

Note: The index is ordered by case number within each section.